AF815696

International Council on Electrocardiology
founded by P. W. Rijlant, Belgium

President	E. Schubert, GDR
President Elect	B. Taccardi, Italy
Honorary Members	H. Abel, FRG
	P. d'Alche, France
	R. Amirov, USSR
	Z. Antaloczy, Hungary
	A. J. Bayes de Luna, Spain
	K. Harumi, Japan
	J. Jagielski, Poland
	F. Kornreich, Belgium
	P. Macfarlane, United Kingdom
	H. Pipberger, USA
	F. de Padua, Portugal
	Z. Pavlov, Bulgaria
	J. C. Rios, USA
	P. Rautaharju, Canada
	I. Ruttkay-Nedecky, CSSR
	R. Selvester, USA
	L.I. Titomir, USSR
	H. Ueda, Japan
	R. Th. van Dam, The Netherlands
	R. Wenger, Austria

He first reported on his method of spatiocardiography in 1952 in Prague, on a session of the Czechoslovak Physiological Society. He was using individually adjusted and corrected orthogonal leads and a device designed and constructed in collaboration with M. Netušil. Vertical amplitudes were superposed on the horizontal plane VCG loop, interrupted with high frequency. Thereafter, several more and more sophisticated models were constructed and complemented by facilities for visual observation, photographing, magnetic tape recording and resolving. He summarized his ideas and results in a monograph "Spatiocardiography. Textbook and Atlas" published in 1964.

Meanwhile, the Laboratory of Higher Nervous Activity has been gradually transformed into a Laboratory of Graphic Diagnostic Methods which moved in 1960 into a new building located within the large hospital area of Bulovka in Prague. The new Laboratory included a ward for in-patients and was equipped for invasive, as well as noninvasive cardiovascular diagnostic procedures. Later it evolved into the present Institute of Physiological Regulations, directed by Laufbergers pupil academician Ctibor Dostálek; the research on the cardiac electric field is here now headed by another of his pupils, Zdeněk Drška. It was in this Institute, where Laufberger was continuing to work daily in his office, up to the age of 95 years, involved in devising a practical and theoretically sound system of vectorcardiographic classification, suitable for computerized and automated data acquisition and processing.

Laufbergers personality and active interest have been of great importance for the iniciation and maintenance of international cooperation in our field of research. He took a very active part in the scientific program of the 2nd Colloquium Vectorcardiographicum held in 1961 in Stary Smokovec (Czechoslovakia). In 1963 he organized and chaired the 4th Colloquium at Liblice and the next year he co-organized the 5th Colloquium in Prague, within the frame of the 4th European Congress on Cardiology. He participated in our meetings regularly until 1975. In 1970 an International Conference was held at the Castle of Smolenice to celebrate his 80th birthsday. He was again with us in 1983 in Bratislava, as President of the 10th International Congress on Electrocardiology.

Academician Vilém Laufberger devoted his life to Physiology. He was a forerunner in several of its fields. He had an admirably inventive mind, sparkling with ideas, but he was also a dedicated and tenacious researcher, who not unlike a Phoenix managed several times to begin anew. He was very informal and sincerely kind. He will be remembered forever by all of us.

Ivan Ruttkay-Nedecký

C O N T E N T S

BODY SURFACE MAPPING - CLINICAL APPLICATION

RHYTHM AND RHYTHM DISTURBANCES

PLENARY LECTURES

First decisive positions were reached by the work of W. Einthoven, who knew the investigations of Waller by his own inspection. His main merits are the construction of a string galvanometer and the expansion of the vectorial theory. The string galvanometer (Einthoven 1901) is the first instrument for the exact direct record of the ecg without any need for corrections, as it was necessary for the capillary electrometer. This instrument enabled the application of electrocardiography to clinical problems and was utilized till to the 1950th. It provided also the first telemetric information transfer in medicine, the "telecardiography" (Einthoven 1906). Einthoven's theoretical work resulted in the Einthoven-Triangle (Einthoven et al. 1913) expressing connections between cardiac potentials and leads, thus giving useful theoretical help for the clinical interpretation of the ecg.
The inventions of Einthoven very soon provoked a vide echo among physiologits and clinicians. Electrocardiography became introduced into clinics, among the first by Kraus and Nicolai at the Berlin Charité in 1907. Clinical data were collected and the first textbooks of electrocardiography appeared (e. g. Samojloff 1909, Kraus and Nicolai 1910, Th. Lewis 1913).
The following development of electrocardiography was concentrated on three main problems: i. the excitation in the heart and its pathways. ii. the electric field of the heart and its relations to the positions of leads and iii. methods of displaying the electrocardiographic measurements. The interpretation of ecg signs became qualified by comparison with data from other cardiological methods and with results of autopsies.
Classical contributions to the knowledge of the spread of excitation in the heart have been given by Th. Lewis (Lewis and Rothschild). His measurements of epicardial activation established hypotheses on the activation of the myocardium, for a long time valid as the characteristics of the source of the cardiac electric field. The main accentuation was laid upon the function of the specific conducting system in consequence of the contemporary morphological results of Aschoff, Tawara, Keith, Flack and His jr.. By this way first exact data about the conduction velocities in the heart could be derived, which opened ways for the understanding of conduction and its disturbances, of the problems of atrioventricular conduction in connection with the provocation of rhythm anomalies and the complex of bundle branch blocks.
From these starting points theoretical an clinical research produced new informations of the cardiac activity. The occupation with conduction and its disturbances resulted in systematic knowledge of rhythm and rhythm anomalies from which highlights are put down in the classical works of Wenckebach and Winterberg (1927) and Wolff, Parkinson and White (1930).
Since than after the definition of the myocardium as a functional syncytium and the detection of the intercalated disks as conduction

P L E N A R Y   L E C T U R E S

One Century Electrocardiography in man

E. SCHUBERT

Institute of Physiology, Humboldt-University,
1040 Berlin, Hessische Straße 3/4, GDR

In the J. of Physiology, Vol. VIII, 1887 (p. 229-234) Augustus D. Waller, at that time physiologist at the St. Mary's hospital in London presented a report about a registration of the electrocardiogram in man under the title "a demonstration on man of electromotive changes accompanying the heart's beat" (Waller 1887). The records are made by means of a Lippmann's capillary electrometer and depict a curve with two phases clearly beginning before the start of the deviation in the mechanical registration of the heart's movement. The electrodes are placed at front and back of the chest, a lead similiar to the modern NEHB J (inferior). A calibration of voltage is not given. In the paper are also demonstrated other leads, e. g. right hand to right foot or mouth to left foot. This is the first publication of a registration of ecg in man and is reported to be done in May 1887.
The records have been decisive enough for causing Waller to present in following publications (Waller 1889, 1893) a discussion about the physical fundamentals of leading off the electrocardiogram from the body surface. With this the conceptions of the cardiac electric field and of vector presentations of the ecg were established. In these contributions the work of A. D. Waller has pronounced all important problems of electrocardiology.
Primarily Waller's interest was turned towards the heart's electrical activity in the isolated organ. He followed the first direct electrocardiographic records performed by means of the rheoscopic frog by Kölliker and Müller in 1856 and the measurements of Marchand, of Engelmann and of Burdon - Sanderson and Page in the 1870th. They used the rheotom - an instrument invented by Dubois-Reymond - for the elucidation of the shape and nature of the electrocardiogram. Being founded on this Waller for the first time was measuring remote from the heart and on the intact body of man.
In consequence of the investigations of A. D. Waller research work began for the establishment of electrocardiography as a method of clinical examination. The work was performed into different directions and reached progress by several great inventive personalities. As the guiding tendencies of the development persisted all over the time improvements in the techniques of measurement, recording, interpretation and modelling as well as the elaboration and corroboration of theories contributing to the widening and refining of the theoretic backgrounds of electrocardiology.

First decisive positions were reached by the work of W. Einthoven, who knew the investigations of Waller by his own inspection. His main merits are the construction of a string galvanometer and the expansion of the vectorial theory. The string galvanometer (Einthoven 1901) is the first instrument for the exact direct record of the ecg without any need for corrections, as it was necessary for the capillary electrometer. This instrument enabled the application of electrocardiography to clinical problems and was utilized till to the 1950th. It provided also the first telemetric information transfer in medicine, the "telecardiography" (Einthoven 1906). Einthoven's theoretical work resulted in the Einthoven-Triangle (Einthoven et al. 1913) expressing connections between cardiac potentials and leads, thus giving useful theoretical help for the clinical interpretation of the ecg.
The inventions of Einthoven very soon provoked a vide echo among physiologits and clinicians. Electrocardiography became introduced into clinics, among the first by Kraus and Nicolai at the Berlin Charité in 1907. Clinical data were collected and the first textbooks of electrocardiography appeared (e. g. Samojloff 1909, Kraus and Nicolai 1910, Th. Lewis 1913).
The following development of electrocardiography was concentrated on three main problems: i. the excitation in the heart and its pathways. ii. the electric field of the heart and its relations to the positions of leads and iii. methods of displaying the electrocardiographic measurements. The interpretation of ecg signs became qualified by comparison with data from other cardiological methods and with results of autopsies.
Classical contributions to the knowledge of the spread of excitation in the heart have been given by Th. Lewis (Lewis and Rothschild). His measurements of epicardial activation established hypotheses on the activation of the myocardium, for a long time valid as the characteristics of the source of the cardiac electric field. The main accentuation was laid upon the function of the specific conducting system in consequence of the contemporary morphological results of Aschoff, Tawara, Keith, Flack and His jr.. By this way first exact data about the conduction velocities in the heart could be derived, which opened ways for the understanding of conduction and its disturbances, of the problems of atrioventricular conduction in connection with the provocation of rhythm anomalies and the complex of bundle branch blocks.
From these starting points theoretical an clinical research produced new informations of the cardiac activity. The occupation with conduction and its disturbances resulted in systematic knowledge of rhythm and rhythm anomalies from which highlights are put down in the classical works of Wenckebach and Winterberg (1927) and Wolff, Parkinson and White (1930).
Since than after the definition of the myocardium as a functional syncytium and the detection of the intercalated disks as conduction

inhomogeneitis new approaches have been found for the determination of the excitation wave within the complete myocardium and for its cellular mechanisms. These results extended the theories based on the experiments of Lewis. As new methods for the support of the results the mikroelectrode technique and special multielectrode measurements became employed in the surviving heart. Standard data originated from the work of the groups of Scher (1953) and of Durrer and van Dam (1970). They demonstrated the exact way of activation running over the atria and the ventricles in a typical cooperation of specific and myocardial conduction and in concordance to the inhomogeneous conduction through the intercalated discs.

New lead techniques allowed to grasp data from limited areas within the heart and started the expansion from conventional electrocardiology to the intracardiac electrocardiography. This opened the access to the examinations of the a-v- and His-Bundleconduction especially in the cooperation with pacing interventions. The combination of the averaging technique with high resolution amplifiers in a very high signal to noise ratio allowed the detection of late potentials as important signs of excitation abnormalities.

Parallel to these technical and clinical developments modelling procedures became more widely available. Thinking started from Waller's and Einthoven's vectorial presentation of the excitation and experimental and mathematical work was accomplished to characterize the spatial spread of activation by the dipol modell. Preliminary theoretical contributions are the two component modell of Schütz (1936) and the theory of the "Momentanvektor" by Koch (1936). Going out from more improved experimental backgrounds Geselowitz (1960) and other groups expanded it to multipolar components.

Beginning with pure mathematical conceptions and tending to contribute to a physical interpretation of the cardiac electric field or components of it the spatial spread of excitation in the regions of bundle branches or even in the whole heart became modelled by means of computers. The results of the work of different groups, among others by Baum (1980), Ruttkay-Nedecky (1980) or Macchi and Taccardi (1980) demonstrate the progress of the efforts in the completion of the models and in the abilities for practical use of these models as program algorithms for computing procedures for the BSM.

The consideration of the influence of the electric field of the heart for clinical purposes of electrocardiography started with the work of F. Wilson in 1930. His theoretical research about "potential differences produced by the heart within the body and at its surface" Wilson (1930), lead to the practical results of the central-terminal electrode and the chest leads which are utilized till today. Their benefit is the widening of the information with respect to the spatial nature of the heart and its field. Many data with importance for clinical diagnostics could be obtained from these new leads.

By that time the investigations brought forth several corrections of the Einthoven-triangle and an improvement of the theory of the relations between leads and the field on the body surface. Theoretical extentions were given by H. C. Burgers developments of the "lead vectors" and the "image surface" (Burger a. van Milaan 1946/7). The attempts to reach exact numerical solutions and physical formulations of the field within the body and at the body surface were put forwarth by the theoretical considerations intended by Nelson (1957). In the way the problems of the formal building up of a unique theory connecting the activation processes inside the heart with its reflexion on the body surface became clear. Important influences of the excentricity of the heart, of the electrical inhomogeneity of the body's tissues and of the short circuiting effect of the blood in the ventricles were defined and taken into consideration. The directions of the inverse and the forward solution in the theory of the cardiac electric field became thus established and are under investigation till now.

Important contributions in the early period of these investigations are the comparative examinations of vectorial representations and the actions of lead networks given by Rijlant (1972).

The theoretical research on the heart's electrical field was accompanied by efforts having in view the practical solution of the task of an exact measurement of the field on the body surface. Early attempts with simple methods done mostly by hand out of single ecg-records were started by Groedel (1934/1940). Results with substantial insights into the real reflexion of the excitatory fronts came out from measurements by Karolczak (1953), Amirow (1961), Taccardi (1963) a. o. In particular the work of Taccardi and many contributors to its scientific conceptions and investigations advanced the general knowledge about the body surface field of the heart. The introduction of computing techniques, inavoidable in crowded quantities of data, contributed remarkably to these advances. Special improvement was reached, when investigations were put together with the results of the examination of the intracardiac excitatory pathways, as for instance in the Nijmegen conference in 1985 (R. Th. van Dam & A.van Oosterom 1986).

Another way of logics in the representation of the myocardial excitatory cycle was its demonstration as vectorcardiogramm. It started from the vectorial interpretation of the ecg. First instruments were devised e. g. by Schellong (1936), who created the term "Vectorcardiogramm". This method improved the understanding of the dynamics of the "cardiac dipol" and can be considered as starting point for a more technically based interpretation of the ecg. After world war II in many laboratories vectorcardiography was carried out for clinical purposes and became an important background for the funcional understanding of the ecg. In this field contacts among scientists of many countries arouse promoted by the organisation of the international colloquium vectorcardiographicum by H. and S. Kowarzyk and W. Laufberger starting in

1959. Since than this meeting, today under the title "International congress on electrocardiology" has been continously working. The dynamics of the growing and disappearing of main topics mirror the development in the scientific field of electrocardiology.

Besides theoretical and experimental investigations in electrocardiography also statistical methods and attempts for the improvement of the complete exhausting of the information contained in electrocardiological registrations became more and more involved. Comparisons of interpretations of clinical electrocardiograms have been the first steps and tended to decisions about the most informative lead combinations as done by F. Kornreich in contributions to many of the ecg-congresses. The development of different leads, above all for the correctet lead systems, and the contrasts between theoretical postulates and clinical possibilities in multilead registrations for BSM provoked accurate and extensive studies. Pionier work is to be owed to H. Pipberger and his coworkers and to P. Rautaharju. The results of these efforts are presented not only in comparative analyses, but the new field of validation and an approach to classified and standardized criteria for ecg signs of clinical relevance of the electrocardiologic methods could be derived. The analysing procedures were completed by leading off the ecg under conditions of load tests. Thus exercise electrocardiography became an important subject for clinical examination and much effort was made for standardized load protocols and analysing criteria. In this way the different diagnostic evidence of pattern recognition of one ecg-curve in contrast to the rhythm analysis of sinusrhythm and extra excitations was realized.

All the different directions of the development in electrocardiology which were pursued during its centennial history demonstrate clearly the prosperous way of the interdisciplinary cooperation of the different specialities which took part in it. Important questions of the clinicians could be brought to a solution by new results of physiological and biophysical research. Innovative ways of receiving information about general or local events in the activation of the myocardium were opened by the utilization of new technical procedures and methods of statistics and mathematics, of modelling and computer techniques, of amplification, data processing, and displaying. Thus from the single ecg-curve, recorded as reflexion of the heart's electrical activity 100 years ago by Waller today the broad spectrum of methods as standard electrocardiography, vectorcardiography, body surface mapping, intracardial His-bundle electrocardiography a. o. arose. These are the instruments for the noninvasive diagnostics of general or local events in the heart and can help the clinician to treat general or localized disturbances of the heart's funcion. Some of these ways seem to be just in its childhood and promise further progress.

References:

(1) Waller, A. D.: J. Physiol. 8, 229 (1887);

(2) Waller, A. D.: Philos. Trans. 180, 169 (1889) and "An introduction into human physiology" 2nd ed. Longmans, Green and Co., New York 1893, 394;

(3) Einthoven, W.: Arch. neerl. sci. Ser. II, 6, 625 (1901);

(4) Einthoven, W.: Arch. int. physiol. 4, 132 (1906);

(5) Einthoven, W. et al.: Pflüg. Arch. ges. Physiol. 150, 275 (1913);

(6) Samoiloff, A. F.: Elektrokardiogramme, Fischer, Jena 1909; Kraus, F. and Nicolai, G.: Das Elektrokardiogramm des gesunden und kranken Menschen, Veit u. Co., Leipzig 1910; Lewis, T.: The mechanism and graphic registration of the heart beat, Shaw, London 1913;

(7) Lewis, T. and Rothschild, M. A.: Phil. Trans. B 206, 181 (1915);

(8) Wenckebach, K. F. and Winterberg, H.: Die unregelmäßige Herztätigkeit, Engelmann, Leipzig (1927);

(9) Wolff, L., Parkinson, J. and White, P. D.: Am. Heart J. 5, 685 (1930)

(10) Scher, A. M. et al.: Circ. Res. 1, 539 (1953);

(11) Durrer, D. et al.: Circulation 41, 899 (1970);

(12) Schütz, E.: Erg. Physiol. 38, 493 (1936);

(13) Koch, E.: Z. Kreisl.forsch. 28, 200 (1936);

(14) Geselowitz, D.: Proc. IRE 48, 75 (1960);

(15) Baum, O. V.: Ruttkay-Nedecky, I. et al. and Macchi, E. et al. in: Models and Measurements of the Cardiac electric field pp. 11, 35, 49, E. Schubert (ed), Plenum New York 1982;

(16) Wilson, F. N.: Am. Heart J. 5, 599 (1930);

(17) Burger, H. C. and van Milaan, J. B.: Brit. Heart J. 8, 157 (1946) and 9, 154 (1947);

(18) Nelson, C. V.: Ann. N. Y. Acad. Sci. 65, 1014 (1957) cf.: The theoretical basis of electrocardiology, Nelson C. V. and Geselowitz, D. B. (eds.) Clarendon Press, Oxford 1976;

(19) Rijlant, P. W. Survey in: Bull. acad. roy. med. belg. 12, 711 (1972);

(20) Groedel, F. M.: Das Extremitäten-, Thorax- und Partialelektrokardiogramm des Menschen, Steinkopf, Dresden 1934 and Cardiologia 4, 1 (1940);

(21) Karolczak, B.: Cardiol. polska 1, 74 (1954) Amirow, R. S.: Elektrokardiotopografia, Medicina, Moskwa 1965; Taccardi, B.: Circ. Res. 12, 341 (1963);

(22) Electrocardiographic Body Surface Mapping, van Dam, R. Th. and van Oosterom, A. (Eds.) M. Nijhoff Publ. Dordrecht 1986; Advances in Body Surface Potential Mapping, Jamada, K., Harumi, K. and Musha, T. (Eds.) University Press Nagoya 1983;

(23) Schellong, F.: Verh. dt. Ges. inn. Med. 48, 288 (1936);

(24) Spatial Vectorcardiography, Kowarzyk, H. and Z. (Eds.) Pol. Med. Publ. Warszawa 1961.

My first 25 years in electrocardiology

R.TH. VAN DAM

Department of Cardiology
Sint Radboudziekenhuis, University of Nijmegen
P.O. Box 9101 6500 HB Nijmegen, The Netherlands

In the fourth year of my medical studies at the University of Amsterdam, in 1949, I became an assistant instructor in physiology at the University of Amsterdam. Professor ten Cate, a pupil of Pavlov, encouraged me to do research work. My first project was on the action of curare on isolated intestines of rabbits. Recordings were made on an smoked drum. My next study on the effect of constant load on the resting excitability of isolated cat papillary muscle introduced me into the field of cardiac electrophysiology. Then, in 1954, started my collaboration with Durrer that would last for 25 years. This period coincides with the rapid and extensive development of knowledge and technological methods that completely has changed the scene of cardiology (of medicine in general) and of our subspecialty of electrocardiology in particular. I have been fortunate as to witness and to some extent actively participate in this evolution and in the expansive development of modern electrocardiology. My main interests were in the fields of the changes in excitability and conduction throughout the cardiac cycle in various conditions, of activation patterns, of peroperative and of interventional electrocardiology. Our steadily growing group continuously developed new experimental approaches, using the latest advances in technology, in collaboration with van der Tweel's Department of Medical Physics at Amsterdam. During this time, our department (officially founded in 1958) became a very active center in the development of cardiac electrophysiology, and attracted scientists and clinicians from all over the world, some of them visiting, others participating in research projects on basic and/or clinically relevant electrocardiology. Howard Burchell was a regular visitor. Since we were working on several lines of research simultaneously during the years in the following summary I will -of necessity- have to jump back and forth in time and not observe a consistent chronological sequence.

In my first years, we studied, with extracellular methods, the sinus node and the spread of activation in the atria and ventricles in dogs, using epicardial and intramural recordings. For the latter purpose, the needle-electrodes served excellently and without causing more than short-lived injury to the myocardium. By these methods, we discovered low voltage signals in acute and chronic myocardial infarctions, indicating the occurrence of fractionnated and asynchronous activation of surviving myocardial fibers. In the late seventies I observed an active participation by the subendocardial Purkinje network in the propagation and

In the laboratory I started, in 1964 a long lasting coöperation with Pozzi from Florence on the effects of experimental chronic bilateral bundle branch block in dogs. He brought in the pathologist Rossi from Milan, who did confirm histologically our two-stage complete sectionings of both bundles and in one case of persistent AV-conduction demonstrated the presence of an intact bundle of Mahaim.

In an experimental study with Goodman, of atrial activation in dogs, I confirmed some preferential conduction along anatomical structures between SA- and AV node, but found no evidence for the participation of specialised conduction tissue as had been claimed by James.

In a human case of atrial flutter we recorded, during operation, an independent activation of Bachmann's bundle.
I became interested again in the differences in refractoriness between myocardium and the His-Purkinjesystem. At first, I studied the effects of Paired Stimulation in the canine heart. In the steady state, with a minimal time-interval between both stimuli, every second stimulus -although augmenting contractility- results in myocardial conduction only, as the conduction system still is blocked by its longer lasting refractory period.
Later on, Janse and I investigated the changes in refractoriness that follow abrupt changes in heart rate. We found astonishing differences between the adaptions of myocardium and of the conduction system, that seemed particularly important if seen against the background of clinical arrhythmias.

Since the late fifties, Meyler had been studying contractility on Langendorff perfused hearts of rats. Together with our biochemist Willebrands, we adapted this technique for the perfusion of larger mammalian hearts during a prolonged period of time and perfected it in many of the canine experiments described so far. Eventually we came to use the main elements of surgical heart-lung machines, and had washed erythrocytes as oxygen-carriers. In 1964, we were at last ready for the "physiological autopsy" studying the isolated human heart. The first became available in Januari 1965, by bequest of a patient who did not survive his second heart attack. Although the experiment was relatively short, we managed to demonstrate abnormal ventricular activation and fractionnated intra-infarction conduction. In the following years, the neurosurgeons provided us with normal hearts from victims of traffic accidents, in a legal way. Although there were some failures, this resulted in a number of good experiments on the spread of activation in the human heart.

In one of our last experiments of this series in 1977, Janse and I produced an acute myocardial infarction by coronary ligation and recorded the first human transmembrane action potentials of acute myocardial ischemia. We also collected some endocardial maps. The human conduction system, however, proved to be much more vulnerable to touch than that of the canine heart, so I had to proceed very carefully during these recordings.

The main objectives of these human heart experiments have been: a contribution to the insight into the distribution of the activation process in the human heart, and a corroboration for the human heart of most of our findings in animal experiments. Also, they provide a basis for modelling of the electrical field of the human heart during its activation, which in the end may contribute to improvement of diagnostic systems.

Several mathematical models of cardiac excitation and its resulting electrical field have been developed throughout the years, in our country by van Oosterom who, together with Strackee and Schoo has contributed a good deal to our advanced electronic technology.Together, we did some measurements of myocardial resistance in the intact heart. Recently, after solving some fundamental mathemical problems, he succeeded in reconstructing from a model that is based on our human heart data and on anatomical analysis by N.M.R., the 12 lead electrocardiograms of some of our present teammates with a high degree of accuracy. These developments may in the near future, contribute greatly to the interpretation of electrocardiographic recordings, as models may provide us with a quantitative and fundamental basis for their diagnostic analysis.

In summary, during this quarter of a century, between the smoked drum and computerised tape recordings, I witnessed a rapid expansion and proliferation of our knowledge and application of electrocardiology. I feel proud to have been one of the shipmates on this voyage into an unknown and territory, seeing "with the eyes of discovery".

Looking forward: what to expect?

I think that a proper place for diagnostical and curative electrocardiology will have to be fought for amidst the rapid and overwhelming growth of other technologies that provide us with facilities for obtaining very exact diagnostic information on cardiac anatomy, contractility and perfusion, such as echo-Doppler, cardiac catheterisation, angiography, scintigraphy, Nuclear Magnetic Resonance and for curative applications, such as laser ablation, PTCA etc. Invasive electrophysiological diagnostic testing and maybe antiarrhythmic interventional stimulation will be developed further for diagnostical and therapeutical purposes. Pacemaker technology will be perfected even more. Instant analysis of peroperative exploration will play an important role in the surgical ablation of arrhythmogenic foci.

Electrocardiogram and vectorcardiogram in the present form are rapidly becoming more or less obsolete, at least less important in the rapidly expanding array of diagnostic methods. In fact, electrocardiography, since the introduction of the 12-lead system, has by the simplicity of its routine use and its worldwide uniform application, more or less contributed to its own downfall. We know now very well that much more abundant and relevant electrocardiographical information is available, that is not routinely collected or used. Of course, the 12-lead ECG will stay for first-order diagnostical use in ischemia, infarction, arrhythmia's and disturbances of conduction. For the renaissance of electrocardiography as an important clinical tool we will need additional and more sophisticated electrocardiographic techniques for the precise recognition and the localisation of myocardial abnormalities. These techniques should be sensitive to the multipolarity of the cardiac electrical field, which is inadequately sampled by ECG and VCG. Probably we will have to combine an easy-to-apply method for extensive mapping with rapid and sophisticated diagnostic computer-interpretation programs. There should be based on models and on the results of verification procedures, that utilise the other available diagnostic techniques.
In the near future, such computerised methods will be - no doubt - increasingly available, everywhere and at low cost, but only if we electrocardiologists make a cooperative effort and do fight for our proper place.

References to all studies mentioned are to be found in:
Meyler, F.L., and H.B. Burchell: Professor Dirk Durrer, 35 years of Cardiology in Amsterdam.
North-Holland Publishing Company, Amsterdam, p.640 - 666 (1986).

Gating properties of cardiac sodium channels

B. NILIUS

Julius Bernstein Institute of Physiology, Martin Luther University, GDR-4020 Halle (Saale)

SUMMARY

Excitation in cardiac muscle can now be approached at the level of Na channel proteins. The following gating behaviour is normally responsible for the fast upstroke of cardiac action potentials and the fast spread of excitation over the myocardium: the channel openings appear clustered at the very beginning of a depolarizing voltage step. Only exceptionally long lasting openings and multiple reopenings (bursts) can be observed. This second type of gating seems to be responsible for i) a partial control of the duration of the cardiac action potential, ii) the slow inactivation of macroscopic Na currents, and iii) can explain the action of some cardioactive drugs. In a third mode of gating the channel is not available to open. The cardiotonic compound DPI 201-106 shifts the Na channel gating towards the mode showing long and multiple reopenings. The arrhythmogenic compound Aconitine favours the "bursting" mode of channel gating. Lidocaine stabilizes the channel in an unavailable mode. It is discussed that the gating of cardiac Na channels can be described as fluctuation between different modes of gating that can be modulated by cardioactive tools.

INTRODUCTION

Excitation in cardiac muscle is generated by a voltage-dependent activation of Na channels. The patch clamp method (Hamill et al. 1981) as used in this study provides a deeper insight into the mechanisms of the gating of single Na channels. It will be shown that cardiac Na channels open in kinetically different modes that can be stabilized by cardioactive tools.

METHODS

Experiments were performed on isolated ventricular cell of guinea pig hearts (Nilius et al. 1986). A standard patch clamp method was used to measure single Na channel currents. The cells were incubated in a bath solution containing (mM): 140 K-aspartate, 10 EGTA, 1 $MgCl_2$, 5 Hepes, pH titrated to 7.4 with KOH. Patch pipettes used to measure single Na channel currents were extremely small (resistance more than 25 MΩ, filled with (mM): 140 NaCl, 2.5 $CaCl_2$, 0.5 $MgCl_2$, 11 glucose, 5 Hepes, titrated with NaOH to pH 7.4, 21 ± 1 °C). The used methods and analysis were described in detail elsewhere (Nilius et al. 1987a).

RESULTS AND DISCUSSION

Figure 1 gives a typical example of the normal gating behaviour of cardiac Na channel in a cell attached membrane patch. The channel (only one channel is in the patch) respond to the voltage step with short openings (inward currents) that cluster at the very beginning of the step. The 4th sweep shows a series of reopenings, the 7th and 8th sweep show no opening (blanks or nulls).

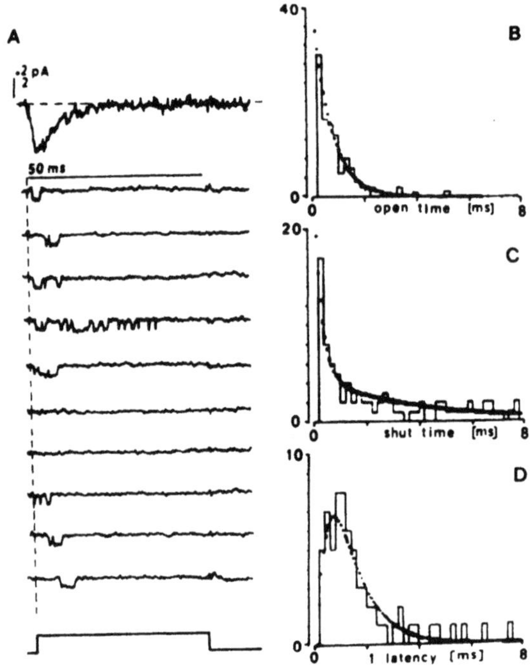

Figure 1. Normal gating behaviour of a cardiac Na channel in a cell attached patch. A: the response to a step from -140 to -50 mV is shown. The 4th sweep shows a burst of openings. The averaged current is from 76 sweeps (current calibrations above for the averaged current, bottom for the single channel current). B: distribution of the open times. The histogram could be fitted with only one exponential, mean open time to = 0.6 ms. C: distribution of the closed (shut) times of the channel. The histogram was fitted with two exponentials, the short mean shut time is 0.3 ms, the long mean shut time is 6.4 ms. D: distribution of the waiting time to the first opening (1. latency). The histogram is fitted with a function $y = a \cdot (1-\exp(-t/t_1) \cdot \exp(-t/t_2)$. The two time constants are $t_1 = 0.9$ ms, $t_2 = 1.2$ ms (sampling rate 10 kHz, 2 kHz filter).

The averaged current from 76 sweeps reveals the transient time course of the probability of the channel to open: the probability is high at the very beginning of the step and tends to zero during the maintained depolarization. This signal represents the macroscopic Na current and matches its time course exactly (figure 1A). A more quantitative analysis is shown in figure 1 B-D. The distribution of the open times can be monoexponentially fitted indicating that the channel protein has only one open (conducting) state. The distribution of the closed (shut) times can be described with two exponentials that refer to at least two closed states of the channel. The waiting time from the onset of depolarization to the first opening (1. latency) shows a maximum indicating that the closed states are in series. From single channel data and the averaged currents (Kunze et al. 1986) one can describe the gating of a single Na channel with the following scheme:

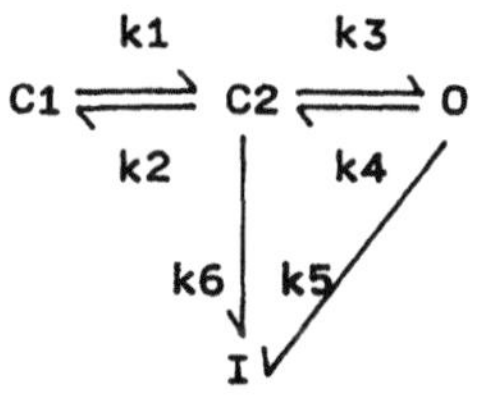

(I)

where k1-k6 are the rate constants that describe the transition between the two closed states of the channel (C1, C2), the open state (O), and the absorbing (inactivated) state (I). If the channel is in state I it cannot reopen in the same sweep. The transition from O to I represent the microscopic inactivation. The pathway C1→C2→I explains a null. A typical set of rate coefficients for a step from -140 to -40 mV is: k1 = 9000, k2 = 1600, k3 = 7000, k4 = 1500, k5 = 850, k6 = 1200 all in (1/s). These values describe the probability of a transition from C1 to I without entering the conducting state to 0.14, the probability that the channel can reopen is 0.67. The coefficients k4 and k5 show an opposite voltage dependence resulting in an only weak voltage dependent mean open time (mean open time: to = 1/(k4+k5)). This scheme nicely describes the normal gating behaviour of cardiac Na channels that can be seen in the majority of sweeps. Figure 2 shows a typical example of Na channel gating that can be observed in membrane patches after removing the patch from the cell (excised, cell free patch). Normally, long lasting openings or bursts can be observed in less than 1% of the sweeps. After excision the probability that the channel opens in a burst or show long lasting openings is strikingly increased. Besides the short voltage independent openings (mean open time about 0.4 ms) long openings appear with a voltage dependent mean open time (at -20 mV, mean open time about 3 ms; to is increased with stronger depolarizations). Sweep 47-49, 51-54 show such long openings, sweep 46, 58-62 show short openings, the sweeps 55-57 are nulls (at least 3 channels are in the patch). A similar gating behaviour can also be observed after application of the arrhythmogenic compound Aconitine (Nilius et al. 1986). Application of lidocaine sensitively abolished the long lasting openings and bursts of openings (figure 3) resulting in a faster decay of the

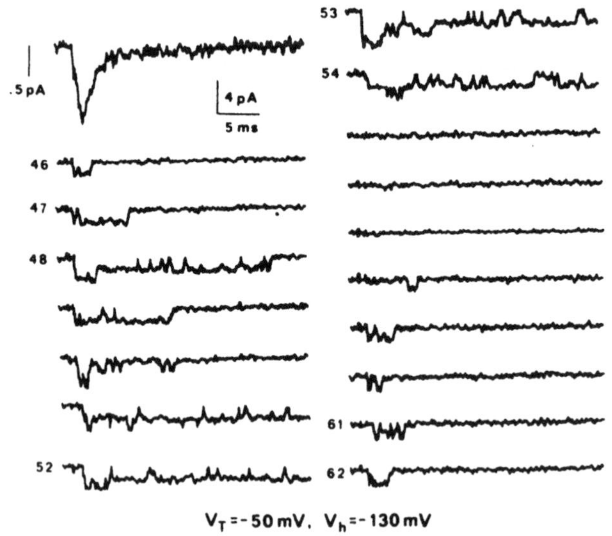

Figure 2. Appearance of long lasting openings and bursts of openings in a patch that has been manually excised for more than 25 minutes. 17 consecutive sweeps are plotted exhibiting 3 nulls, 8 sweeps with long openings, 6 sweeps with short openings. Note, that the different kinds of gating behaviour do not appear randomly but grouped. This non-random appearance of sweeps with only short-, long openings, or nulls, respectively, can be statistically verified (10 kHz sampling, 2 kHz filter).

macroscopic Na currents and a shortening of the action potentials (e.g. Sheu and Lederer 1985, Nilius et al. 1987b). An earmark of a basic property of Na channel gating in heart muscle can be unveiled after application of the new cardiotonic compound DPI 201-106 (Sandoz AG, Basle). In the presence of the positive inotropic drug the Na channel respond to a depolarizing voltage step with both short and long lasting openings (figure 4). Short openings at the very beginning of the depolarizing pulse generate the transient early part in the averaged current. The long lasting openings, however, correlate to the maintained current. It could be proved that both types of openings and also the nulls appear in clustered sweeps (Nilius 1987). These results can be interpreted as a gating property of cardiac Na channels: the channel can spent a time of seconds (several sweeps) in a certain kinetic scheme and can randomly leave this mode of gating jumping into another scheme. Under normal conditions the probability to find the channel in a conformation that allows it to respond to a depolarizing pulse in the way as sketched in the kinetic scheme (I) is near to 1. This is the reason for the fast upstroke of the action potential and the fast spread of the excitation wave over the myocardium. Under special con-

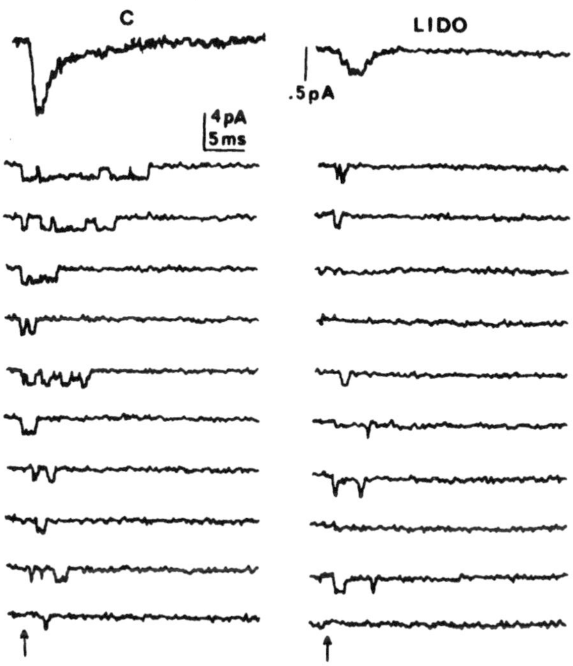

Figure 3. Effects of lidocaine on the gating of cardiac Na channels. At the left hand side the response of a single Na channel to a voltage step from -120 to -50 mV is shown. The patch was excised. The first two sweeps show long lasting openings. After application of 5 μM lidocaine to the same patch from inside only short openings appear. The number of nulls is dramatically increased resulting in a decreased averaged peak current. The slow decay as seen in the control disappeared due to a complete block of long openings. Lidocaine stabilizes the channel in a non-available mode (sampling 10 kHz, 2 kHz filter). The arrow marks the onset of depolarization.

dition the probability of the channel to stay in another mode of gating can be sensitively changed. Two examples have been demonstrated. Cardiac Na channels can skip to a mode of gating characterized by a defect in the inactivation (hibernating inactivation, h_h). The absorbing state I cannot be entered, therefore, long lasting openings or multiple reopenings can be observed. Aconitine and DPI can stabilize the Na channel in such a mode with hibernating inactivation. DPI dramatically decreases the rate coefficients k3 and k4. Within a certain scheme of gating (mode) the rate coefficients can considerably fluctuate (Patlak et al. 1986). Figure 5 shows a possible scheme of gating modes of the cardiac Na channel. The normal gating behaviour is shown in the S-mode. Short openings at the very beginning of a voltage step and a fast transition into an absorbing state characterize this mode of gating (scheme I). A longer stay of the channel in a conformation in which the channel cannot open is called O-mode. After application of lidocain (increased number of nulls, Reuter et al. 1985, Nilius et al. 1987b) the channel is supposed to stay in this state

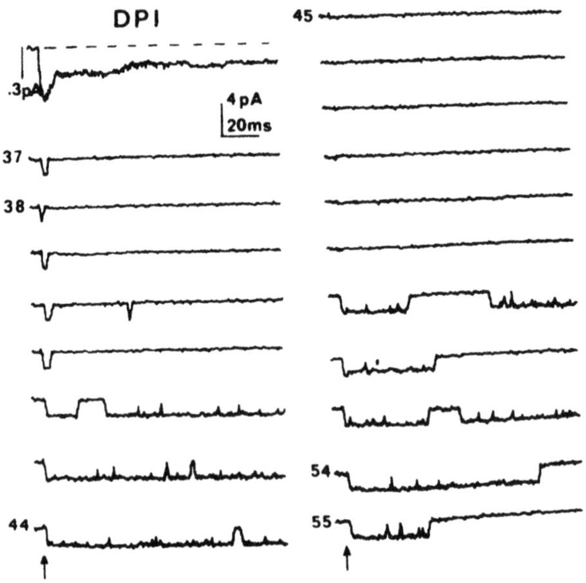

Figure 4. Appearance of different modes of gating behaviour of a single cardiac Na channel after application of 5 µM DPI. Sweep 37 to 41 show short openings as under control conditions. Extremely long openings can be seen in sweep 42-44, and 51-55. Sweeps 45-50 are nulls. The different types of openings appear high significantly non-random (Nilius 1987) (sampling 2.5 kHz, 1 kHz filter, note the change in the time calibration).

unvailable to open (hibernating activation, m_h, O-mode, figure 5). Whith a low probability the channel can enter a state with a defect in the inactivation (hibernating inactivation, h_h). In this gating mode the channel can reopen and shows long openings in dependence on the actual rate coefficients (L-mode, figure 5). It can be entered with a high probability under certain conditions (Aconitine: Nilius et al. 1986; DPI: Kohlhardt et al. 1986, Nilius et al. 1987a; excision: Horn and Vandenberg 1986, Nilius 1987). Normally, less than 1% of the sweeps show this type of openings (Patlak and Ortiz 1986, Nilius et al. 1986, Nilius 1987). The normal gating behaviour of cardiac Na channel is characterized by a fluctuation between the different modes of gating, however, its transfer probabilities sensitively depend on the actual situation.

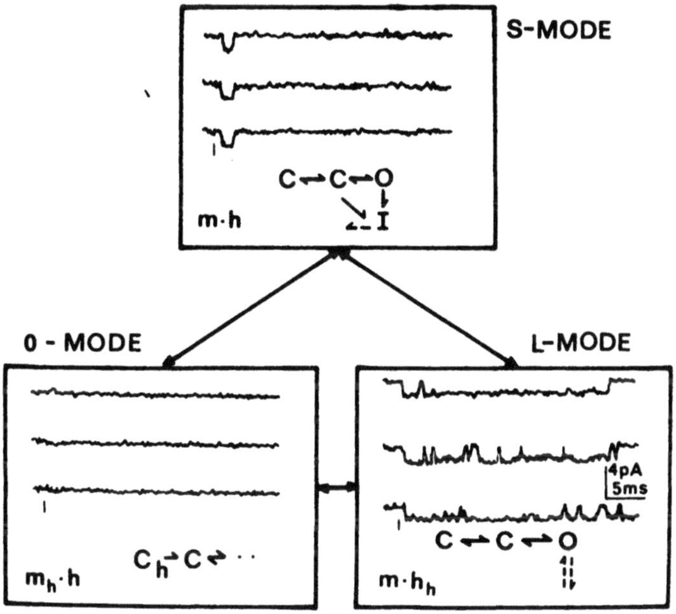

Figure 5. Scheme of different modes of Na channel gating. The subscript h means that the activation (m) or inactivation (h) is "hibernating". Gating is supposed as fluctuation between the shown different kinetic schemes.

REFERENCES

/1/ Hamill, O.P., A. Marty, E. Neher, B. Sakmann, and F.J. Sigworth: Pflügers Archiv 391, 85-100 (1981)
/2/ Nilius, B., K. Benndorf, and F. Markwardt: Pflügers Archiv 407, 691-693 (1986)
/3/ Nilius, B., K. Benndorf, F. Markwardt, and T. Franke: Gen. Physiol. Biophys. 6 (in press) (1987a)
/4/ Kunze, D.L., A.E. Lacerda, D.L. Wilson, and A.M. Brown: J. Gen. Physiol. 86, 691-719 (1985)
/5/ Nilius, B.: Biomed. Biochim. Acta 46 (in press) (1987)
/6/ Patlak, J.B., M. Ortiz, and R. Horn: Biophys. J. 49, 773-777 (1986)

/7/ Sheu, S.-S., and W.J. Lederer: Circ. Res. 57, 578-590 (1985)
/8/ Reuter, H., A.B. Chachelin, J.E. de Peyer, and S. Kokubun: in "Cardiac Electrophysiology and Arrhythmias", ed. D.P. Zipes, J. Jalife, Grune & Stratton, London - New York, 13-17 (1985)
/9/ Nilius, B., K. Benndorf, and F. Markwardt: J. Mol. Cell. Cardiol. (in press) (1987b)
/10/ Kohlhardt, M., U. Fröbe, and J.W. Herzig: J. Membrane Biol. 89, 163-172 (1986)
/11/ Horn, R., and C.A. Vandenberg: in "Ion Channels in Neural Membranes", ed. J.M. Ritchie, Alan Liss, Inc., New York, 71-83 (1986)
/12/ Patlak, J.B., and M. Ortiz: J. Gen. Physiol. 87, 305-326 (1986)

Computer Modelling in Cardiac Electrophysiology

MAREK MALIK

Department of Computer Science, Charles Univesity
Malostranske namesti 25, CS-118 00 Praha 1, Czechoslovakia

SUMMARY

The so called 'Anterograde Electrocardiographical Problem' (1) means the artificial production of electrocardiograph recors corresponding to any given condition of the heart and surrounding thorax tissues. Computer modelling (2) has previously been employed to solve this problem. Computer models are able to reproduce the behaviour of separate components of the heart and to imitate the process of ECG generation.

During past fifteen years, a variety of ECG models have been created. None of these models covers completely all features which contribute to the generation of electrocardiogram. Each existing model emphasises some mechanisms and omits or simplifies others. Moreover, some important electrophysiological aspects are not known sufficiently well to enable their accurate simulation.

The following paper present a brief survey of ECG modelling, describes two different modelling approaches and shows their results. The aim of the paper is to demonstrate the possibilities offered by ECG modelling and to point out some unsolved problems in this field.

A SURVEY OF ECG MODELLING

First attempts to create artificially an ECG pattern were based on mechanoelectrical models (3) or simple multidipole models (4). At the same time, more sophisticated concepts were also suggested (5), but they had no appropriate computational background. The early multidipole models considered a division of the ventricular myocardium into a small number of segments and treated each of them like an independent dipole. The computer was only used to calculate the main QRS axis from the parameters of separate dipoles. The input of the model has to contain the description how each dipole contributes the ECG and how the separate dipoles have to be synchronized. The later point became important when improving the accuracy of multidipole models by increasing the number of dipoles. The most developed model of Geselowitz et al (6,7) considers several thousand muscle elements and synchronizes their depolarisation by data based on laboratory measurement. This restrict the model to simulation of pathological situations in which musculature elements do not act properly but in which the activation sequence is not damaged. For studies involving impaired synchronization (8) the model requires special input data to be obtained.

A different approach is necessary for the simulation of pathological situations in which the model follows an abnormal excitation sequence. Some models study particular aspects of intracardiac synchronisation (9), while others enhance the modelled transmission apparatus and activation sequence (10,11).

The objective in both these approaches is to construct the exact form of ECG wave or complex. However, computer models can also be used to reproduce and study different cardiac rhythm disturbances. For this purpose, the model need not mirror the main procedure of electropotential changes, but must imitate the processes of excitation transmission between heart structures (12,13). Rhythm modelling requires also the rate

Fig. 1. Simulation results of the Shell Model: a physiological heart beat (a) and two pre-excited beats (b,c) in which an abnormal connection bypassing the AV node is present. The pre-excitation fibre links together the right atrium and the right ventricle.

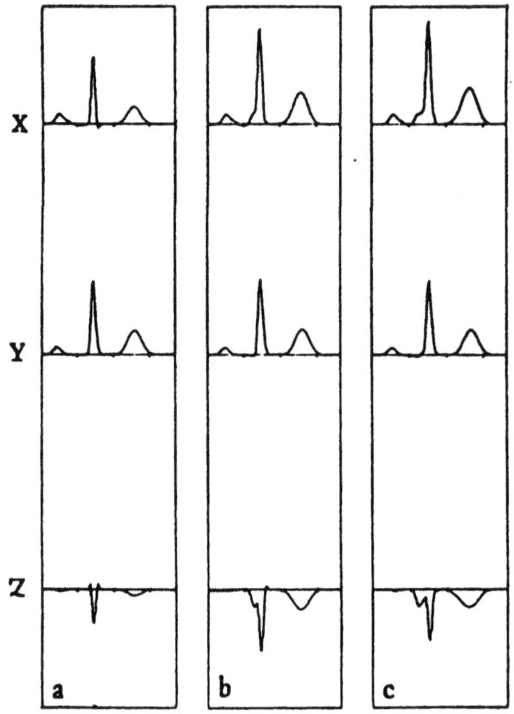

dependences of refractoriness and of the AV nodal conduction velocity, as well as the antero-retrograde anisotropy in excitation transmission, etc. to be taken into account. Computer testing of pacemaker algorithms (14,15) is an important application of these rhythm models.

MODELLING OF ECG MORPHOLOGY

In brief, we shall present the so called "Shell Heart Model" (11,16), which enhances the excitation transmission properties. The model represents the heart muscle by a three dimensional hollow shell with a central septal plane. The shell and the septal plane consit of more than 6000 basic myocardium elements. Depolarised and resting states are introduced for these elements, depolarisation of each of them contributes to the modelled ECG output signal. This contribution is also influenced by the direction in which the excitation wave radiates along the heart wall.

The model contains special structures representing the sinus and AV nodes and the conduction system. The image of the conduction apparatus has the form of a network built up from more than 200 linear fibres. The modelled excitation originates in the sinus node or, when an ectopic beat is simulated in an accessory centre and radiates along the conduction fibres. Each of the final ramifications of the network represents a Purkinje fibre and contacts a myocardium element. Different anterograde and retrograde conduction speeds are introduced for transmission fibres.

The organization of the model renders it possible to simulate very different pathologies of the conduction process. Figure 1. presents results obtained when physiological and pre-excited heart beats were simulated.

HEART RHYTHM MODEL

The models reproducing heart rhythms only, do not need to comprehend a large number of separate elements. For the rhythm studies, including most artificial pacamaker rhythm problems, a small set of different heart structures (nodes, ectopic centres, bypass tracts, muscle elements, etc.) is sufficient for the model.

We have introduced a very simple configuration into the so called "Mecanno Rhythm Model" (17) to study a standard DDD pacemaker mode and its two modifications designed to prevent the so called pacemaker mediated reentry tachycardia (PMRT) (Fig. 2,3.).

COMBINED RESULTS

The division of electrophysiology studies into rhythm problems and single beat morphology problems does not cover those cases in which both aspects must be combined. For instance, interference between two independent rhythms producing heart contractions in which excitation waves radiating from different sources fuse. Appropriate modelling of this case involves both morphology and rhythm aspects.

Fig. 2. and 3. Modelled actions of a standard DDD pacemaker (a) and of its two modifications (b,c). A premature ventricular beat initiates PMRT under the standard DDD mode while the modified pulsers prevent the tachycardia (left - see the modelled marker channels). However, the standard DDD mode is able to follow an accelerating sinus rhythm (right) but the modifications are not.

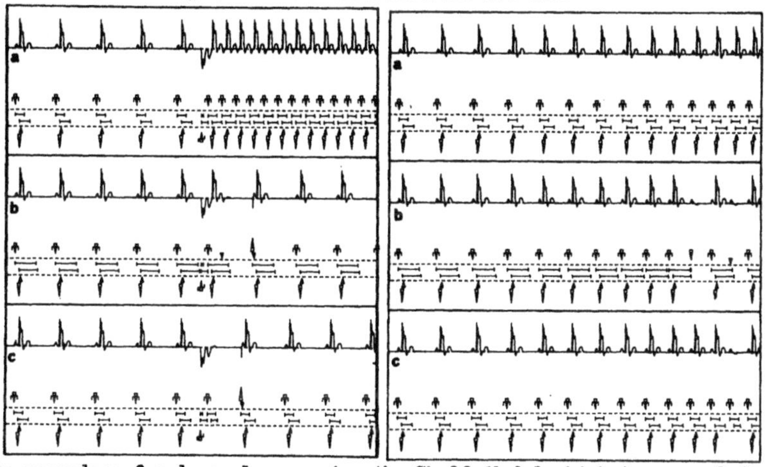

We were able to reproduce fused complexes using the Shell Model which is a complete heart model allowing both rhythm and morphology disturbances to be simulated (Fig. 4.). However, the current version omits for instance the cycle rate dependences.

The Shell Model was also used for modelling some possible pathophysiological mechanism of torsade de pointes tachycardia (18) (Fig. 5.). However, the model is not able to reflect changing repolarisation periods in different areas of the heart muscle, which should be certainly taken into account.

DISCUSSION

The present models cover quite large areas of cardiac electrophysiological problems. It might seem that the best way for future development of ECG models is to compound all three approaches (dipole representation, conduction properties, rhythm features) and to create a model covering both local musculature changes and conduction apparatus affections and the complex rhythm features. Nevertheless, such an ides has some serious drawbacks.

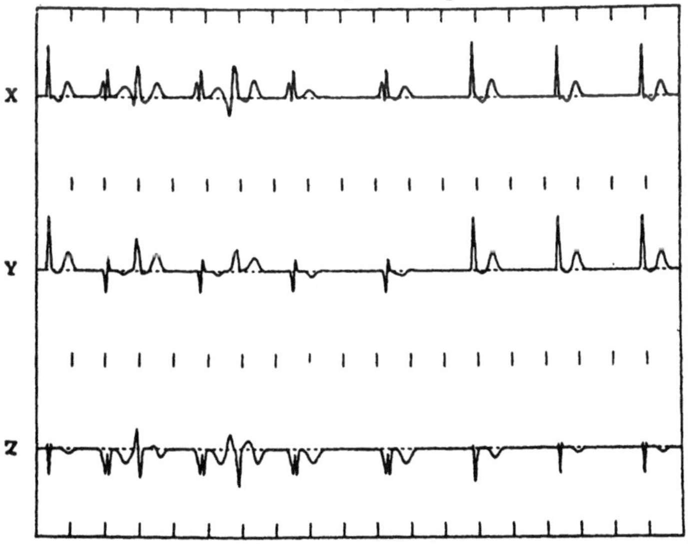

Fig. 4. Interfaces of AV nodal rhythm with an ectopic ventricular rhythm simulated by the Shell Model. The odd forms of QRS complexes correspond to fusion of excitation waves.

Current morphology models simplify the musculature image assuming a point like structure of fundamental elements.

Although the myocardial anisotropy can be introduced into such a structure, a realistic fibre to fibre conduction process (19) might be very important for modelling of serious disorders (ventricular fibrillation, etc.). Such a detailed morphology of the model based on real histological situation (20) will make the simulation experiments very CPU time intensive. This is not too important for appropriate morphology studies requiring the simulation of a single beat, but it is a serious restriction for using such a universal model for rhythm experiments involving tens or hundreds of heart cycles.

Fig. 5. Simulation of two different pathophysiological processes producing an ECG pattern similar to torsade de pointes: (a) - Combination of two pathological foci (one in the left ventricle, the other in the septum), both with changing rates. (b) - Pathological focus moving along the "edges" of the ventricular septum.

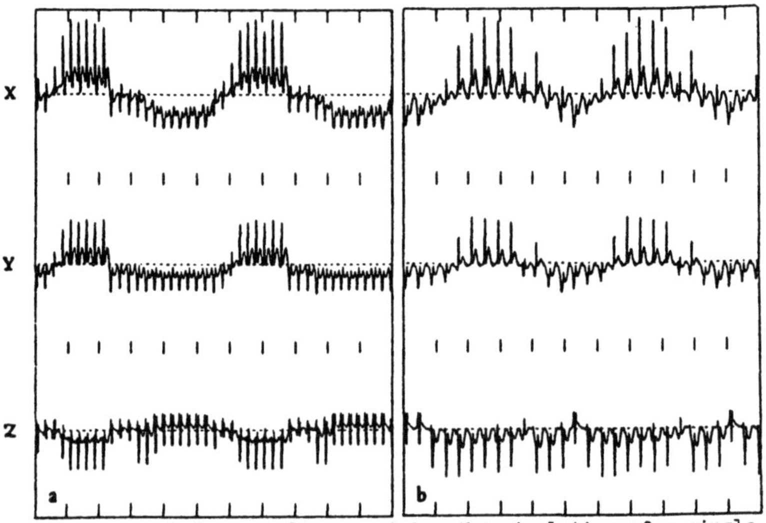

An exact image of separate heart beats is not required for most rhythm studies. Thus a rhythm oriented model can reproduce the ECG patterns approximately only, but it should deal in detail with such aspects as the cycle rate dependences, random frequency and conduction alternations, etc.

Another important area are the repolarisation studies. It is necessary to model accurately the ways in which individual heart elements treat the excitation impulse and change their own state of polarisation.

Consequently, the best way forward in ECG modelling is not the construction of a totally universal model reflecting all known electrophysiological features. It would be much more efficient to develope a library of model segments enabling different problem oriented models to be created. Employment of such purpose-made models would be less costly and more easily accessible.

(1) Nelson CV, Geselowitz DB (eds.): The Theoretical Basis of Electrocardiology, Clarendon, Oxford 1976
(2) Zeigler BP: Theory of Modelling and Simulation, Wiley, New York 1976
(3) d'Alche P, Coraboeuf E: J Electrocardiol. 4, 187 (1971)
(4) Wartak J: Computers in Electrocardiology, C.C.Thomas, Springfield 1970
(5) Baum OV: In: Biofizika sloznych sistem i radiacionnych narushenii (in Russian), Nauka, Moscow 1977, pp119
(6) Cuffin BN, Geselowitz DB: IEEE Trans. Bio. Med. Eng. BME29, 242 (1977)
(7) Miller WT, Geselowitz DB: Circ. Res. 43, 301 (1978)
(8) Lorange M, Gulrajani RM: IEEE Trans. Bio. Med. Eng. BME33, 862 (1986)
(9) Smith JM, Cohen RJ: Proc. Natl. Acad. Sci. 81, 233 (1984)
(10) Malik M, Cochrane T, Camm AJ: Comput. Biomed. Res. 16, 454 (1983)
(11) Malik M, Cochrane T: J. Biomed. Eng. 7, 266 (1985)
(12) Malik M, Cochrane T, Camm AJ: Comput. Biomed. Res. 19, 237 (1986)
(13) Holley L, Uther J: Vectors 14, 14 (1985)
(14) Dassen WRM, van der Steld A, van Braam W, et al: PACE 8, 574 (1985)
(15) Malik M, Davies W, Camm AJ: CPEP 4, 137 (1986)
(16) Malik M, Cochrane T: Simulation 45, 242 (1985)
(17) Malik M, Cochrane T, Davies W, Camm AJ: Med. Biol. Eng. Comput. in press (1987)
(18) Malik M, Camm AJ: Cardiovasc. Res. 20, 436 (1986)
(19) Plonsey R: J. Electrocardiol. 7, 237 (1974)
(20) Greenbaum RA, Yen Ho S, Gibson DG, et al: Brit. Heart J. 45, 248 (1981)

Body Surface Potential Mapping in Children

Jerome Liebman, M.D.
Case Western Reserve University and Rainbow Babies and Children's Hospital
Cleveland, Ohio U.S.A.

Electrocardiography can be divided into two major areas, that related to dysrhythmias, and that related to hypertrophy. We are in the midst of a magnificent period in the area of arrhythmias, for the basic science is constantly being infused into the clinical arena, while the basic investigators and the clinical cardiologists are in constant communication. On the other hand, those same electrocardiographers, often remarkable sophisticated related to dysrhythmias, appear to have little understanding when hypertrophy is the issue. Interpretation related to hypertrophy (and bundle branch block as well) are usually based upon pattern reading, and are loosely based upon Frank Wilson's teachings from the 1930's[1] and 1940's,[2] as though the great Dr. Wilson could not have continued learning had he lived.

There is intensive research into the nature of the cardiac electric source in the myocardium[3,4,5,6] and about activation sequences[7] although little is yet known in pathological states. (There is also little yet known about how the sources project onto the epicardium).[8] There is also intensive research into the secondary sources due to the various inhomogeneities within the volume conductor,[9,10,11] and there is an increasing awareness of the major effects of proximity.[12] The non cardiac effects upon the electrocardiogram, in fact, contribute perhaps as much to the surface electrocardiogram as does the myocardial source itself. We need also to develop accurate "forward problem" solutions[13] from known pathology using realistic torso models; and we need to develop accurate solutions to the inverse problem[14] in order to predict the epicardial potentials (and eventually myocardial potentials) from the potentials on the torso. In order to accomplish these difficult tasks and test out their accuracy, we need large numbers of surface electrodes, and we need accurately <u>measured</u> epicardial potentials in order to prove the worth of the <u>calculation</u> of those potentials.

Our work on Body Surface Potential Mapping (BSPM) has been developed hand in glove with theoretical electrocardiographers, first with Dr. Robert Plonsey,[8] now at Duke, and in recent years with Dr. Yoram Rudy.[11] Our lead system (developed under the guidance of Dr. Cecil Thomas)[15] has 180 dry electrodes, encased in various sized vests (described at the 12th International Congress on Electrocardiography at Minsk)[16] and is displayed color calibrated. Our major interest has been in cardiac hypertrophy (hypertrophy in the child is likely to be "pure", not contaminated by coronary disease), - although many of our papers have been involved in studies of ventricular conduction defects, which have also needed a new look.

In this brief presentation on BSPM in children, we will present PSPM's on various aspects of hypertrophy and conduction abnormalities of children with various congenital heart defects (ending with a few remarks about the WPW syndrome).

In recent years we have studied a series of children, normal[17,18] and abnormal[19,20] and have included various quantifications of both time and magnitudes. In children after infancy evidence for epicardial right ventricular (RV) breakthrough (indicative of activation of the right ventricle through the normal bundle branch system) is present in 100 %. In normals the right ventricle is not recognized separately from the left ventricle until late in activation. In right bundle branch block (RBBB) RV breakthrough is not recognized even when the block is partial;[20] right ventricular activation is via a fusion from the left ventricle and through the normal conduction system. There is a great spectrum within both partial and advanced RBBB,[19,20] but in advanced RBBB, evidence for left ventricular breakthrough is always present, manifested by rapidly moving negative potentials from above and below which separate the left ventricle from the right. In partial RBBB we have recognized left ventricular breakthrough in approximately three quarters of cases. In advanced RBBB activation of the left ventricle is on the way to completion by the time there has been slow conduction across the upper part of the septum to activate the right ventricle. In our series of children who have had a ventriculotomy involving the moderator band as part of surgery for tetralogy of Fallot,[19] it then took an average of 100.8 ms to complete activation of the right ventricle consistent with slow cell to cell conduction not utilizing the Purkinje system. When partial RBBB was created, the average was 51.1 ms in our study group, consistent with fusion.

In a group of patients with right volume overload (atrial septal defect)[20] RV breakthrough occured, usually late, from the left anterior superior (as in normal newborns).[21] Once the right ventricle was recognized to the right and anterior, it took as long to complete activation of the RV (average 48.2 ms) as it does in partial RBBB. Terminal RV conduction delay can occur in normals as well, and can also occur in the RVH due to pressure overload (PS); (in both cases of course with evidence for RV breakthrough). With increasing severity of the hypertrophy due to pressure overload, RV breakthrough is often from the superior to the left of the sternum as in right volume overload, and may or may not be late. (The breakthrough time and place surprisingly can even be as in normals). However, positive magnitudes anterior are very increased, after which peak to peak magnitudes right and anterior may be extremely high. In severe cases, the peak "vector" of initial QRS activation is often to the left;[22] the mechanism is not known. Initial QRS activation includes activation of the left posterior septum, left posterior free wall near the septum, the right septum and the right ventricular endocardium (as well as activation up the septum stimulated by the left anterior branch of the left bundle). In severe PS it can only be postulated that the abnormal early negative potentials to the right anterior (often inferior) in the BSPM are due to activation of a thick right septum plus RV endocardium to the left and inferior of where initial activation normally begins.

Investigations are just beginning into the nature of the BSPM in LVH. In left ventricular volume overload the "vector" of initial activation usually remains right anterior superior and is often of increased magnitude to the right superior (commonly interpreted as indicating left septal hypertrophy. After normal RV breakthrough greatly increased peak to peak magnitudes develop with the maximum anterior left, then posterior left. In the last part of the QRS there is usually a straight posterior, or right posterior superior maximum, but anterior superior positive potentials can be recognized as well. In patients with pressure overload, (aortic stenosis (AS)) there are differences. Initial maxima and minima are usually normal in mild to moderate cases, but in severe cases the "vector" of initial activation is usually left anterior (and frequently inferior). The most common manifestation in the BSPM is for the early maximum to be abnormally left anterior, but we have seen an abnormal position of the minimum as well. The postulate as to cause of the initial "vector" of activation to the left is hypertrophy of the free posterior wall of the left ventricle near where left posterior septal activation normally begins. After normal RV breakthrough there is then greatly increased peak to peak magnitudes left anterior then posterior, as in severe volume overload. Our preliminary data indicates another possible difference from volume overload in that the last maximum recognized at the end of the QRS is frequently right posterior superior (presumably from posterobasal LVH). In standard ECG and VCG a large terminal vector posterior and to the right is common, although more so in the presence of coarctation of the aorta than in aortic stenosis. In patients with coarctation after infancy, it is often difficult to differentiate pure LVH including posterobasal, from LVH plus partial RBBB or LVH plus RVH.[23] In the BSPM we have seen all three, and believe we can differentiate. A surprising number show LVH plus RVH even though right ventricular pressure is normal at the time. We speculate that the RVH is reflecting previous hemodynamics during utero and in early infancy when the right ventricle has had a hemodynamic load. It is believed that both hypertrophy and hyperplasia are stimulated to occur at that time, so that it is postulated that the larger number of cells may remian throughout life. The BSPM in the initial part of QRS usually does not demonstrate the abnormal positions of minima and maxima seen in severe AS.

There are congenital (perhaps acquired as well) conduction abnormalities which are quite specific for certain congenital cardiac abnormalities.[24] Particularly common is the "abnormally superior vector" (formerly called left axis deviation)[25] present at birth in the presence of an endocardial cushion defect (ECD). "The abnormally superior vector" is present even when the ECD is part of a more complex lesion such as tricuspid atresia (TA) or double outlet right ventricle. It is manifested in standard ECG and VCG with an initial QRS inferior after which most of the vector is superior. Left anterior hemiblock, an acquired condition, has the same frontal plane ECG. The initial QRS is inferior because the normal initial superior activation is stimulated by the left anterior branch of the left bundle. Durrer's studies give evidence that the abnormally superior vector results from early activation of the posterobasal left ventricle.[26] The early BSPM is striking in that potentials are negative superior and positive inferior. Then there is rapid change to the negative potentials inferior and the positive potentials superior. What appears likely to be RV breakthrough then may occur from the inferior rather than the superior. Even in so complex a condition as complete AV canal with a hypoplastic left ventricle, where there is severe RVH, the BSPM is characteristic.

Of particular interest is the BSPM in the hypoplastic right ventricle (HRV) which includes three clearcut types. In the HRV with pulmonary atresia a ventricular septal defect (VSD) is not present, so that the characteristic BSPM of an ECD is also not present. The RV pressure may be very high and, though hypoplastic, the wall would be hypertrophied. Therefore, in the BSPM, characteristic positive potentials presumably originating in the RV are recognized anteriorly after straightforward late RV breakthrough from the superior, as seen in RVH. There is no evidence of conduction abnormality. In TA there is a VSD which is usually posterior, an endocardial cushion defect. The characteristic potentials of "the abnormally superior vector" are recognized and in addition there is abnormally early RV breakthrough (12 ms in a recently studied patient). Of great interest is another conduction abnormality which simulates left lateral wall infarction on the VCG in that the initial QRS extends posterior and to the right before extending left, after which there is often evidence for considerable intraventricular slowing. (In the standard ECG only LVH is diagnosed).[23] In the BSPM, myocardial infarction is not suggested. After RV breakthrough the relatively inferior minimum is right anterior near the sternum and the relatively superior maximum is left anterior slightly to the left. These potentials then remain relatively stable for a very long time. The peak to peak magnitude is very large, perhaps 11,000 , before the postive potentials extend more posterior. When TA is associated with transposition of the great arteries the VSD is usually more anterior, not in the endocardial cushion position. Thus the characteristic BSPM of the early part of QRS in the latter is not present. But abnormally early RV breakthrough is present and the remainder of the BSPM may be similar, suggesting a similar intraventricular conduction abnormality.

In all of the above cases described we hypothesize pathogeneses to explain the BSPM. But often we are on "soft footing". We have ideas as to mechanisms but confirmation, or presumably changes in concept, must come from direct epicardial mapping in humans.

Much more proof has been available of course with the BSPM in WPW syndrome, where predictions of locations of bypass tracts are becoming very reliable. (26,27,28) We have been disappointed in the use of the ST-T as well as the rigid use of 40 ms into the QRS as the time of reference. We have learned to follow the positive and negative potentials of the early QRS until a virtually unchanging location of the minimum and maximum are definite. Recently reported independently was a modification, where the location of the tract was judged when the minimum reached 150 ,(29) an excellent way of quantitating our similar technique. Confirmation with surgical tract location has been very encouraging for we have even been able to predict paraseptal tracts. More pertinent to this paper has been the BSPM's excellent way of tracking cell to cell conduction plus the ability to clearly recognize exactly when RV breakthrough occurs as part of study of fusion in WPW.

References

(1) Wilson, F.N. et al.: Am Heart J. 10, 46 (1934)

(2) Wilson, F.N. et al.: Am Heart J. 32, 277 (1946)

(3) Plonsey, R., Rudy, Y.: Med Biol Eng Comput. 18, 87 (1980)

(4) Rudy, Y., and Quan, W.L.: Circ Res (in press, 1987)

(5) Spach, M.S. and Kootsey, J.M.: IEEE Tran Bio Eng BME. 32, 743 (1985)

(6) Ramsey, R., and Barr, R.C.: Biophys J. 51, 548 (1987)

(7) Durrer, D. et al.: Circulation 41, 899 (1970)

(8) Plonsey, R.: Chapter 3 in Pediatric Electrocardiography, Liebman, et al., Williams and Wilkens publ. (1982)

(9) Rudy, Y.: Chapter 4 in Pediatric and Fundamental Electrocardiography, ed. Liebman, et al., Martinus Nijhoff publ. (1987)

(10) Gulrajani, R.M., and Mailloux, G.E.: Circ Res. 52, 45 (1983)

(11) Rudy, Y. et al.: Circ Res 44, 104 (1979)

(12) Rush, S.: Univ Press of New England (1975)

(13) Rudy, Y.: Chapter 20 in Simulation and Imaging of the Cardiac System, ed. Sideman, Beyar; Martinus Nijhoff publ. (1985)

(14) Messinger-Rapport, B.J., and Rudy, Y.: IEEE Trans Biomed Eng BME. 33, 667 (1986)

(15) Thomas, C.W., and Lee, D.: Chapter 16 in Pediatric and Fundamental Electrocardiography, ed. Liebman, et al., Martinus Nijhoff publ. (1987)

(16) Kavuru, M. et al.: Chapter 15 in Pediatric and Fundamental Electrocardiography, ed. Liebman, et al.., Martinus Nijhoff publ. (1987)

(17) Liebman, J. et al.: J Electrocardiol 14, 249 (1981)

(18) Liebman, J. et al.: Chapter 19 in Pediatric and Fundamental Electrocardiography, ed. Liebman, et al., Martinus Nijhoff publ. (1987)

(19) Liebman, J. et al.: J Electrocardiol 17, 329 (1984)

(20) Liebman, J. et al.: Chapter 20 in Pediatric and Fundamental Electrocardiography, ed. Liebman, et al., Martinus Nijhoff publ. (1987)

(21) Spekhorst, H., et al.: Chapter 3 in Electrocardiographic Body Surface Mapping, ed. Van Dam and Van Oosterom, publ. Martinus Nijhoff (1986)

(22) Liebman, J., et al.: Jap Heart J. 23 (suppl), 480 (1982)

(23) Liebman, J.: Chapter 11 in Pediatric Electrocardiography, Liebman, et al., Williams and Wilkens publ. (1982)

(24) Liebman, J.: Chapter 2 in Pediatric Electrocardiography, Liebman, et al., Williams and Wilkens publ. (1982)

(25) Liebman, J. and Nadas, A.S.: Am J Cardiol. 27, 577 (1971)

(26) Durrer, D. et al.: Am Heart J. 71, 642 (1966)

(27) Benson, W. et al.: Circulation 65, 1259 (1982)

(28) Iwa, T. and Magara, T.: Japan Circ J. 45, 1192 (1981)

(29) Kamakura, S. et al.: Circulation 74, 89 (1986)

Features of ventricular septal activation in the cardiac electric field

I.RUTTKAY-NEDECKÝ

Institute of Normal and Pathological Physiology,Centre of Physiological Sciences,Slovak Academy of Sciences,Sienkiewiczova 1, 81371,Bratislava

Early explanation of ECG waveforms related the Q deflection to activation of papillary muscles(1).The direction of the instantaneous Q axis was ascribed to greater mass of papillary muscles in the left ventricle with respect to the right one (2).In compliance with the scheme published by Lewis and Rothschild(3),the depolarization wave was thought to invade the septum from above downward,and from the septal surfaces on each side to the interior.This of course did not give any clue to the identification of features of septal activation in the initial portion of the QRS complex.

Re-examination of the activation sequence of the dog ventricular myocardium by improved techniques in the early fifties (4,5,6) has shown that the first region in the ventricle to be activated was on the mid-left septal surface and the major direction of early depolarization in the septum was from left to right.Extrapolation from experimental data obtained in dogs and from the known position of the human heart in the chest led to the concept of a septal vector directed rightward,anteriorly and superiorly,giving rise to an initial positive deflection in V_1, a negative dflection in V_{5-6} and producing the Q deflections in the standard limb leads.This conceptual scheme has been accepted in clinical electrocardiology.

While canine ventricular activation sequence is similar to that of man, they are not identical.Therefore,substantial progress in our understanding of the shaping of the cardiac electric field in man has been achieved by investigation of isolated and perfused human adult and fetal hearts (7,8).In man,in contrast to canine experiments,not one,but three regions of synchronous early activity were found on the left endocardial surface.One,like in the dog,was located on the central portion of the left middle third of the septum,another area was high on the parietal endocardium,near the base of the left anterior free wall,and finally,a third one in the parietal endocardium was located in the middle lower part of the posterior paraseptal region.The basal endocardium and the septum just below the pulmonic walves were activated last.In the human septum,like in the canine septum,activation proceeds in general from left to right and in an apical-basal direction.A right-to-left component is present in a varying degree,since on the right septal surface activity initiated from the right bundle branch is always later than the earliest activity on the left septal surface.In man,the earliest vectors are then a resultant of at least three component vectors,orginating not only in the septum,but also in the subendocardial regions of the left ventricular wall.In spite of this composite picture and in contradiction to expectation,the normal intra- and interindividual variability of the earliest vectorcardiographic vectors is lowest in the whole course of ventricular activation,as documented by recording in deep inspiration (9),by investigating sexual differences (10),as well as interindividual variability.

As shown on Fig.1 areas occupied by vector termini until the 10th ms after beginning of QRS are a rather monotonously and symmetrically growing function of time.Thereafter appears a tendency to disperse first in the leftward and then also in the inferior directions.

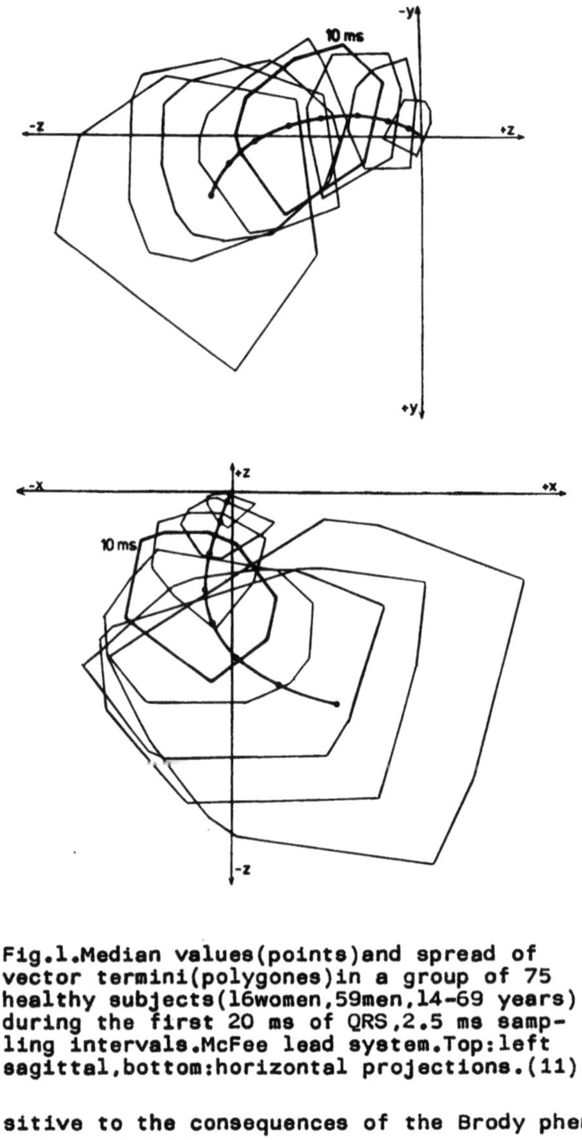

Fig.1.Median values(points)and spread of vector termini(polygones)in a group of 75 healthy subjects(16women,59men,14-69 years) during the first 20 ms of QRS,2.5 ms sampling intervals.McFee lead system.Top:left sagittal,bottom:horizontal projections.(11).

It seems that the paraseptal free ventricular wall activation front begins to play an evident role in the shaping of the external potential field only after 10 ms. There may be various explanations for this phenomenon. The septum usually curves so as to function as a part of the left ventricle but is thinner and flatter than the free wall.The maximal curvature of the left ventricular wall is in the transverse plane of the free wall and the least curvature in the apex-to-base plane of the septum.This may result in more internal cancellation of the activation fronts propagated across the left free ventricular wall,than across the septum.In addition,the lower two thirds of the septum and ventricular walls are ridged by interlacing muscular trabeculae cowered by Purkinje strands creating an anatomical framework for collisions and mutual cancellations of propagating wavefronts,Moreower,the subendocardial regions are more sensitive to the consequences of the Brody phenomenon,accentuating the external manifestation of radially oriented dipoles of the concentrically propagated activation front originating on the smoother and flatter left septal surface,and at the same time suppressing the manifestation of the

tangentially propagating wavefronts in the trabeculae carneae. According to Chou et al.(12) forces generated by the endocardial to epicardial activation of the anterior and posterior paraseptal regions neutralize each other, then the net effect of early left ventricular excitation is determined in most instances by the activation of the midseptal region. These events are manifested in the body surface potential distribution by appearance of a positivity in the upper or midsternal area, developing its maximum first in a left-to-right direction and then moving as a whole downward and to the left(13).
It is also interesting to note that there is a comeback of ideas concerning the role of papillary muscle activation. Epicardial mapping of about 7 months old fetal hearts (14) showed deepest Q waves coinciding with the beginning of left ventricular cavity potential on the posterior attachment of the ventricular septum and near the attachment of the posterior papillary muscles of the right and left ventricles. Since the relation of the Q and the papillary muscles is evident, activation of papillary muscles from their base to apex plays an additional role in the genesis of the Q deflection. It is of interest that Muraki (15) found also in the isolated dog heart immersed in a volume conductor, after dissection of free left and right ventricular walls, that these contributed to the early forward and to the right oriented vectors.

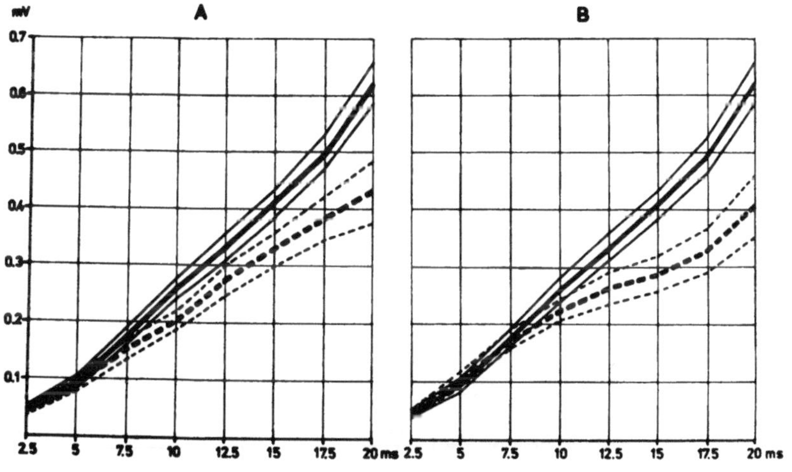

Fig.2. Mean and 2xS.E. of spatial magnitude in 75 normals (full line), 39 pts with anteroseptal myocardial infarction (A, broken lines) and 46 pts with anterolateral infarction(B). Abscissa: time from beginning of QRS.

The role of the left ventricular free wall activation in the genesis of the initial portion of the QRS complex may explain unexpected behavior of early depolarization vectors in some cardiac pathologies. In spite of the involvement of the septum in left ventricular hypertrophy, significant negative correlation was found between the spatial magnitude of the 10ms QRS vector (McFee lead system) and the left ventricular peak systolic pressure in cases of congenital aortic stenosis .This may be explained by the increasing role played by activation fronts in the left ventricular free wall.In left ventricular volume overload,on the contrary,the spatial magnitude of the 10 ms vector is increased,maybe as a consequence of the Brody phenomenon (16).In right ventricular pressure overload,the magnitude of the 10ms vector,while in average less than in left ventricular volume overload,correlates positively to right ventricular peak systolic pressure ($r= 0,3341$, $p< 0,05$),in contrast to its behavior in left ventricular pressure overload.This may be explained by the delay of the right ventricular free wall excitation.As regards the orientation of the early QRS vectors,it was shown by Kawai et al.(17) that there is a significant correlation between the azimuth values of the 10 to 26 ms instantaneous QRS vectors and the spatial orientation of the septum estimated by transmission computed tomography,this relation being best expressed in cases of ventricular volume overload,explaining the left anterior orientation of early QRS vectors often found in right ventricular hypertrophy and dilatation.In anteroseptal and anterolateral myocardial infarction,the decrease of the spatial magnitude of the abnormally posteriorly oriented initial QRS vectors as compared to normal controls, begins only about 7 ms after QRS onset (Fig.2).This delay and the extent of the change may be due to anterior free wall involvment.

In conclusion,in man at least,while the features of septal activation are from the onset on hidden in the composite pattern produced by the practically simultaneous activation of the septum,the papillary muscles and adjacent free ventricular wall,septal activation seems to play a decisive role in the genesis of this pattern during the first 10ms of QRS duration.

References

(1) Hering,H.E.:Z.exp.Path.Ther.7,363-378(1910)

(2) Zárday,J.:Az elektrokardiogramm,Rényi,Budapest 1944,p.275

(3) Lewis,T.and M.A.Rothschild:Phil.Trans.roy.Soc.Lond.B206,181-226(1915)

(4) Sodi-Pallares,D.,M.J.Rodriguez,L.O.Chait and R.Zuckermann:Am.Heart J. 41,569-583(1951)

(5) Scher,A.M.and A.C.Young:Circulation Res.4;461-469(1956)

(6) Durrer,D.,L.H.van der Twool,G.Derroklouw and L.P.van der Way:Am.Heart J.50,860-872(1955)

(7) Durrer,D.,T.Th.van Dam,G.E.Freud,M.J.Janse,F.Z.Meijler and R.C.Arzbaecher:Circulation,41,899-911(1970)

(8) Brusca,A.and E.Rosettani:Am.Heart J.86,79-87(1973)

(9) Ruttkay-Nedecký,I.in:Rijlant,P.(ed.)The Electrical Field of the Heart Presses Académiques Européennes,Bruxelles 1972,p.462-465

(10) Groeben,von der J.,D.D.Fisher and J.G.Toole:Am.Heart J.75,487-509(1968)

(11) Ruttkay-Nedecký,I.,Le ngoc Trong,V.Szathmáry:Bratisl.lek.Listy.87,15-24(1987)

(12) Chou,T.C.,R.A.Helm and S.Kaplan:Clinical Vectorcardiography,Grune and Stratton,New York 1974,p.465

(13) Taccardi,B.,L.DeAmbroggi and G.Viganotti in:Nelson,C.V.and D.B.Geselowitz(ed.):The theoretical bases of electrocardiology,Clarendon,Oxford 1975,p.544

(14) Durrer,D.et al.:Am.Heart J.61,303-314(1961)

(15) Muraki,H.:Japan.Circulation J.31;995-1005(1967)

(16) Ruttkay-Nedecký et al.:Electrocardiology'83,Excerpta Med.Amsterdam 1984

(17) Kawai,N.et al.:J.Electrocardiology,17,401-408(1984)

Mechanisms of antiarrhythmics

EDWARD CARMELIET

Laboratory of Physiology,
University of Leuven, 3000 Leuven, Belgium

Classification of antiarrhythmic drugs.

Antiarrhythmics have been classified into four groups[1]. Because of the increasing number of drugs available at the present time, there may be a need to adapt this classification. The criteria used by Vaughan Williams furthermore were not comparable: class I and IV were determined by the type of ionic current blocked, class II by the type of transmitter receptor and class III by the change in action potential duration. Since all electrophysiological effects are primarily determined by changes in ionic currents, it seems logical to use the type of channel with which a drug interferes as the decisive criterium. In such case however, beta-receptor blockers cannot be categorized. As an alternative one could distinguish between drugs interfering directly with channels and drugs interfering indirectly via receptor activation and stimulation of an intracellular messenger (Table 1).

Table 1. Antiarrhythmic drugs and channels

1. Direct interaction : i_{Na}, i_{Ca}, $i_{K(V)}$, $i_{K(ATP)}$, $i_{K(Ca)}$, $i_{K(ACh)}$, i_f, $i_{cat(Ca)}$
2. Indirect interaction : via transmitter receptor and intracellular messenger (e.g. : beta receptor and cAMP).

Channels that are directly affected include the Na and Ca channel, different K channels, sensitive to voltage (V), ATP, Ca or acetylcholine (ACh), the pacemaker channel (i_f) and a non-specific cation permeable channel activated by internal Ca ions (i_{cat}). The K channel, activated when ATP decreases below a given level, may play a role in ischemia-related arrhythmias, and can be blocked by substances belonging to the sulphonylureas[2]. A specific blocking substance for the pacemaker current, i_f has recently been developed: alinidine shifts the activation curve in the hyperpolarizing direction and reduces the fully-activated conductance[3]. Specific blockers may also soon be available for the i_{cat} current, which is responsible for the delayed after depolarizations (unpublished observation with the experimental drug R56865).
Beta-receptor blockers are given as an example of drugs with indirect interaction. At the present time no other drugs can be added to this group but it seems quite possible that antiarrhythmic drugs will be developed which interact with receptors coupled to the metabolism of inositol-phospholipids.

Use-dependency. Activation and Inactivation trapping.

The remaining of this overview will be limited to drugs acting on the Na and Ca channel. In general a drug can modify the gating or the ion transfer mechanism of a channel. The distinction between these two functions is based on the Hodgking-Huxley model of an ionic channel. According to this model the channel's permeability is determined by a selectivity filter, the actual flow of current by the state of activation and inactivation gates.

A characteristic of the block by certain local anesthetics and Ca channel antagonists is its use-dependency. At elevated frequencies of stimulation, i.e. when the channels are used, block is facilitated. Two conditions have to be fulfilled: preferential binding to activated-inactivated channels and slow recovery during the rest period. The phenomenon of use-dependence has been explained in the framework of the "modulated receptor" hypothesis[4]. According to this hypothesis the affinity of the channel depends on the state of the channel (resting, activated, inactivated) and as a necessary correlarium, drug-associated channels have their inactivation curve shifted in the hyperpolarizing direction (inactivation trapping). In accord with this hypothesis many local anesthetics (for the Na channel) and dihydropyridines (for the Ca channel) are more effective in depolarized tissue. They cause a shift in the voltage sensitivity of the inactivation gate, with the result that the channel already shuts at slightly depolarized levels. Recovery from block for these drugs will be favoured by hyperpolarization. However, this scheme does not apply to all blocking drugs. In the case of disopyramide and penticainide the inactivation curve is not shifted and recovery from block is not facilitated but slowed by hyperpolarization[5]. The phenomenon can be explained in terms of the "guarded-receptor" hypothesis[6]. According to this hypothesis hydrophylic, electrically charged drugs are trapped when the activation gate closes on hyperpolarization. In confirmation, acidosis was found to slow recovery from block[5].

Combination of drugs.

In order to improve therapeutic efficiency combination of drugs may be used. Different schemes can be proposed. 1) Combination of drugs acting on separate channels: a drug acting on the K channel may prolong the action potential, allowing in such way the fuller development of an inactivation block by a Na channel antagonist. 2) Combination of drugs acting on the same channel may result in competitive behaviour. Experimentally lidocaine (with fast kinetics) has been shown to displace bupivacaine (slower kinetics) from the receptor of the Na channel[7]. Competitive behaviour has also been shown to exist between lidocaine and quinidine or lorcainide for the activated channel. For the inactivated channel however, the hypothesis of competition could not be verified: the faster acting drug seemed rather to exclude the slower drug from interaction with the receptor[8].

References

1. Vaughan Williams, E.M. In Symposium on cardiac arrhythmias. E.Sandoe, E.Flensted-Jensen & K.H.Olesen, Eds: 449 - 472. Astra. Sweden (1970).
2. Beller, B., J. Hescheler, G. Trube. Pflüg. Arch. (in press, 1987)
3. Snijders, D.J., P.-P. van Bogaert. Pflüg. Arch. (in press, 1987)
4. Hondeghem, L.M., B. G. Katzung. Ann. Rev. Pharmacol. Toxicol. 24, 37 - 423 (1984)
5. Gruber, R., E. Carmeliet. Arch. int. Pharmacodyn. (in press, 1987)
6. Starmer, C.F., K. R. Courtney. Amer. J. Physiol. 251, H848 - H856 (1986)
7. Hondeghem, L.M. Circulation, 75, 514 - 520
8. Fransen, P. Doctoral thesis (Leuven, 1987)

Clinical Application of Magnetocardiographic Measurements*

FENICI R.R., MASSELLI M., LOPEZ L., MELILLO. G.

Clinical Physiology-Biomagnetism Unit, Catholic University
Lg. A. Gemelli 8, 00168 Rome, Italy

SUMMARY

A superconducting instrumentation is used, in our unshielded hospital laboratory for clinical, magnetocardiographic (MCG) measurements. Equivalent Current Dipole (ECD) inverse solution has proven to be useful for threedimensional (3D) localization of cardiac sources like His-Purkinje system , Kent bundles or arrhythmic foci. So far 72 patients, all affected by different kinds of cardiac arrhythmias, have been magnetically investigated. Simultaneous MCG and electrophysiological measurements have been performed as well in order to validate the accuracy of biomagnetic localization. In all cases both preexcited areas as well as atrial and ventricular ectopic activity were reproducibly localized by the MCG method. The accuracy of MCG 3D localization has been also tested by "MCG pace-mapping" . ECD localization of the artificial dipole satisfactorly corresponded to the anatomical position of the pacing electrodes, provided that the catheter didn't move during the procedure, probably being sequential mapping the main source of error.

INTRODUCTION

So far clinical usefulness of magnetocardiography has been widely questioned and still very few cardiologits are involved in this field. However, as the antiarrhythmic therapy is changing with the advent of effective surgical procedures, new techniques are required for preoperative, reproducible localization of the pathologic structures to be ablated (Cox, 1985). The number of potential candidates to antiarrhythmic surgery is largely increasing as a function of the improvement of surgical results. Moreover, as the clinical conditions of these patients can be severe, expecially when arrhythmias are due to ischemic heart disease, non invasive methods are desirable to define with maximal accuracy the site of origin of the arrhythmia preliminarly to any invasive procedure. Such an approach can minimize the time required for invasive localization and the risk of prolonged intervention, which could impair the clinical outcome of surgery.

In this perspective magnetocardiography has been developed in our laboratory as an independent method for functional localization of cardiac electrophysiological phenomena, and present research is adressed to quantify its accuracy and diagnostic power. Two years ago, the first validation of magnetocardiographic localization of Kent bundles in patients with Wolff-Parkinson-White Syndrome was reported by our group (Fenici et al, 1985). Simultaneous invasive electrophysiology and surface electrocardiographic recordings were used as reference goldstandards to test the accuracy of magnetocardiographic threedimensional (3D) localization. Intracardiac mapping and direct recording of Kent bundle electrogram were used to identify the atrial insertions of the accessory pathway. Magnetocardiographic mapping under direct pacing close to the preexcited area was proposed as a more accurate method to calibrate the magnetic system. Since then the research protocols have been adapted to study different kinds of arrhytmias. For space limitation only the highlights of our experience will be summarized here. The interested reader is referred to recent papers for a more detailed review on this topic (Fenici et al, 1987 a,b).

---

*The work was partially supported by National Research Council (CNR) contracts N. PF 85.01473.57, 85.00462.04, 86.00062.04, and by a grant (60%) from the Italian Ministery of Education.

MATERIAL AND METHODS

Magnetocardiographic mapping is performed with the prototype of a commercial biomagnetic instrumentation (BIOMAG I, Elettronica S.p.A., Rome, Italy), featuring a symmetric second order gradiometer with a pick-up coil diameter of 3 cm (1985-86) or 1.5 cm (1986-87). A baseline of 5 cm was adopted as the best compromise between optimal sensitivity to the investigated field and rejection of the environmental noise (Barbanera et al, 1981).
The output of the SQUID is preamplified and coupled to a COMB filter to reject power line interferences (50Hz) and harmonics. The final amplification and filtering before A/D conversion is provided by a custom made four channel signal conditioning unit for both magnetocardiographic and surface electric signals (recording bandwidth .016-250 Hz).

MCG computer processing is performed, after 12 bits resolution A/D conversion, with an HP A700 minicomputer. The software programs allow analysis of the recordings in the time domain at various level of resolution, isofield contour map drawing and automatic computation of the equivalent current dipole (ECD) parameters when a magnetic field distribution of dipolar configuration is experimentally found (Erne' and Fenici 1984). Further off-line processing provides bidimensional as well as three-dimensional displays of cardiac activation pathways, given by the movement of the ECD in function of time within the X-ray obtained heart silhouette (Fenici et al, 1987b).

Fluoroscopic imaging of the heart in any projection is provided by a mobile X-ray unit with image intensifier and double digital memory TV (SIAS 9C1/U Bologna, Italy). Radiopaque references are placed on the chest surface as well as in the esophagus both during cardiac catheterization and MCG recordings to define, in individual patients, the position and size of the heart as well as that of the catheters, with respect to the MCG recording grid (Fenici et al, 1986).

A programmable four channel MINGOGRAF 4 (Siemens-Elema AB, Sweden) is used for conventional intracardiac mapping and standard surface ECG recordings. Cardiac pacing is performed with a programmable stimulator SAP 40 (cb Bioelettronica S.p.A. Firenze, Italy). To avoid artefacts when performing simultaneous MCG and intracardiac recordings or MCG mapping under cardiac pacing, custom non ferromagnetic electrocatheters expecially designed to provide an artificial current dipolar source for the pacemapping technique were developed (Fenici et al, 1986). All signals are stored in a 14 channel Racal FM tape recorder for further analysis.

So far 72 subjects (53 males and 19 females, aging between 11 and 83 years) have been studied, 12 normals (control group) and 60 affected by different kinds of cardiac arrhythmias associated with WPW, ischemic or other organic cardiomyopaties. When clinically indicated, invasive electrophysiologic study was performed and a validation of MCG localization was possible by comparison with endocardial catheter mapping. The recording procedures have been extensively described elsewere (Fenici et al 1987 a,b). The reproducibility of the measurements carried out with different gradiometers, or during different recording sessions was evaluated. When required, pharmacological tests were used to improve the accuracy of MCG localization. For magnetocardiographic pacemapping the artificial dipole was placed, according to the clinical problem, at different atrial and ventricular sites, to test the amount of localization error for sources located at different depths in the heart (Fenici et al, 1985,1986a,1987a,b,c).

RESULTS

In figures 1 and 2, Typical examples are given of respectively left posterolateral and right lateral Kent bundles MCG localization in patients with stable ventricular preexcitation.
The opposite distribution of the magnetic field generated during the delta wave is evident. The ECD inverse solution is adequate to localize both preexcited areas on the frontal projection of the patient heart .

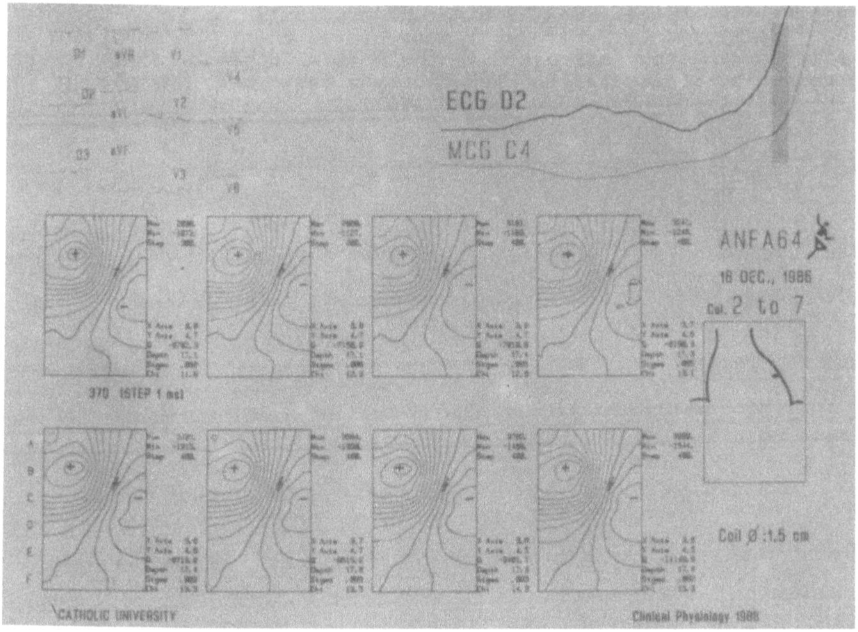

Fig. 1: WPW syndrome: Left postero-lateral Kent bundle. The site of initial ventricular preexcitation is indicated by the asterisk on the heart silhouette. Each map represents the magnetic field distribution over the anterior chest wall (36 positions recording grid). The field leaves the chest from the negative area.

These figures are representative of the results of an extensive prospective magnetic study on WPW syndrome (Fenici et al, 1986b, 1987b,c). In all patient with stable preexcitation an accurate localization was possible at the beginning or within the first 20 msec. of the delta wave. Four types of ventricular preexcitation were magnetically classifiable. No MCG pattern was found suggestive for left sided paraseptal accessory pathways.
In all cases invasively investigated, a satisfactory agreement was observed between MCG and catheter localization.
A reasonable localization accuracy was observed also in patients with focal tachycardias originating either in the left atrium or in the right ventricle (Fenici et al, 1987a,b).
The localization error of a pacing dipole was quantifiable as a sphere of diameter in between 7 and 20 millimeters around the actual position of the source (Fenici et al, 1986a, 1987b).

DISCUSSION

The spatial resolution of catheter mapping for source localization has not yet been quantified. In the order of one or two centimeters, it may be sometime insufficient to define exactely the origin of an arrhythmia. However epicardial and endocardial mapping during open chest surgery are usually capable to provide adequate localization of the arrhythmogenic tissue. The need therefore for preoperative non invasive localization is at present mainly related to the potential risk that the clinical arrhythmia may be sometimes not reproducible at the operation theatre. This could imply higher risk and poor outcome of surgical treatment. On the other hand catheter ablation techniques are under development, which will need closed chest three-dimensional localization imaging adequate to the spatial discrimination of the microscopic surgical lesion produced by a laser beam (Narula et al, 1986) or radiofrequency probe (Huang 1987).

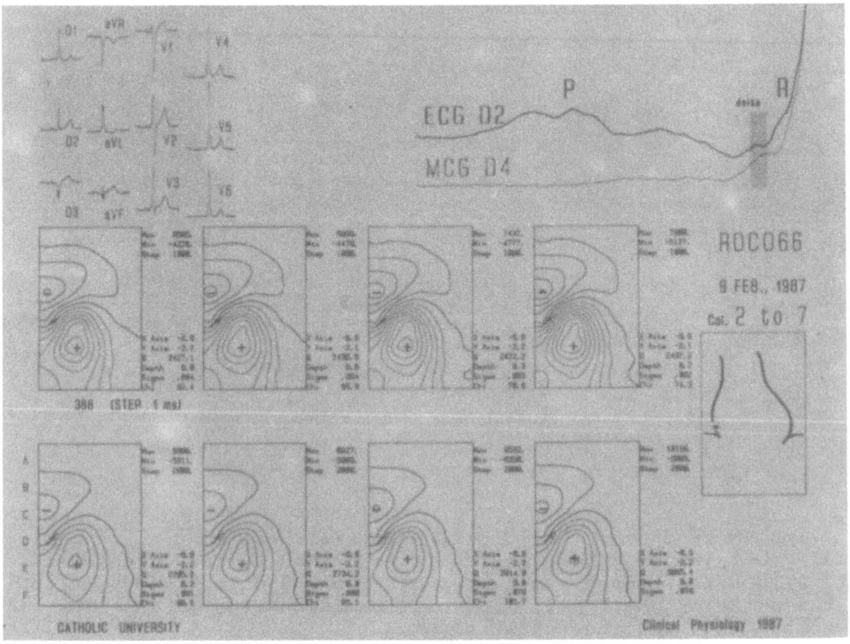

Fig. 2: WPW syndrome: Right lateral Kent bundle.

A good agreement was found between magnetocardiographic and endocardial catheter localization of preexcitation in all patients undergoing invasive electrophysiology, and with epicardial localization and cryoablation in one patient recently operated for a left postero-lateral Kent bundle with very short refractory period (Fenici et al 1987b). MCG localization in the latter case was well within the accuracy range of the epicardial mapping. This suggest that with future technological improvements magnetocardiography could provide a preoperative and intraoperative three dimensional imaging of arrhythmogenic structures for magnetically guided catheter ablation of cardiac arrhythmias.

REFERENCES

1) Barbanera S, Carelli P, Fenici RR, Leoni R, Modena I, Romani GL: Use of superconducting instrumentation for biomagnetic measurements performed in a hospital. IEEE Trans Magn MAG-17: 849-852, (1981).

2) Cox JL: The status of surgery for cardiac arrhythmias. Circulation, 71, 413, (1985).

3) Erne' SN, Fenici RR: The present state of Magnetocardiography. In Collan H, Berglund P, Krusius M (eds), Proc. of the Tenth International Cryogenic Engineering Conference, Helsinki, Butterworth, Westbury House, 329-338, (1984).

4) Fenici RR, Masselli M, Lopez L, Sabetta F: First simultaneous MCG and invasive Kent bundle localization in man. New trends in arrhythmias 1: 455-460, (1985).

5) Fenici RR, Masselli M, Lopez L, Sabetta F: Simultaneous MCG mapping and invasive electrophysiology to evaluate the accuracy of the equivalent current dipole inverse solution for the localization of human cardiac sources. New trends in arrhythmias 2, 357-369, (1986a).

6)* Fenici RR, Masselli M: Magnetocardiography: localization of accessory pathways (WPW). In Proc of the IEEE Engineeering in Medicine and Biology Society 8th Annual Conference, 437-438, Dallas, Nov. 7-10, (1986b).

7) Fenici RR, Masselli M., Lopez L., Melillo G: Clinical Value of Magnetocardiography. In "What's new in Electrocardiography and Drug Therapy", Ed by Hombach V. Hilger HH, Martinus Nijhoff Publishers, Boston. In press (1987a).

8) Fenici RR, Masselli M., Lopez L., Melillo G: Clinical Magnetocardiography: Localization of arrhythmogenic structures. Proceedings of the I.S.I. Workshop on "Functional localization : a challenge for Biomagnetism" , Torino 1986. In press, (1987b).

9) Fenici RR, Masselli M., Lopez L., Melillo G: Magnetocardiographic Localization of Arrhythmogenic Sources, (Abs.) PACE, Vol. 10, Part I, 600, (1987c).

10) Huang SKS: Use of radiofrequency energy for catheter ablation of the endomyocardium: a prospective energy source, J Electrophysiology, 1, 1, 78-91, (1987).

11) Narula OS, Bharati S, Chan MC, et al: Microtransection of the His bundle with laser radiation through a pervenous catheter: correlation of histologic and electrophysiologic data. Am J Cardiol 54:186, (1986).

Comparison of mathematical and geometrical approach in spacecraft and in our triaxicardiometric (Polarcardiographic) programs

Zoltán ANTALÓCZY, Gábor ENDRŐCZI *

2nd Medical Clinic of Postgraduate Medical School, H-1389 Budapest, POB.112.Hungary
* Central Research Institute for Physics, H-1525 Budapest, POB.49.Hungary

The human being takes an intermediate place between the microcosmos and macrocosmos and has formed a continuously changing image of its own world and of the surroundings from the time of its first realization. Galileo Galilei observs the universe and in his famous book "Assayer" draws "triangles,circles and geometrical figures" instead of numbers. But must be noted, that Descartes just about that time put geometry into a quantitative form. If Galileo had used the method of analytical geometry he would be able to talk about algebraic equations instead of triangles, circles and lines. The nuclear, air-space and computer engineering and modern electronics were developed during and after the 2nd World War. The world learned the name of Gagarin who was the first space-explorer on the board of the first spaceship of the world named "VOSTOK-1". Later, the firsts Moon Walk Neil Armstrong's "giant leap for mankind", and the planetary probes came - toward the Mercury, Mars, Venus, Jupiter, Saturn and so on... The Sojuz-Apollo program had been realized the American and Russian spacecrafts were coupled, we have learned to orientate in the air and space. The program of the onboard computer of the spaceship Apollo named "set state vector" shows that this orientation can only be realized through the use of Cartesian coordinates X, Y, Z and the Vx Vy and Vz parameters.

The location determination of the space-shuttle as well as other man-carrying spacecrafts is made on the Earth. The geometrical relation of this operation is shown on the first figure.

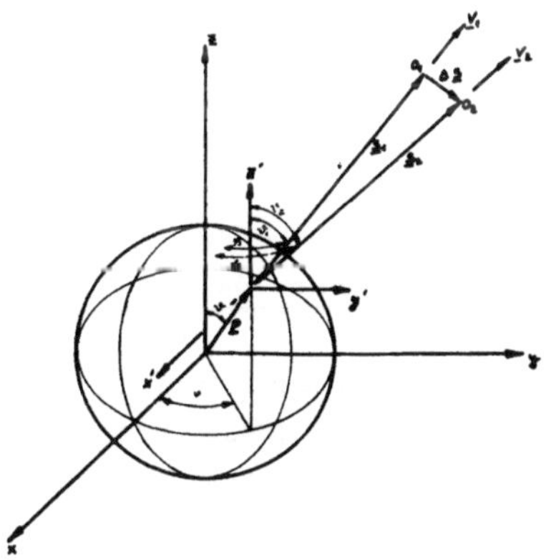

In the earth-linked coordinate system xyz where x, y and z axes go through the midpoint of the Earth, the P vector shows the place of the observer upon the surface of the Earth. The coordinate system is originally determined so, that the γ and φ angles are to be corresponded to the degrees of longitude and latitude. The coordinate system x' - y' - z' linked with the terrestrial observer, is parallel to the x-y-z coordinate system.

The z axis is coincided with the rotation axis of the Earth. It is worth mentioning that this arrangement has great significance in the astrology. One moving axis of the telescopes is always coinciding with z' - and the rotation of the telescope around this axis makes possible to take star-photographes with an exposition time of more than one hour. The basic task of location determination is to measure the distannce, the angle-position and velocity of a sky object in the time point $\underline{t}_1$, compared with the terrestrial observation post. The angle position of the antenna, receiving the signals of the spacecraft, gives directly the φ_1 and γ_1 angles. The space of time, elapsed between the radiation of a signal from the terrestrial observation post and return from the spacecraft - gives the distance of them. The $\underline{S}_1$ vector can be calculated from the distance and the angles. Thus - the position of the spaceship in $\underline{t}_1$ timepoint - is $\underline{P} + \underline{S}_1$. This is expressed in coordinates:

$$x = P\sin\gamma\cos\varphi + S\sin\gamma'\cos\varphi'_1\underline{i}$$
$$y = P\sin\gamma\sin\varphi + S\sin\gamma'_1\sin\varphi'_1\underline{j}$$
$$z = P\cos\gamma + S\cos\gamma_1\underline{k}$$

where

P - is the distance of the observation post from the midpoint of the Earth

S - is the distance of the spacecraft from the terrestrial observation post

In the t_1 point of time only that component of the velocity vector of the spacecraft can be measured from the Doppler displacement (frequency difference) between the originally radiated and the object-reflected signal - which is in the direction of the $\underline{S}_1$ vector. The direction of the real velocity can be calculated if the position of the speceship is measured in the $\underline{t}_2$ timepoint, after a short time. The changing position of the cpacecraft is equal to $\underline{S}_2-\underline{S}_1$ vector (ΔS), thus the vectorial velocity of the object is approximately $\Delta \underline{S}/\Delta t$, or $(\underline{S}_2-\underline{S}_1)(t_2-t_1)$. The above given value is corrected with the supposition that the $\underline{S}_2$ directed component of the velocity is identical with V_2. In practice however, for sake of adequate accuracy these data are very frequently measured on different points of the Earth and the mean of these values determines the real position. Frequency of the measurements is more than $1/\sec^{-2}$. The whole process of the determination of the location of the spacecraft is given on the following scheme:

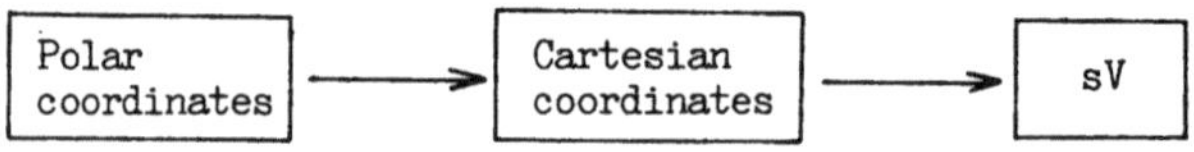

It was the great Ampere who in 1834 while analyzing different branches of scince and technology formulated the ideas of isomorphism which give evidence that e.g. biology and botany have the same structure. However a century had to pass until the founder of modern cybernetics Norbert Wiener took use of the ideas of isomorphism emphasizing the necessity to analyze different systems with the help of the same methods.
Therefore the same mathematics, geometry and computer-technics is to be employed by the medical engineering for the determination and characterization of the human heart potential vectors as in the determination of the location of a spaceship. The magnitude and orientation of heart potential vector is determined by the number of simultaneously active muscle fibers, their divergency and the magnitude of action potential. The generated heart potential vectors spread out in the space. The frontal plane projections of heart potential vectors was first determined by Einthoven in 1903 with the help of the so-called Einthoven-triangle. Since 1942 the Goldberger-like unipolar leads determine also the projections of the spatial heart vector in the frontal plane. Wilson and his collaborators introduced the precordial unipolar ECG leads in 1934 for the representation of potential vectors in the horizontal plane. For the representation of sagittal planal vectors unipolar paravertebral ECG leads were used by us in Hungary in 1963.
Our investigations have shown that the 12 conventional leads completed with three

paravertebral (VD_{1-3}) unipolar dorsal leads could form a triaxial system in which the direction of the X, Y, Z vector components can be defined. Frank described in 1956 which being well-proved, spread all over the world. The spatial X, Y and Z vector components of the Cartesian coordinates are registered in the form of orthogonally taken bipolar leads and orthogonal vector-cardiograms (frontal, horizontal and sagittal Lisajous loops). The Frank ECG leads are axial projections, the Lissajous loops are the planal projections of the spatial vectors. In polar-coordinate system it is possible to determine the spatial vector itself instead of its axial or planar projections. Polarcardiography or triaxicardiometry is a new branch of vectorcardiography taking its origin in the works of McFee, Abildskov, Sayers, Pipberger, Moore and Dover. Polar-coordinates are characterized by the spatial magnitude (M), by the azimuth (H^o) and elevation (V^o) angles. There has been a close mathematical correlation between the Cartesian and the polar-coordinates. If anyone wishes to convert Cartesian coordinates into polar ones the following equations are to be used by him $M = \sqrt{Mx^2 + My^2 + Mz^2}$ $H^o = \text{arc.sin}\,\frac{Mz}{Mxz}$ $V^o = \text{arc.sin}\,\frac{My}{M}$. If the term is reversed the equation will be as follows: $X = M\cos V^o \cos H^o$ $Z = M\cos V^o \sin H^o$ $Y = M\sin V^o$. In mathematical sense the information content of Cartesian and polar-coordinates are the same. Spatial velocity (sV) means the velocity of spread of impulse computed or derived from the coordinates X, Y, Z. Quantification of spatial velocity is based on the formula where X, Y Z represent Cartesian coordinates, ($sV = \sqrt{\left(\frac{dx}{dt}\right)^2 + \left(\frac{dy}{dt}\right)^2 + \left(\frac{dz}{dt}\right)^2}$) while dx, dy and dz are their changes in the function of dt, Spatial velocity was first defined by Hellerstein and Hamlin, in 1960. In the Pipberger program the data for both spatial magnitude and spatial velocity are computed by automatic analysis from the numerical data of the Cartesian X, Y, Z coordinate system. We examined in 1974 the quantification of spatial magnitude and velocity of normal and abnormal QRS. One normal and 19 abnormal groups were formed out of the 440 subjects studied. We concluded that sV ECG itself is of little informative vaalue. According to Yano and Pipberger "spatial velocity did not contribute more than 1,5% in diagnostic recognition rates". Oppositely, in location determination of spacecrafts spatial velocity has a 100% informative value.(Fig.2)

Fig.2.

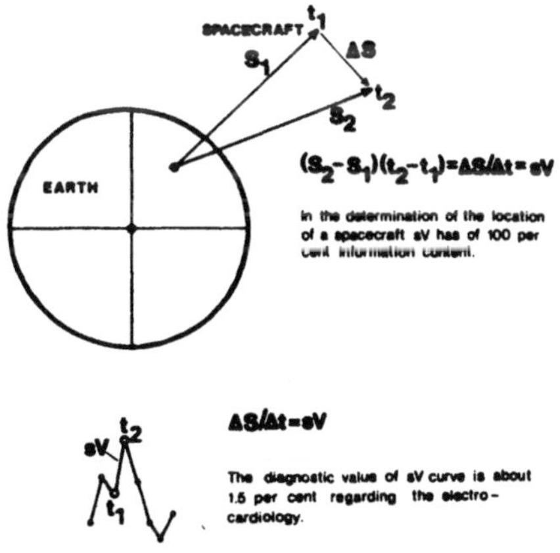

In the location determination process of spacecrafts the original xyz coordinate-system (which is drawn through the midpoint of the Earth) is transposed to the observation posts and the transposed x'y'z' system determined so that the azimuth and elevation angles are to be automatically corresponded with the longitude and latitude grades.(Fig.3) During the electrocardiological measurements the source of information are the Cartesian coordinates (Frank leads) which are drawn through the centre of thorax (Fig.4). The centre of thorax, however - is not identical with the dipole centre of the heart, like the observer post of the spacecrafts is not identical with the centre of Earth. The x'y'z' electrical coordinates drawn through the continuously changing dipole centres, and not the employed xyz space-coordinates i.e. Frank leads were that "observer posts", from where the real dipole centres of the heart would be determined. The dipole centre is the realization

Fig.3.

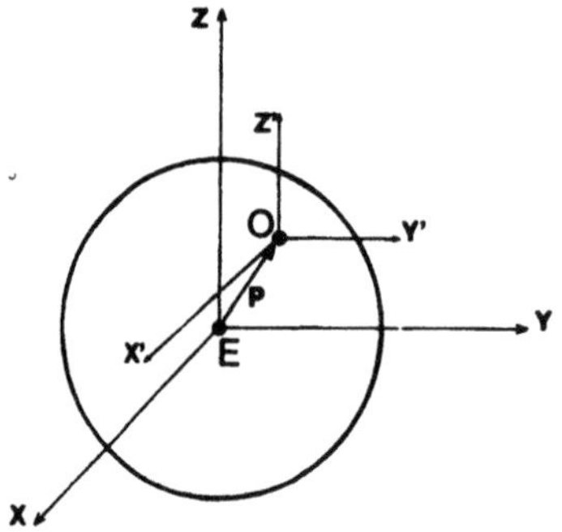

E = mid-point of Earth
O = observer post

of the electrical symmetry in the heart electrical field, the principle of its determination is the mirror image phenomenon of ECG, which is attached to the names of Duchosal, Laufberger and others. The automatical determination of that continuously changing dipole-centres has been failed up to this time.

This woodout from the 16th century (Fig.5) demonstrates the beginning of the algorhythmic view. Pythagoras and Boetius are competing in the presence of the goddess of arithmetics. The solution is symbolic from one side, numeric by help of an abacus from the other side.

Polar-coordinates are derivational amounts, counted either manually or analogically or digitally by computer out of the Cartesian coordinates. The analogue computer used for this purpose is the Triaxicardiometer (TCM) which was developed in Hungary by us in 1968. According to our triaxicardiometric method the Vx, Vy and Vz biopotentials of the triaxial Frank leads are fed directly into the calculating units of the Triaxicardiometer, which forms the polar-coordinates (triaxicardiograms). These functions are continuously given on the output of our device and are registered in the form of diagrams. This is the on-line operational mode.

The triaxicardiograms may also be stored in off-line mode for indirect analysis.

Fig.4.

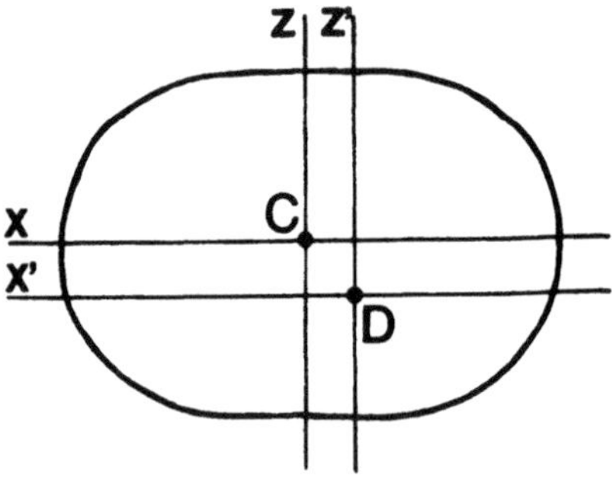

C = thorax center
D = dipol. center

Fig.5.

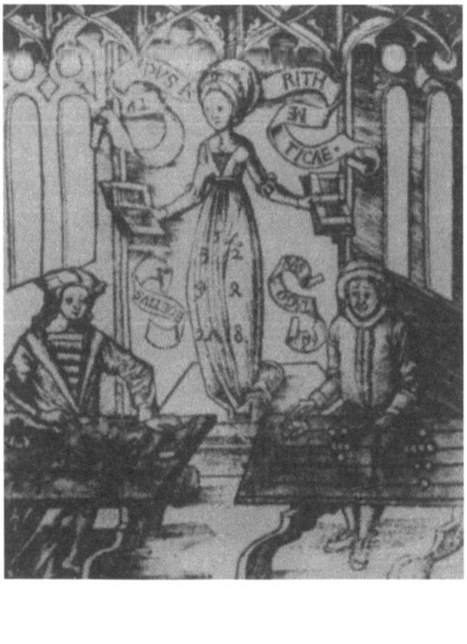

Polarcoordinates can also be determined by computer in a digital form. After having developed the Triaxicardiometer analogue computer we established the Budapest computer ECG diagnostic system.

Galilao Galilei in his above mentioned famous book wrote about "triangles, circles and geometrical figures" instead of numbers.

The performance of the dipolar electrical forces of the heart may also be represented "in triangles, circles and other geometric figures" either in Einthoven's triangle or in Cartesian planal and spatial coordinates.

All of them are members of an interrelation system.

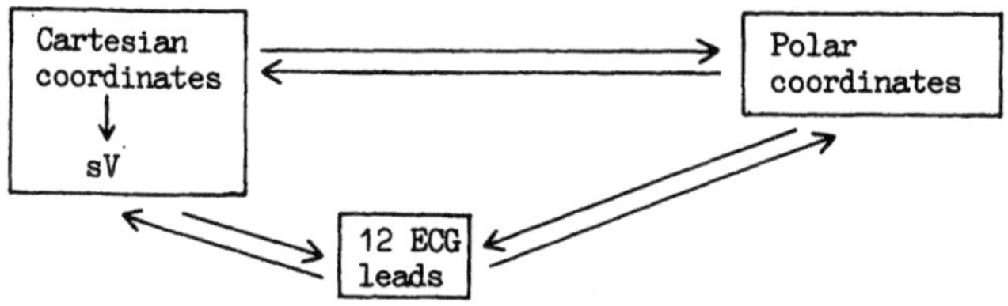

Out of the data of other members any of them can be computed. For example - our Budapest computer ECG diagnostic system is able to display the different vector positions either as Cartesian coordinates (Frank leads), Lissajous loops, or polar-coordinates, and even in the form of the 12 conventional leads. Finally it prints out the ECG diagnosis.
The twentieth century is marked by the tendency of integrating different branches of sciences. As a result of the gradual extension of the applicability of its methods, physics incorporates an ever increasing number of disciplines. That is why the location determination of our spacecrafts and the description of our heart's electrical vectors are made according to the same mathematical, geometrical and computational principles and relations.
One can have the impression that the organizing principles in the macrocosmos and our biological microcosmos are comparable and similar. Both of them and their sciences have the same methodology, the language of which are mathematics and geometry.

YOUNG INVESTIGATORS AWARD

Transcavitary Conduction and the Mean Frontal QRS Axis.

J. M. BEATTIE, F. A. GAFFNEY, C.G. BLOMQVIST

University of Texas, Southwestern Medical School, Dallas, Texas, USA.

SUMMARY

To study the possible electrocardiographic effects of variation in the sequence of ventricular activation we compared the echocardiographic morphology of left ventricular false tendons in 12 normal hearts with their respective mean frontal QRS axes.

INTRODUCTION

Left ventricular false tendons are fibromuscular structures invested in endocardium and they contain elements of the Purkinje network. They represent intracavitary ramification of the peripheral conduction system of the heart and contribute to ventricular activation. They show much anatomic variation and the purpose of this study was to compare variations in the echocardiographic morphology with the resultant mean frontal QRS axis.

METHODS

The study population consisted of 12 normal subjects 14-53 (mean 29) years, 10 of whom were women and 5 Caucasian. They comprised a heterogeneous group of laboratory volunteers and hospital clinic patients all of whom were considered to have clinically normal hearts with normal electrocardiograms. The unifying feature of this group was the presence of a single false tendon of varying morphology on echocardiography.

ECHOCARDIOGRAPHY

Echocardiograms were performed using a 90° phased array imaging system (Hewlett-Packard 77020A). Real-time images were displayed using focused 2.5 MH_z or 3.5 MH_z transducers and permanent records retained on 0.5 inch videotape. Four orthogonal imaging planes were sampled in all subjects for the supine or semi left lateral position. Views included the parasternal long-axis (PLA), parasternal short-axis (PSA), apical-4-chamber (Ap4Ch) and the apical-2-chamber (Ap2Ch). For diagnosis, false tendons had to be evident in at least two of these views. To facilitate classification of tendon morphology, left ventricular regions were defined by criteria of the American Society of Echocardiography (ASE, 1980). Fig. 1.

False tendons arising and inserting within the same ventricular region were classified as transverse and those connecting adjacent ventricular regions as diagonal.

ELECTROCARDIOGRAPHY

Standard 12-lead electrocardiograms were recorded with the subjects resting supine using a Marquette Series 4000 System. The limb **leads I, II and III** were recorded simultaneously and the mean frontal QRS axis estimated conventionally by comparing the relative amptitudes of the Q, R and S waves for these bipolar leads within a triaxial reference system.

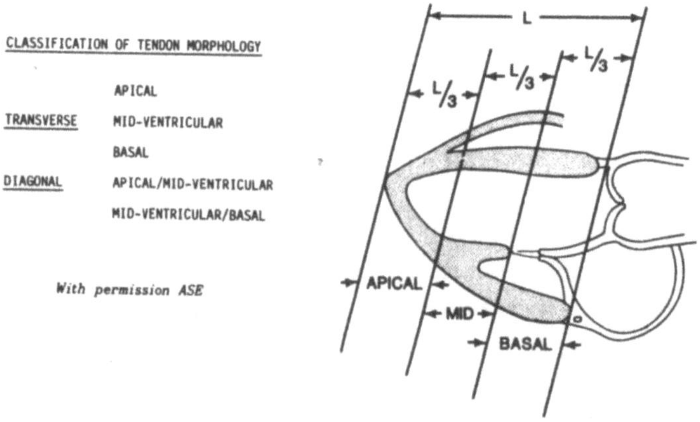

Figure 1 Nomenclature of ventricular regions.

RESULTS

The echocardiographic features of left ventricular false tendons of various morphology are demonstrated in figure 2. Two subjects exhibited apical tendons of transverse orientation. In 7 subjects, a mid-ventricular transverse tendon was evident and in 3, a diagonal tendon passed between the base of the heart and the mid ventricular region. Derived mean frontal QRS axes associated with specific tendon groups are shown in Table 1.

Table 1 False tendon morphological groups and their respective mean frontal QRS axes.

TENDON MORPHOLOGY	SUBJECTS (n)	MEAN FRONTAL QRS AXIS Degrees	(SD)
Apical transverse	2	+75	(16)
Mid-ventricular transverse	7	+37	(14)
Mid-ventricular/basal diagonal	3	+47	(20)

In the presence of apical transverse tendons, the axis appears to be directed more inferiorly while with mid-ventricular/basal diagonal and mid-ventricular transverse tendons, the axis shifts progressively leftward. All of the axis measurements, however, are within the normal range for the age groups studied.

DISCUSSION

Einthoven was the first to suggest that the complex sequence of electrophysiological events underlying ventricular activation could be summated as a vectorial entity dervided from the surface electrocardiogram (Einthoven et al, 1913). The concept of the electrical axis or manifest orientation, however, has a multifactorial basis (Horan, 1987). Major assumptions are conceded in terms of the uniformity of spread of the wavefront of activation through the ventricular myocardium and its continued propergation through heterogeneous tissues of different conductivities to the sampling electrodes. While the orientation of the heart within the thorax is accepted as a major determinant (Lepeschkin, 1979), little attention has been

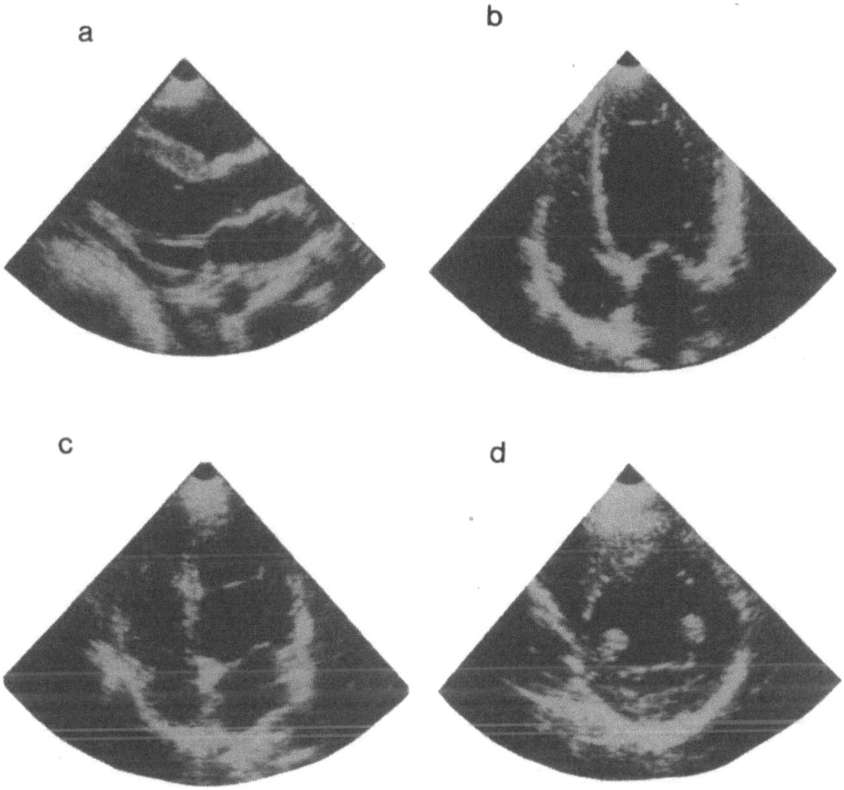

Figure 2 Examples of false tendon morphology.
a) Mid-ventricular/basal diagonal (PLA). b) Apical transverse (Ap4Ch)
c) Mid-ventricular transverse (Ap2Ch). d) Inter-papillary muscle. (PSA).

paid to the effect of anatomic variation in the intracavitary Purkinje network.

The major branches of the intracavitary conduction system are seen as false tendons and their echocardiographic variation has recently been described (Beattie et al, 1986). This technique permits comprehensive evaluation of the geometry and points of attachment of these structures in several orthogonal planes and the use of a system of nomenclature for ventricular regions and myocardial wall segments based on internal cardiac landmarks, provides precise definition of sites of Purkinje-myocardial coupling.

Previous studies in canine hearts have demonstrated the intimate relationship between the anatomy of these specialised conduction bundles and patterns of endocardial activation (Myerburg et al, 1975). Whether such structures contribute to the classic sequences of endocardial activation described by Durrer is a matter of conjecture (Durrer et al, 1970).

It is likely that the presence of false tendons results in early activation of the left ventricular free wall and this in vivo study supports the hypothesis that there is an associated leftward shift in the ventricular axis. The results suggest that the higher the point of free wall activation, the greater will be the contribution to the resultant axis. It is suggested therefore that the anatomic variability of these structures contributes to the spectrum of normality of the mean frontal QRS axis.

REFERENCES

(1) The American Society of Echocardiography Committee on Nomenclature and Standards: Circ. 62, 212 (1980).

(2) Einthoven, W., G. Fahr and A. de Waart: Pfluger's Arch. f.d. ges. Physiol. 150, 275-315 (1913).

(3) Horan, L. G.: J. Am. Coll. Cardiol. 9 1049-56 (1987).

(4) Lepeschkin, E.: in Progress in Electrocardiology (Ed.) P. W. Macfarlane, Pitman Medical, London. 417-20 (1979).

(5) Beattie, J. M., F. A. Gaffney, L. M. Buja and C. G. Blomqvist, Br. Heart J. 55, 525 (1986).

(6) Myerburg, R. J., K. Nilsson, A. Castellanos, R. Lazzara, B. Befeler and H. Gelband: in Recent Advances in Ventricular Conduction (Ed.) M. Cerqueira, Adv. Cardiol., Karger, Basel. 14, 2-14 (1975).

(7) Durrer, D., R. Th. Van Dam, G. E. Freud, M. J. Janse, F. L. Meijler, and C. Arzbaecher: Circ. 41, 899-912 (1970).

Localization of accessory atrioventricular connections and origin of ventricular tachycardia in patients with malignant tachyarrhythmias by electrocardiographic, electrophysiologic and scintigraphic techniques

D.PFEIFFER[1], R.PUNDRICH[2], H.J.OTTO[3], K.J.ROSTOCK[1], H.GUNKEL[3], K.RATHGEN[1]

1: Central Institute of Heart and Circulation Research, Academy of Sciences, Wiltbergstr. 50, Berlin, 1115

2: Medical Clinic, Department of Cardiology, Medical Academy, Leipziger Str. 44, Magdeburg, 3090

3: Radiologic Clinic, Department of Nuclear Medicine, Medical Academy, Leipziger Str. 44, Magdeburg, 3090, GDR

Summary: Localization of accessory atrioventricular pathways (AP) and of the originating side of ventricular tachycardia (VT) is an essential prerequisite for direct treatment by surgery or catheter ablation. To examine accuracy of different invasive and noninvasive mapping methods we investigated 18 patients (pts.) with AP and 5 pts. suffering from VT. The methods used were 12-lead electrocardiogram, 94-lead surface mapping, endocardial catheter mapping and radionuclide angiographic phase imaging (RAPI). RAPI revealed a 2nd AP in two pts. We demonstrated the AP on left side by electrical methods and on right side by RAPI in a further pt. The results in the remaining pts. are in correspondence. RAPI can localize the origin in pts. with VT and normal contraction pattern. RAPI is of less value in pts. suffering from VT because most of them have abnormal wall motion.

Introduction

Localization of accessory atrioventricular pathways (AP) and of the originating side of ventricular tachycardia (VT) is an essential prerequisite for direct treatment by surgery or catheter ablation (1). The topography of the arrhythmia can be revealed by 12-lead surface ECG (2), surface mapping (3), endocardial catheter mapping (4) and epicardial and endocardial mapping during open-chest surgery (5). These electrical mapping techniques are completed by methods of detection of mechanical action of the heart. Whilst kymography (6) and echocardiography (7) give no satisfactory results for detection the first contraction radionuclide angiographic phase imaging (RAPI) proves to be sufficient (8).

We compare different invasive and noninvasive techniques of localizing arrhythmia. The purpose of this study is to investigate usefulness and accuracy of different closed-chest mapping techniques in patients (pts.) with malignant tachyarrhythmias.

Material and methods

We investigated 18 pts. with anterogradely conducting AP and paroxysmal reciprocating tachycardia and/or atrial fibrillation. Localization of the AP in pts. with preexcitation syndrome was performed using 12-lead ECG, 94-lead surface mapping, endocardial catheter mapping and RAPI.

5 pts. suffered from VT. Topographic diagnosis of arrhythmia origin was performed with catheter mapping and RAPI.

For comparison of different mapping techniques of AP location we followed the proposal of the International Society and Federation for Cardiology, suggesting 6 subgroups of preexcitation with the help of 12-lead ECG (9). The technique is based on the polarity of delta wave and QRS complex. Surface mapping was performed with 94 leads from 1st to 7th intercostal space around the chest. We used polarity of delta wave 40 ms after the onset of QRS complex. Both methods were performed during sinus rhythm in pts. with distinct delta wave. In 7 pts. with minimal delta wave or masked forms of preexcitation we applied both techniques during atrial stimulation (fig. 1 and 2). Electrophysiologic methods of AP localization were used during sinus rhythm, atrial or ventricular stimulation and reentry tachycardia. The location of AP can be revealed by the measurement of retrograde conduction in cases with intermittend bundle branch block or ventricular premature beats during reentry tachycardia. The exact position of the AP is found on the point of the shortest anterograde (stimulus-delta-wave with maximal preexcitation) or retrograde conduction time (during ventricular stimulation or reentry tachycardia)(fig.3).

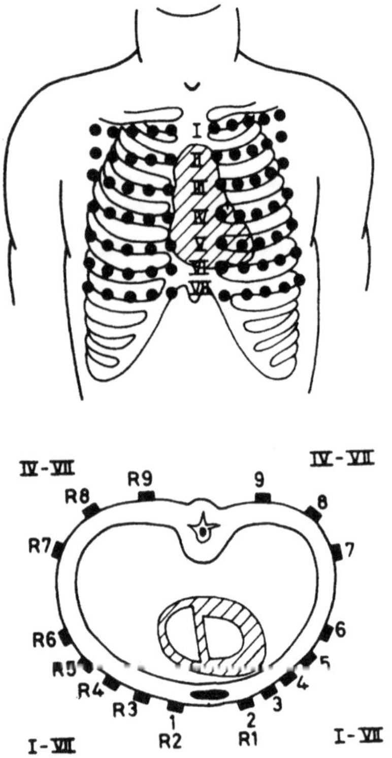

fig.1: Position of 94 leads for surface mapping

Phase analysis of the equilibrium blood pool scintigram was performed by fitting the fundamental Fourier harmonic to the multiple-gated left ventricular counts data in left anterior oblique projections during sinus rhythm, atrial and ventricular stimulation and sustained tachycardia. The study followed the frame mode at 30 frames per cycle. The site of the earliest contraction was determined from phase data displayed as composite static and dynamic images and phase histogram of each visually determined region.

5 pts. with VT were investigated with left and right heart endocar-

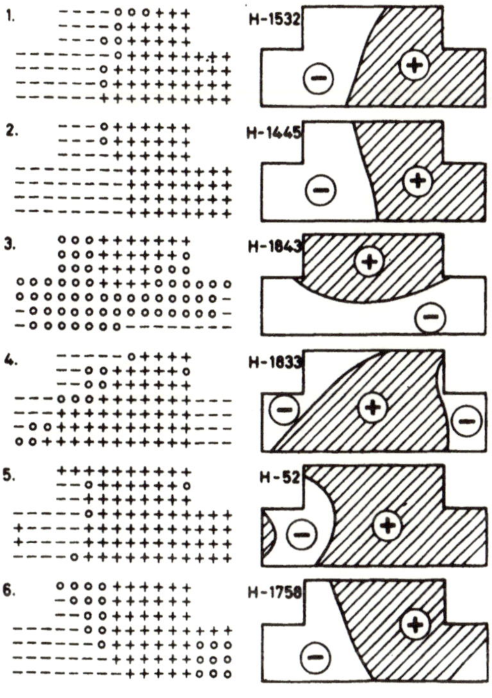

fig.2: Results of 94-lead surface mapping in pts. with AP in anterior right (1.), posterior right (2.), posterior left (3.), left free wall (4.), anterior (5.) and posterior paraseptal positions (6.)

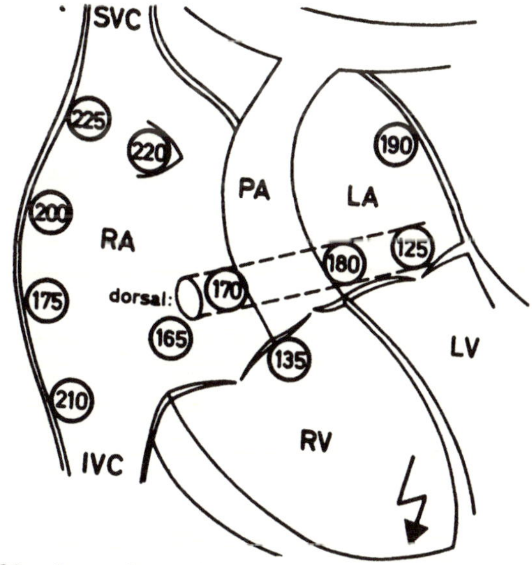

fig.3: endocardial catheter mapping in a pt. with left free wall AP

dial catheter mapping and RAPI.

Results

Determination of location of AP was performed by 12-lead ECG in 11/18, by 94-lead surface mapping in 9/18 cases and by catheter mapping and RAPI in 17/18 cases. Identical results of all methods used were found in 13/18 cases. 2 pts. had two AP as revealed by RAPI (tab. 1).

Best concurrence of different mapping techniques was found in anterior right, posterior left and anterior paraseptal positions of AP.

Pts. with VT suffered from coronary heart disease (n=2) or dilatative cardiomyopathy (n=2). One pt. had an idiopathic VT without evidence of any heart disease. Catheter mapping in right and left ventricle during sustained VT was performed in each pt. as RAPI. The abnormal contraction pattern in 3 pts. revealed a chaotic left ventricular wall motion without evidence of arrhythmia origin. In the 2 remaining pts. the results of catheter mapping and RAPI were in correspondence. The origin of the VT was in the basal interventricular septum (pt. with idiopathic VT) and in the basal posterior left free wall (pt. with cardiomyopathy).

Discussion

Direct treatment of tachyarrhythmias requires topographic diagnosis of arrhythmia origin (1, 2, 4, 8). Different invasive and noninvasive methods are investigated for closed-chest detection of arrhythmia substrates. The comparison of different techniques allows an estimation of the usefulness and precision of each method.

tab. 1: Results of mapping in 18 pts. with preexcitation syndrome

pat.	a/g	ECG	surf.	cath.	RAPI
1. H.H.	17/f	1	1	1	1
2. H.H.	51/m	-	-	4	2
3. F.M.	34/m	3	3	3	3,5
4. H.D.K.	42/m	3	?	3	3
5. E.K.	46/m	-	-	3	3
6. W.K.	34/m	-	-	4	4
7. A.F.	14/f	5	-	4	4
8. H.K.	48/m	3	4	4	4
9. E.K.	51/f	4	-	4	4
10. O.B.	19/m	4	4	4	4
11. M.L.	56/m	-	4	4	4
12. J.B.	41/m	-	-	4	4
13. J.S.	37/m	5	5	5	5
14. G.J.	39/m	1	1	6	6
15. H.S.	31/m	6	6	6	-
16. G.H.	20/f	-	-	6	6
17. M.S.	42/f	-	-	6	6
18. A.K.	48/m	4	1	6	3,6

The location of AP can be realized by surface ECG and surface mapping. Both methods can be used in pts. with visible delta wave. The techniques can not be used in pts. with retrogradely conducting AP. The methods are problematical in pts. with intermittend preexcitation or slow conducting AP. Atrial stimulation can enlarge delta wave in selected pts. In 12/18 pts. of this study (66,7 %) detection of the AP location was possible with surface ECG and surface mapping. The results from 9/12 pts (75,0 %) were in correspondence to other methods.

Catheter endocardial mapping is the method of choice for detection of AP location as well as the origin of VT (4, 10). The results are easy to obtain and reproducible. The difference between catheter mapping and RAPI with regard to the 2nd pt. is not clear. We suppose the presence of a 2nd AP as found in the 3rd and 18th pt.

The method is of high precision in cases with VT. Other techniques are less exact.

RAPI is useful in pts. with normal contraction pattern. In most cases with the preexcitation syndrome the wall motion is normal. In one pt. of this study (15th pt.), who was very anxious, we could not get sufficient results for detecting the site of AP. RAPI detected a 2nd AP in two pts. (3rd and 18th pt.). We do not have further evidence for the existence of two AP in these pts. The surgeons found a 2nd AP in 10-15% surgically treated pts. We believe that assuming further AP might help direct treatment (1, 2).

RAPI is of less value in most pts. with VT because of their abnormal wall motion. The method can control the results of catheter mapping in selected pts. with hemodynamically tolerated VT without underlying heart disease or with less disturbed contraction pattern.

In conclusion of these results we believe that a combined use of the above discussed methods for detecting the origin of VT and the AP location proves to be sufficiently precise. Further studies for estimating posterior paraseptal and lateral left locations of AP are necessary. RAPI is of interest because it is the only method for the detection of more than one AP in this study.

References

1. Gallagher, J.J.: Pace 10, 583-584 (1987)
2. Gallagher, J.J., E.L.C.Pritchett, W.C.Sealy, J.Kasell, A.G.Wallace: Progr.Cardiovasc.Dis. 20, 285-327 (1978)
3. Benson, D.W., R.Sterba, J.J.Gallagher, A.Walston, and M.S.Spach: Circulation 65, 1259-1268 (1982)
4. Miles, W.M., R.Yee, G.J.Klein, D.P.Zipes, and E.N.Prystowsky: Circulation 74, 493-500 (1986)
5. Gallagher, J.J., J.Kasell, J.L.Cox, W.M.Smith, R.E.Ideker, and W.M. Smith: Amer.J.Cardiol. 49, 221-240 (1982)
6. Bandiera, G., and P.F.Atognetti: Circulation 17, 225-229 (1958)
7. Windle, J.R., W.F.Armstrong, H.Feigenbaum, W.M.Miles, and E.N.Prystowsky: J.amer.Coll.Cardiol. 7, 1286-1294 (1986)
8. Nakajima, K., H.Bunko, A.Tada, J.Taki, N.Tonami, K.Hishida, T.Misaki, and T.Iwa: J.Nucl.Med. 25 7-13 (1984)
9. Willems, J.L., E.O.Robles de Medina, R.Bernard, P.Coumel, C.Fish, D.Krikler, N.A.Mazur, F.L.Meijler, L.Mogensen, P.Moret, Z.Pisa, P. M.Rautaharju, B.Surawicz, Y.Watanabe, and H.J.J.Wellens: J.amer. Coll.Cardiol. 5, 1261-1275 (1985)
10. Josephson, M.E., L.N.Horowitz, S.R.Spielman, H.L.Waxman, and A.M. Greenspan: Amer.J.Cardiol. 49, 207-220 (1982)

Correlation between biomagnetic localization of primary cardiac sources obtained by different models and radiographic-echocardiographic images

SICURO M.* and GONNELLI R.**

* Servizio di Cardiologia, Ospedale Valdese, Pomaretto (Torino), Italy
** Dipartimento di Fisica, Politecnico di Torino, Torino, Italy.

Summary
We compared the biomagnetic localization of cardiac sources obtained by the equivalent current dipole model (ECD) and by the current multipole model (CME) with morphological images (echocardiography and Xray teleradiography) during ventricular activation in normals. The results indicate that the CME model locates the primary sources in reliable positions when the ECD model fails (maps not strictly dipolar) and may give new useful informations on the sources depth even when maps have a good dipolar shape.

Introduction
For some years the equivalent current dipole (ECD) has been the only model used for the inverse problem solution and the source localization in cardiomagnetism. It is based on the assumption that the magnetic cardiac field detected outside the chest can be represented, in a first approximation, by the single current dipole generating, in a homogeneous conducting media, the magnetic field which best approximates the measured one.
It is well known that ECD model works well when the magnetic field is produced by small sources (relatively to the distance from the detection coil of the magnetometer) as in the case of His bundle and some accessory atrio-ventricular pathways (Erné and Fenici, 1984). For sources larger and deeper in the thorax, i.e. during the ventricular activation, magnetic field distribution shows, besides the ECD and the volume currents effects, contributions which can be interpreted as produced by other dipolar sources or by higher order components of the current multipole expansion (CME) of the primary sources (Varpula et al., 1985, Gonnelli and Agnello, 1987).
After some theoretical analyses of the CME (Katila and Karp, 1983), only very recently the CME model has been applied to the inverse problem solution in one subject affected by a severe WPW syndrome (Katila et al. 1987).
The purpose of this study is to apply the CME model to the analysis of experimental magnetic maps of normals during ventricular activation, verifying if the source localization so obtained is more realistic than that one obtained by the ECD model.

Materials and methods
Nine subjects aged 30-51 years, without history and clinical evidence of cardiovascular diseases, were studied by magnetocardiographic maps, echocardiography (ECHO) and Xray chest films.

The magnetocardiographic maps were obtained on the standard 36 points chest grid by a SQUID based second order asymmetric gradiometer with a baseline of 8 cm and a pick-up coil diameter of 2.42 cm.
The recording bandwidth was 0.1-100 Hz and the analog MCG signals, together with the ECG lead DII reference signals, were sampled at a frequency of 1 KHz by an A/D converter at 8 bits. Data acquisition and the first on-line analyses (peaks detection, signal periodicity controls, automatic artifact rejection) were performed by a microcomputer Apple IIE. Then data were transferred via an RS 232C interface and a special communication program to a microVAX II computer for subsequent analyses.
The inverse problem solution was obtained by a least square fit of the experimental maps, modeling the sources with the ECD alone (first term of the CME) and with the current multipole expansion truncated at the second term.
Such a procedure, searching for the best matching between theoretical field distribution and the measured one, determines the values of the 5 (ECD) and 8 (CME) parameters of the model. In the CME case they represent the 3 spatial coordinates of the source, the strengths of the first and the second order components and the 3 angles which describe the spatial orientation of these components.
In order to obtain 2D parasternal long-axis and M-mode left ventricle images in the same experimental conditions of the MCG maps, ECHO was performed in supine position by a Diasonics VTR 400 equipment. Interventricular septum (IVS_d) and left ventricular posterior wall (PW_d) diastolic thicknesses were digitized from the echocardiographic images together with the respective distances from the anterior chest surface.
Supine Xray chest teleradiographies were taken with a distance subject-film greater then 130 cm and with radioopaque markers of the limits of the MCG grid. From this films we extract the informations on cardiac silhouettes.

Results

In all the subjects we analysed the magnetic isofield maps at different instants of the QRS: during the early ascent of the R wave, in proximity of the R peak and at the terminal phase.
All the maps, during these instants, show a roughly dipolar structure, but two typical kinds of pattern are usually present.
The first one is visible at the early moments of the R wave onset and at the terminal phase: on the measured map the single dipole contribution is greatly prevalent and the isofield lines distribution is symmetric. Figure 1 shows an example of source localization in this case. The ECD model localizes the dipole, in the frontal plane, always inside the cardiac silhouette in a position consistent with the heart phisiology. In all these cases the source localization obtained by CME model is almost the same on the frontal plane. Nevertheless when we compare the depth of the equivalent sources with the position of cardiac structures (septum and left ventricle posterior wall) we observe that the CME localization is always deeper and physiologically more reliable than ECD localization (see fig. 1, lower right map). Using the CME approach the accuracy of the numerical fit has an appreciable increasing. This is demonstrated by the reduction of the σ parameter which represents a relative standard deviation between the fitted theoretical isofield map and the experimental one (Fig.1).
The second typical pattern is observed in the ascent phase of the R wave and at the R

peak: on the measured map the dipolar structure is still recognizable, but an important asymmetry is noted both in maxima and minima field values and in the extension of the positive and negative areas.

The positive values predominate, so that, at some instants, the map appears almost "monopolar-like".

In 5 out of the 9 subjects ECD analysis of these maps collocates the dipole outside the cardiac silhouette.

When inside, it is often placed in proximity of the apex.

In all the 9 cases the CME analysis localizes the sources inside the left ventricle projection on the frontal plane in positions more central and basal compared to ECD.

In Figure 2 a typical example of these results is shown.

For all the 9 subjects we compared the ECD and CME sources depths with the positions and thicknesses of septum and left ventricle posterior wall as obtained by ECHO.

The CME source location is always deeper in the thorax than the ECD one.

Figure 3 shows this comparison at the instant of maximum ventricular activation. In 7 subjects the ECD position is outside the sagittal projection of the left ventricle while only in 1 case the CME localizes the sources outside it.

Finally, at these instants, the numerical fit accuracy has a big improvement and the decreasing of σ reaches an average value of 56.4% .

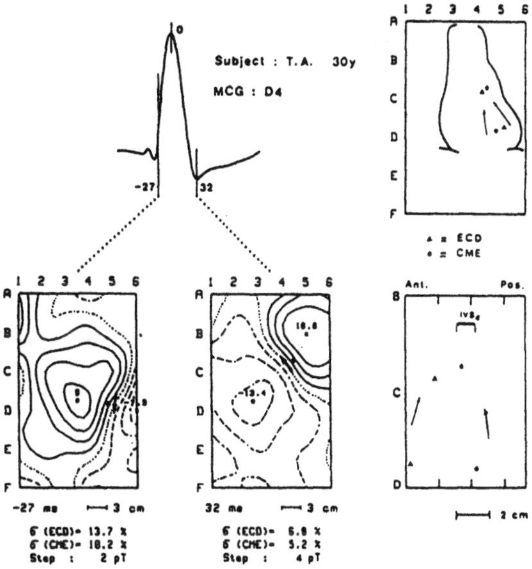

Figure 1. ECD and CME source localizations at two instants of the QRS in a normal subject. Full arrows on the maps indicate position and direction of the fitted ECDs. In the right side maps localizations are compared with cardiac silhouette and with diastolic position of the septum (IVS_d)

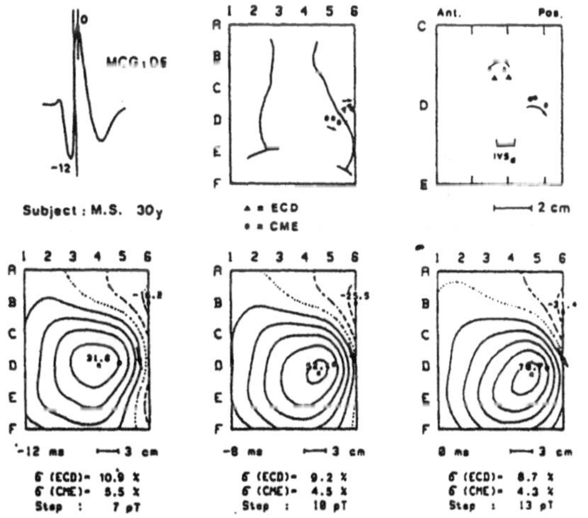

Figure 2. ECD and CME localizations at three instants during the ascent phase of the R wave in a normal subject. All the details are like in Figure 1.

Discussion and Conclusions

It is quite obvious that increasing the number of terms of the multipole expansion increases its numerical accuracy in representing experimental maps but it was not obvious that the parameters of the model so obtained constituted a good representation of the sources from the anatomical and physiological point of view. In fact, it is well known that a good mathematical coherence of a model with the experimental data not

always leads to a source localization consistent with the physiological knowledge.
Our results seem to demonstrate a better consistency of CME source localization with heart physiology when compared with ECD results.
When the portion of the cardiac muscle involved in the depolarization process is relatively limited in the space - in our case, the activation of interventricular septum, apical portion and basal ventricle structures of the heart - the magnetic field distribution outside the thorax can be analyzed with the ECD model. In such cases, CME analysis does not add substantially different informations for source localisation on the frontal plane while seems to give more physiologically reliable results on the sagittal one. When the depolarization wavefront involves greater parts of the cardiac muscle, as in ventricular free wall activation, the magnetic field contains contributions related to the complex and anysotropic fenomenon and, perhaps, to the presence of divergence-free circular primary currents as suggested by our previous theoretical and experimental results (Gonnelli and Agnello, 1987).

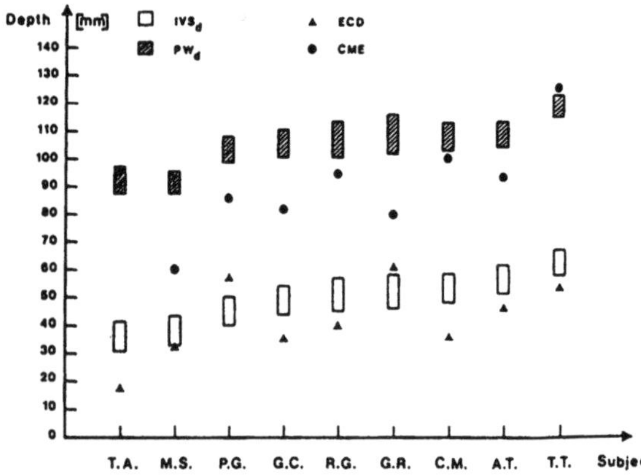

Figure 3. Comparison between source localizations obtained by the two different models and diastolic positions and thicknesses of interventricular septum (IVS_d) and left ventricle posterior wall (PW_d) at the QRS peak instant.

At these instants MCG isofield maps symmetry is lost and the ECD model alone becomes inadequate. CME model seems the only method to obtain a good source localization as is shown by the better correlation with morphological images obtained by other techniques. Generally speaking our results suggest that the CME model can be the best method to treat experimental data when maps are not strictly dipolar or even when they are monopolar but, on the other hand, it seems able to give new useful informations, at least on sources depth, even when maps have a good dipolar structure. Therefore we believe that this model can be also used for localization of normal or pathological sources of small extent like accessory A.V. pathways or arrhytmogenic foci.

References

(1) Erné, S.N. and R.R. Fenici: Proc. 10th ICEC, ed. H. Collan, P. Berglund and M. Krusius, Butterworth, London, 329-338 (1984)
(2) Varpula, T., T. Katila, T. Poutanen, and M. Seppänen : "Biomagnetism: Applications ahd Theory, ed. H.Weinberg, G.Stroink and T.Katila, Pergamon,Oxford, 180-185 (1985)
(3) Gonnelli R.S. and M. Agnello: Phys. Med. Biol. 32, 1, 133-142 (1987)
(4) Katila, T.E. and P.J. Karp : "Biomagnetism: an Interdisciplinary Approach", ed. S.J.Williamson, G.L.Romani, L.Kaufman and I.Modena, Plenum,New York, 237-263 (1983)
(5) Katila, T.E., R. Maniewski, M. Mäkijärvi, J. Nenonen and P. Siltanen: Phys. Med. Biol. 32, 1, 125-131 (1987)

Functional significance of a negative U wave in the exercise electrocardiogram

G.CHRONOPOULOS[1],D.V.COKKINOS[1],G.ATHANASOPOULOS[1],W.MOORE[2],R.D.LEACHMAN[2]

1 Tzanio State Hospital,Pireaus,Greece

2 Texas Heart Institute,Houston,Texas

S U M M A R Y

A negative U wave (nU) in exercise electrocardiography (ExE)signifies significant left anterior descending (LAD) disease.We correlated Ex changes with Tc^{99} radionuclide angiography in 96 patients (pts),all with coronary arteriography.The following significant data were found: Pts with a nU (38/96) compared to those without had a lower resting (0.46±11 vs0.57±7, p<0.01)and exercise (0.47±14 vs 0.61±11,p<0.01)ejection fraction(EF)and a greater incidence ofinferoapical-apical Ex motion abnormalities(p<0.05). Among pts (36/96)who increased their Ex EF those with a nU had a lower increase (p<0.01),of EF and a lesser inprovement of apical and septal motion.Among pts with a nU,those increasing their Ex EF had fewer septal apical abnormalities.

Conclusions : Pts with a Ex nU have a high incidence of LAD>75% stenosis. They increase their Ex EF to a lesser degree and manifest greater motion abnormalities.

I N T R O D U C T I O N

The appearance of a negative U wave in the precordial leads at exercise electrocardiography is a very specific marker of severe stenosis of the left anterior descending artery (LAD)[1,2].No data exists regarding its correlation with alterations of the left venticular (LV) function at exercise.

We investigated this correlation with the use of exercise radionuclide angiography.Additionally we compared the diagnostic value of these two methods for assessing severe LAD stenosis.

P A T I E N T S A N D M E T H O D S

Ninety-six patients (pts) who had :

a. Coronary arteriography with Sones and Judkins method

b. Treadmill exercise electrocardiographic (ECG) test(Bruce protocol,maximal exercise) and

c. Equilibrium (gated) radionuclide angiography, were studied.

The latter study was performed with the injection of 20($^+$Tzanio Hospital) or 30 (* Texas Heart Institute)mCi of Tc^{99m} pertechnetate,at 30^{0+} or 45^{0*} left anterior oblique,at rest,and during exercise,either in supine$^+$ or 45^{0*} sitting position,with the use of an electronically braked bicycle. Graded exercise was performed at 25W(150kpm/min)$^+$ or 100kpm/min* increments every 3 minutes,to the point of chest pain,preater than 1mm ECG ST

-segment depression or extreme fatigue.Data were also collected at 3-6 minutes following the cessation of exercise.

A CGR+ nuclear camera with computer estimation of the wall motion and an Ohio nuclear* camera with observer graded wall motion were used.

A normal study was considered if the LV ejection fraction (EF) increased by 5% at exercise[3],while an abnormal test was defined as no increase or decrease of the EF and/or appearance of LV wall motion abnormalities(hypokinesis,akinesis or dyskinesis).

R E S U L T S

Twenty-six pts had a normal coronary arteriogram and were excluded from further study.

Seventy pts ,who had significant coronary artery disease (CAD),including LAD disease were the subject of the following observations :

1. LAD stenosis ⩾75%

The diagnostic value of a nU,a decrease in EF and LV motion deterioration for LAD stenosis is seen in Table 1.It can be seen that a decrease in EF is a weaker predictor of LAD stenosis (Figure 1).

Table 1. Diagnostic value of various markers for LAD disease

	Sensitivity	Specificity	Pos.Pred.value	Neg.Pred.value	Accuracy
nU	0.62	0.78	0.92	0.34	0.65
↓EF	0.45	0.41	0.70	0.19	0.44*
Septal wall deter.	0.73	0.57	0.87	0.34	0.70
Apical deter.	0.78	0.50	0.86	0.36	0.72

* $p<0.005$

nU : negative U wave

↓EF : decrease in Ejection Fraction

deter : deterioration of motion

Figure 1

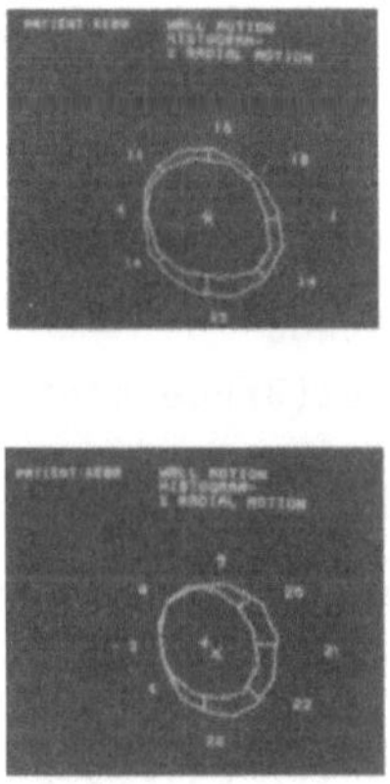

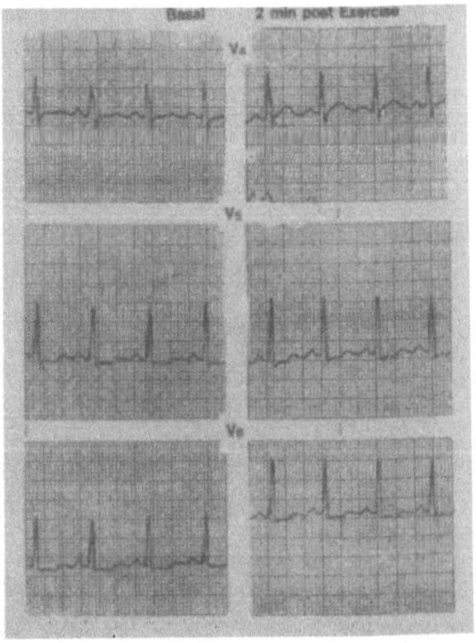

A 53 year old man with exercise precordial negative U waves.At exercise there is a decrease of the EF and septal dyscinesis.

2. <u>Existance of a nU</u>

Pts with a nU at exercise (38/96) compared to those without had a lower resting (0.46 ± 11 vs 0.57 ± 7, $p < 0.01$)and exercise(0.47 ± 14 vs 0.61 ± 11, $p < 0.01$) EF and a lesser % increase of the EF.Moreoever,those with a nU had more frequent inferoapical and apical wall motion deterioration.

3. Among pts with a nU,those with a decrease in EF had a greater incidence of septal and apical LV wall motion deterioration,while among pts with an increase of the EF at exercise,those with a nU had more frequent septal , inferoapical and apical LV wall motion deterioration (Table 2).

A nU has equal validity for predicting a decrease in EF with a positive U for predicting an increase.

<u>Table 2</u>. Segmental wall motion deterioration at exercise %.

	Septal	Inferoapical	Apical	Posterolateral
nU – EF↑	36	50	43	50
	*		+	
nU – EF↓	71	71	87.5	54
↑EF – nU	47	53	74	37
	*	+	*	
↑EF – pos U	10	8	30	30
segm.deter. – nU	58	74	84	39
		*	+	
segm.deter. – posU	69	44	50	12.5

* $p < 0.05$
+ $p < 0.01$

D I S C U S S I O N - C O N C L U S I O N S

From our results a nU appears to be a more valuable technique than a de - crease in EF or septal wall motion deterioration.Athough many authors have found sensitivity of the EF at 86% and of the regional wall motion deterioration at 56-73% for CAD in general[3,5],few give actual data for LAD[6].. Altogether a nU signifies a lesser increase in EF and LV wall motion deterioration even when the EF increases.Thus our results are similar to those of Gerson et al as regards the validity of a nU for predicting LAD disease and to those of Kishida et al[7] and Choo et al[8],who found more significant LV dysfunction.

This sign is obtained by simple exercise electrocardiography and schould be scrutinized more closely.

R E F E R E N C E S

1. Gerson MC,JF Phillips,SN Morris,PL McHenry:Circulation 60,1014-20(1979)
2. Salmasi A-M,SN Salmasi,AN Nicolaldes et al:Eur.Heart J.6,437-43(1985)
3. Lindsay J,NG Nolan,SA Goldstein,JM Bacos:Am.Heart J.106,271-78(1983)
4. Iskandrian AS,A-H Hakki,NL De Pace et al:JACC 1,1518-29(1983)
5. Jones RH,P McEwan,GE Newman et al:Circulation 64,586-601(1981)
6. Borer JS,KM Kent,SL Bacharach et al:Circulation 60,572(1979)
7. Kishida H,JS Cole,B Surawicz:Am.J.Cardiol. 49,2030-6(1982)
8. Choo MH,DG Gibson :Br.Heart J.55,428-33 (1986)

COMPONENTS OF THE HEART RATE POWER SPECTRUM DURING INDIVIDUAL SLEEP STAGES AND THEIR ASSOCIATION TO CENTRAL HEMODYNAMICS

G. Varoneckas

Palanga Dept., Inst. Cardiovasc. Res., 4 Vydūno St., Palanga 235720, Lithuanian SSR, USSR

SUMMARY. An analysis of heart rate (HR) power spectrum components in association with central hemodynamics during individual sleep stages demonstrated reduced HR parasympathetic control paralleled by deterioration of central hemodynamics in IHD patients. The most unfavourable situation was found to be REM sleep, characteristic by markedly reduced parasympathetic control and low level of cardiac output, which both might be responsible for appearance of cardiac abnormalities in this sleep stage.

INTRODUCTION

The heart rate (HR) power spectrum contains there major oscillatory components: low frequency component (LFC), associated with thermal-metabolic regulation, medium frequency component (MFC), reflecting predominantly sympathetic control, and high frequency component (HFC), reflecting parasympathetic control. There are data (Eckoldt et al., 1983; Žemaitytė et al., 1984) advocating for reduction of autonomic HR control by an impairment of IHD patients functional cardiovascular reserve. Reduced autonomic HR control have been found to be reflected by relative constancy of HR pattern throughout all the stages of sleep (so called reduced HR sleep pattern (HRSP)), as compared with patients, having typical HRSP, characterized by a decrease of HR and its variance with augmentation of respiratory arrhythmia during non-REM sleep and opposite their changes in REM sleep (Žemaitytė et al., 1984).

The aim of this study was an analysis of HR power spectrum components in association with central hemodynamics in IHD patients and in reference group of healthy subjects during sleep stages.

MATERIAL AND METHODS

The subjects were 30 healthy males, aged 29.8 (SEM 9.92) yrs, and 130 male IHD patients, aged 52.6 (SEM 8.68) yrs, including 32 patients with reduced HRSP, aged 59.9 (SEM 5.88) yrs. The patients with reduced HRSP were the ones with the worst cardiac functional status, the most of them with evidence of heart failure or previous myocardial infarction, NYHA class III. The polygraphic recordings of EMG, EOG, EEG, ECG, and rhythmogram (RG) were performed continuously throughout the night using conventional techniques (Žemaitytė et al., 1984). The impedance cardiography was used in stroke volume (SV) and cardiac output (CO) evaluation. RG and SV values were simultaneously fed into a Hewlett Packard computer throughout the night. The sleep stages were identified visually according Rechtschaffen and Kales' criteria (1968). An average HR (RR interval), SV, and CO were calculated by computer with respect to wakefulness and individual sleep stages. The HR power spectrum was evaluated using a Hamming window and divided into 3 major oscillatory components (Žemaitytė et al., 1986) (Fig.1.). The relative contribution by each oscillatory component to the HR power spectrum was calculated as relation of the power of each component to the total spectral power.

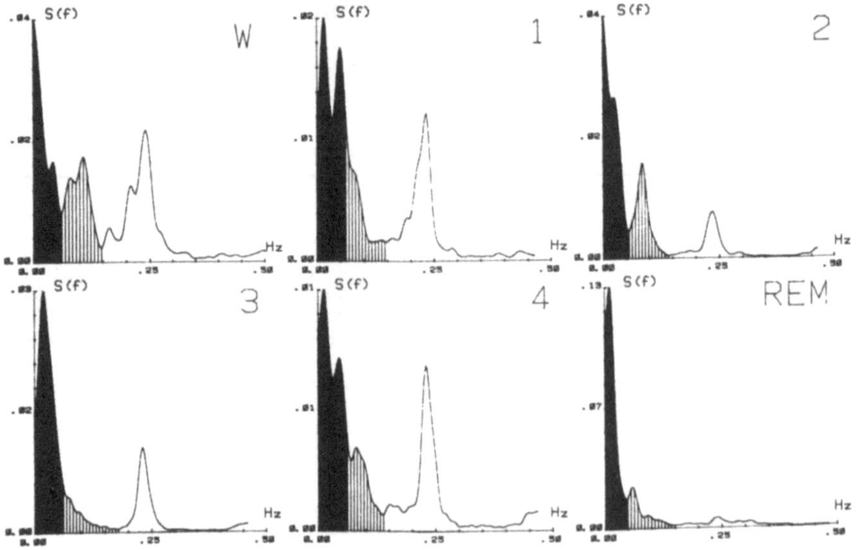

Fig.1. An example of the HR power spectra during wakefulness and sleep in a healthy subject. *W*, wakefulness; *1, 2, 3, 4*, and *REM*, stages of sleep. *Black area*, the share of LFC; *shaded area*, the share of MFC; *unshaded area*, the share of HFC.

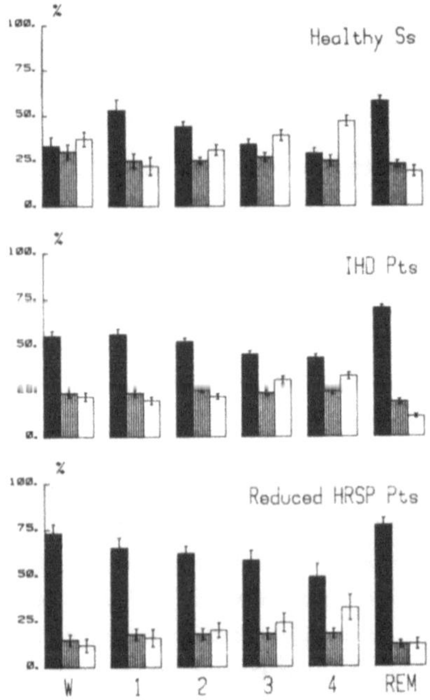

Fig.2. The relative values of the oscillatory components of the HR power spectrum during wakefulness and sleep in healthy subjects, IHD patients, and reduced HRSP patients. For designations see Fig.1.

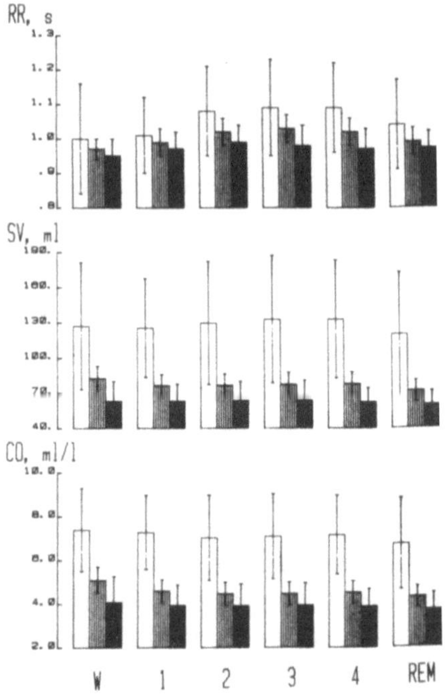

Fig.3. Means and SEMs for RR interval (*RR*), stroke volume (*SV*), and cardiac output (*CO*) as functions of individual sleep stages in healthy subjects, IHD patients, and reduced HRSP patients. For designations see Fig.1.

RESULTS

Heart Rate Power Spectrum during Sleep. The absolute values for individual oscillatory components of the HR power spectrum in a healthy subject were equal during wakefulness (Fig.1.). The deepening of sleep was paralleled by a decrease in total spectral power, largely accountable for by LFC. During stage 4 the total spectral power was at its nadir, contrasted by an increased contribution by HFC with lowered values of LFC and MFC, REM sleep was characterized by an increase in total spectral power largely accountable for by marked prevalence of LFC due to relatively small contribution of MFC and HFC. Similar results were observed in the group of healthy subjects (Fig.2.). The contribution of LFC in the HR power spectrum, rising in stage 1, gradually diminished by deepening of sleep and increased again in REM sleep. MFC contribution remains relatively constant during all sleep stages. HFC, gradually rising during progress of non-REM sleep, dropped markedly in REM sleep.

In IHD patients, as compared with healthy subjects, wakefulness state was characterized by a lower total spectral power, especially of HFC and MFC, being responsible for relative increase of LFC contribution and diminution of HFC and MFC ones to HR power spectrum (Fig.2.). The sleep dependent dynamics of relative contributions by the oscillatory components to the HR power spectrum, however, was similar in healthy subjects and IHD patients. Reduced HRSP patients were characterized by a more marked decrease in the total spectral power and all oscillatory components in wakefulness. The relative contribution by MFC in this group was nearly constant during non-REM sleep, but it was decreased in REM sleep only in parallel to diminution of HFC. LFC decreased and HFC increased during slow wave sleep and opposite was true in REM sleep.

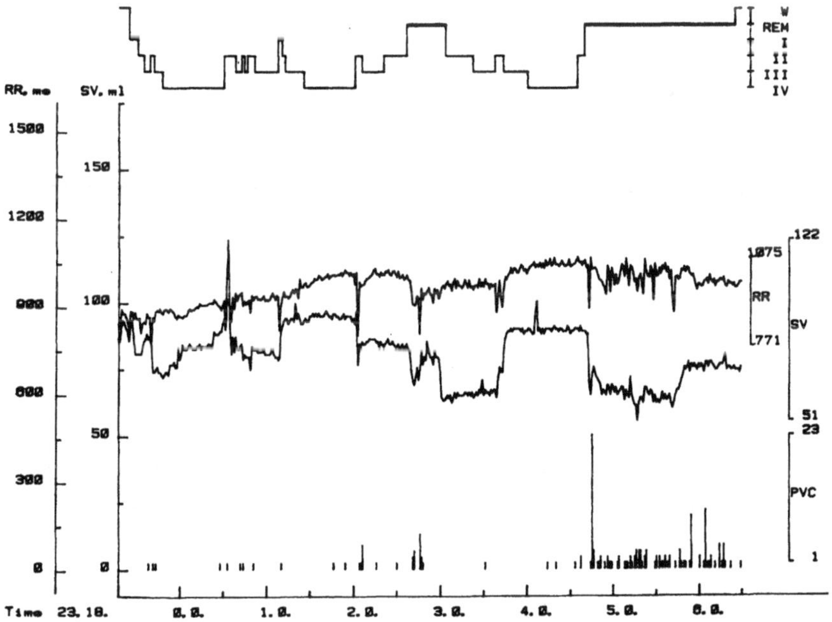

Fig.4. An example of HR and central hemodynamics analysis during sleep demonstrating an increase of premature ventricular contractions (*PVC*) associated with a decrease of stroke volume (*SV*) during REM sleep. *Abscissa,* time *ordinate,* RR interval (*RR*), SV and PVC averaged in 1-min periods. A hypnogram which shows scores of sleep stages also is given.

Central Hemodynamics Changes during Sleep. Wakefulness state of IHD patients, as compared with healthy subjects, was characterized by a lowered baseline level of SV and CO without the difference in HR frequency of both groups (Fig.3.). HR decreased in IHD patients as well as in healthy subjects during non-REM sleep and increased in REM sleep. The group of reduced HRSP was characterized by relatively constant HR values. In healthy subjects, SV gradually rising during non-REM sleep dropped in REM sleep. CO remained nearly constant during all the stages of sleep. In IHD patients, SV slightly diminishing during non-REM sleep decreased additionally in REM sleep. CO progressively dropped during all sleep stages, especially REM sleep. In reduced HRSP patients, SV and CO were nearly constant during non-REM sleep, although they had the lowest level of CO in REM sleep because of more expressed drop of SV without evident changes in HR during this sleep stage. Thus, REM sleep is the very situation with the mostly reduced central hemodynamics, especially in patients with reduced HRSP. Cardiac abnormalities, such as a depression of the ST segment of ECG and dangerous dysrhythmias, predominantly occurring in REM sleep, were characteristic to IHD patients, especially to the patients with reduced HRSP. An example of a marked increase of premature ventricular contractions during sleep, associated with the onset of REM sleep and diminution of central hemodynamics is presented in Figure 4.

DISCUSSION

Diminution of CO followed by reduction of parasympathetic control during REM sleep in IHD patients, especially with reduced HRSP, might be seen as mostly responsible for occurrence of dangerous cardiac abnormalities during this sleep stage as a result of low level of central hemodynamics paralleled by lack of protective role from parasympathetic control. Mechanism of the association between the reduction of autonomic HR control and deterioration of central hemodynamics in IHD patients remains to be explained. It is still not clear if those changes are occurring anly as parallel but independent, or the reduction of autonomic HR control is the result of changes in central hemodynamics, particularly through influence from increased resistance in small blood vesels. Nevertheless, an evaluation of HR power spectrum and its components might be suggested as a noninvasive indication of functional cardiovascular reserve.

CONCLUSIONS

IHD patients, as compared with healthy subjects, were characterized by reduced HR control, predominantly parasympathetic one, evident from decreased HR total spectral power, especially from reduction of HFC contribution. The reduction of HR control is paralleled by diminution of stroke volume and cardiac output, especially in patients with reduced HRSP. Reduced parasympathetic HR control and diminished central hemodynamics, particularly during REM sleep, in IHD patients with reduced HRSP might be seen as responsible for more frequent appearence of dangerous cardiac abnormalities occurring during this stage of sleep.

REFERENCES

1. Eckoldt, K., H. Cammann, and U. Manthey: 10th International Congress on Electrocardiology, Bratislava, 68 (1983).
2. Žemaitytė, D., G. Varoneckas, and E. Sokolov: Psychophysiology 21, 290-298 (1984).
3. Žemaitytė, D., G. Varoneckas, K. Plauška, and J. Kaukėnas: Int. J. Psychophysiology 4, 129-141 (1986).

Nondipolarity Estimation - an Additional Diagnostic Information in Myocardial Infarction ?

ROBERT HATALA and MICHAL MACO

Departments of Internal Medicine and Clinical Pathophysiology, Comenius University School of Medicine, Bratislava, Czechoslovakia

Summary

With progressive deviation of ventricular activation process from the "ideal" dipolar behaviour the contribution of nondipolarity (ND) in CEF increases. For it´s estimation the MEHG model was used. In healthy persons a typical ND time course pattern during QRS complex was observed, in patients with MI a close relation of the timing of ND peak in QRS complex to MI location was found. The proposed method might offer a new additional diagnostic information concerning MI localization and extent.

Present clinical interpretation of ECG is still based on the concept of dipole representation of the cardioelectric field (CEF). However, today there is sufficient evidence obtained by different methods that the real CEF contains already under physiological conditions a significant contribution of nondipolar (or extradipolar) information (Taccardi, 1963, Horan et al., 1972, Harumi et al., 1986). This fact might be explained by physiological deformation of the myocardial activation wave spread, which becomes more prominent under pathological conditions, especially with focal myocardial lesions. It was the purpose of our study to quantify the nondipolar (ND) content in CEF during ventricular activation in normal men and in patients with myocardial infarction (MI).

Our method of ND estimation is based on the model of multipole equivalent heart generator (MEHG) comprising dipole, quadripole and octapole. The data necessary for the calculation of successive components of the multipole expansion were obtained by body surface potential mapping from 190 electrodes on the chest and by measuring of the chest geometry, both with the EKKG-80 system (Kneppo and Titomir, 1979). By means of the previously described mathematical formulas using the surface integration (Kneppo and Titomir, 1979, Maco et al., 1984) we have calculated the first 15 components of the MEHG (A_{nm}, B_{nm}). The magnitude of contributions from individual multipoles was evaluated as the root mean square potential calculated on spherical surface enveloping the heart. Nd contribution was defined as the ratio of summed quadripolar and octapolar contributions to the dipolar contribution :

$$K_{oq/d} = \frac{1}{RD} \sqrt{\frac{3}{5} Q^2 + \frac{3}{7} O^2}$$

where R is the sphere radius and D,Q and O characterize the contributions of dipolar, quadripolar and octapolar components, respectively, defined by the relations :

$$D = \sqrt{A_{11}^2 + B_{11}^2 + A_{10}^2}$$

$$Q = \sqrt{A_{20}^2 + 3(A_{21}^2 + B_{21}^2) + 12(A_{22}^2 + B_{22}^2)}$$

$$O = \sqrt{A_{30}^2 + 6(A_{31}^2 + B_{31}^2) + 60(A_{32}^2 + B_{32}^2) + 360(A_{33}^2 + B_{33}^2)}$$

We have estimated the ND contribution in a control group of 28 healthy men of 23 to 35 years age (mean age 27.3 ± 3.7 years) and in a group of 21 men of 44 to 64 years age with MI (mean age 55.2 ± 6.6 years). The patients were examined 3 weeks to 3 months after the acute coronary event, the localization of the MI as determined by 12 leads ECG, VCG and BSPM was anterior in 9 cases (AMI), infero-posterior in 7 cases (IMI) and circular in 5 cases (CMI).

Results

1. ND during ventricular activation in healthy subjects

The mean value of the ND contribution during QRS complex was 31.8 ± 8 % and 26.6 ± 5.9 % during T wave. In the time course of the ND contribution in QRS complex two characteristic minima were observed (Fig.1).

2. ND during ventricular activation in patients with MI

In patients with MI a significant increase in overall ND level during the entire ventricular complex was observed. The mean value of the ND contribution during QRS complex and T wave reached 39.3 ± 12.7 % and 42.1 ± 11.4 % , respectively. In the time course of ND contribution in QRS complex considerable alterations of it´s pattern were observed. The character of these changes was in close relation to MI location (Fig.2).

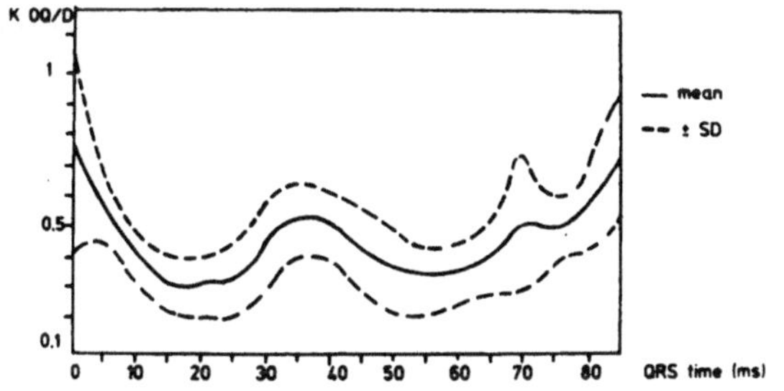

FIG.1 Time course of ND contribution estimated my means of the Koq/d ratio during QRS complex in the control group. Two typical minima are observed, appearing 15-25 ms and 50-60 ms after QRS onset, respectively. For all fig. the abscisa is the QRS time axis measured from QRS onset, the ordinate represents Koq/d values (see text for definition).

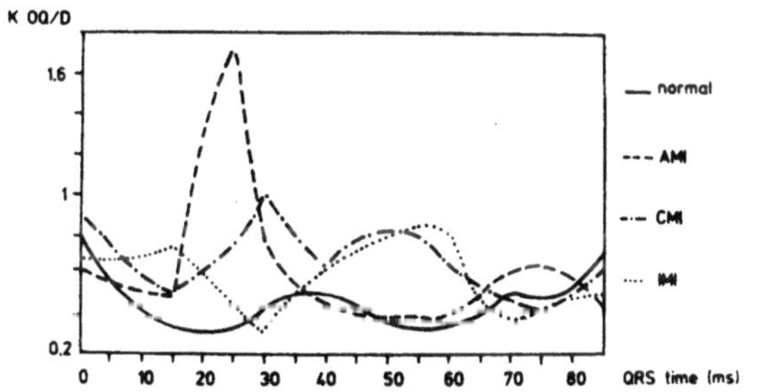

FIG.2 Time course of ND during QRS complex in selected pts. with MI in different locations (anterior-AMI, circular-CMI, inferoposterior-IMI) compared with the mean control ND pattern. Note the significant alterations of the ND pattern and their timing: major peak in AMI 25 ms after QRS onset, in IMI 55 ms after QRS onset and in CMI a continual rise of ND level throughout the QRS complex.

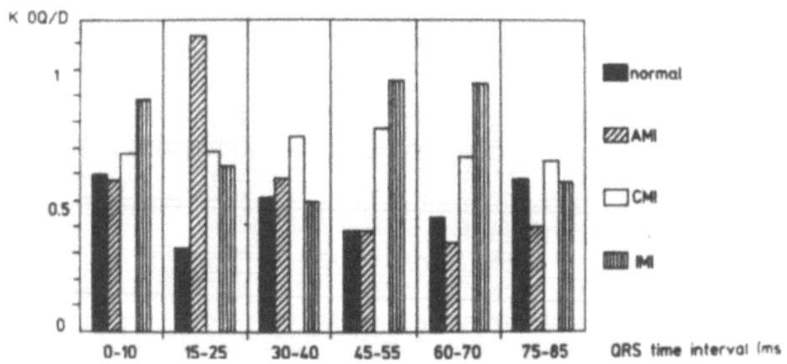

FIG.3 ND level during QRS in controls and MI patients expressed by time integration in selected QRS time-intervals. The bars represent the mean ND level in the concerned "time-window" (see text for further comments).

Discussion

Our findings concerning the time course of ND contribution during QRS complex are consistent with the presently accepted knowledge of ventricular activation sequence (Durrer et al., 1970). The initially high ND content might be the consequence of multifocal initiation of septal and paraseptal endocardial activation. The subsequent rise of the rather homogenous activation front is reflected in the dominantly dipolar character of the CEF. A further increase of ND contribution 25-35 ms after QRS onset might be explained, in agreement with published data (Taccardi, 1963, Harumi et al., 1986), with the occurence of right (area pretrabecularis) and, later, left epicardial breakthroughs. Terminal increase of ND content might be due to the coexistence of tangential and transmural activation spread in distant, anatomically separated ventricular regions (posterobasal regions of both ventricles, LV lateral region, conus pulmonalis). In patients with MI a marked increase of the ND contribution was observed, with peak levels in the time intervals corresponding to the time of normal activation of the infarcted area (i.e. time instance during which the concerned area would be activated if it were not infarcted). In cases with AMI the maximum of ND contribution was observed 15-30 ms after QRS onset, in IMI 45-75 ms after QRS onset and for CMI a relatively continual increase of ND level during the entire QRS complex was found (Fig.3).

Conclusions

The proposed method of ND estimation in CEF might provide further insight into both physiologic and pathologic ventricular activation process. In patients with MI it might offer a new additional diagnostic information concerning MI localization and extent, it´s clinical value has to established by further studies.

References

1. Taccardi, B.: Circulation, Res.12, 341-352 (1963)
2. Horan, L., Flowers, N.C., Miller, C.B.: J.Electrocardiol. 5, 211-224 (1972)
3. Harumi, K., Tsunakawa, H., Kanesaka, S., Nishiyama, G. in van Dam, R.Th. and van Osteroom, A.: Electrocardiographic Body Surface Mapping, 283-288, Martinus Nijhoff Publ., Dordrecht (1986)
4. Kneppo, P., Titomir, L.I.: IEEE Trans. Biomed. Eng. 26, 21-28 (1979)
5. Maco, M., Kneppo, P., Hatala, R., Kužmová, J. in Ruttkay-Nedecký, I. and Macfarlane, P.: Electrocardiology ´83, 104-109, Excerpta Medica (1984)
6. Durrer, D., van Dam, R.Th., Freud, G.E., Janse, M.J., Meijler, F.L., Arzbaecher, R.C.: Circulation 41, 899-912 (1970)

FUNDAMENTALS OF CARDIAC EXITATION

Transient outward current in mammalian ventricular fibres and its role in the control of action potential configuration

J. ŠIMURDA, M. ŠIMURDOVÁ

Department of Biophysics, Research Institute of Medical Engineering (Chirana), Brno, Czechoslovakia

Summary

The inhibition of slow inward current (I_{Ca}) in dog ventricular muscle unmasks a transient outward current (I_{to}) which is activated by depolarizing steps above 40 mV from resting voltage. The suppression of this current by 4-aminopyridine (1 mM) has a striking effect on the course of repolarization phase of action potential (AP). In addition to I_{Ca}, I_{to} plays a role in the mechanism of rhythm-induced variations of AP configuration. Both currents contribute to the increase of plateau level and prolongation of premature APs.

Introduction

The transient outward current was identified in response to depolarizing steps of membrane voltage in nerves and muscles. It has been long believed that in the heart a similar current is inherent only in Purkyně fibres. Two different components of I_{to} have been separated. One of them is probably controlled by activating and inactivating gating mechanism, the other is related to changes of intracellular Ca concentration. The existence of I_{to} in atrial muscle has been demonstrated by voltage clamp experiments in different species. In ventricular muscle the presence of I_{to} is controversial. I_{to} has been identified in rabbit (Kukushkin et al., 1983) and rat (Josephson et al., 1984), however, these species are atypical as far as the repolarization phase of AP and its rhythm-induced variations are concerned. On the other hand, the existence of I_{to} was questioned in guinea-pig (Josephson et al., 1984) and cat (Ten Eick and Robertson, 1983). Thus, the question of ubiquity and functional significance of this current system in the heart remains open. In our experiments I_{to} was identified in dog ventricular muscle. It is suggested that both I_{Ca} and I_{to} are responsible for supernormal premature action potentials.

Material and methods

Thin trabeculae (less than 0.7 mm in diameter) without branches and residual Purkyně fibres were excised from right ventricle of adult dogs under deep urethan anaesthesia and mounted into a double sucrose gap chamber provided with five compartments. Muscles were stimulated by short (1 ms) current pulses and APs were recorded. In voltage clamp experiments membrane currents were recorded in response to rectangular pulses of membrane voltage (for detailes see Šimurda et al., 1981). To inhibit I_{Ca} verapamil (Isoptin Lek) was added into the Tyrode solution in concentration of 10^{-5} M. I_{to} was depressed by addition of 4-amino-pyridine (4-AP) 10^{-3} M. The pH and temperature of solutions were 7.3 ± 0.1 and 30 ± 0.2°C, respectively.

Results

Under normal conditions in current responses to depolarizing clamp steps I_{to} is not discernible because it overlaps with much larger I_{Ca} (Fig.1,a). Only after an effective block of I_{Ca} a surge of transient outward current appears on the current trace (b) following the decay of rapid inward current (I_{Na}). This current is partially or completely depressed after the addition 1 mM 4-AP (c), an inhibitor of Ca_i-independent component of I_{to} in Purkyně fibres. I_{to} appears at depolarizing

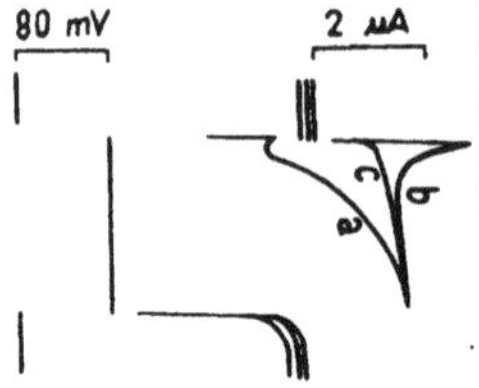

Fig. 1 Transient outward current in dog ventricular muscle. Responses of membrane current to voltage pulse 300 ms, 80 mV from holding voltage = resting voltage. a: normal Tyrode solution; b: Tyrode + verapamil; c: Tyrode + verapamil + 4-AP. The difference of current traces (b - c) is considered I_{to}.

steps above 40 mV (from holding voltage = resting voltage) and increases progressively with the magnitude of steps. Rapid activation of I_{to} is followed by slower inactivation with the time constant of about 25 ms which is not clearly related to membrane voltage. At the resting voltage the recovery from inactivation proceeds with the time constant of approximately 400 ms (not illustrated).

Farmacological analysis makes it possible to estimate the contribution of the transient currents I_{Ca} and I_{to} to the rhythm-induced variations of AP repolarization (Fig.2). The muscles were stimulated with suprathreshold pulses (0.5 Hz) and APs were recorded. Excitations with variable prematurity (T) were interpolated under steady state conditions. In Fig.2 the time course of electrical restitution is characterized by the dependence of duration of AP (D) on its prematurity T. D was measured on the level of membrane depolarization by 50 mV. Under control conditions (Tyrode solution) the AP duration rapidly increases in time to a maximum at about 0.35 s and then slowly declines to a steady state value (curve a). This overshoot is only partly abolished by 4-AP (b). The verapamil induced block of I_{Ca} causes a substantial shortening of AP, however, the region of the prolonged premature APs (supernormal AP) still remains (c). Only if I_{Ca} and I_{to} are blocked simultaneously (by verapamil + 4-AP) the overshoot on the electrical restitution curve disappears completely (d).

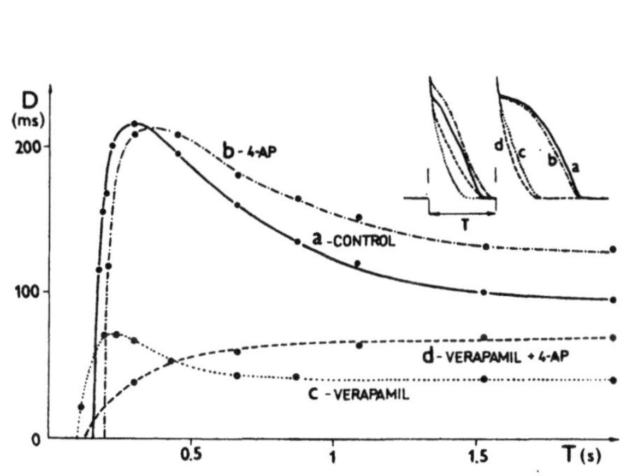

Fig.2 The dependence of action potential duration (D) on the prematurity of excitation (T) in normal Tyrode solution (a), in Tyrode + 4-AP (b), in Tyrode + verapamil (c), and in Tyrode + verapamil + 4-AP (d). The rate of stimulation was 0.5 Hz. The inset above illustrates the steady state AP (T = 2 s) and the ensuing premature AP (T = 0.3 s).

In the following experiments the last steady state and the premature APs were substituted by clamped rectangular pulses (Fig.3) and ionic membrane currents were recorded. I_{Ca} and I_{to} were estimated under the effect of 4-AP and verapamil, respectively, and measured as illustra-

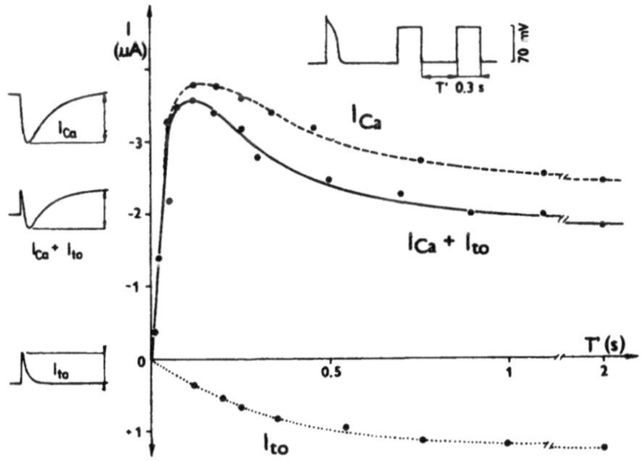

Fig.3 The relationships between the components of membrane current and duration of premature interval in normal Tyrode solution (I_{Ca} + I_{to}), in Tyrode + 4-AP (I_{Ca}), and in Tyrode + verapamil (I_{to}).

ted on the left part of Fig.3. The control current measured in normal Tyrode solution (frequently but inaccurately considered net I_{Ca}) is labelled $I_{Ca} + I_{to}$.

The relationships between magnitudes of current components and intervals between clamped pulses (T) clearly show that either I_{Ca} or I_{to} are able to constitute the the overshoot on the electrical restitution curve. The resulting effect becomes more pronounced with simultaneous operation of both factors.

Discussion

Unlike in Purkyně fibres, I_{to} in dog ventricular muscles is masked by the slow inward current. Therefore, it could easily remain unnoticed in earlier voltage clamp experiments. I_{to} tends to accelerate membrane repolarization namely during its early phase resulting in a depression of plateau and AP duration. Thus, the gradual recovery of I_{to} from inactivation after preceding excitation is manifested by gradual shortening of APs. It might seem that the course of electrical restitution curve with the region of prolonged APs may be explained by approximately exponential recovery of two transient currents with the opposite effect on plateau level and AP duration. The recovery of I_{Ca} results in prolongation while a slower recovery of I_{to} in shortening of AP. Nevertheless, as demonstrated in Fig.3, even the interval-dependence of net I_{Ca} exhibits a maximum, thus supporting our earlier observations (Šimurda et al., 1984). Hence, two independent mechanisms are responsible for electrical restitution curve with the region of prolonged APs.

Cohen et al. (1976) have shown that the progressive shortening of AP between endocardial and epicardial layers (which is closely related to the polarity of T wave of ECG) is rate-dependent and that the electrical restitution curve with overshoot exists in endocardial but not in epicardial region of a sheep ventricle. It remains to demonstrate whether the mechanism responsible for this heterogeneity of ventricular tissue includes also I_{to}.

References

(1) Kukushkin, N.I., R.Z. Gainullin, and E.A. Sosunov: Pflügers Arch. 322, 87 - 92 (1983)
(2) Josephson, I.R., J. Sanchez-Chapula, and A.M. Brown: Circ. Res. 54, 157 - 162 (1984)
(3) Ten Eick, R.E. and L. Robertson: Federation Proc. 42, 730 (1983)
(4) Šimurda, J., M. Šimurdová, P. Bravený, and J. Šumbera: Pflügers Arch. 391, 277 - 283 (1981)
(5) Šimurda, J., M. Šimurdová, P. Čupera, A.A. Freydin, and J. Šumbera: In: Electrocardiology '83. Eds. I. Ruttkay-Nedecký and P. Macfarlane, Excerpta Medica, Amsterodam-Oxford-Princeton, 22 - 26 (1984)
(6) Cohen, I., W. Giles, and D. Noble: Nature 262, 657 - 661 (1976)

Bioelectric activity of frog atrium cells with non-typical impulse activity

KAMKIN A.G., KISELEVA I.S., KIRCHEIS R., KOSITZKY G.I.

2nd Pirogov's Medical Institute,
Ostrovityanova St., 1, Moscow 117437, USSR.

Summary

Atrium cells of the isolated frog heart perfused with physiological solution were investigated using microelectrode technique. Beside the known cells of the working myocardium and conduction system in the greater-trabecula and smaller-trabecula layers the cells were studied from the deeper transverse fine-fibred layer containing smooth muscle elements. It is shown that membrane potential value of this layer's cells ranges within -25mV and action potential amplitude from -5mV to 25mV or not detected at all. Induced intracellular hyperpolarization caused linear action potential amplitude increase up to 180mV. In a number of cases spontaneous hyperpolarization interchanging with spontaneous depolarization occurred with corresponding action potential amplitude change The assumption is made that the cells under consideration are involved in heart function control.

Introduction

While investigating intercellular interaction in frog atrium we managed to implant microelectrodes in the deeper myocardium layers and detect bioelectrical activity of the cells of this layer. The cardyomyocytes on the inner side of the atrium showed typical bioelectric potentials. When deeper advanced, microelectrodes reached layer of cells with non-typical impulse activity. Finally, when microelectrodes were advanced close to the exit from tissue on the atrium outer side cardiomyocytes again showed typical bioelectric potentials. We found it interesting to investigate the cell layer posessing non-typical impulse activity.

Material and methods

The work was done using microelectrode technique and electronic measuring equipment with high-resistance measuring current-stabilization components that enables induced intracellular membrane polarization with simultaneous bioelectric activity monitoring using only one microelectrode. Preparations of the open isolated heart of the brown frog were made up for the experiments, thus enabling access to the endocardial surface of the atrium. The preparation was fixed in the perfusion chamber and perfused with physiological solution during the experiment.

Results

The revealed cells with non-typical impulse activity feature membrane potential value of -25 ± 2mV. The action potential amplitude of

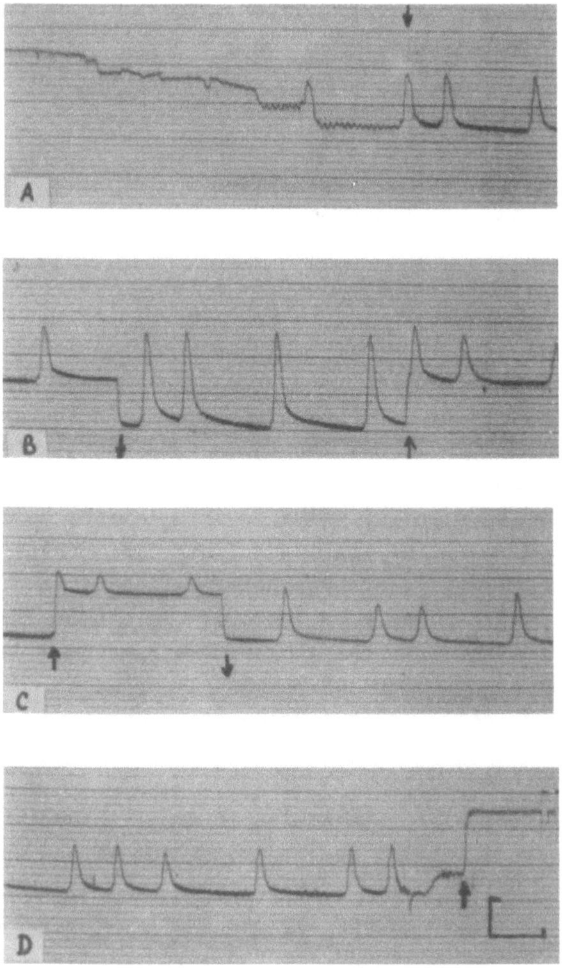

Fig.1. Induced membrane polarization effect on bioelectric potentials of the cells with non-typical impulse actyvity.
A - implanting micro-elecrrode in the cell. Implanting moment is marked with symbol (↓); B - induced intracellular membrane hyperpolarization. Set off by symbols (↓↑); C - induced intracellular membrane depolarization. Set off by symbols (↑↓); D - withdrawing microelectrode from the cell. Withdrawall moment is marked with symbol (↑). Calibration: 25mV, 1,5s

these cells ranges from 5mV to 25mV. In a number of cases action potential is not detected at all. The action potential frequency in cells with non-typical impulse activity equals action potential generation frequency of cardiomyocytes within 100mkm from detection point.

It was shown that induced membrane potential shift in cells with non-typical impulse activity leads to action potential amplitude change but not impulse activity frequency (Fig.1). Membrane hyperpolarization causes action potential amplitude increase, the value being linearly dependent on membrane potential shift and may reach 180 ± 10mV. Membrane depolarization causes decrease of action potential amplitude or complete termination of its generation.

The tests have shown that cells with non-typical impulse activity are found in the deeper atrium myocardial layers, especially in the area adjacent to sino-atrial foramen, they are less in number closer to the ventricle, practically not found in its myocardium. These cells are also found on the heart outer surface in the sinus venosus area, where they appear in locuses.

In the experiments we registered spontaneous membrane potential shift of such cells with respective action potential amplitude change. In a number of cases we detected significant membrane potential increase with respective action potential amplitude increase in heart arrest settings with only few contracting trabeculae (Fig.2). In these cases the heart either stopped beating completely with termination of these cells' action potential generation and pronounced membrane hyperpolarization, or regained its initial rate when steady contractions in the presence of significant action potential values extended to all trabeculae. After this membrane depolarization was observed and membrane potential and action potential reversion to initial level.

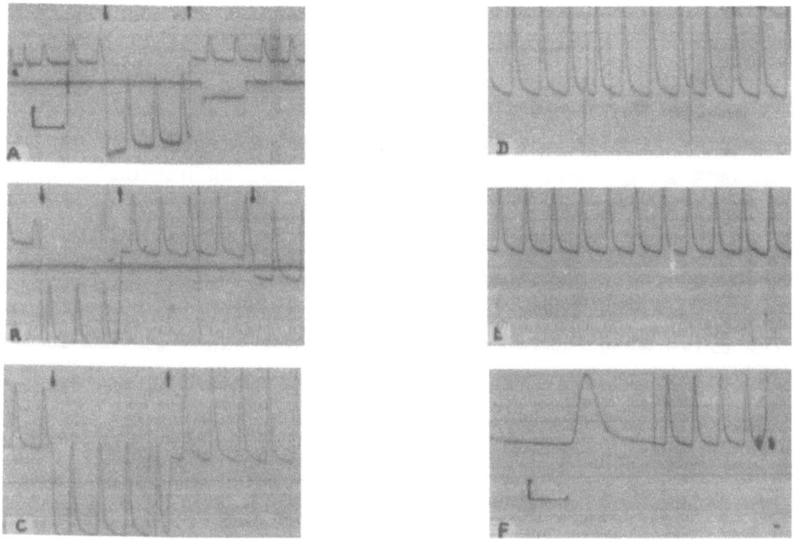

Fig.2. Spontaneous membrane potential shift with resulting action potential amplitude change in cells with non-typical impulse activity in heart arrest settings.
A - implanting microelectrode in the cell; B -, C -, D -, E - spontaneous cell membrane potential shift with corresponding action potential amplitude change; F - withdrawing microelectrode from the cell.
Symbols (↓↑) off set induced membrane hyperpolarization.
Calibration: 30mV,

Discussion

We bring several arguments favouring the idea that the phenomenon we discovered is not an artifact. Firstly, there might be an assumption that low membrane potential and action potential values of these cells might be the result of the broken microelectrode tip. However, with perpendicular microelectrode advance, after it passes through the layer of these cells, we detect standard cell action potentials in the working myocardis. Similar cells are also found on the heart's outer surface, the probability of the tip breaking being lower in this case. Besides, in spite of equal opportunities for breaking microelectrode tip in all parts of the heart, these cells are found only in specific areas. Finally, it can hardly be assumed that extra-cellular polarization may affect extra-cellular potentials. Secondly, it might be assumed, that these cells are non-viable, damaged in this or other way. However, we detected these cells not only in the deeper myocardium layers but also on the upopen isolated heart, on the atrium outer surface of non-isolated heart, where they appear in locuses. It can hardly be assumed that in the deep of the myocardium exist a whole layer of perishing cells and on atrium outer side their locuses. Finally, we have registered their spontaneous hyperpolarization and action potential increase effect. Thirdly, published information identify six layers in frog atrium (Шидловский В.Н. и Дауэ Н.С) with the deepest-transverse fine-fibred layer, containing smooth-muscle elements - being practically unexplored. There are only indications that spots of this layer may appear in locuses on the outer atrium surface. And this is consistent with our findings.

We may assume that described cells unified in the transverse fine-fibred layer play significant role in the heart's regulatory control, which is evident in generating significant values of action potentials when hyperpolarized (Камкин А.Г. и соавторы). Apparently, any functional change in the body causing, for example, compound formation that hyperpolarizes membranes of these cells leads to their action potential amplitude increase that, in turn, forms electric excitation focus in the heart drive area. This may either disturb heart rhythm or even stop it, or, vice versa, serve as a natural pacemaker.

References

(1) Шидловский В.Н., Дауэ Н.С. В сб.: Материалы по экспериментально-клинической электрокардиологии. Москва, 24 - 31 (1953)

(2) Камкин А.Г., Киселёва И.С., Косицкий Г.И. Физиология и патофизиология сердца и коронарного кровообращения. 2 Всесоюзный симпозиум, Киев, 67 - 68 (1987)

Antiarrhythmic effects of Ca channel blockers on canine Purkinje fibers

KYOKO ENDOU, YOSHIHIRO NARA, HAREAKI YAMAMOTO, AND TOSHIRO SATO
Dept. of Medicine, School of Medicine, Kitasato University,
1-15-1, Kitasato, Sagamihara, Kanagawa, 228 Japan

<Summary>

Among Ca channel blockers, 1.0×10^{-6}M verapamil decreased conduction velocity (n=10) significantly($p<0.05$). $\dot{V}$max and amplitude(n=4) were decreased significantly in the preparations which slowed conduction velocity. 1.0×10^{-6}M nifedipine also decreased conduction velocity(n=5), and had tendency to decrease Vmax and amplitude(n=3). Diltiazem(n=8) and nicardipine(n=4) did not show any changes. Therefore, verapamil and diltiazem may have effect to depress fast Na channel as class I antiarrhythmic drug. Passive electrical properties (space constant, internal resistance, and membrane resistance) were not changed by any Ca antagonists. Delayed afterdepolarizations induced by acetylstrophanthidin were depressed by 2×10^{-7}M verapamil, diltiazem and nifedipine. This effect may be due to blocking Ca channel which was also
represented by shortening of APD50.

<Introduction>

Ca channel blockers have rescently been used in clinical practice for their anti-hypertensive, anti-anginal and anti-arrhythmic effects.

Among these Ca channel blockers, verapamil is frequently used to treat arrhythmia. Diltiazem and nifedipine are also reported to depress triggered arrythmia in dogs.

A slowing of the conduction velocity is one result of anti-arrhythmic effects, decreasing SA and AV node conduction has been well documented. In this experiments, we compared the effects of Ca channel blockers, verapamil, diltiazem, nicardipine, and nifedipine on the conduction of Purkinje fiber. Both active and passive properties were studied because these properties have effects on conduction velocity.

The effects of Ca channel blockeres to the delayed afterdepolarization, abbreviated as DAD, which caused triggered arrhythmia, were also compared.

<Methods>

A false tendon of canine Purkinje fiber was excised and was mounted in a lucite chamber, in which 4 mM K Tyrode's solution was perfused. The temperature of the solution was 35.5°-36.5° C. PH was 7.3. The microelectrodes method was employed to record membrane potential.

Measurement of action potential characteristics and conduction velocity

The preparations were stimulated at 1 HZ. The amplified

membrane potentials were recorded on a digital data recorder. The conduction velocity was calculated using camera film. The distance between the two microelectrodes was divided by the time delay.

1.0×10^{-6}M Calcium channel blockers were administered for 20 minutes.

<u>Measurement of passive electrical properties</u>

Fig. 1 reveals the method to obtain electrotonic properties for passive electrical properties. A constant current with a 250 msec duration at 0.5 HZ was conducted into compartment A. The current flowed through the tissue into compartment B. The two electrotonic potentials were used for the calculation of passive electrical properties, space constant, λ, internal resistance, ri, and membrane resistance, rm.

<u>Measrement of delayead afterdepolarization</u>

The Purkinje fiber was stimulated at 1 HZ. At five minutes before the erug exposure, the stimulus was switched to 2HZ and continued during the drug exposure. The fiber was superfused with Tyrode's solution containing 2.4×10^{-7}M acetylstrophanthidin (AS) for 20 to 25 minutes. After washing out the AS for 40 minutes, the preparation was then perfused with Tyrode's solution containing AS and Ca channel blockers. Every 5 minutes during AS administratio, Purkinje fiber was submitted to a current with a cycle lengths of 1000 msec, 10 times, followed by a 5 sec. pause. AS administration for 10 to 25 minutes induced DAD. Concentration of Ca channel blocker was 2.0×10^{-6}M.
Paired t test was used for the statistical analysis.

<Result>

<u>Conduction velocity</u> (Fig.2)

With Verapamil (n=10), represented by the open circle, conduction velocity by almost 35% significantly ($p<0.05$). Nifedipine (n=5) also significantly depressed the conduction velocity by almost 20%. Diltiazem (n=4) did not have any effects on the conduction velocity. Since maximum diastolic potential in all of the preparations were more negative than -76mV, the slowing of the conduction velocity by verapamil and nifedipine is not due to Ca channel blocking effects. Therefore, this effect was not caused by the blocking Calcium channel. So, we examined the action potential characteristics and passive electrical properties.

<u>Active electrical properties</u>

Table 1. reveals changes of the maximum rising velocity of phase 0 of the action potential ($\dot{V}max$), amplitude of action potential, and action potential duration at 50% of the amplitude (APD50). Means of the maximum diastolic potentials (MDP) were between 84 and 92mV. $\dot{V}max$ was signifimantly decreased by verapamil for 20 min. administration in the preparations which showed decrese in conduction velocity. Nifedipine had tendency

Table 1

	n	MDP mean+ SE	Vmax (V/sec) before	10 min.	20	wash-out
Verapamil	4	85+37	333+48	295+32	260+62*	313+72
Diltiazem	5	84+ 2	348+58	354+54	323+46	380+38
Nicardipine	4	84+ 2	240+53	267+43	242+63	240+43
Nifedipine	3	92+ 2	313+46	295+68	284+51	282+27

	Amplitude (mV) before	10	20	w-o	APD50 (msec) before	10	20	w-o
Ver	102+5	100+6	78+10	97+7	245+27	205+26*	197+36	238+47
Dil	114+6	118+4	120+4	122+6	215+17	178+15	171+13*	221+18
Nic	108+7	123+20	121+36	124+15	182+5	189+9	197+17	224+22
Nif	121+8	116+11	110+9	131+17	185+31	136+7	135+10	179+8

Fig.1

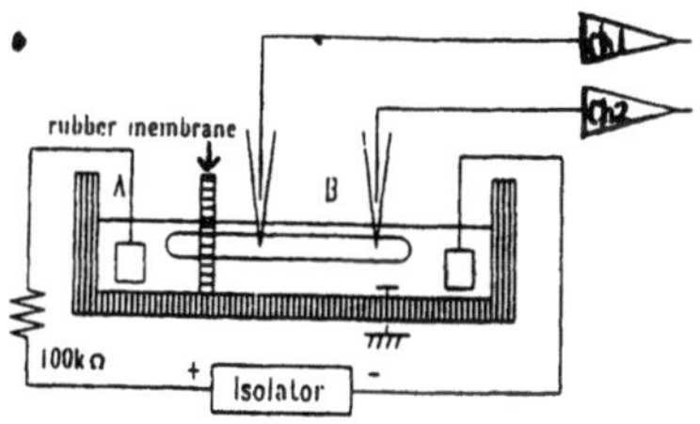

Fig.2 Conduction Velocity

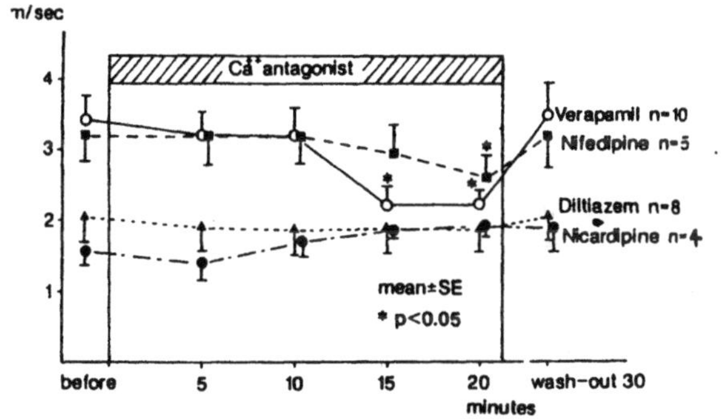

Fig.3 % Change of Space Constant, λ

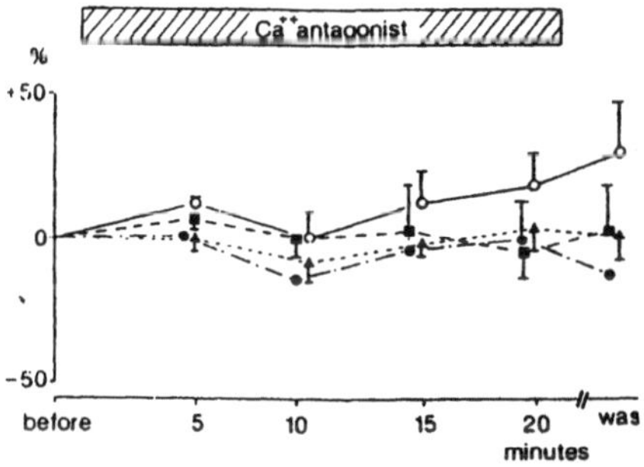

Fig.4 % Change of internal resistance ,ri

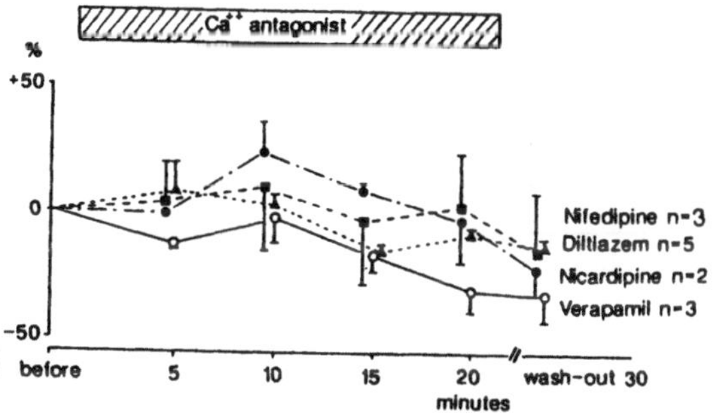

Fig.5 % Change of membrane resistance, rm

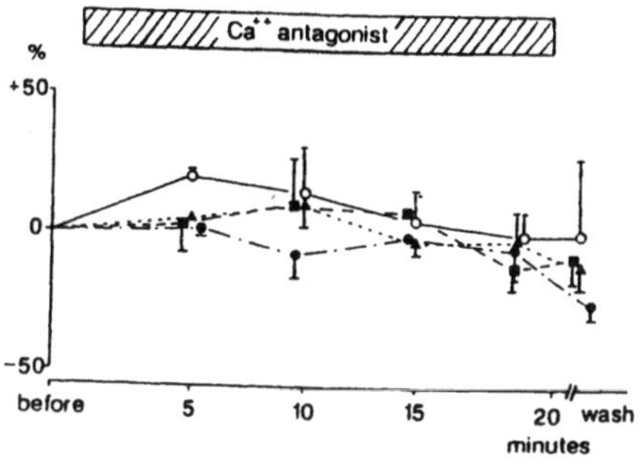

Fig.6 Change of DAD amplitude

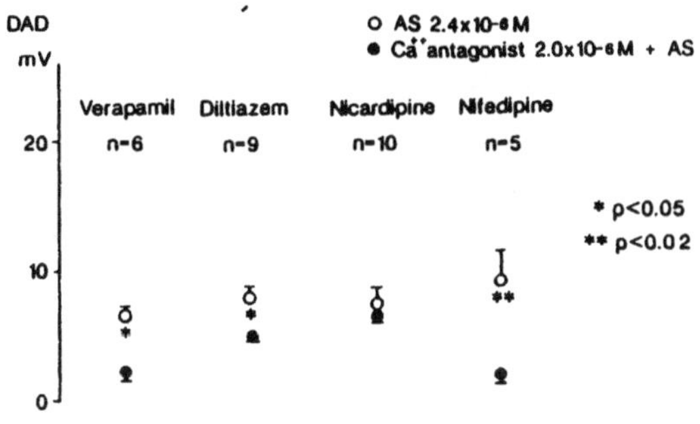

of decreasing $\dot{V}max$. Nicardipine and nifedipine did not show any changes. Amplitude of action potential was depressed by verapamil for 15 min. administration significantly. Nifedipine had tendency to depress amplitude. Nicardipine and diltiazem did not show decrease. APD50 was significanlty shortened by verapamil and diltiazem. Nifedipine had tendency to decrease APD50. Nicardipine did not show any changes.

Passive electrical properties (Fig.3,4,5)
λ, ri and rm were not increased by any Ca antagonists. Space constant, , was not changed.

Delayed afterdepolarization (DAD)(Fig.6)
Verapamil, diltiazem and nifedipine depressed acetylstrophanthidin-induced DAD significantly. Nicardipine did not have any effect on Purkinje fiber.

<Discussion and conclusion>

We compared the antiarrhythmic effects of Ca channel blockers, verapamil, diltiazem, nicardipine and nifedipine on Purkinje fibers. Conduction velocity was decreased by $1.0x10^{-6}M$ verapamil and nifedipine significantly. $\dot{V}max$ and amplitude were decreased by these drugs. Therefore, these effects may be due to decreasing fast Na channel as class I antiarrhythmic drug. Rosen et al(1) reported $6x10^{-6}M$ verapamil decreased coduction velocity, Vmax and amplitude. $1x10^{-6}M$ might be a critical concentration. We examined 10 preparations, while they examined in 6 preparations. Nifedipine also decreased conduction velocity significantly, and had tendency to decrease Vmax and amplitude. Dangman et al (2) reported $0.9x10^{-6}M$ nifedipine did not decrease $\dot{V}max$ in 2.7mM K Tyrode's solusion, while we used 4 mM Tyrode's solution. We need further study to confirm this results. As other result to influence conduction velocity, passive electrical properties were examined. However, verapamil did not change, ri, and rm, as Pressler et al(3) reported. Nifedipine, nicardipine, and diltiazem also did not change λ, ri, and rm.

Triggered arrhythmia is caused by DAD. Therefore, we compared the effects of Ca antagoniost on DAD. Verapamil, nifedipine, and diltiazem depressed amplitude of DAD. This effect was almost same as those of Ca channel blocking as shown by shortening of APD50.

In clinical use, nifedipine has indirect effect that it stimulates the sympathetic nerve causing a marked decrease in blood pressure. Therefore, the antiarrhythmic effect of nifedipine is not manifested.

<References>

(1) Rosen, M.R., J.P.Ilvento, H.Gelband, and C.Merker: J.Pharmacol. Exp. Ther. 189,414-422 (1974)

(2) Dangman,K.H., and B.F.Hoffman: Am. J. Cardiol. 46, 1059-1067(1980)

(3) Pressler, M.L., V.Elharrar, and J.C.Bailey: Circ. Res. 51,637-651 (1982)

Antiarrhythmic effects of Ca antagonists

Intercellular interaction in frog heart

KISELEVA I.S., KAMKIN A.G., KIRCHEIS R., KOSITZKY G.I.

2nd Pirogov's Medical Institute,
Ostrovityanova St., 1, Moscow 117437, USSR.

Summary

To investigate intercellular electrotonic interaction in the beating heart directly through cardiomyocyte membrane high-permeable contacts paired microelectrodes off set by 40 to 50 mkm were used and an electronic measuring circuit that enables biopotential monitoring with induced intracellular polarization using one microelectrode. Two-way pulse conduction between cardiomyocytes of isolated open frog heart was found. In atria transfer ratio mean value was 0.12 in either direction. However, intercellular interaction was not uniformly detected. In a number of cases electrotonic interaction between the cells was lacking. Part of the tests registered one-way electrotonic interaction between the cells. The wide range of control tests permist assuming heterogeneity in myocardiac functional pattern.

Introduction

Excitation in the myocardial tissue propagates through high-permeable contacts between the cells and is determined by cardiomyocyte membrane properties, the arrangement and functional properties of high-permeable contacts and geometry of their interconnections (Беркинблит М.Б.) At the same time each heart's compartment is different in its anatomic composition, cell structure and intercellular interaction. Hence, the difference in high-permeable contact functioning and role in different heart compartments. This permits assuming heterogeneity in myocardium functional pattern. The present-day view of the myocardium as functional syncytium results from experiments based on electrotonic potential propagation evaluation, induced by extra-cellular electric current application to a strip of myocardial tissue by means of suction-electrode. The applied current, however, is high and membrane potential shift may be detected even in the cells offset from the source and lacking high-permeable contacts. Besides, in this case the current reaches both inside the cell and extra-cellular pathways, which makes it more difficult to evaluate its travel efficiency through high-permeable contacts.

Material and methods

The most adequate method that, as we think, enables investigating intercellular interaction in the intact beating heart is intracellular membrane polarization of one cell by means of a microelectrode with simultaneous monitoring of its passive electric properties and membrane potential shift in the nearby cells. Glass microelectrodes offset by 40 to 50 mkm were used for the experiments. Since the distance was standard for each test we may assume that between the cells under consideration always lay a defifnite quantity of intermediate cells and, hence, a definite quantity of high-permeable contacts. This enables us to estimate electric pulse transfer ratio as K = V2/V1, where V1 - membrane potential of artificially polarized cell and V2 - membrane potential shift in the nearby cell. The ratio's relativity in this case would have to be considered, if intercellular interaction of the two nearby cells were modelled. But we are conserned with system approach to intercellular interaction at the organ level with all interconnections between the studied cells. The offered study was done on the open isolated heart of brown frog perfused with physiological solution.

Results

First of all, induced intracellular polarization effect on the cells of the beating heart's working myocardium was studied. It was shown that atrium cardiomyocyte membrane hyperpolarization using standard 10^{-9}A microelectrode did not cause changes of action potential's amplitude, its form and adhesive activity frequency (Fig. 1). This may be due to the fact that myocardial cells generate themselves current reaching 10^{-7}A during action potential phase. At the same time, use of sharpened microelectrodes enabled application of high-value currents and detect action potential amplitude increase and its form change in response to membrane hyperpolarization. However, impulse activity frequency did not change (Fig. 2).

In tests on the cells of the atrium working myocardium intracellular square pulse travel was detected, conducted through high-permeable contacts, that had a two-way character in most cases. K1 = K2 = 0.12 ± 0.01 (Fig. 3). A number of cases registered one-way square pulse transmission, also in a number of cases intracellular interaction was not detected.

Direct electrotonic interaction between atrium cells is witnessed by control experiments which show absence of conduction in case both

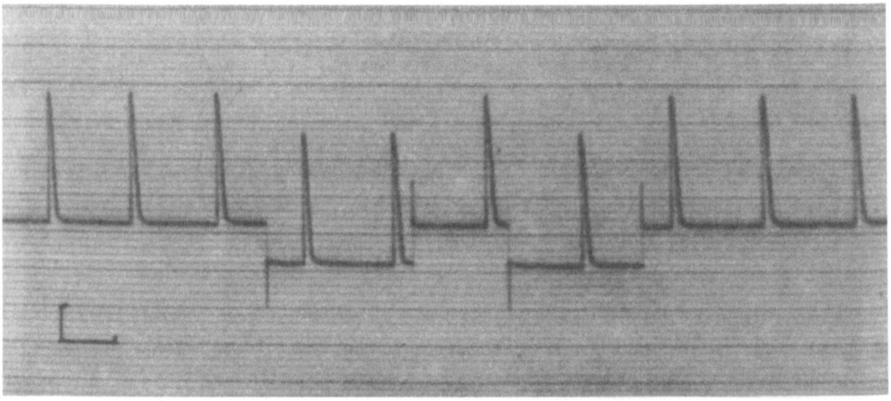

Fig. 1. Induced intracellular hyperpolarization of the atrium working myecardium cell using standard microelectrode.
Calibration: 40mV

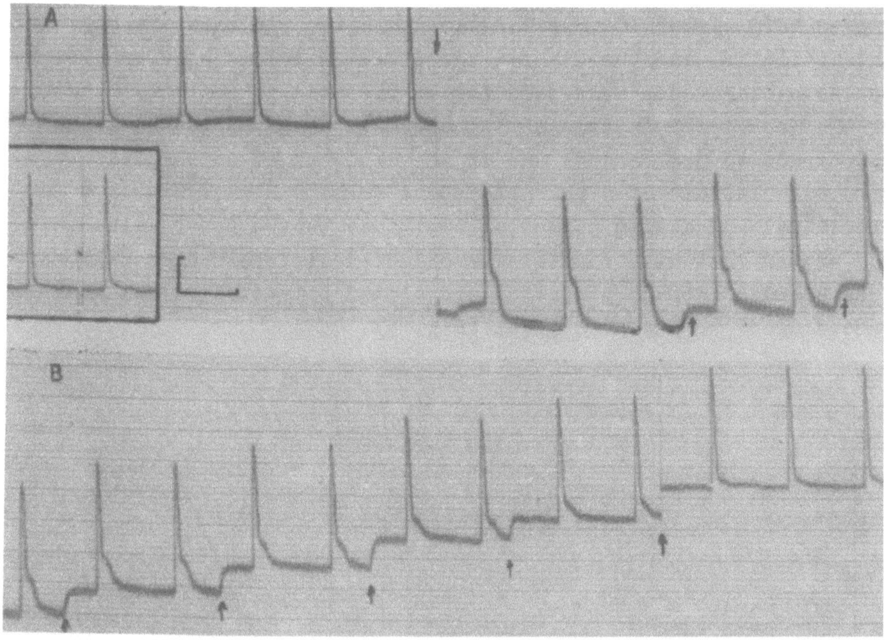

Fig. 2. Induced intracellular hyperpolarization of the atrium working myocardium cell using sharpened microelectrode.
A - the beginning of the curve. Induced intracellular membrane hyperpolarization. Set off by symbol (↓).
B - the continuation of the curve. Induced intracellular membrane hyperpolarization reduced. Set off by symbol (↑).
Calibration: 40mV

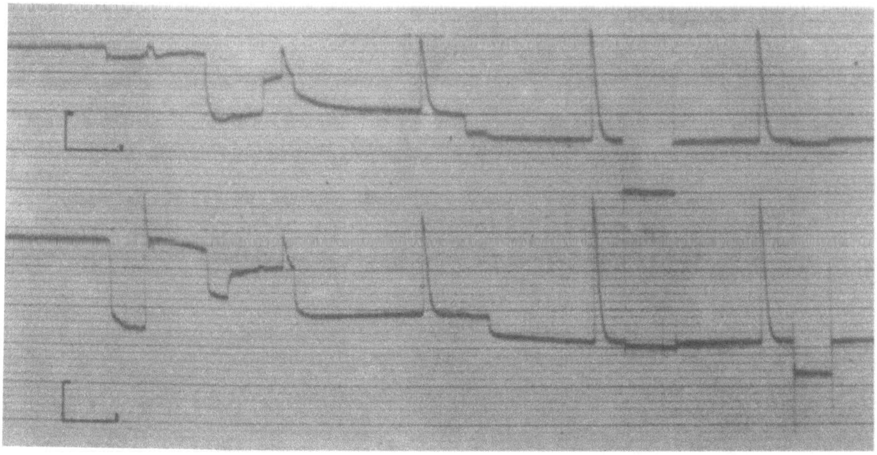

Fig. 3. Two-way electrotonic pulse transmission between atrium cells. Induced hyperpolarization of the first cell (upper curve) causes membrane potential shift in the second cell (lower curve) and vice versa
Calibration: 60 mkm; 40mV (upper curve), 32.5mV (lower curve)

electrodes were placed in physiological solution, in case one was used for intracellular, and the other - for extra-cellular activity detection in case both electrodes were used for extra-cellular activity detection. As for the one-way conduction or its complete absence, the shunting of microelectrode to membrane of one of the cells might be suggested. However, calculations of a possible shunt value and analysis of membrane potential and action potential amplitude versus shunt value that we made showed that with shunts even slightly different from cell membrane resistance membrane potential and action potential values show pronounced drops to the zero level (Fig. 4).

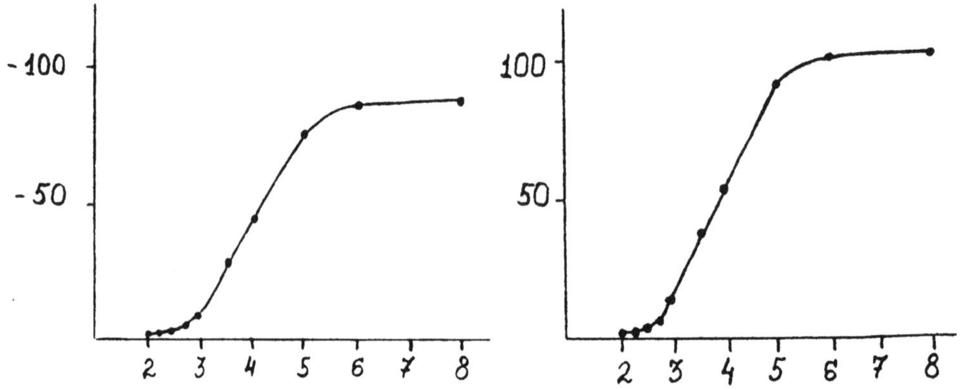

Fig. 4. Membrane potential change versus shunt value (A), action potential amplitude change versus shunt value (B).
X - shunt resistance value logarithm (MOm); Y - membrane potential and action potential amplitude values (mV).

Discussion

Thus, presented results may serve as evidence of myocardium heterogeneity and permit disapprobation of treating myocardium structure as a functional syncytuim, and the fact of one-way transmission needs further checking.

References

(1) Беркинблит М.Б. Высокопроницаемые контактные мембраны. Москва, Наука I - 464 (I98I).

Technical aspects of intercellular electrotonic interaction investigation in the myocardium

KAMKIN A.G., KISELEVA I.S.

2nd Pirogov's Medical Institute,
Ostrovityanova St., 1, Moscow 117437, USSR.

Summary

Electronic measuring circuit is discussed, using high-resistance current-stabilization components in its measuring part, that enables induced intracellular membrane polarization with simultaneous bioelectrical activity monitoring using only one microelectrode. The equipment is successfully used in cell bioelectric parameter testing in the beating heart and intercellular interaction investigation through high-permeable cardiomyocyte membrane contacts.

Introduction

Myocardic electrotonic interaction studies through cell high-permeable membrane contacts were conducted using various methods, the major ones being saccharose bridge technique (Barr L.), electric current application through suctionelectrode (Букаускас Ф.Ф.) and others. The method that won the broadest acceptance is electrotonic potential propagation assessment induced by extra-cellular square-pulse application through suction electrode with simultaneous membrane potential shift monitoring at different distances. However, the method enables only indirect assessment of high-permeable contact functioning, since strong current is applied in these cases and membrane potential shift may be detected even in the cells lacking high-permeable contact connections. The suction area extends to both intact and damaged cells. Moreover, with extra-cellular polarization applied current reaches both inside the cell and extra-cellular pathways which impedes current travel efficiency assessment through high-permeable contacts (Sperelakis N.). On the whole, the approach does not allow investigation of high-permeable contact functioning and their regulation in the intact, beating heart.

Material and methods

The most adequate procedure that enables investigation of intercellular interaction in the intact beating heart and specify cardiomyocyte contact functioning is intracellular membrane polarization of single cell through microelectrode with simultaneous monitoring of its passive electric properties and membrane potential shift in the nearby cells. Attempts of the kind were made using bridge circuits that enable applying one microelectrode for both cell biopotential monitoring and its simultaneous membrane polarization. However, since relatively high-resistance microelectrodes are used on the myocardial cells having low membrane time constant and also the need for strong microelectrode currents, tangible difficulties were encountered with respect to proper bridge balancing. Precise balance is feasible only in case of constant microelectrode resistance value. The actual electrodes display non-linear properties when current is applied. Moreover, the electrode's resistance changes when it is implanted in the cell. Finaly, the cell's input resistance also changes with the action potential generation which makes overall bridge balancing still more difficult and results in significant errors.

Results

We designed an electronic measuring circuit using high-resistance current stabilization components in its measuring part that enables cell biopotential monitoring and simultaneous intracellular membrane polarization applying only one microelectrode. Since 1979 (Камкин А.Г. и соавторы) we successfully used the circuit for investigating nervous system intercellular electrotonic interaction and, of late, we use its modified version for investigating intercellular interaction in the intact beating heart (Fig. 1). The offered circuit is made up of several loops

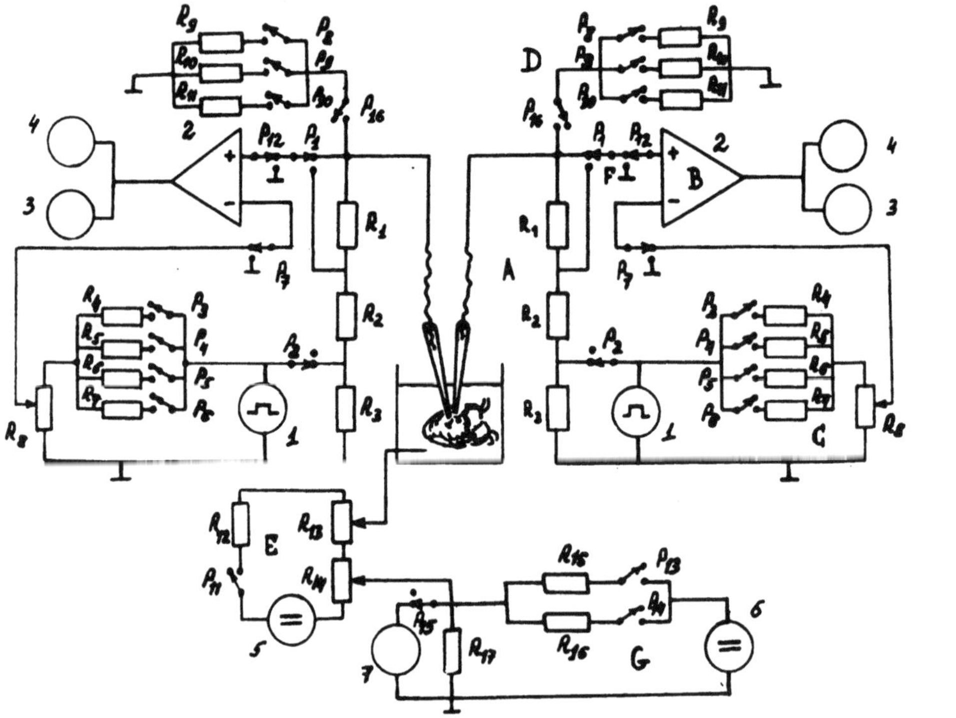

Fig. 1. The electronic measuring circuit.
A - The circuit current stabilization and measuring unit; B - Biopotential amplifier; C - Microelectrode voltage drop compensation unit; D - Microelectrode resistance measuring unit; E - Potential constant component adjustment unit; F - Amplifier input grounding unit; G - Voltage calibration unit,
1 - generator, 2 - biopotential amplifier, 3 - oscillograph, 4 - mirror-galvanometer, 5 -, 6 - direct current source, 7 - digital voltmeter.

each of which combines:

- The circuit current stabilization and measuring unit using high-resistance components R1 and R2, resistor R3 and relays P1 and P2. Resistor R1 rating at $2{,}2 \cdot 10^9$ ohm ensures generator-1 current stabilization that induces intracellular membrane polarization. Resistor R2 ($18 \cdot 10^6$ ohm) produces this current's measurements with required accuracy. Switching is provided by relay P1. Relay P2 starts the square pulse gene rator-1.

- Biopotential amplifier-2 outfitted with oscillograph-3 outputs for visual process monitoring and mirror-galvanometer-4 cell impulse activity recording.

- Microelectrode voltage drop compensation unit using resistors R4-R7, variable resistance R8 and relays P3-P6. Introducing microelectrode voltage drop compensation unit appears necessary since generator-1 pulse is advanced towards the cell through the microelectrode. In this case amplifier-detected signal comprises the microelectrode voltage drop and cell membrane potential change induced by pulse current. Resistors R4-R7 connected through relays P3-P6 are employed for coarse, and resistor R8 - continuous compensation. The unit is connected using relay P7.

- Microelectrode resistance measuring unit containing resistors R9-R11 and relays P8-P10. The combined output of relays P8-P10 is connected to the amplifier input with other sides of the relays employed for connecting resistors R9-R11 of known values. They are connected in series to amplifier input in parallel to microelectrode.

- Potential constant component adjustment unit comprising resistors R12, variable resistances R13, R14, direct current source-5, relay P11. The unit enables constant potential shift compensation, resulting from microelectrode potentials and other sources of circuit electrochemical asymmetry.

- Amplifier input grounding unit comprising relay P12 which, when is turned on, grounds the positive amplifier input.

- Voltage calibration unit is formed of resistors R15-R17, direct current source-6, digital voltmeter-7, relays P13-P15.

The system operates as follows. When microelectrodes submerge in physiological solution the loops' measuring zeros are defined by means of amplifier input grounding unit relay P12. Relay P11 is then turned on and using variable resistances R13, R14 from potential constant component adjustment unit constant potential shift is compensated, resulting from circuit electrochemical asymmetry. Then relay P16 connects microelectrode resistance measuring unit, the measuring being done in the first and second loops of the system by connecting subsequetly resistors R9-R11. Then microelectrode voltage drop compensation unit is connected through relays P7 of both loops. When relay P2 is turned on and generator pulses are connected oscillograph's zero line registration with respect to generator pulses is obtained connecting subsequently resistors R4-R7 and variable resistance R8. After this loops' voltage is calibrated using relays P13-P14 connecting resistors R15, R16, the voltage value being defined by digital voltmeter connected through relay P15. Finally, each loop's current is determined by relay P1 connecting resistor R2.

Discussion

The circuit enables any stimulator pulse duration. Besides, when starting pulse generation the current, in fact, does not depend on microelectrode resistance. Moreover, radioelectronic component resistance of the $5 \cdot 10^9$ ohm order (three times over the cell input resistance) enables preventing current leakage from the cell in between the stimulator pulses. The basic problem, when using this circuit, is that the potential detected by the amplifier is composed of two components: microelectrode voltage drop and cell stimulation-induced membrane potential change. It is evident, that the first component must be excluded from amplifier input signal which may be attained through electronic subtraction or direct compensation. Finally, when using this circuit, high demands are imposed on switching elements whose contact insulation resistance should be as high as 10^{12} ohm. The soldered joints' thermo-emf should also be taken into account.

The equipment is successfully used in cell bioelectric parameter testing in the beating heart and intercellular interaction investigation through high-permeable cardiomyocyte membrane contacts.

References

(1) Barr L. Comparative Physiology of the Heart. A Satellite of the XX1V Internation Congress Union of Physiological Sciences, Birkhäuser Verlay, Basel and Stuttgart, 102 - 110 (1969).

(2) Букаускас Ф.Ф. Межклеточное электрическое взаимодействие и процессы распространения возбуждения в сердце в норме и при гипоксии. Автореф. докт дисс. Купавна, I - 40, (I982).

(3) Sperelakis N. Comparative Physiology of the Heart. A Satellite Symposium of the XX1V International Congress Union of Physiological Sciences, Birkhaüser Verlay, Basel and Stuttgart, 135 - 141 (1969).

(4) Камкин А.Г. и Дергачев В.В. В сб.: Физиологическая кибернетика. Москва, 354 - 355 (I98I)

Extracellular K^+ and Ca^{2+} activities ($a^o_{K^+}$, $a^o_{Ca^{2+}}$) at the region of suction electrode placed on the ventral wall of frog ventricular epicardium during the development of monophasic action potential (MAP) caused by the negative pressure

SLAVÍČEK, J., STOJAN, M., VYSKOČIL, F., +)

Laboratory of Cardiology, 2nd Department of Medicine, Faculty of Medicine, Charles University, U nemocnice 2, 128 08 Prague 2, ČSSR, and Institute of Physiology, Czechoslovak Academy of Sciences, Vídeňská 1083, 142 20 Prague 4, ČSSR +)

Summary

The $a^o_{K^+}$, $a^o_{Ca^{2+}}$ and membrane potential (MP) were measured before, during and after action of negative pressure under a suction electrode placed on the surface of frog heart ventricle in situ beating spontaneously. The application of negative pressure from -5 to -40 kPa for 10 min. changed the maximum diastolic $a^o_{K^+}$ in three phases: a phase of rapidly rising $a^o_{K^+}$, a slowly decaying phase and a phase of slowly rising $a^o_{K^+}$. The $a^o_{K^+}$ changed together with the change of MP. The changes reversed when the suction was discontinued during the rapidly rising and decaying phase, but were not reversed during the slowly rising phase. The $a^o_{Ca^{2+}}$ decreased between -5 and -13 kPa, but increased during higher negative pressures. The results showed the depolarization, the elevation of K^+_e and the changes of Ca^{2+}_e during the action of negative pressure under the suction electrode.

Introduction

Since 1932 (Schütz) the negative pressure under a suction electrode has been used for inducing injury currents on the surface of the heart both experimentally and clinically in the studies of repolarization (Burgess, 1979). But the changes of membrane permeability and ion activities under a suction electrode have not so far been investigated (Franz et al., 1986). In our laboratory we found the depolarization under the suction electrode in frog ventricular epicardium (Slavíček et al., 1979). In the present work we studied the extracellular K^+ and Ca^{2+} activities by the method of ion-selective electrodes. The purpose of the contribution was to obtain the preliminary information about the contributions of K^+ and Ca^{2+} for the development of MAP. Some of our results have been published recently (Slavíček et al., 1984a, 1984b, 1985, 1988, Slavíček and Vyskočil, 1985).

Material and methods

Fifty frogs (Rana esculenta) were pithed (brain and spinal cord) and the thorax was opened. A suction glass capillary electrode (1,0 mm tip diameter) was applied to the surface of ventral wall on the base, middle part or apex of the heart ventricle during spontaneous contractions

(f_{min}=40$\pm$ 5;temperature +20°C)(Fig.1A,left). The detailed description of measurement of ion activities was made formerly (Slavíček and Vyskočil, 1985). Briefly, the suction capillary contained another small capillary (a tip diameter of 0,5 mm) in the central part filled with the liquid ion-exchanger for measurement of a^{o}_{K}+ or a^{o}_{Ca}2+.The reference channel (suction capillary) was filled with conventional frog Ringer solution (0,1 ml). The electrodes were connected with Ag/AgCl wires to the input of high impedance DC amplifier and the ion activity measured from the potential differences between the extracellular ion-selective electrode and the reference electrode placed in the Ringer solution in the suction capillary (during T-Q segment of ECG). To measure the MP, a floating microelectrode filled with 3 mol.l^{-1} KCl was placed inside the suction electrode and inserted into the cell(Fig.1A,right). The reference was placed in the suction capillary.

Results

Potassium changes (Fig.1B).On the surface of the ventricle base, the maximum diastolic a^{o}_{K}+ was 5,0$\pm$0,8 (S.E.M.) mmol.l^{-1}. The first phase characterized by rapidly rising a^{o}_{K}+ was observed within several seconds after beginning suction of -40 kPa. This increase reached 11,0$\pm$0,6mmol. .l^{-1}in the 1^{rst} min. The more negative pressure from -5 to -40 kPa,the more pronounced the 1^{rst} phase of rapidly rising a^{o}_{K}+ was observed. The second phase of small compensatory decrease of a^{o}_{K}+ lasted about 5 min. and a^{o}_{K}+ decreased during this time from 11,0 to 7,7$\pm$0,8 mmol.l^{-1}. This phase was suppressed by ouabain, by cooling the tissue to +2^{o} C and in absence of spontaneous beating. The phase was more pronounced in the base than in the apex. The 3rd phase of slowly rising a^{o}_{K}+ began in the 7th min. of suction and reached 10,0$\pm$ 0,9 mmol.l^{-1} in 4 min. The change of a^{o}_{K}+ could be reversed by discontinuing suction during the initial rapidly rising and the 2nd decaying phase (dashed line in the 6thmin. of Fig.1B), but was not reversible during the 3rd slowly rising phase (Fig.1B,10th min.). The MP changed in parallel with the a^{o}_{K}+ changes (Fig.1C): during the 1^{rst} rising phase of a^{o}_{K}+ the MP decreased from -68 $\pm$1,3 to -52,0$\pm$1,5 mV. Then, between the 2nd and 6th min. of experiment (slowly decaying a^{o}_{K}+ phase) the membrane polarization increased to -60 $\pm$0,8 mV and finally the MP decreased again to -52,0$\pm$0,5 mV, starting from the 6th min. of experiment. The calculated potassium equilibrium potential (E_{K}+)(open circles in Fig. 1C) was more negative (-71,9 mV) than MP (-68,0 mV) before suction. But the differences of E_{K}+ and MP were insignificant during the experiment. Calcium changes (Fig.2). During the action of negative pressure of -5 kPa, the a^{o}_{Ca}2+ measured under the suction electrode slowly decreased from 2,0$\pm$0,1 to 1,8$\pm$0,1 mmol.l^{-1} within 2 min. The subsequent increase of negative pressure to -13 kPa decreased the a^{o}_{Ca}2+ further to 1,1$\pm$0,1 mmol.l^{-1} in two min. But the subsequent increase of the negative pressure to -26 kPa had the opposite effect and an a^{o}_{Ca}2+ increase to 1,7mmol.l^{-1} was obsrerved after 4 min. When the negative pressure was lowered from -26,6 kPa to -13 kPa, it

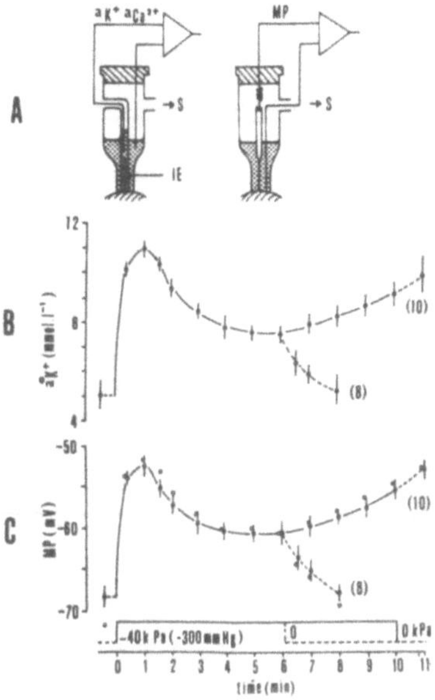

Fig.1

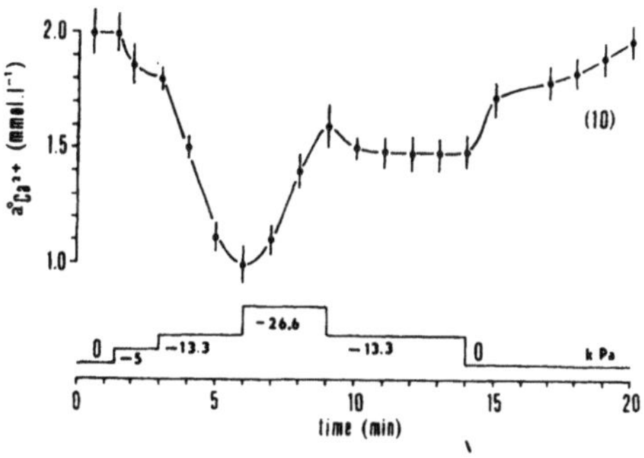

Fig.2

Fig.1. Scheme of a suction electrode (A) for measurement of $a^o_{K^+}$ or $a^o_{Ca^{2+}}$ (left part) and MP (right part). S-suction, IE-ion exchanger. $a^o_{K^+}$(B) and MP (C) measured during maximum diastolic potential (T-Q) with an ion-selective electrode before, during and after the action of negative pressure -40 kPa under the suction electrode placed on the base of ventral wall of the frog heart ventricle. Open circles: calculated potassium equilibrium potential (E_{K^+}). In the lower part, the time and value of negative pressure is schematically indicated. Broken lines: values after suction had been discontinued. Numbers in brackets- numbers of experiments. The results are mean$\pm$ S.E.M.

Fig.2. $a^o_{Ca^{2+}}$ measured before, during and after applying various negative pressures from -5 to -26,6 kPa. Mean values of 10 experiments$\pm$S.E.M. are given. In the lower part, the time course and values of negative pressure are schematically indicated.

again caused a slow decrease of $a^o_{Ca^{2+}}$ to 1,5$\pm$0,1 mmol.l^{-1} in 5 min. Complete release of suction in the 14th min. of the experiment let to slow $a^o_{Ca^{2+}}$recovery to 1,9$\pm$0,08 mmol.l^{-1} within 6 min.

Discussion and conclusions

The decrease of MP (Fig.1C) confirmed the former hypotheses about the partial depolarization under the suction electrode (Hoffman et al.,1959, Burgess, 1979). The $a^o_{K^+}$ changed together with the change of MP; it also proved the previous hypotheses. While the rapid increase of $a^o_{K^+}$ is apparently due to the pasive movement of K^+ from the cell interior along the electrochemical gradients, the 2nd phase is probably due to the activation of Na^+-K^+ transmembrane pump. It was proved indirectly in the presence of ouabain or after cooling of tissue, the well known factors blocking the Na^+ pump, where the 2nd phase of compensatory decrease of $a^o_{K^+}$ was absent (Slavíček et al.,1984a,b). The higher Na^+-K^+-ATPase activity was observed in sarcolemmal vesicles of the base, where the 2nd phase of compensatory decrease of $a^o_{K^+}$ was high (Slavíček et al.,1985). It would be due to the higher Na^+ pump activity in the base than in the apex. The 3rd phase of irreversible increase of $a^o_{K^+}$ is probably due to the damage of membrane structure by the negative pressure. The similar changes of $a^o_{K^+}$ during the negative pressure have been obtained in rat ventricular epicardium in situ (unpublished). The explanation of the changes in $a^{o}_{Ca^{2+}}$ in our experiments remains still open. The lower negative pressure caused the Ca^{2+} influx similarly as in the experimental ischemia provoked by the ligature of the coronary artery. But it is impossible to explain which mechanism is responsible for the Ca^{2+} efflux in the higher negative pressure. For this reason the experiments from the table 1 have been performed showing that in the beginning of suction there are the changes in the permeability of Na^{+},K^{+}, and Ca^{2+},which develop under the suction electrode.It would be convenient to study the

Table 1

Influence of Na^{+},K^{+}, and Ca^{2+} current blockers placed in the tip of suction electrode (0,1 ml) on the epicardial ECG measured under the suction electrode in frog ventricular epicardium before and during the introduction of negative pressure (suction) -40 kPa.

Agent (0,1 ml)	Before suction	During suction
Tetrodotoxin 1,6.10^{-4} mol.l^{-1} or sucrose 200-800mmol.l^{-1}	Spontaneous MAP	Unchanged
4-aminopyridine 20 mmol.l^{-1} or tetraethylammonium 40--800 mmol.l^{-1}	Small elevation of ST-T	MAP as in controls (the effect of agents was suppressed)
Verapamil 0,25 mg	Unchanged	MAP of different plateau shape than in controls
Controls (Ringer)	Normal ECG	MAP

ionic currents under the suction electrodes to explain more exactly this problem. In conclusion, our results proved the depolarization, potassium outflow, and Ca^{2+} changes during the development of MAP under the suction electrode placed in frog ventricular epicardium when the negative pressure was introduced.

References

(1) Schütz,E.: Klin.Wochenschr. 10, 1454-1457 (1931)
(2) Burgess,M.J.: Amer.J Physiol. 236, H391-H402 (1979)
(3) Franz,M.R.,Burkhoff,D.,Spurgeon,H.,Weisfeldt,M.L.,Lakatta,E.G.:Eur. HeartJ. 7,34-41 (1986)
(4) Slavíček,J.,Stojan,M.,Netušil,M.,Bělohlávek,M.: Physiol.Bohemoslov. 28,469 (1979)
(5) Slavíček,J.,Vyskočil,F.,Stojan,M.; Physiol.Bohemoslov.33,560 (1984a)
(6) Slavíček,J.,Netušil,M.,Stojan,M.,Teisinger,J.,Vítek,V.,Vyskočil,F.: J.Physiol.Paris 79, 85A (1984b)
(7) Slavíček,J.,Vyskočil,F.: Physiol.Bohemoslov. 34,2o1-207 (1985)
(8) Slavíček,J.,Teisinger,J.,Vítek,V.,Stojan,M.,Vyskočil,F.: Physiol. Bohemoslov. 37, In press (1988)
(9) Hoffman,B.F.,Cranefield,P.F.,Lepeschkin,E.,Surawicz,B.,Herrlich,H. C.: Amer.J.Physiol. 196, 1297-1301 (1959)

The histology of the atrioventricular nodal cells in the human heart

KAZUHIKO SHIMIZU, KENICHI HARUMI, MASAHIRO TOHAYA, KOH GOTOH*, FUMIAKI SAGAWA*

Division of Cardiology, *Division of Hospital Pathology, Showa University Fujigaoka Hospital, 1-30 Fujigaoka, Midori-ku, Yokohama 227, Japan

Summary

The new method to make the semi-thin preparations of the human atrioventricular (AV) node from ordinal autopsied hearts was developed, and the three types of cells were classified and their distribution was studied. The subjects were 25 autopsy cases with no cardiac diseases and normal PR interval (0.14-0.18 sec. 0.15±0.011). The AV nodal area was dissected by the modified Lev's method. The selected sections were embedded in epon polymer and cut into 1µm thickness specimens. The three types of the AV nodal cells were classified. (1) The cell with coarse myofibrils (the width: 8.8±1.2µm, 20.5% of the total cell) (2) The slender cell (4.8±1.1.µm, 4.2%) (3) The cell with rich myofibrils (9.5±1.2µm, 75.3%).(1) showed the structure resembled the sinoatrial (SA) nodal cell, and was distributed mainly in the lower part and nearby the His bundle portion of the AV node. (2) was distributed mainly in the nearby approach portion. (3) was distributed generally in the AV node. These results suggested that the AV nodal area has the possibility of automaticity in general.

Introduction

There has been conflicting discussion on classification and distribution of the human AV nodal cells. One of the reasons is that the fine structure of cells has been obtained only by the thin preparation of electron microscopy. We developed the semi-thin preparation of the human AV node from ordinal autopsied hearts and made it possible to differentiate the AV nodal cells from their fine structure.

Materials and Methods

The subjects were 25 autopsy cases (15 men and 10 women) with no cardiac disease, with normal PR interval (range 0.14 to 0.18, mean 0.15± 0.011), and their average age was 40.4 years (range 10 to 55).

The AV nodal area was removed by the modified Lev's method and was cut into 10 serial sections about 1mm thickness each. These sections were embedded in the 10 serial paraffin blocks. The ordinal 6µm specimen of Elastica-van-Gieson stain was used to identify the AV node, and a minute block of the AV node was cut away from the residual paraffin blocks.(Fig.1)

The process of making the semi-thin sectins (1μm) by epon embedding were deparaffinize, dexylenize, exchange, immersion, epon embedding, section and stain. The total procedure took about two weeks. We divided the AV node into six segments, and examined by light microscopy. Five visual fields were selected from each segments. Each field was 100μm x 100μm at 1000 x magnification in size, and cells were classfied and counted in each of the five visual fields. The distribution rate of the cells in a segment was calculated by averaging the number of cells in five visual fields.

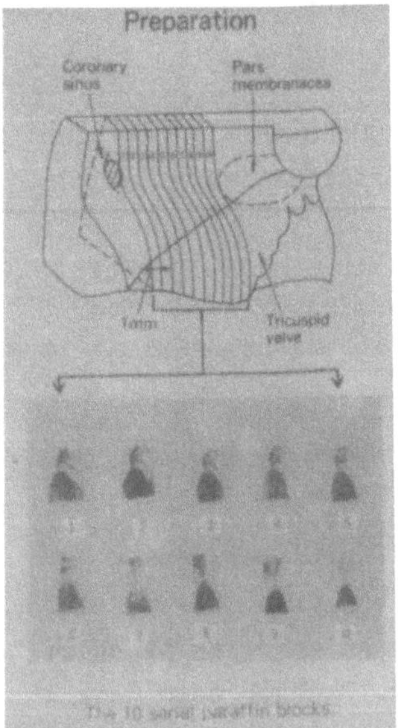

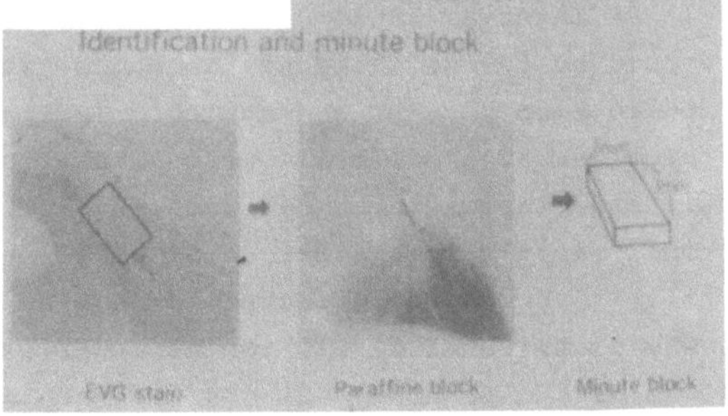

Fig.1

Results

(1) Classification (Fig.2)

Fig.2 showed the three types of the AV nodal cells, these classified by the semi-thin section speciments.

I: The cell with coarse myofibrils. The mean width of the cell was 8.8±1.2μm and the cell occupied 20.5% of the total cell. This cell contained scanty and thin myofibrils, and resembled the SA nodal cell.

II: The slender cell. 4.8±1.1μm, and 4.2%. This cell contained abundant and thick myofibrils. III: The cell with rich myofibrils. 9.5±1.2μm, and 75.3%. This cell contained abundant and thick myofibrils. IV: Unclassified cells were excluded in this study.

(2) Distribution (Fig.3, Fig.4)

Fig.3 showed the typical case of each six segments, and the distribution rate of three classified cells was shown in Fig.4. Seg.1 and 2 were the nearby approach portion. Seg.3 and 4 were the central portion, and seg.5 and 6 were the nearby His bundle portion of the AV node. In seg.1, the slender cells were overlayer and were connected to the cells with rich myofibrils. Seg.2, the cells with rich myofibrils were in layers which were shown in cross stratum and longitudinal stratum. There were some cells with coarse myofibrils in the lower part. Seg.3, branching of the cells with rich myofibrils were shown. Seg.3 was similar cell distribution rate to seg.2. Seg.4, the frame network of the cells with rich myofibrils, where the cell with rich myofibrils and the cells with coarse myofibrils were scattered in a group. Seg.5, its distribution rate was similar to seg.4. Seg.6, the cell with coarse myofibrils were

Fig. 2

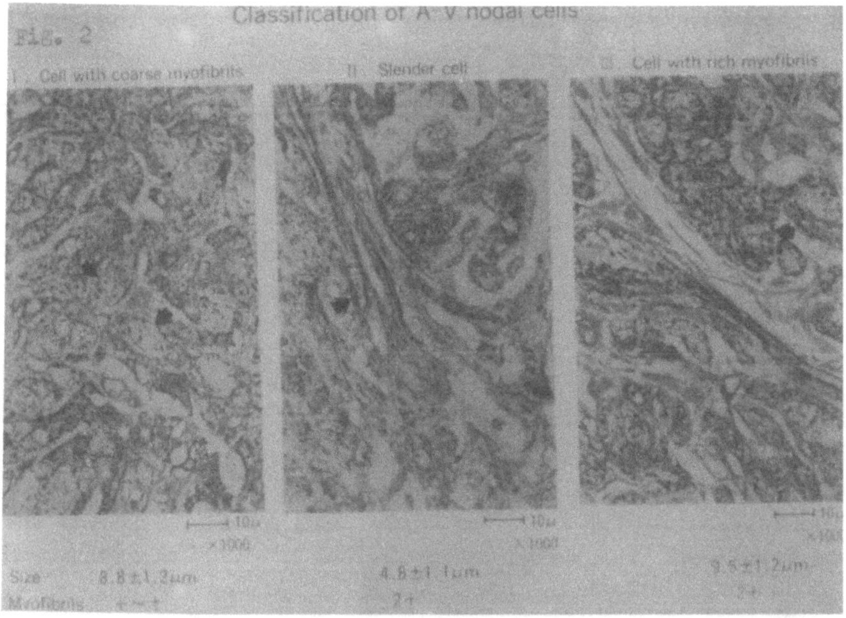

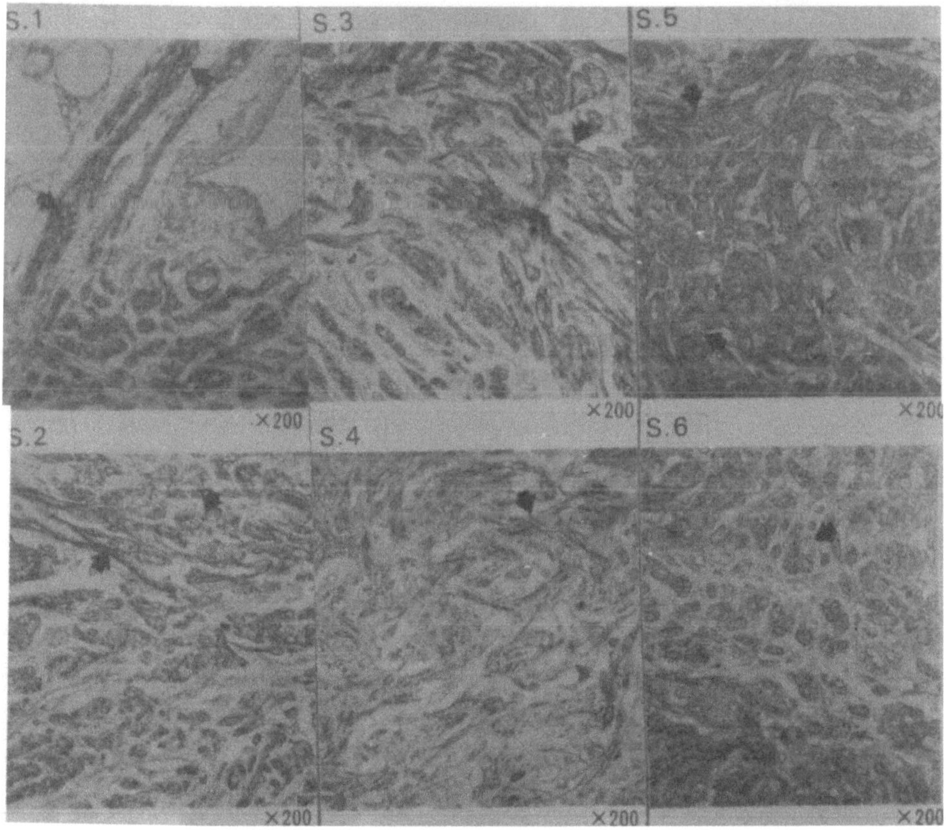

Fig.3 Distribution of AV nodal cells

markedly increased and the cells with rich myofibrils were scattered among them.

Discussion

Preparations of the semi-thin sections of the human AV node from ordinal autopsied hearts made it possible to differentiate the individual AV nodal cells from their fine structures.

Previously a few studies of the isolated human AV node was done by James and Sherf,[1) 2)] Vassall-Adams.[4)] James and Sherf described the canine AV node as containing four different types of cells. They were (1) P cell, (2) the three types of transitional cells; slender, oblong and oval cells.[3)] Vassall-Adams described that a spectrum of the human AV nodal cells which ranged widely in size and in myofibril content from slim cells and packed with myofibrils to wide empty cells.[4)]

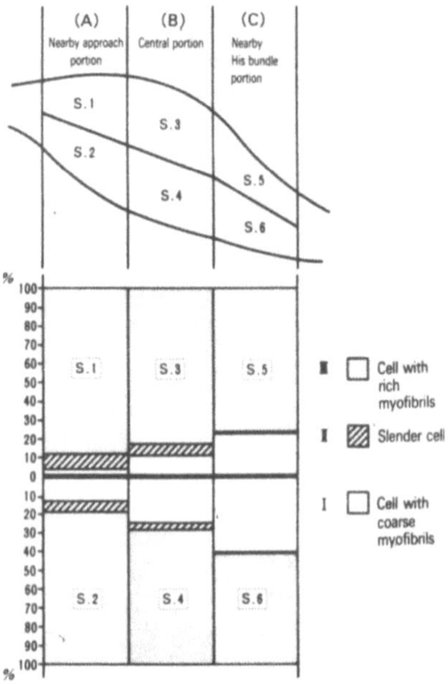

Fig.4 Distribution

We classified three types of the human AV nodal cells. They were (1) the cell with coarse myofibrils, (2) the slender cell and (3) the cell with rich myofibrils. (1) cell resembled the SA nodal cell and corresponded to P cell by James and to wide empty cell by Vassall-Adams. This type cell had a high distribution in the lower part and the nearby His bundle portion, but had a slight distribution in the higher part and the approach portion of the AV node. These results were compatible with that of Kokubun and Irisawa who observed the spontaneous action potential in rabbit AV node in general.[5)]

Finally, the present method provides a useful preparation for the histological study of the human AV node.

References

1) James,T.N., et al: Am.Heart J. 62, 756 - 771 (1961)
2) James,T.N., et al: Circulation 37, 1049 - 1070 (1968)
3) Sherf,L., et al: J.Am.Coll.Cardiol. 5, 770 - 780 (1985)
4) Vassall-Adams,P.R.: Europ.Heart J. 4, 449 - 460 (1983)
5) Kokubun,S., et al: Jpn.J.Physiol. 30, 529 - 540 (1980)

Structural and functional organization of atrioventricular conducting system in the avian heart

PROSHEVA V., RAPOTA I.

Institute of Biology, Academy of Sciences of the USSR, Komi Branch, Syktyvkar, USSR

SUMMARY
The topography of atrioventricular conducting system in the heart of an adult pigeon and chicken was studied by morphological and electrophysiological methods. It was stated that in the heart of these animals considerable prolongation of a pacemaker area of atrioventricular node takes place. A pacemaker zone found in the muscle valve creates functional discontinuity between the right atrium and right ventricle. It was shown that in the subendocardium, deep layers of myocardium and close to the epicardium Purkinje fibers of various diameters occur simultaneously. A scheme of structural-functional organization of atrioventricular conducting system in the bird heart suggested.

INTRODUCTION
Though there are many papers devoted to the study of conducting system in the bird heart,still in literature there is much discrepancy concerning topographical location of atrioventricular(A-V) conducting system in the bird heart (Kim, Yasuda, 1979; Vassall-Adams, 1982). A specific feature of A-V conducting system of the bird is the right ring of specialized fibers which takes its start immediately from the A-V node and locates in the right muscle A-V valve.But functional role of this ring of specialized fibers is still obscure. By this work we tried to answer the following questions: 1) What types of specialized cells can be observed in the right A-V valve and what is their topography in it?
2) What is the moment of electrical activation of the muscle valve during the cardiac cycle? 3) In what way are Purkinje fibers distributed in the free walls of the ventricles of the bird heart?

MATERIAL AND METHODS
The object of our investigation was 30 adult pigeons both male and female(mass 288-396 g)and 22 adult white Leghorns(mass 1.1-1.5 kg). We used generally accepted histilogical methods,multipolar technique and the method of microelectrode mapping previously described(Prosheva,1986) The results are expressed as mean values$\pm$standard error of the mean.

RESULTS
Action potential distribution of conducting system cells in the muscle valve and its activation. Fig.1 gives the configurations of three main types of action potentials(APs) registered from the atrial side of the muscle chicken valve:APs of pacemaker cells(Fig.1, B,C), APs of Pur-

kinje cells(Fig.1, A,E,F)and APs of working myocardium cells(Fig.1, D). For the purpose of description we distinguished five main parts of the valve(Fig.1, 1-5). Action potentials of pacemaker cells are always registered at the basis of the valve along the whole of its path from dorsal to ventral attachment to interventricular septum, but only on its atrial side, i.e. they are strictly localized. The width of pacemaker zone is about 600 μm and its length coincides with the length of the valve of the investigated subject and is equal on the average to 12.8±0.6 mm(n=10)for pigeons and 19.5±0.4 mm(n=15) for chicken. Action potentials of Purkinje cells on the atrial as well as on the ventricular side are usually registered from the part of the free edge of the valve, attached to the right ventricle wall and also from the areas adjacent to dorsal and ventral sides of the interventricular septum. At the basis of the valve on its atrial side Purkinje cells are found only in four preparations. Unlike this there are rather many Purkinje cells at the basis of the valve on the ventricular side and here they are located in the main in false tendons. Action potentials of Purkinje cells are also registered from the free edge of the valve (on both sides) but not so often as in the regions mentioned above.

There is a literature hypothesis that early distribution of conducting system fibers immediately to the muscle valve is a specific feature letting this valve actively contract in the initial moment of ventricu-

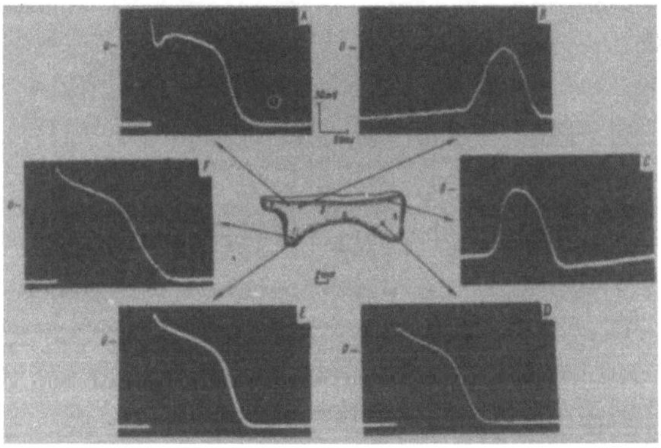

Fig.1. Transmembrane action potentials of the atrial side cells of the right atrioventricular valve in chicken heart. In the center of this picture there is a scheme of the isolated valve with the adjacent atrial tissue. 1 - part of the free edge of the valve, attached to the right ventricle wall, 2 - region of the valve junction with the ventral side of the interventricular septum, 3 - the basis of the valve, 4 - the region of the valve junction with the dorsal side of the interventricular septum, 5 - free edge of the valve; A-F - typical action potentials registered in different parts of the valve.Points show to the places of these action potentials registrations.

lar activity. In connection with this we made an attempt to find the exact moment of exctation of the muscle valve of pigeons and chicken within the whole cardiac cycle. It appeared that electrical activation of the muscle valve in chicken takes place on the average on the (8.8±0.4)msec (the mean duration of the initial ventricular complex - 25 msec;n=7) but in pigeons it happens on the (5.2±0.3)msec (the mean duration of the initial ventricular complex - 17 msec;n=8) from the start of ventricle depolarization, in the period of excitation of the myocardium main mass of the right ventricle free wall.

Distribution of Purkinje fibers in the free walls of ventricles in the pigeon heart(n=12). In the apex of the heart Purkinje fibers(P.F.)occur close to the blood vessels at the distance of about 800 μm from epicardium. Diameters of P.F. may be 13.0-20.8 μm. In the region of the left ventricle bottom P.F. are not numerous. In the subendocardium their diameters are from 9 to 33 μm, in the myocardium thickness they are from 9 to 21 μm and concentrate in the ventral part locating in its deeper layers. At the level of the apical third of the interventricular septum under the endocardium of the free left ventricle wall we observe P.F. of a small diameter of 6-9 μm. In the myocardium thickness they are located in its deep layers, distributing not evenly along the whole layer but concentrating in lateral, ventral and partly in dorsal regions. On the free wall of the right ventricle P.F. occur in the main in the deep myocardium layers concentrating in the lateral region. At the level of the middle third of the interventricular septum under the endocardium of the free left ventricle wall P.F. are from 6 to 21 μm in diameter. In the myocardium thickness P.F. are located in the main closer to ventral and dorsal parts of the free left ventricle wall, concentrating in its deeper layers. In the myocardium thickness of the free right ventricle wall P.F. of various diameters(9-18 μm) are observed in the main in the deep myocardium layers, concentrating in the lateral region. At the level of basal third of the interventricular septum under the endocardium of the free left ventricle wall alongside with large(24-30 μm)P.F. there occur some smaller(6 μm)ones. In the myocardium thickness P.F. of various diameters(9-24 μm)are located in ventral and dorsal regions, in their deeper layers. In the myocardium of the free right ventricle wall P.F. occur in the layers adjacent to endo- and epicardium, and in deep layers they are absent.

DISCUSSION AND CONCLUSIONS

Thus, the results of our electrophysiological and morphological investigations and literature data(Kim, Yasuda, 1979; Prosheva, 1981) give the possibility to present structural-functional organization of A-V conducting system in the bird heart in the following way. The presence of the muscle valve in the bird heart causes a considerable prolongation of the pacemaker area of the A-V node(i.e. the pacemaker zone in the muscle valve is also included into the structure of the node). The right A-V ring of specialized fibers in the bird heart has the structure and plays the functional role which are similar to those of the A-V node in mam-

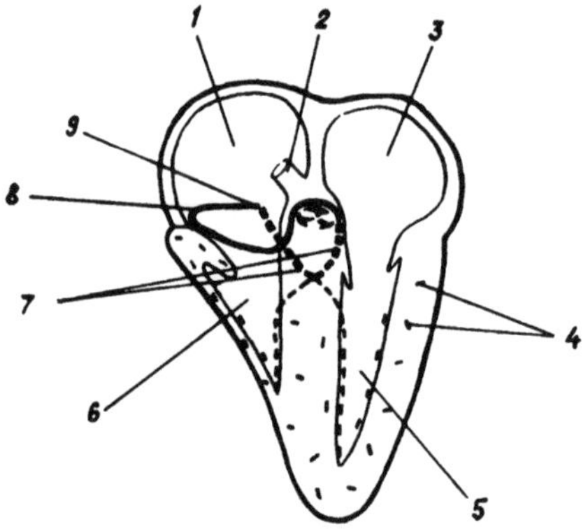

Fig.2. The scheme of topography of atrioventricular conducting system in the bird heart. 1 - right atrium, 2 - aorta, 3 - left atrium, 4 - Purkinje fibers, 5 - left ventricle, 6 - right ventricle, 7 - atrioventricular bundle, 8 - pacemaker area, 9 - atrioventricular node.

mals. Thanks to the great prolongation of the A-V node in the bird heart from our point of view it should be named an "A-V junction", but not a "node" or "ring". Accordingly the A-V bundle is highly branched.A primary branching takes place: the branch taking its start from the right dorsolateral side of interatrial and interventricular septum(similar in topography to the A-V bundle of mammals)and the branch taking its start on the right side of the aorta basis. The latter corresponds to the recurrent branch(Davies,1930)or to the middle branch(Gossrau,1969)or to the fasciculus truncobulbaris(Kim, Yasuda,1979)or septal and retroaortal components of the right A-V ring(Vassall-Adams,1982). In the area which is at the distance of about one fourth from the basis to the apex of the interventricular septum there occur a secondary branching,the bundle is divided into the right and left limbs. Its terminal ramifications, P.F., penetrate deep into the myocardium thickness of the free ventricles walls,but their density both in subendocardial as well as in intramural layers is rather low. Though the network of Purkinje terminals is rare their electrotonic junctions with contracting myocardium cells is of a discrete character.

REFERENCES

(1) Kim, Y., M. Yasuda: Zbl. Veterinärmed. 8, 138 -150 (1979).(2) Vassal-Adams, P: J. Anat. 134, 169 - 183 (1982). (3) Prosheva, V: Physiol. J. of the USSR. 72, 940 - 946 (1986). (4) Davies, F: J. Anat. 64, 129 - 146 (1930). (5) Prosheva, V: In Comparative Electrocardiology, Leningrad, Nauka, 45 - 49 (1981)(in Russian). (6) Gossrau, R: Z. Anat. Entwick-Gesch. 128, 163 - 184 (1969).

MODELLING OF HEART ACTIVITY

Modelling of isopotential and field strength distribution in the human thorax

by HAUG, T. and MALDENER, K.

Klinik Wonneberg, Am Wonneberg 7, D 6748 Bad Bergzabern
Federal Republic of Germany

SUMMARY: In a plane model, for two cross-sections through the human torso isopotential lines as well as field strength lines have been computed assuming non-conducting finite medium between heart surface and body surface. With respect to reciprocity of isopotential lines and field lines, the model can also be used for any physiological distribution of potential maxima, minima and zero positions on the heart's surface. A qualitative extension was made for homogeneously conducting media. Reciprocal use of trajectories needs in this case new notions of "isoratio lines of potential" instead of "isopotential lines" and of "ratio field lines" instead of "field lines".

INTRODUCTION: The purpose of the study is to find a simple and descriptive representation of the field lines and isopotential lines which are spread from the heart's electrically active surface through the chest space to the body surface. As a first trial, several years ago an electrostatic experiment was carried out. It showed some interesting details with field strength lines, but was difficult to interpret. The physical arrangement of electrodes was used to find a mathematical solution.

MATERIALS AND METHOD: From an anatomical atlas, a horizontal and a vertical cross-section through the human torso were taken as plane models for a finite electrical space, delimited by the heart's contour H (inside) and the contour T of the torso (outside).

A) Assuming isopotential surfaces I+ in H and I- in T, a dense set of isopotential lines was computed by equidistant dividing of intermediate space and smoothing with spline interpolation. After that, field lines were computed starting orthogonally at regular distances from H. Field line trajectories are drawn by means of a shortest-way-algorithm (figs. 1 and 2). In this model, field lines run radially from H to T, and isopotential lines I are stepped at equal distances like shells around the heart.

B) Field lines and isopotential lines being defined as reciprocal (= orthogonal) to each other, we are authorized to exchange the physical denomination of both sets of curves. Now - without any change in the trajectories! - the isopotential lines run radially from H to T, and field lines F are shell-like grouped around the heart. This configuration is much closer to any physiological distribution characterized by potential maximum, minimum and zero located around the heart's surface. The isopotential lines are ending in corresponding positions of MAX, MIN and 0 on the body surface T (fig. 3).

RESULTS: Figs. 1 and 2 show, that to every point on the heart's surface there is corresponding just one other point on the body surface: The mecanism of field transfer results in a kind of projecting the heart's surface to the body surface. The projection is systematically distorted by the excentric position of the heart. The density of projection lines arriving on the body surface varies considerably: High density in precordial area, low density in dorsal and right-lateral areas. But the density of projection lines is also strongly depending from accidental peculiarities of the heart's shape. - The diaphragmatical face of the heart is projected to a subdiaphragmatical circular band around the torso. - Fig. 3 shows clearly the correspondence between heart and torso with respect to typical electro-physiological data: Maximum, minimum and zero positions of potential are distinctively projected from the heart surface to the body surface. Any other thinkable configuration of potential distributions will be transferred in the same true manner to the body surface.

EXTENSION: The more realistic case of a finite homogeneously conducting medium in the space between heart and body surface is difficult for computation, but can be qualitatively estimated by the mecanisms shown in (A) and (B):

C) In the same arrangement as described in (A), an electric current is flowing from H to T through the conducting medium. The decrease of potential being proportional to the current density, isopotential lines I are generally condensed closer to high-density field ranges near the heart. Only in the precordial area exhibiting nearly constant current density, isopotential lines keep approximately their previous positions. In dorsal and right-lateral ranges, current density decreases considerably from inside to outside, as can be seen from field lines in fig. 1. In these ranges, isopotential lines are stepped with increasing distances from inside to outside. (Both statements - equidistant precordial stepping as well as condensed stepping in other regions - have been confirmed by a rough experiment on a graphite plated paper model). But the general arrangement of trajectories remains similar to case (A): Field lines are running radially from inside to outside, and isopotential lines are shell-like grouped in the intermediate space around the heart.

D) If now again - similar to case (B) - we make an exchange of the physical meaning between both groups of potential and field lines, there will be an important difference: With exception of the zero lines, the radial group of trajectories is no longer an "iso"-potential group! But every relative position in the configuration of potential distribution remains the same as well on the heart as on the body: The decreased maximum "max" on the body surface is still on the same potential line than the original maximum "MAX" on the heart's surface, and the same mecanisme applies to the minimum and also to each other ratio V/Vmax (resp. V/Vmin) of potential (e. g. 50% / 20% / 5% of maximum or of minimum). The trajectories are still the same, but now they represent "isoratio" lines of potential, not "isopotential" lines (fig. 4). In the same manner, the other group of lines being orthogonal to the isoratio-group now will represent a "ratio field" (i. e. the reciprocal of isoratio lines) instead of the original field strength. The meaning of the ratio field is to indicate the shortest-way-trajectories between two different isoratio lines along their extent. The ratio field lines are shell-like grouped around the heart and parallel to the heart's surface (while the real field lines are running obliquely between heart and torso).

DISCUSSION and CONCLUSIONS: The model presented in this report is quantitatively computed only for the case of a non-conducting medium in a finite space between two isopotential surfaces (case "A" with radial field lines). Just the same, the description of the reciprocal field arrangement (case "B" with radial isopotential lines) claims the same degree of accuracy, since reciprocity between field lines and isopotential lines is set up by definition. Case (B) is a better approximation to physiological conditions than case (A). The model (A) is qualitatively extended for conducting media in the finite space between heart surface and body surface (case "C"). Both groups of lines (isopotential lines as well as field lines) are displaced in a specific way depending upon the conductivity of the medium, but the general character of each group remains the same: Radial trajectories of field lines, shell-like trajectories of isopotential lines. The application of reciprocity to case (C) - still authorized by definition - reveals the necessity of a new understanding of both kinds of trajectories (case "D"): The potential group of radial trajectories represents in this case not a constant potential but a constant ratio V/Vmax (resp. V/Vmin) of potential, whereas the field group of shell-like trajectories can be understood as the gradient of the constant-ratio lines. Therefore it is suggested to introduce new denominations: "Isoratio lines of potential" and "ratio field lines". The use of these new types of trajectories will lead to a better understanding of the mecanism of field transfer from an inner surface with given distribution of electric sources through finite conductive media to the outer border surface. The application of reciprocity and of "isoratio" and "ratio field" notions may initiate the use of simple mathematical tools for exact calculations even in cases of non-homogeneous conductive media in complicated geometric arrangements.

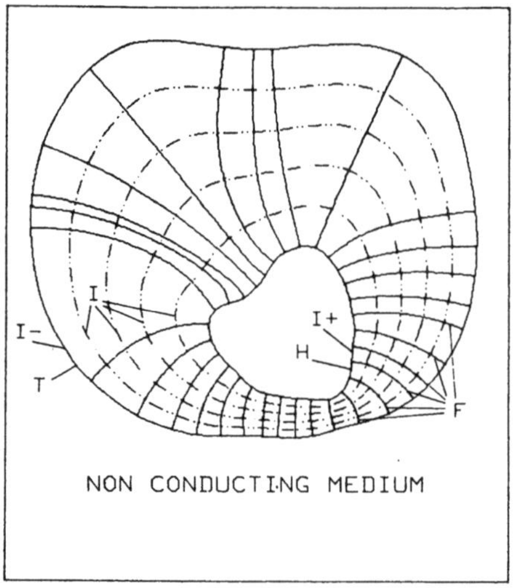

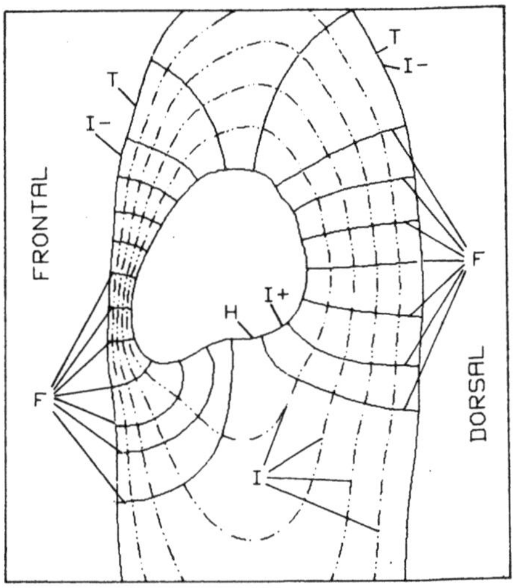

Fig.1. Computed isopotential lines I and field strength lines F in a horizontal cross-section through the human thorax. H, T = isopotential contour lines on the heart resp. the torso; non-conducting medium between H and T.

Fig.2. Computed isopotential lines I and field strength lines F in a vertical cross-section through the human thorax. H, T = isopotential contour lines on the heart resp. the torso; non-conducting medium between H and T.

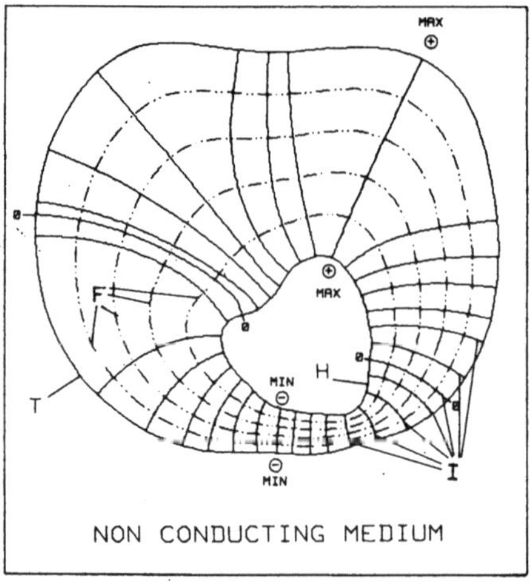

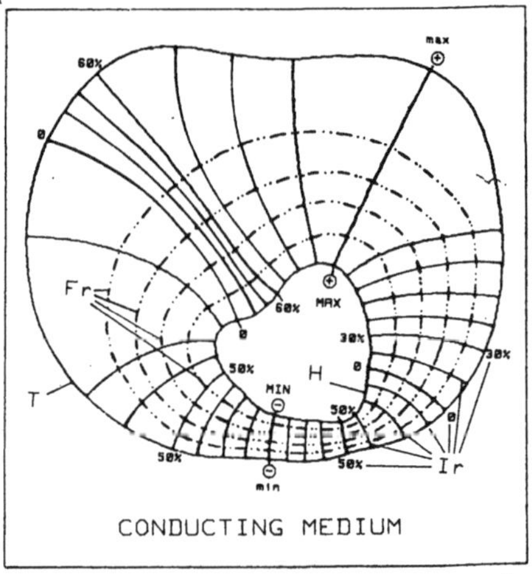

Fig.3. Reciprocal field lines F and isopotential lines I in the same horizontal cross-section of fig.1. H = field contour line on the heart's surface with potential MAX, MIN and 0; T = field contour line on the body with corresponding positions of potential maximum, minimum and zero. Non-conducting medium.

Fig.4. Reciprocal "ratio field lines" Fr and "isoratio lines of potential" Ir in the horizontal cross-section of fig.3. H = ratio field contour line on the heart's surface with potential MAX, MIN and 0; T = ratio field contour line on the body with corresponding positions of potential max, min and 0. The isoratio lines are the trajectories of constant ratio V/Vmax (resp. V/Vmin) of potential V, the ratio field lines are their orthogonals. Extended from figs.1 and 3 for conductive medium.

Theoretical analysis of magnetic fields resulting from heart activity

W. HABERKORN and G. ALBRECHT

ZWG, Academy of Sciences of the GDR, Rudower Chaussee 6,
Berlin, 1199, GDR

Summary

The magnetic fields arising from current dipole models of the sources in the heart are studied. Analytical expressions are presented for a linear source and current dipole layers with elementary shapes. The magnetic heart vector is derived for planar current dipole layers and the effect of circulating currents is analysed.

Introduction

Appropriate heart models are needed for the understanding and the detailed analysis of magnetocardiograms. The purpose of the present study is to provide the analytical solutions for the magnetic field of basic models which approximate cardiac sources and to analyse the magnetic heart vector. Furthermore, the effects of circulating currents are investigated. If such currents exist, they contribute nothing to the electrocardiogram.

Methods

Following (1), the magnetic field of cellular cardiac sources embedded in a homogeneous, isotropic, and infinite volume conductor is given by the expression

$$\frac{4\pi}{\mu_0}\vec{B}(\vec{r}) = \int_V \vec{j}^{\,i}(\vec{r}\,') \times \frac{(\vec{r}-\vec{r}\,')}{|\vec{r}-\vec{r}\,'|^3}\,dv' + \sum_m \int_{F_m} g_m(\vec{r}\,')\,\frac{(\vec{r}-\vec{r}\,')}{|\vec{r}-\vec{r}\,'|^3} \times d\vec{f}_m' \,, \qquad (1)$$

$$g_m(\vec{r}\,') = \sigma_i^m U_i(\vec{r}\,') - \sigma_e^m U_e(\vec{r}\,') \;.$$

In the first contribution, $\vec{j}^i$ is the impressed current density which is zero outside the active cellular membranes. The second term describes the effects at the membranes represented by surfaces F_m, where σ_i^m and σ_e^m are the intracellular and extracellular conductivities, respectively, and U_i and U_e are the corresponding potentials.
Considering the case of a circular cylindrical fibre, the application of Eq. (1) leads to the results of (2) for the nerve axon. It can be shown that the contribution to the magnetic field from the impressed current density can be neglected for the cardiac tissue (1) and the nerve axon (2). Furthermore, from Eq. (1) we have that at a distance an active cell behaves like a single current dipole having the moment

$$\vec{p}_m = -\int_{F_m} g_m(\vec{r}')\,d\vec{f}_m' \quad . \tag{2}$$

Increasing the distance from the heart model, a multicellular region can also be represented by a single current dipole having a moment which is obtained by summing all cellular moments of the complex. These considerations provide the basis for the current dipole models of the heart. Using the discrete description of cardiac sources, the magnetic heart vector is given by

$$\vec{m}_H = \frac{\mu_0}{2} \sum_n \vec{r}_n \times \vec{p}_n \quad , \tag{3}$$

where $\vec{r}_n$ is the vector from the heart center to the current dipole $\vec{p}_n$.

Results

First the theory presented above is used to calculate the magnetic field of a linear source lying on the x axis. For a uniform distribution of current dipoles pointing in the x direction, we obtain the expression

$$\frac{4\pi}{\mu_0}\vec{B}(\vec{r}) = q\,\frac{\vec{e}_x \times \vec{r}}{y^2+z^2}\left\{\frac{x+l}{[(x+l)^2+y^2+z^2]^{1/2}} - \frac{x-l}{[(x-l)^2+y^2+z^2]^{1/2}}\right\} \quad , \tag{4}$$

where q is the constant dipole density and $\pm$ l are the dimensions of the line along the x axis.
The next application is the case of a planar sheet of uniformly distributed current dipoles which are perpendicular to the layer. For a rectangular shaped sheet lying in the x = 0 plane, the magnetic field

is given by

$$\frac{4\pi}{\mu_0}\vec{B}(\vec{r}) = \tau\vec{e}_z \sum_{\sigma=\pm}\left\{\operatorname{arsinh}\frac{z-\sigma b}{[x^2+(y+\sigma a)^2]^{1/2}} - \operatorname{arsinh}\frac{z+\sigma b}{[x^2+(y+\sigma a)^2]^{1/2}}\right\} \tag{5}$$

$$- \tau\vec{e}_y \sum_{\sigma=\pm}\left\{\operatorname{arsinh}\frac{y-\sigma a}{[x^2+(z+\sigma b)^2]^{1/2}} - \operatorname{arsinh}\frac{y+\sigma a}{[x^2+(z+\sigma b)^2]^{1/2}}\right\},$$

where τ is the constant dipole density and $\pm$ a, $\pm$ b are the dimensions of the layer in y and z direction, respectively.

A similar calculation for the circular current dipole layer leads to complete elliptic integrals.

For the planar current dipole layer, the magnetic heart vector can be shown to be

$$\vec{m}_H = \frac{\mu_0}{2}(\vec{r}_0 \times \vec{p}_H) - \frac{\mu_0\tau}{6}\int_0^{2\pi} d\varphi\, \vec{\varrho}^{\,3}(\varphi)\vec{e}_\varphi \quad , \quad \vec{p}_H = \tau\vec{F} \,, \tag{6}$$

where $\vec{p}_H$ is the corresponding electric heart vector, τ is the dipole density, $\vec{\varrho}$ is the curve enclosing the layer of area F, and $\vec{r}_0$ is the vector from the heart center to the layer center. It can be seen that $\vec{m}_H$ and $\vec{p}_H$ are perpendicular.

Finally, the magnetic field of circulating currents arising from ring-shaped arrangements of current dipoles is given by

$$\vec{B}(\vec{r}) = \frac{\mu_0}{4\pi}\sum_n I_n \oint_{L_n} \frac{\vec{dl}_n \times (\vec{r}-\vec{r}_n)}{|\vec{r}-\vec{r}_n|^3} \,, \tag{7}$$

where L_n is the closed path/way of the current I_n. Note that at a distance such a current behaves like a magnetic dipole.

For the planar current dipole layer enclosed by a circulating current I, the magnetic heart vector becomes

$$\vec{m}_H' = \vec{m}_H + \mu_0 I\vec{F} \,, \tag{8}$$

where the second contribution is the moment of the magnetic dipole arising from the current I.

Discussion

The model of the current dipole line can serve as a basic element for studies of the fields produced by the His-Purkinje system and an accessory conducting path. The rectangular shaped and the circular current dipole layers represent models of the myocardial activity.

For these basic models, the analytical expressions for the magnetic field were presented above. Note that the results can also be used to determine the conditions for the approximation of the sources by a single current dipole. Considering the case of the linear source, the lowest-order nonzero term of the expansion of the magnetic field with respect to the source length is given by

$$\vec{B}^{(1)}(\vec{r}) = \frac{\mu_0}{4\pi} \frac{\vec{p} \times \vec{r}}{r^3} \quad , \quad \vec{p} = (2ql, 0, 0) . \tag{9}$$

The first deviations from this behaviour of a single current dipole having the moment $\vec{p}$ can be shown to be proportional to l^3. Similar considerations can also be made for the current dipole layers.
Note that the presence of circulating currents cannot be ruled out in cardiac activation (3). On the basis of Eq. (7) the behaviour of such currents can be compared with the magnetic field of other cardiac sources. For a circular current path/way, the calculation of the magnetic field leads to complete elliptic integrals.
Finally, we remark that for the planar current dipole layer enclosed by a circulating current the relationship between the heart vectors becomes

$$\vec{m}_H' \vec{P}_H = \mu_0 \tau I F^2 . \tag{10}$$

It can be seen that the presence of a circulating current leads to deviations from the orthogonality. This result can serve as a basis for the detection of circulating currents.

References

(1) Plonsey, R.: Biophys. J. 39, 309-312 (1982)
(2) Swinney, K. R., and J. P. Wikswo, Jr.: Biophys. J. 32, 719-732 (1980)
(3) Wikswo, Jr., J. P., and J. P. Barach: J. theor. Biol. 95, 721-729 (1982)

Computer Simulation of the Electrical and Magnetical Heart Field

BRAUER, H.[+], FUNKE, TH.[++]
[+] Institute of Technology, P.O.B. 327, 6300 Ilmenau, GDR
[++]District Hospital, A.-Schweitzer-Str. 3, 6013 Suhl, GDR

Introduction

The purpose of the investigations is an as real as possible mathematical-physical description of the relations of the field distributions on the heart and outside the thorax. Based on an epicardial heart generator model /1/ will be analysed the effects of epicardial fields on the field distributions at the thorax surface including pathological excitation spreads /2,3/.
The same algorithm was chosen for the inverse problem, founded upon the results of Yamashita /4/ who has shown that for the epicardial potential model an unique solution exists.

Mathematical-physical model

The mathematical description founds on the assumption of a piecewise homogeneous volume conductor approximating the real torso geometry (fig. 1) and supposes linear and isotropic material parameters /3/. Both electrical and magnetic field can be assumed to be stationary.

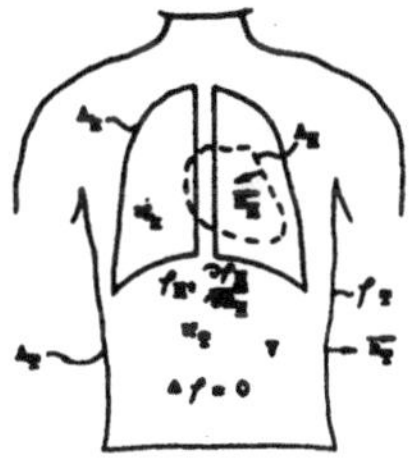

Fig.1: Volume conductor and boundary conditions

Electrical field

forward problem

$$\Delta \varphi = 0 \quad \text{in } V$$
$$\varphi = \varphi_H \quad \text{on } A_H$$
$$\partial \varphi_T / \partial n = 0 \quad \text{on } A_T$$

inverse problem

$$\Delta \varphi = 0 \quad \text{in } V$$
$$\varphi = \varphi_T \quad \text{on } A_T$$
$$\partial \varphi_T / \partial n = 0 \quad \text{on } A_T$$

Using the second Green's theorem equivalent integral equation system can be deduced which give the following matrix equations ($\alpha_H = \partial \varphi_H / \partial n$) :

$$\begin{bmatrix} \underset{\sim}{A} & \underset{\sim}{B} \\ \underset{\sim}{C} & \underset{\sim}{D} \end{bmatrix} \cdot \begin{bmatrix} \underline{\varphi}_T \\ \underline{\alpha}_H \end{bmatrix} = \begin{bmatrix} \underset{\sim}{E} \\ \underset{\sim}{F} \end{bmatrix} \underline{\varphi}_H \qquad \begin{bmatrix} \underset{\sim}{G} & \underset{\sim}{H} \\ \underset{\sim}{I} & \underset{\sim}{J} \end{bmatrix} \cdot \begin{bmatrix} \underline{\varphi}_H \\ \underline{\alpha}_H \end{bmatrix} = \begin{bmatrix} \underset{\sim}{K} \\ \underset{\sim}{L} \end{bmatrix} \underline{\varphi}_T$$

The submatrices A to L contain coefficients which represent integrals over discrete surface elements of volume conductor boundaries. They depend on geometrical configuration and material parameters at the boundaries only and can obtained by numerical quadrature /3,5/.

Magnetic field

An impressed current density $\vec{J_i}$ generates an electrical field described by the integral equation

$$4\pi x \rho + \sum_j \int_{S_j} (x_i - x_a) \rho \cdot \nabla (\frac{1}{r}) \, \vec{dS_j} = \int_V \vec{J_i} \cdot \nabla (\frac{1}{r}) \, dV$$

and a magnetic field

$$4\pi \vec{B} = \sum_j \mu_0 \int_{S_j} (x_i - x_a) \rho \cdot \nabla (\frac{1}{r}) \times \vec{dS_j} + \mu_0 \int_V \vec{J_i} \times \nabla (\frac{1}{r}) \, dV .$$

Thus the electrical and magnetic field are closed coupled through the potential distribution on the boundaries S_j (or the socalled secondary sources)/6/.

Numerical model

The torso model consists of a thorax surface, approximated by a cylinder with a realistic cross section and added caps to the end, the lungs and the heart surface (fig. 2). These boundaries were approximated by bicubic or 2D parametric spline functions and than discretised into square surface elements, 130 for the thorax surface, 144 for each of the lung surfaces and 324 for the heart surface.

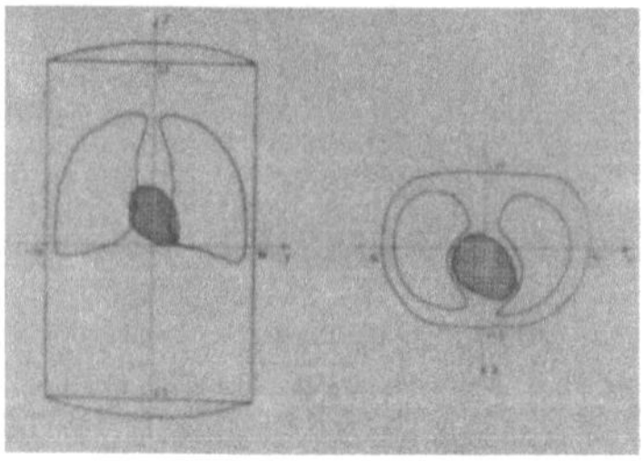

Fig.2: Torso model and cross section

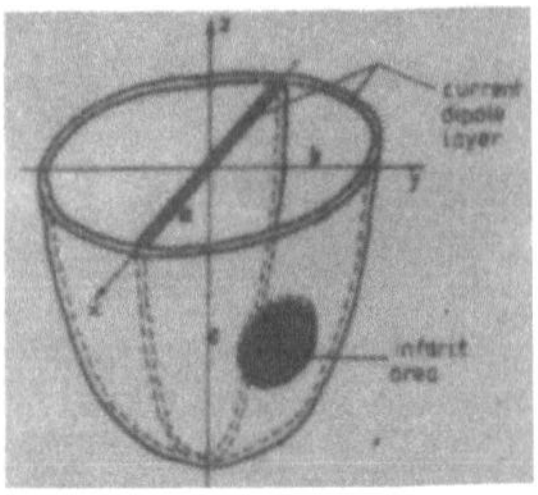

Fig.3: half ellipsoid shaped cup model

Equivalent heart generators for the electrical field are epicardial potential distributions at several moments of the ECG cycle /7/ and a cup carriing an uniform current dipole layer /6,8/ for the magnetic field (fig. 3).

Results

The electric forward problem was solved for homogeneous and inhomogeneous torso models with epicardial potential distributions (from /1/) as equivalent generators (fig. 4,5). Fig. 6 shows the effect of pathological myocardial excitation spread, an anterior wall infarction of

about 6 cm^2 area. It can be noticed decreasing potential values as well as a displacement of the potential minimum which dimension depends on size and location of the infarct area.
Fig. 7 shows as a result of the inverse solution a numerical simulated epicardial potential distribution. The apical located infarct area reflected by a considerably potential decrease (shaded area) embedded in the positive excited sorroundings /3/.

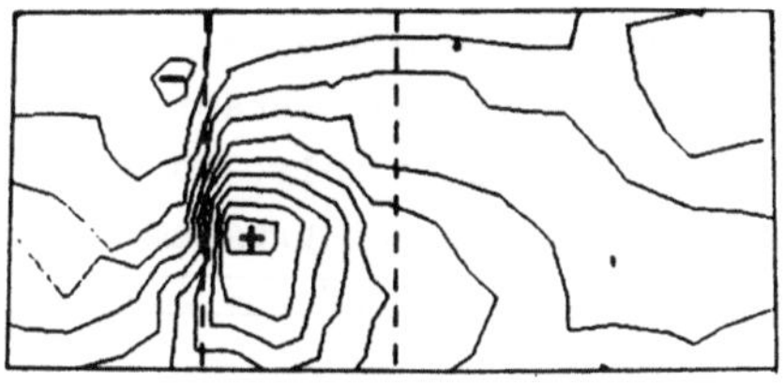

Fig.4: Isopotential map of a homogeneous torso model (R-peak)

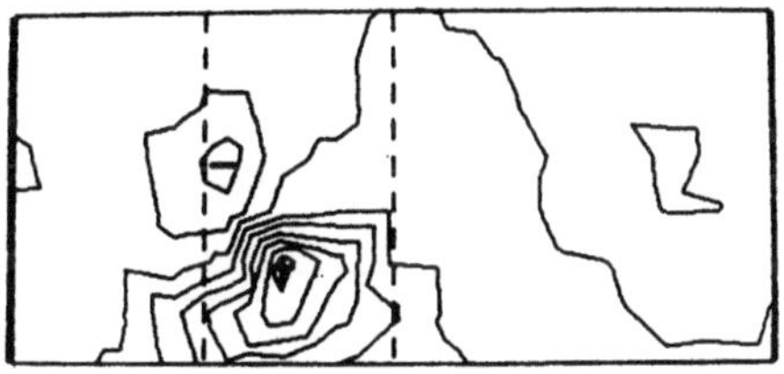

Fig.5: Isopotential map of a inhomogeneous torso model (R-peak)

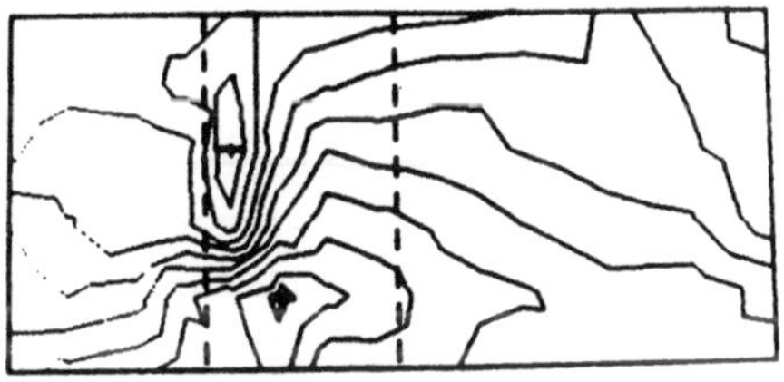

Fig.6: Forward simulation of an anterior wall infarction

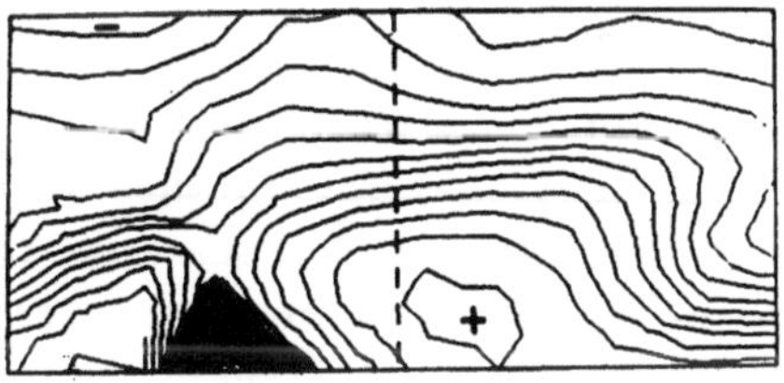

Fig.7: Inverse simulation of the epicardial potential distribution containing infarction

Fig.8: Isomagnetic map for uniform cup model (component B_x)
a) without infarction b) with infarction

The magnetic field in front of the chest of the torso model which contains a cup model like fig. 3 are shown in fig. 8.

The computer simulation makes clear that all components of the magnetic induction are effected by the electrical secondary sources, hence they has to be considered. It follows also that it seems to be not allowed to use only simple current dipoles as sources of biomagnetic fields. It is rather necessary to develope other equivalent generator models for instance like the epicardial potential model for the electrical field.

Conclusions

The boundary integral equation method has proved to be suitable for computer simulation of bioelectric and biomagnetic fields, especially if there are available computers of small or middle size only, so that implementation of a possibly more efficient finite-element program would be not sensible. That's also true for the solution of the inverse problem.

The introduced numerical torso model joint with the epicardial potential generator model provides in a relative simple way surface mappings for normal as well as for pathological excitation spreads on myocard. The magnetic field simulation explains the closed connections with the electrical field and indicates the necessity of using improved generator models compared to usual current configurations.

General important for further investigations would be arrangements about the criteria for the interpretation of simulated or measured surface mappings, also in connection with questions of possibilities for standardization and classification of such data as supposition for computer aided pattern recognition and diagnosis systems. These problems must be solved in the next future.

Literatur

/1/ Wach, P. et al.; Biomed. Technik, 31(1986)11, 255-260

/2/ Barr, R. et al.; IEEE Trans. BME-24(1977)10, 1-11

/3/ Funke, Th.; Thesis, TH Ilmenau, 1987

/4/ Yamashita, Y.; IEEE Trans. BME-29(1982)11, 719-725

/5/ Brauer, H. et al.; Biomed. Technik, 32(1987)3, 34-40

/6/ Brauer, H.; 18. Internat. Symp. TTP, Georgenthal/GDR, 1986

/7/ Durrer, D. et al.; Circulation, 41(1970)6, 899-912

/8/ Peters, M. J. et al.; Il Nuovo Cimento, 20(1983)2, 324-339

DECARTO: A new concept for analyzing and presenting orthogonal electrocardiographic signals

I.RUTTKAY-NEDECKÝ, L.I.TITOMIR, O.V.BAUM, L.BACHÁROVÁ
Inst.of Normal and Pathol.Physiology,Centre of Physiol.Sci.,Slovak Acad. Sci.,Sienkiewiczova 1,81371,Bratislava,CSSR;Inst.of Problems of Information Transmission,Acad.Sci.USSR; Inst.of Biological Physics,Acad.Sci. USSR; Inst.of Medical Bionics,CSSR.

Summary

In dipolar electrocardiotopography (DECARTO), orthogonal ECG signals are transformed by means of a simple mathematical model to represent the equivalent generator of the cardiac electric field as a uniform double layer with time varying size and localization on a spherical surface approximating the ventricular wall,called image sphere.Objective topical probabilities were computed from groups of healthy subjects in order to construct reference image spheres of activation for signals recorded by either Frank or McFee-Parungao lead systems. Individual data were expressed as a fuzzy set with membership characteristic functions equal to the probability that the element will be normally in activated state. Then the associated membership set of the fuzzy set quantifies the degree of individual normality. Data are expressed as a series of maps of activation at predetermined instants of time during ventricular depolarization,as well as chronotopograms showing the sequence of freshly activated areas on a single image sphere.

Introduction

The advantage of physically corrected orthogonal leads is the biophysically based approach and a rletively small volume of input data, allowing meaningful mathematical treatment. An important prerequisite for optimal diagnostic evaluation is their proper mathematical treatment and adequate graphic representation. A simple mathematical model of the cardiac generator may be obtained by assuming that the generator is an uniform double layer shaped as a spherical segment on the spherical surface approximating the ventricular walls,called image sphere. The vector of total dipole moment of the double layer is perpendicular to the plane of its border and oriented outwards,i.e.it coincides with the radius vector of the centre of the double layer in the coordinate system with origin at the centre of the sphere. It should be noted that according to the well known theorem of electrodynamics, uniform double layers of any shape,having identical borders and intensity will have the same magnitudes of dipole moments.Then the change of the dipole moment magnitude of the cardiac generator will be determined solely by the radius of the border of the double layer of the spherical segment. In the model under consideration, the dipole moment is maximal if the radius is equal to that of the image sphere. The localization of any point on the image sphere within the boundaries of the spherical segment modelling the front of activation is the criterion that at the given instant of time the point is activated (1, 2, 3).

Material and methods

For graphical visualization of the maps of ventricular wall excitation, the image sphere was discretised into 264 points and unwrapped together with projected anatomical landmarks onto a rectangular planar surface in such a way,that the distances along horizontal directions are proportional to latitudes and along vertical direction to polar distances of the spherical coordinate system. The left and right borders of the rectangular map coincide with the meridian of the sphere, viewing the right axillary region of the subject.Ventricular activation is represented by time series of maps of activated points on the image surface.
More compact, but also easily percepted visualization of the same data may be obtained in the form of summary maps of cardiac excitation, or chronotopocardiograms. They present the distribution of two basic electrophysiologic parameters, those of activation delay (time from onset of ventricular depolarization up to the instant when the respective point is activated), and of activation duration on the aforementioned image sphere.
A computer program was developed for visualization of ECG data based on the above described method. The program computes and graphically presents instantaneous DECARTO maps of activation, as well as DECARTO chrono topocardiograms. The probability of being activated was computed for each of the 264 points on the spherical image surface at 10 ms time intervals of QRS for orthogonal ECGs recorded in a sample of 145 healthy subjects (81 men,64 women,aged 11 to 72 years) with the McFee lead system and in another sample of 123 subjects (69 men, 54 women, aged 9 to 72 years) with the Frank lead system.

Results

Fig.1 shows areas of activation with $p > 0{,}05$ probability and with maximum probability on instantaneous DECARTO topograms.
Fig.2 displays trajectories of maximum probabilities for the McFee and Frank lead systems, respectively.
The ordinary set of discrete elements (points) on the image surface may be treated as consisting of two fuzzy subsets at any instant of time, those of activated and those of non-activated elements. Attributing to each element of the reference spherical surface the probability of being activated at a given instant of time as its characteristic membership function,we obtain the reference fuzzy subset of activated elements at time t expressed in symbols as follows:

$$\underset{\sim}{A}_t \subseteq H;\ \forall a_t \in \underset{\sim}{A}_t:\ \mu_{\underset{\sim}{A}_t}(a_t) \in \langle 0,1 \rangle \qquad /1/$$

where $\underset{\sim}{A}$ is the fuzzy subset of activated elements (points) belonging to the ordinary set H of all elements on the image surface. μ denotes the set of membership characteristic functions of the fuzzy set $\underset{\sim}{A}$. The index t stands for time.
The cardiac electric activity of a subject may then be expressed as

time series of fuzzy subsets, each representing the activated elements of the spherical image surface at predetermined instants of time with membership functions obtained from the reference fuzzy subset. After having computed in our reference sample the individual sums of membership functions for each 10th ms of QRS duration, we may define the following criterion of normality in terms of fuzzy mathematics:

$\underset{\sim}{A}_t \neq \emptyset \mid t \leqq 60$ ms; $\quad \sum \mu_{\underset{\sim}{A}_t} (a_t) \geq k$

t(ms)	10	20	30	40	50	60
k	0,05	2,61	25,81	46,91	10,68	1,92

Lower limits of the sums of membership functions were determined from the reference sample as arithmetic mean minus two standard deviations. Subjects having no zero membership function but not attaining the required minimum level of their sums may be regarded as borderline normals.

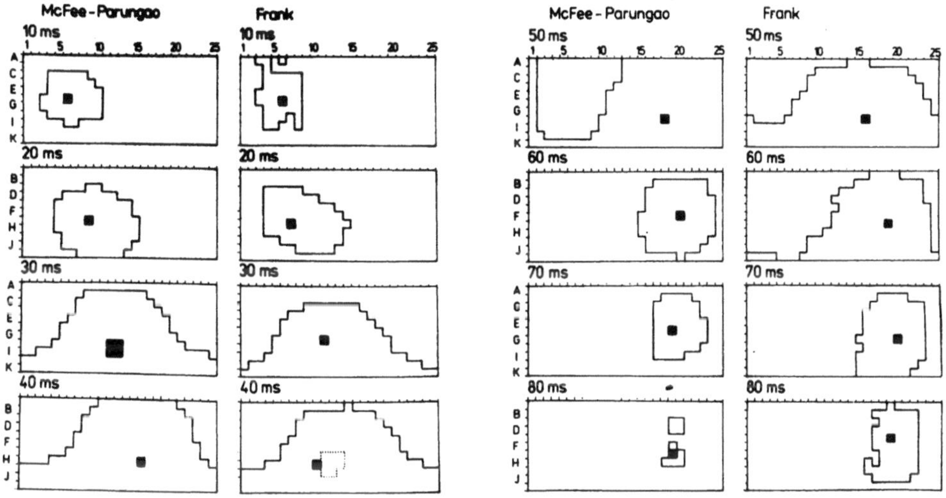

Fig.1. Areas of activated points on the spherical image surface with $p > 0{,}05$ probability (empty) and with maximum probability (black) during QRS (10th to 80th ms) obtained with the McFee (left) and Frank (right) lead systems in normal subjects. Each point on the sphere is represented by a square on the rectangular surface. Lateral borders: right midaxillary line, 1 - 12 anterior, 13 - 25 posterior hemisphere.

Discussion and conclusions

Medical diagnostic is decision making in fuzzy environment and so fuzzy sets help to handle our data in mathematical modelling (4,5), as well as in diagnostic utilization of the cardiac electric field.

This approach gives the possibility not only to show that the subject under consideration eventually does not have any element with zero membership function, differently stated, with zero probability of normality, but it expresses in a quantitative manner also the degree of its normality, e.g. as the sum of its membership functions.

The topography of elements with zero membership function on the image surface is then an important feature of differential diagnostics.

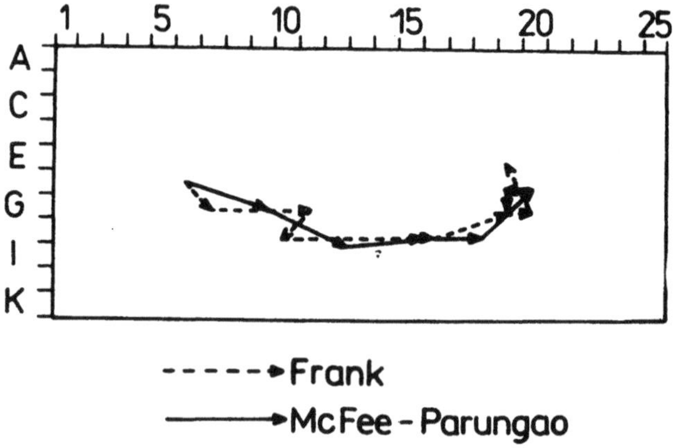

Fig.2.Trajectory of points with maximum probability of activation (10th to 80th ms during QRS). Broken line: Frank lead system, full line: McFee lead system. See also description of Fig.1.

The transformation of ECG data into patterns of activation on the image surface may undergo statistical treatment of any type and may be evaluated by algorithms of mathematical pattern recognition.
These approaches together with qualitative visual evaluation may provide for a more effective way of diagnostic utilization of orthogonal electrocardiographic information.

References

(1) Ruttkay-Nedecký,I.,L.I.Titomir and L.Bachárová,in: XII Int.Congress on Electrocardiology.Abstract Book.Minsk, Vysheishaia Skhola 1985.

(2) Titomir,L.I.:Obraznoie predstavlenie vektorkardiograficheskich dannych.Preprint.Akademia NaukSSSR,Moskva 1985, p.56.

(3) Titomir,L.I. and I.Ruttkay-Nedecký: Int.J.Bio-Medical Computing 20, 275-282(1987).

(4) Ruttkay-Nedecký,I.,in:S.Reuse-Blom(ed.):Le Coeur et l´Esprit.Editions de l´Université de Bruxelles,Bruxelles 1977,p.877.

(5) Ruttkay-Nedecký,I.,in: Z.Antalóczy (ed.):Modern Electrocardiology, Akadémiai kiadó,Budapest 1978, p.567.

Computer Simulation of Cardiac Excitation in the Hypertrophic Heart

EIFRIG, Th. (1); SZATHMARY, V. (2)

Institute of Pathological Physiology, Karl Marx University, Leipzig, GDR, (1); and Institute of Normal and Pathological Physiology, Slovak Academy of Sciences, Bratislava, CSSR, (2)

Summary

Model calculations were performed to determine the ventricular activation sequence in the hypertrophic heart. The excitation spreading was simulated on a digital computer. The dimensions of both the ventricles were fitted to anatomically realistic values. Concentric cardiac hypertrophy was investigated as well as excentric hypertrophy of the heart.

Cardiac hypertrophy results in an increase of the magnitude of the maximal vector of the VCG only if the increase of cardiac mass is caused by an enlargement of the ventricles, that is in the case of excentric hypertrophy. Concentric hypertrophy produces characteristic alterations of the vector magnitude towards the end of the QRS complex.

Introduction

Cardiac hypertrophy is frequently indicated by an increase of the magnitude or of particular components of the maximal spatial vector of the VCG. Such a connection was proved experimentally in many cases, e.g. in the humans hypertrophic heart developed by dynamical physical training, the so-called athletes heart (1). During the normal growth period of animals the maximal dipole moment of the heart develops proportionally to the increasing cardiac mass (2), as it was found by comparison of adult animals of various species with very different cardiac masses (3), too. On the other hand the development of a considerable left ventricular hypertrophy is not necessarily connected with an increase of the maximal vector of the VCG (4). The aim of our model calculation is to elucidate the effects of different patterns of cardiac hypertrophy on the VCG.

Method

The ventricular activation sequence was determined by means of a digital computer. The calculations are based on an algorithm worked out at the Academy of Sciences in Bratislava and described earlier (5). The procedure consists of two steps: First the continuous geometrical model of the heart is discretized by inserting in a spatial point lattice. In that way a discrete spatial pattern of the heart arises the points of which are either excitable if they are located inside the cardiac walls, or nonexcitable if they are located outside the heart. In the second step the cardiac activation is initiated at selected points and the activated region spreads step by step over the whole heart by means of the activation of neighbouring points. Following up this process the activation front can be determined at each time.

The geometrical model of the heart was constructed approximating its shape by concentric ellipsoids (Fig.1). The dimensions of both the ventricles were fitted to anatomically realistic data from the adult human (5, 6). A distance of 1 mm between the points was chosen so that the number of points inside the heart is about 165000. The calculations were carried out on the computer EC1055 requiring a memory of 700 KBytes.

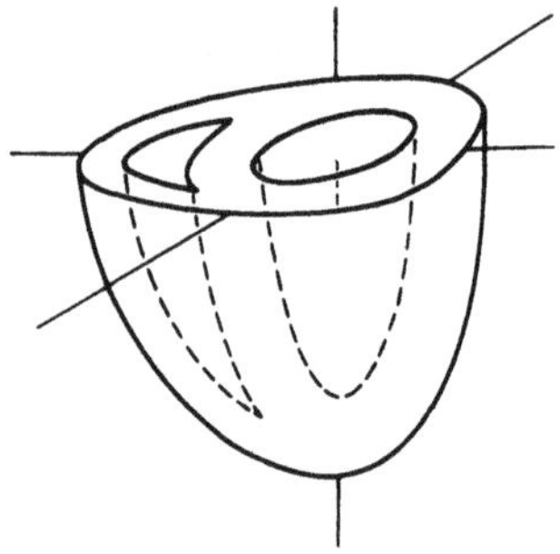

Fig. 1: Geometrical model of the heart

Results

Two different patterns of cardiac hypertrophy were investigated.

i) The model of a concentric hypertrophy is characterized by an increase of wall thickness without any increase of ventricular volume. In this case the ratio ventricular volume/volume of ventricular walls, V_v/V_w is shifted to lower values. We calculated the case of an increase of the thickness of both ventricular walls by the factor 1.2, hence it follows a ratio $V_v/V_w = 0.25$. Fig. 2 shows the carthesian components D_x, D_y, D_z, and the magnitude D of the resultant cardiac dipole moment during the whole excitation spreading period.

The duration of the excitation spreading, T_{QRS}, is prolonged by 15% in the hypertrophic heart compared to the normal heart. However, there is no essential deviation of the dipole components and accordingly of the dipole magnitude from the normal up to a time $t = 0.9\ T_{QRS}$. Especially the maximal vector is not changed significantly.

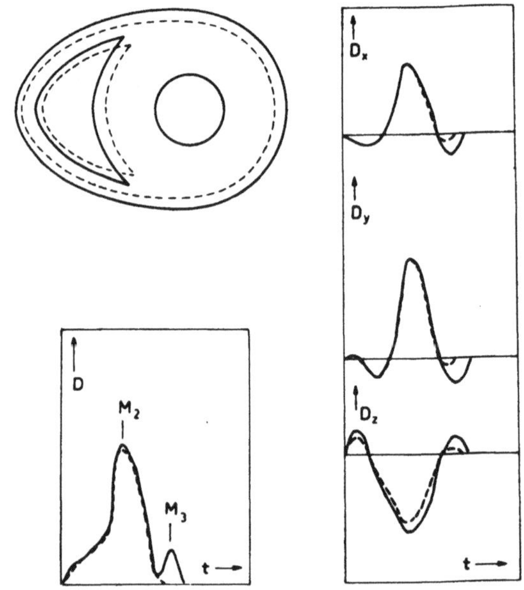

Fig. 2: Concentric cardiac hypertrophy. Horizontal cross section of the model heart, carthesian components D_x, D_y, D_z and vector magnitude D of the resultant dipole moment during the QRS complex. Broken lines give the results for normal geometry.

A characteristic sign of a concentric hypertrophy is an additional peak in the vector magnitude towards the end of the QRS complex (denoted by M_3 in Fig. 2), caused by increased S waves of all three dipole components.

ii) We investigated the case of an excentric cardiac hypertrophy that is an increase of ventricular wall thickness connected with an increase of ventricular volume. In that case the ratio $V_v/V_w = 0.3$ remains normal. We calculated an isometrical enlargement of the whole heart by the factor 1.2 (Fig. 3).

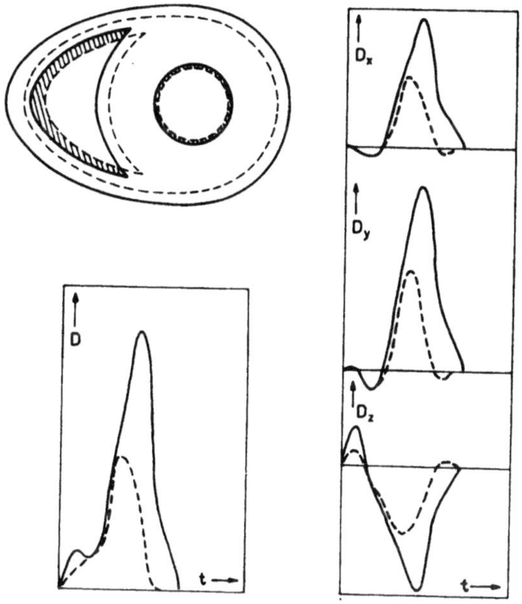

Fig. 3: Excentric cardiac hypertrophy. Horizontal cross section of the model heart, carthesian components D_x, D_y, D_z, and vector magnitude D of the resultant dipole moment during the QRS complex. Broken lines give the results for normal geometry.

Also in this case the duration of the excitation spreading is prolonged. However, unlike the above described case the dipole moment is greater than in the normal heart already from the beginning of the activation. The maximal values of all three dipole components and accordingly the maximal vector magnitude increase to the twice of the normal value.

Discussion

In both calculated examples of hypertrophy an increase of the cardiac mass to an amount of 135-150% occurs. However, the alteration of the VCG doesn't simply reflect the change in cardiac mass but it depends strongly on the cardiac mass distribution. Only an enlargement of the whole heart causes an increase of the maximale dipole moment. Therefore, cardiac hypertrophy without significant increase of ventricular volume should not cause any increase of the maximal vector despite of an increase of cardiac mass. This conclusion agrees with the results of Hodgkin et al. (4) for the concentric hypertrophic rat heart. Instead of an increase of the maximal vector they found an increase of the vector amplitude towards the end of the QRS complex which is in accordance with our model calculations. This peak is created at a time where the most parts of the heart are already activated and the activation front still spreads over the apex of the hypertrophic heart.

The here described possibility to attribute characteristic changes in the VCG to definite alterations of the cardiac geometry instead of changes of cardiac mass should be of interest for clinical application,too.

References

(1) Chignon, J.C., R. Distel, and B. Courtois: Proc. Sat. Symp. 25th Intern. Congr. Physiol. Sci. and 12th Coll. Vectorcard., Bruxelles, 1972.

(2) Joel, A., and Th. Eifrig: Gegenbaurs morph. Jahrb. 129, 419-424 (1983)

(3) Hodgkin, B.C., and P.R. Gastonguay: Ann. Biomed. Engineer. 3, 308-314 (1975)

(4) Hodgkin, B.C., C.V. Nelson, and E.T. Angelakos: Am. J. Physiol. 241, H541-H546 (1981)

(5) Ruttkay-Nedecky, I., A. Drkosova, and V. Szathmary: Simulation of systems in biology and medicine, Proc. 3rd Intern. Symp., Dum techniky CSVTS Praha, 1982

(6) Hutchins, G.M., B.H. Bulkley, G.W. Moore, M.A. Piasio, and F.T. Lohr: Am. J. Cardiol. 41, 646-654 (1978).

A Study of the Diagnostic Informativity of BSPM Based on a Multipolar Cardiac Source Model

E.NYSSEN †, J.CORNELIS †, P.DE MUYNCK †, M.NYSSEN◊, P.BLOCK*
Vrije Universiteit Brussel VUB ; †Electronics dept.ETRO ; ◊ Medical Informatics dept. MINF; *Cardiovascular Research Unit HART - Pleinlaan 2 - B-1050 Brussels - Belgium

Summary

This paper is related to the study of the diagnostic informativity of features extracted from Body Surface Potential Maps (BSPM). One of the data reduction techniques is based on the orthogonal expansion of the spatial potential distribution in terms of spherical multipole moments. If this model is restricted to the three dipole moments, it is equivalent to a classical measurement method: Frank's vectorcardiogram (VCG) - based on measurements on 7 electrodes. The first part of the paper motivates the use of the multipolar source model and describes a comparative study - based on numerical simulation - of two multipole moment estimation techniques. The second part describes a comparative study of the diagnostic information content of Frank's VCG on one hand and BSPM's on the other hand. The two clinical groups involved in this study are normals and MI patients. The values of the dipole moments appear to carry a significant diagnostic information. A significant increase of the classification performance was noticed when quadrupolar diagnostic variables were added to the dipole variables confirming the superior diagnostic informativity of BSPM and validating the use of multipole moments as diagnostic variables. The software developed for these studies is running under UNIX®(4.3 BSD) and is available on request.

Introduction

One can show that there is no unique relation between the potentials measured at the outer surface of a conductor - like the human thorax - and the embedded (cardiac) current source. It is therefore necessary to design a model for the latter, characterised by parameters which can be determined uniquely from geometrically restricted potential measurements.

The general approach for modeling the sources is to consider them as a weighted superposition of some n base sources J_{Ii}:

$$J_I = \sum_{i=1}^{n} a_i J_{Ii}$$

The coefficients are used to characterise the source distribution. The heart vector is a special case of this model: n=3 and the sources are the unit current dipoles in -resp. the X,Y and Z-direction. Assuming that the potential in a point $\mathbf{r}$ generated by the i-th source is $\Phi(\mathbf{r},J_{Ii})$, we have - according to the superposition principle:

$$\Phi(\mathbf{r},J_I) = \sum_{i=1}^{n} a_i \Phi(\mathbf{r},J_{Ii}) + \varepsilon(\mathbf{r})$$

The term $\varepsilon(\mathbf{r})$ represents an error signal which can not be explained by the source model. In a procedure where the potentials are measured at a set of m independent measurement sites $\mathbf{r}_j$ on the surface of a conductor, the coefficients a_i can be estimated, when $m >= n$, when $\Phi(\mathbf{r}_j,J_{Ii})$ are known and when the potential distributions $\Phi(\mathbf{r},J_{Ii})$ are linearly independent. The estimation procedure may be a linear regression, where the a_i are least

®Registered trademark of AT&T in the USA and other countries

square estimations of the model parameters, i.e. their value minimises:

$$\sum_{j=1}^{m} \varepsilon^2(\mathbf{r}_j)$$

An important source model is the multipolar model. Let $\Phi_\infty(\mathbf{r})$ be the potential that would be generated by a current source distribution in a homogeneous medium of infinite extent. Since it can be shown that

$$\left[\frac{1}{r}\right]^{n+1} P_n^m(\cos\theta)\cos m\phi \quad \text{and} \quad \left[\frac{1}{r}\right]^{n+1} P_n^m(\cos\theta)\sin m\phi$$

- where P_n^m is the n-th degree, m-th order Legendre function - have all characteristics of potential functions (analyticity and harmonicity) in a source-free region, they may be considered as independent potentials, generated by some reference sources in the origin and $\Phi_\infty(\mathbf{r})$ may be written as a series:

$$\frac{1}{4\pi\sigma r}\sum_{n=0}^{\infty}\sum_{m=0}^{n}\left[\frac{1}{r}\right]^{n} P_n^m(\cos\theta)\,(a_{nm}\cos m\phi + b_{nm}\sin m\phi)$$

The coefficients a_{nm} and b_{nm} are the so-called spherical multipole moments of the sources. The multipolar source model has several advantages:

- The moments are uniquely determined by the source distribution once a system of rectangular coordinates has been chosen. For other source models it is often necessary to specify a number of constant parameters to characterise the basic sources - like for example, the position and occasionally the orientation of the dipoles in the multiple dipole model; in the spherical multipolar model, only the reference system needs to be specified.
- The model provides us with a complete set of base functions; the potentials generated outside a bounded region containing the current sources can be approximated to an arbitrary precision by a linear combination of multipolar base functions.
- The first three (spherical) multipole moments correspond to the heart dipole moments, given by Frank's VCG; in other words: the higher degree multipole moments represent that part of the signal information which can not be explained by the model of Frank.
- One can show that - unlike the cartesian multipolar moments - the spherical multipolar moments are uniquely related to the potentials generated in (a subregion of) an infinite medium or at the outer boundary of an insulated homogeneous conductor, containing the sources.
- If the geometry of the external surface S of a finite, insulated and homogeneous conductor is known and also the potential distribution on S, the spherical multipole moments of the enclosed sources can be computed from this information. Moreover the spherical multipole moments characterise the infinite medium potential outside the region containing all sources. Since there is no unique relation between the surface potentials and the current source distribution, this property of the multipolar model means that the spherical multipoles characterise the maximal information that can be observed at the surface of a conductor.

The integral equations published by Geselowitz in 1960 (Geselowitz) allow the computation of the unknown model parameters - the multipole moments - from the knowledge of any physically realisable source distribution as well as from the knowledge of the potential distribution on the outer surface of an insulated, bounded homogeneous conductor enclosing the sources and from the geometry of the conductor. To compute the multipole moments on the basis of a surface potential distribution, an alternative method to the integration technique of Geselowitz can be considered: a regression technique based on the superposition principle, described earlier. First, the potential distributions are computed for a set of (lowest degree) basis multipole sources, using a numerical procedure (Lynn and Timlake). The multipole moments of an unknown source, generating potentials on the same conductor, can then be determined by performing a linear regression analysis: the moments are the weight factors by which the computed basis potential distributions have to be multiplied to match the measured potentials.

Methods

We tried the two multipole moment estimation methods on a homogeneous cylinder model containing a dipolar current source. The regression approach appeared to be more accurate and robust than the integration approach for all three dipole moments.

For multipole moments, synthesised from the thoracic potential distribution, we designed and validated criteria for an automatic diagnosis, in order to make conclusions about their diagnostic information contents. The stastical study was based on diagnostic variables extracted from the dipolar and quadrupolar moments of the cardiac current distribution, estimated with the regression method described earlier, on the basis of the homogeneous torso model derived from Horacek's model (Horacek). The values of these variables were determined for the times 1 up to 8 during ventricular depolarisation, in a time scale having a unity corresponding to 1/8 of the duration of depolarisation and having an origin corresponding to the onset of depolarisation. The two clinical groups, involved in the study were the normal patients and the infarction patients. The data originated from the Dalhousie university (Halifax - Canada). For each statistical experiment, we applied the following procedure:

- Synthesis of a set of candidate-diagnostic variables
- Design of a classification function, based on the values of the candidate-diagnostic variables for some training group (discriminant analysis)
- Application of the discriminant function to the cases of an independent test group
- Test of the statistical hypothesis on the significance of classification of the test group

Results

The values of the dipole moments appeared to carry a significant (χ^2-test, $p<0.001$) diagnostic information. The classification results are shown in next table:

		normal	infarction
training group	normal	49	9
	infarction	2	31
test group	normal	32	6
	infarction	5	13

A significant increase (binomial test, $p<0.05$) of the classification performance was noticed when quadrupolar diagnostic variables were added to the dipolar variables: from the patients of the test group, classified incorrectly on the basis of the VCG, 9 were classified correctly on the basis of dipole + quadrupole components, while only 2 patients were classified correctly by the first classifier and incorrect by the second one. The classification results are shown in the next table.

		normal	infarction
training group	normal	52	6
	infarction	2	31
test group	normal	35	3
	infarction	1	17

Discussion and conclusions

The study of the multipole moment estimation methods demonstrates the relatively great power of the regression method: not only is a partial knowledge of the potential distribution sufficient but also, it is not necessary to know potentials on surface points where the normal vector has components, parallel to the Y-axis, to determine the Y-directed dipole components of the sources. In the integration technique, only the surface elements, having a normal vector which is not perpendicular to the Y-axis contribute to the determination of the Y-dipolar component.

Also from a practical standpoint, it is possible to formulate arguments in favour of the regression technique: Both methods can be used for the estimation of the multipole moments and both methods are based on some model for the conductor - like Horacek's torso model (Horacek). This model however is truncated at the level of the head, the arms and the lower part of the body. To obtain a complete knowledge of the parameters of the current source distribution, it is necessary to take into account all surface elements of the model when the integration method is used to determine the multipole moments - even in zones where these elements do not exist for a real torso. This problem can be avoided in the regression method. Note that in the latter method the knowledge of the potentials in a discrete set of points (e.g. electrode positions) is sufficient.

When potentials are measured at a large number of electrode positions the loss of a number of channels (due to hardware problems, bad skin-electrode contacts ...etc.) is a common event. Events of that kind have no implications for the application of the regression method when there enough redundancy in the measurements.

The comparison between the heart dipole moments estimated with the regression technique and the VCG of Frank did not reveal a significant difference in diagnostic information content. A remarkable fact however was the elimination from the test group of two patients during the discriminant analysis of the VCG data due to the absence of measurement data for some of the 7 leads used to synthesise Frank's leads. This confirms the practical advantages of the use of the regression method.

It has been demonstrated that the quadrupole moments of the cardiac potential distribution carry supplementary diagnostic information about the heart condition in comparison with Frank's VCG. This confirms the superior diagnostic informativity of BSPM's and is in agreement with earlier studies which have demonstrated that Frank's VCG does not contain the total ECG information (Taccardi).

References

(1) D.B.Geselowitz, "Multipole representation for an equivalent cardiac generator," *Proc. IRE.* 48, 75-79, (1960)

(2) M.S.Lynn and W.P.Timlake, "The use of multiple deflations in the numerical solution of singular systems of equations with applications to potential theory," Publication 37.017, IBM Data Processing division, Houston, january 4 (1967)

(3) M.Horacek, "Numerical model of an inhomogeneous human torso," *Adv. Card.* 10, 51-57, Karger, Basel (1974)

(3) B.Taccardi, "Distribution of heart potentials on the thoracic surface of normal human subjects," *Circ.Res.* 12, 341 (1963)

The usefulness of multipoles in differentiation of human cardiac electric fields

MACO, M., KNEPPO, P., KRIČFALUŠI, M.

Department of Clinical Pathophysiology, School of Medicine, Comenius University, Bratislava, Czechoslovakia

Summary

Human cardiac electric field (HCEF) is represented by 24 multipole components (MC), dipole, quadripole, octapole and hexadecapole. Etalons of each MC were calculated during QRS complex and T-wave for three different groups of persons. Standard statistics was used to differentiate HCEF by etalons of MC.

Introduction

It is useful to transform surface potentials induced by cardiac currents into a direct description of human heart electric properties or into an equivalent cardiac generator. Our effort was devoted to the utilization of multipole equivalent electric generator for cardiac electric activity description. Components of multipole expansion (dipole, quadripole, octapole, hexadecapole) can be determined from ECG-surface potential distribution and human torso geometry by means of surface integration (SI) over the human torso using formulas derived previously (Geselowitz, 1960; Maco et al, 1984).

Material and methods

Body surface potential mapping together with direct torso geometry measurement of each person was performed by an automated measuring and computing system EKKG-80 (Kneppo et al, 1979) from 152 points of the thoracic surface during two cardiac cycles with 4 ms sampling rate.
By this way we have studied three groups of healthy persons:

- M: group of 25 males (21 - 30 years old)
- W: group of 15 females (20 - 29 years old)
- S: group of 9 intensively trained sportsmen (21 - 26 years old)

By the method of SI 24 MC were calculated for each person. Then the etalons for each group as well as for each MC were calculated as arithmetical means for each time sample. Normal sample distribution for each time instance, MC, and studied group, respectively, was examined by standard statistics. Using three statistic methods (t-statistic for two means, one sample test statistic for the mean, variance statistic test) we have compared by computer etalons of corresponding MC between M and W, M and S.

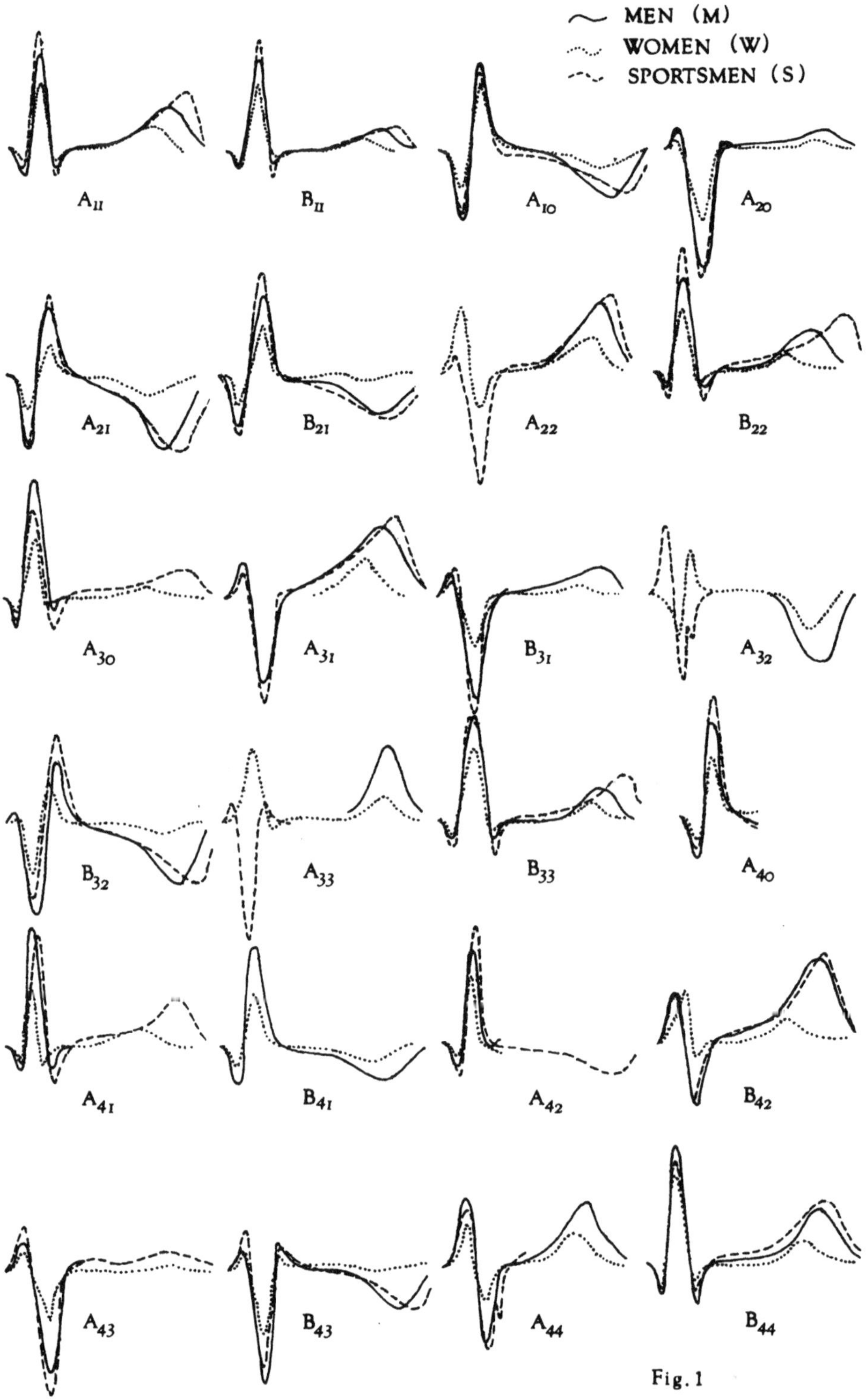
MEN (M)
WOMEN (W)
SPORTSMEN (S)
A_{11}
B_{11}
A_{10}
A_{20}
A_{21}
B_{21}
A_{22}
B_{22}
A_{30}
A_{31}
B_{31}
A_{32}
B_{32}
A_{33}
B_{33}
A_{40}
A_{41}
B_{41}
A_{42}
B_{42}
A_{43}
B_{43}
A_{44}
B_{44}

Fig. 1

Results

The samples of all MC have normal distribution during QRS in 94,2 % of time instances and during T-wave in 98,0 % of time instances. Graphical results, time courses of MC etalons, are in fig. 1. Etalons were not calculated when the average dispersion of samples during QRS or T-wave was more than 60 %. It concerns the following etalons of MCs: for the M group A_{22}, A_{32}, A_{33} during QRS complex and A_{30}, A_{40}, A_{41}, A_{42}, A_{43} during T-wave; for the W group A_{31} during QRS and A_{40}, A_{42} during T-wave and for the S group B_{41} during QRS and A_{20}, B_{31}, A_{32}, A_{33}, A_{40}, B_{41}, A_{44} during T-wave. By means of the cited statistics and calculated MCs it is possible to differentiate HCEF of healthy men and women at high level of reliability. All three used statistic tests equally differentiated M and W group by etalons of dipole components (DC) in 34 % of time instances (TI) during QRS and in 40 % during T-wave, by etalons of quadripolar components (QC) in 49 % during QRS and in 100 % during T-wave, by etalons of octapolar components (OC) in 60 % during QRS and in 100 % during T-wave and by etalons of hexadecapolar components (HC) in 54 % during QRS and in 95 % during T-wave. By means of at least two simultaneously used statistic tests it is possible to differentiate HCEF of men and sportsmen with following success rates: by DC in 3 % TI of QRS and in 18 % of T-wave, by QC in 17 % TI of QRS and in 34 % TI of T-wave, by OC in 15 % TI of QRS and in 13 % TI of T-wave, by HC in 10 % of QRS and in 5 % TI of T-wave.

Conclusion

Supposing adequate number of measuring points and successful solution of the capping problem, the method of SI permits a sufficiently accurate MC evaluation. Higher multipolar terms (octapole, hexadecapole) are measurable and calculable and yield new information. For the chosen group of healthy persons with similar somatic characteristics it is possible to calculate the MC etalons characterizing their HCEF. The etalons might be useful as a source of information relevant especially for computer based ECG differential diagnostics.

References

(1) Geselowitz, D.B.: Proc. IRE, 48, 75-79 (1960)

(2) Maco, M., P. Kneppo, R. Hatala, J. Kužmová: In Electrocardiology ´83, 104-109 (1984), edts.: I. Ruttkay-Nedecký, P. MacFarlane, Excerpta Medica, Amsterdam - Oxford - Princeton

(3) Kneppo, P., V. Rosík, M. Tyšler: In Progress in Electrocardiology, Pitman Medical Press, Glasgow, 212-214 (1979)

A Computer Model of Cardiac Rhythm and Heart - Pacemaker Interface

MAREK MALIK, A. JOHN CAMM

Department of Computer Science, Charles University
Malostranske namesti 25, CS-118 00 Praha 1, Czechoslovakia

SUMMARY

A computer simulation model of cardiac rhythm disturbances and of the heart - pacemaker interaction has been created and implemented on different mini- and microcomputers. The model has a form of an open library of simulation segments. It enables different configurations of heart images to be created using special modelling structures of two kinds: model elements represent separate parts of cardiac tissues, model connectors link the element together and perform the modelled excitation radiation. This enables different parts of the heart to be modelled with different accuracy. The computer implementation of the model contains also a large library of pacemaker algorithms including both clinically realistic and experimental modes.

The model incorporates important electrophysiological properties of the cardiac structures, including appropriate cycle length dependence of the refractory periods and of the atrioventricular nodal conduction.

Computational experiments of the model produce an explicit time table of polarisation changes, a simulated one channel electrocardiographic record and, when a pacemaker is considered, a pacemaker marker channel.

The model has been employed in various experiments which validated its clinical relevance.

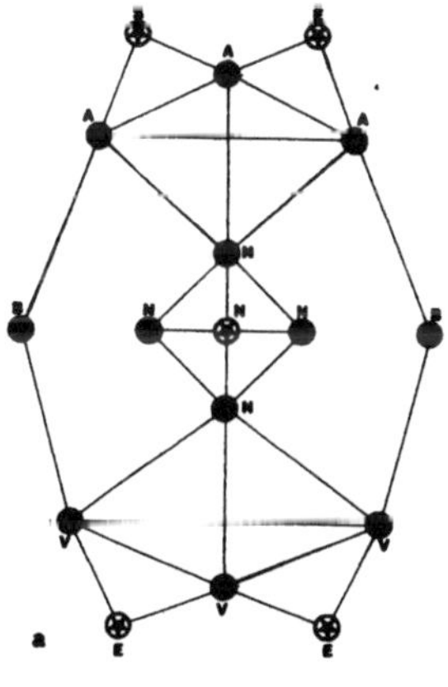

Fig. 1. Example of a model structure, S - sinus node, A - atria, V - ventricles, N - AV node, B - bypass tracts, E - ectopic centres. The elements marked by asterisks are able to generate the depolarisation wave.

INTRODUCTION

Computer modelling has previously been used to solve the Anterograde Electrocardiographical Problem, the objective of which is an artificial production of electrocardiograph records corresponding to given conditions of the heart. An important area of these studies is created by models addressing specifically the cardiac rhythm disturbances (1,2). This also includes testing of pacemaker algorithms (3,4) and prediction of their behaviour under complex circumstances (5).

METHOD - CARDIAC RHYTHM MODEL

Computer simulation studies of cardiac rhythms and heart-pacemaker interface require that representation of all relevant parts of the heart are incorporated into the model. Thus atrial and ventricular myocardium, sinus and atrioventricular (AV) nodes, pathological centres emitting ectopic impulses, pathological tracts bypassing the AV node, etc. must be inserted.

The model under description introduces either one or a small number of the so called 'elements' to represent each part of the heart. The number of elements modelling different cardiac tissues or their different parts may be different. Hence, variuos heart structures can be simulated with different accuracies according to the need of each modelling study. Some elements can generate excitation signals and radiate them to neighbouring structures, other elements only transmit the depolarisation wavefront. For all elements, the model distinguishes depolarised and resting states, and comprehends the changes between these states to be instantaneous.

The interactions between neighbouring elements are not direct. Other model elements called the 'connectors' link pairs of elements together and create uni- or bidirectional conduction pathways. A conduction delay, i.e. the time necessary to transmit an excitation pulse, is considered for each conector, but depolarised and resting states are not introduced. Using the concept of elements and connectors, different images of the artificial heart may be created. (Fig. 1).

Fig. 2. Example of a time table tracing the polarisation and excitation transmission events of model elements.

TIME :	4133 ms :	element	(A)	depolarized
TIME :	4136 ms :	element	(AVJ)	signal transmitted
TIME :	4143 ms :	element	(A)	signal transmitted
TIME :	4144 ms :	element	(AV1)	depolarized
TIME :	4144 ms :	element	(AVA)	depolarized
TIME :	4153 ms :	element	(AV6)	repolarized
TIME :	4170 ms :	element	(AVG)	repolarized
TIME :	4173 ms :	element	(AV1)	signal transmitted
TIME :	4174 ms :	element	(AV2)	depolarized
TIME :	4181 ms :	element	(AV7)	repolarized
TIME :	4183 ms :	element	(AVA)	signal transmitted
TIME :	4184 ms :	element	(AV8)	depolarized
TIME :	4203 ms :	element	(AV2)	signal transmitted
TIME :	4204 ms :	element	(AV3)	depolarized
TIME :	4209 ms :	element	(AV8)	repolarized
TIME :	4210 ms :	element	(AVH)	repolarized
TIME :	4222 ms :	element	(AV8)	signal transmitted
TIME :	4223 ms :	element	(AVC)	depolarized
TIME :	4232 ms :	element	(AV3)	signal transmitted
TIME :	4233 ms :	element	(AV4)	depolarized
TIME :	4238 ms :	element	(AV9)	repolarized
TIME :	4250 ms :	element	(AVI)	repolarized
TIME :	4261 ms :	element	(AVC)	signal transmitted
TIME :	4261 ms :	element	(AV4)	signal transmitted
TIME :	4262 ms :	element	(AVD)	depolarized
TIME :	4262 ms :	element	(AV5)	depolarized
TIME :	4266 ms :	element	(AV0)	repolarized
TIME :	4289 ms :	element	(AVJ)	repolarized
TIME :	4290 ms :	element	(AV5)	signal transmitted
TIME :	4291 ms :	element	(AV6)	depolarized
TIME :	4300 ms :	element	(AVD)	signal transmitted
TIME :	4301 ms :	element	(AVE)	depolarized
TIME :	4319 ms :	element	(AV6)	signal transmitted
TIME :	4320 ms :	element	(AV7)	depolarized
TIME :	4328 ms :	element	(A)	repolarized
TIME :	4339 ms :	element	(AVE)	signal transmitted
TIME :	4340 ms :	element	(AVA)	repolarized
TIME :	4340 ms :	element	(AVF)	depolarized
TIME :	4348 ms :	element	(AV7)	signal transmitted
TIME :	4349 ms :	element	(AV8)	depolarized
TIME :	4354 ms :	element	(V)	repolarized

Some rhythm studies, especially those dealing with supraventricular tachycardias, require the cycle length dependences of repolarisation periods to be considered. Similarly, the influence of cycle length on AV nodal conduction delay must be introduced. The way in which ventricular recovery depends on the heart rate has been the subject of many studies (6,7) and different mathematical formulae have been suggested to express this dependence (8,9). However, all formulae only approximate the results of clinical and laboratory experiments. For these reasons, the duration of repolarisation of each element is determined by a numerical table, which represents a piecewise linear curve describing the relationship between refractoriness and cycle length. The average cycle length of several recent cycles is computed for each element and used to correct its repolarisation. Characteristic prolongation of the AV nodal recovery and shortening of myocardial recovery with increasing heart rate can be reproduced in this way. AV nodal conduction dely is treated similarly although it depends on only the last cycle.

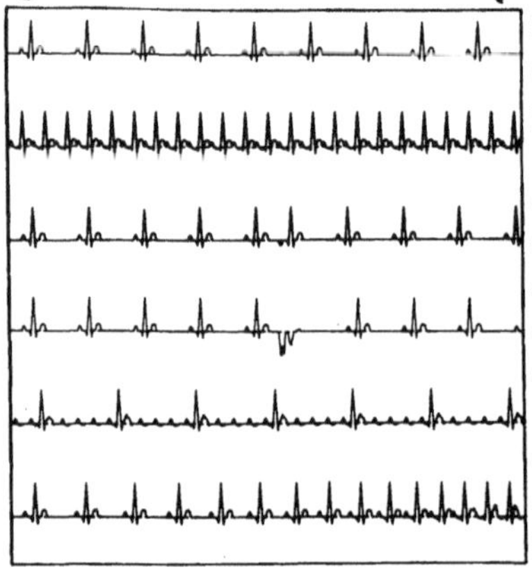

Fig. 3. Simulated physiological rhythm (top) and different rhythm disorders modelled by simple changing the parameters of elements creating the artificial cardiac structure.

Pacemaker algorithm may be connected to the cardiac conduction model. Atrial and ventricular sensing and pacing areas are defined as sets of elements. The depolarisation of a sensing area is recognised by the device, while the pacing stimuli are sent to all elements of the corresponding pacing area. The current version of the model includes a library of pacemaker algorithms which contains both clinically realistic and experimental modes. Using special predefined means, additional pacing modes can also be described and modelled.

Computational results are offered in several different forms. A trace of polarisation changes and signal transmission events of model elements, and of pacemaker actions is generated in the form of an exact

Fig. 4. Models of different patters in AV nodal rhythm. The retrograde (negative) P waves precede (top), fuse with (middle) and follow (bottom) the ventricular QRS complexes.

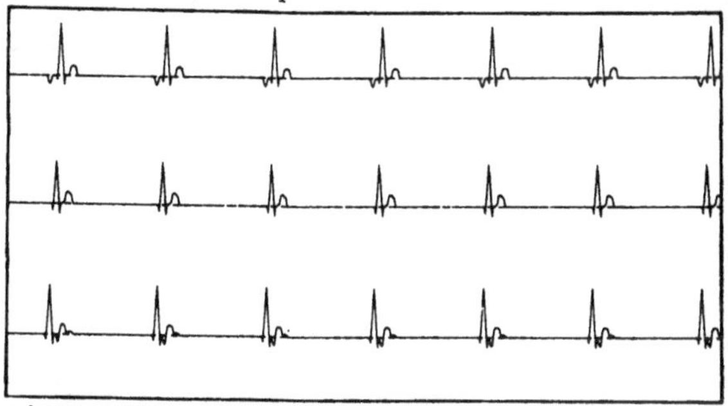

time table (Fig. 2.). An easily interpretable display of results is produced in the form of simulated single lead ECG record. The simplified structure of the modelled heart does not allow the natural ECG generation process to be simulated. Therefore, the model uses several predefined patterns of P-Ta and QRS-T complexes. The output patern depends on the connector which transmits the excitation to the central atrial or ventricular element. This mirrors the reality that the shape of P waves and QRS complexes is mainly determined by the way in which the excitation wavefront radiates through the myocardium. Pacing artefacts are also modelled. Models with pacemaker algorithms may also produce a marker channel, which is common with recent pacemakers. The exact form of the simulated marker channel is variable and depends on the model's input data. The time table tracing the excitation waves may be used for computer generation of the ladder diagrams explaining the AV conduction disorders in a medically acceptable form.

Fig. 5. Modelled AV reentry tachycardia : top - preexcited rhythm; middle strip - atrial premature beat initiates an orthodromic tachycardia; bottom - ventricular premature beat initiates an antidromic tachycardia.

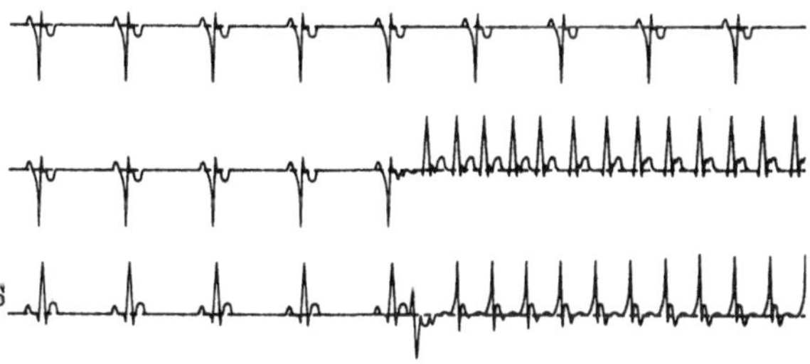

MODEL IMPLEMENTATION AND RESULTS

The model is based on disrete event simulation (10,11). The most complete version is written in FORTRAN 77 and its source text has approximately 11000 lines. Currently, a new version of the model is under development for the IBM PC AT computer and a distributable version written in Turbo Pascal should be available in the near future.

The model has been employed in various experimental studies. By simple changing the parameters of the heart model, basic rhythm disturbances may be reproduced (Fig. 3. and 4.). Figure 5. presents a model of different patterns of AV reentrant tachycardia. Figure 6. shows the results of a study examining the capability of the dual chamber pacemakers with short AV delay to prevent an AV reentrant tachycardia intiated by an atrial premature beat. Figures 7. and 8. models intra AV nodal oscilations which terminate the AV reentry tachycardia or change its rhythm.

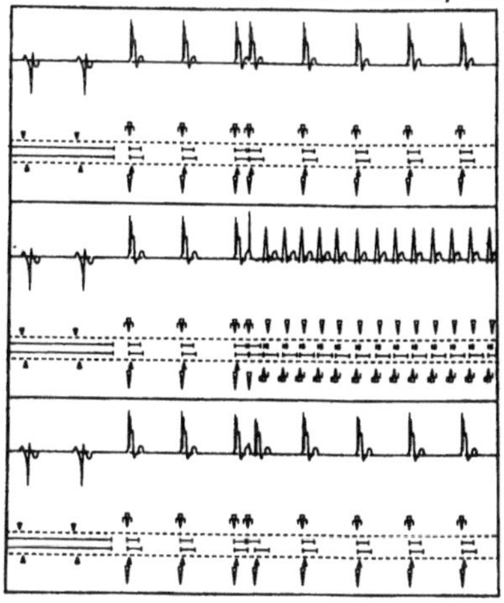

Fig. 6. Computer experiments examining the capability of the dual chamber pacemakers with short AV delay to prevent an AV reentrant tachycardia initiated by an atrial premature beat: a constant short AV delay pacing prevents the tachycardia when the refractory period of ventricles is short (top), but fails when it is prolonged (middle). In this case, the Wenckebach-prolonged AV delay mode has to be used (bottom).

DISCUSSION

The present model seems to operate satisfactorily and its simulation results are realistic. At the same time, the simplified heart structure with reduced properties does not allow many important pathophysiological features to be comprehended. For instance, atrial flutter and fibrillation and their interrelationship with other pathologies are out of modelling possibilities of the current version.

In spite of the important simplifications, the experiments perfomed with the model show that its potential application and investigation-support possibilities are extensive. Computer modelling of heart-pacemaker interactions may also enable individual characteristics of particular patients to be used as input data to problem oriented simulation studies (5). Obviously, more experience is necessary before fully accepting the results from models oriented to individual patients.

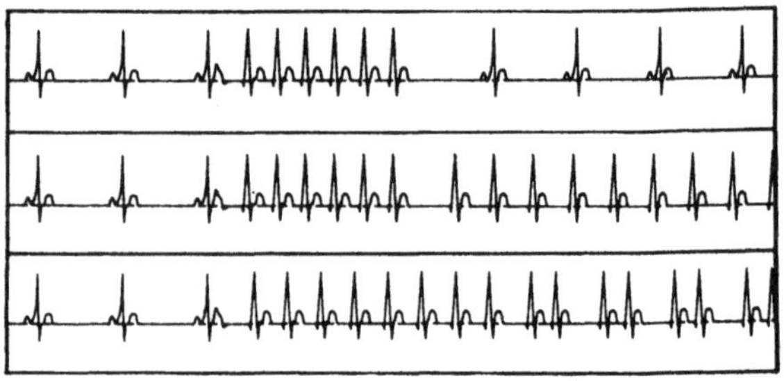

Fig. 7. Intra AV nodal oscillations terminate the AV reentry tachycardia (top), switch it to a slower cycle (middle) or produce a rhythm alternation (bottom).

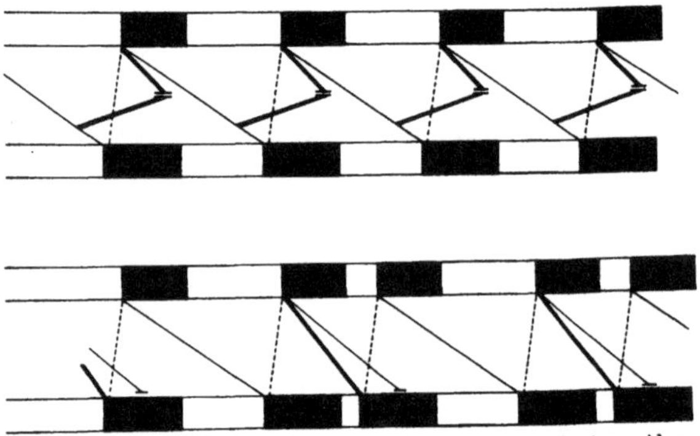

Fig. 8. Modelled ladder diagrams explaining the tachycardia rhythm changes shown in Fig. 7. A fast and a slow intra nodal path are supposed. (top) - slower tachycardia cycle, (bottom) - rhythm alternation.

REFERENCES

(1) Hagen CT, Dassen WRM, Bump TE, et al: In: Ripley KL (ed.): Computers in Cardiology, IEEE, Silver Springs, 1983, pp. 217
(2) Malik M, Cochrane T, Davies DW, Camm AJ: Med. Biol. Eng. Comput. in press (1987)
(3) Dassen WRM, van der Steld A, van Braam W, et al: PACE 8, 574 (1985)
(4) Malik M, Davies DW, Camm AJ: PACE, in press (1987)
(5) Malik M, Davies DW, Camm AJ: CPEP 4, 137 (1986)
(6) Rickards AF, Norman J: Br. Heart J. 45, 56 (1981)
(7) Ahnve S, Vallin H: Circulation 65, 435 (1982)
(8) Kawataki M, Kashima T, Toda H: J. Electrocardiol. 17, 371 (1984)
(9) Dorveaux L, Heddle W, Jones M, et al: PACE 8, 646 (1985)
(10) Zeigler BP: Theory of Modelling and Simulation, Wiley, New York 1976
(11) Franta WR: The Process View of Simulation, Elsevier, New York 1977

Higher Degree Multidipolar Components Sum on the VCG Spherical Surface

DRŠKA Z., VALOVÁ D., MÁLKOVÁ A.

Institute of Physiological Regulations, Czechoslovak Academy of Sciences, Bulovka, Pav. 11, Prague 8, Czechoslovakia

Sumary

The procedure to transform BSPD onto the surface with unit transfer coefficients, derived from Frank VCG leads (Drška Z.), was used for differentiation of main dipolar component from other dipolar components sum of equivalent multidipole.

Introduction: importance of higher degree components of equivalent source is assumed on both theoretical and clinical levels of interpretation of body surface potential distribution (BSPD). Methods for their extraction developed at this time are technically difficult and time consumpting because of necessity of lead points coordinates measuring.

Materials and methods: Solving the system of 3 (x,y,z) linear equations for every ECG, the matrix of ECGs VM(ij) measured from the chest surface in a regular grid was synthetized from orthonormal ECGs of Frank VCG system. Least squares fit method was used. Synthetized ECGs correspond to the measured signals with known (estimated) precision given by the SEE and by the value of correlation coefficient in regression.

The non-dimensional source is assumed and also that Frank VCG system is sufficiently urthonormal and representing dominant dipolar component of equivalent source. Then it is possible the result of subtraction of measured ECG (VMijt) and ECG synthetized from VCG orthonormal ECG to interpret as ECG of other dipolar components sum of equivalent multidipole (RES(ijt)):

$$VM(ijt) = VD(ijt) + RES(ijt)$$, where

$$VD(ijt) = A(ij).x(t) + B(ij).y(t) + C(ij).z(t) + D(ij)$$

Values of coefficients correspond to the x,y,z components (in the VCG system) of the transfer coefficient of individual lead of measured ECG matrix. By the normalization of coefficients this equation can be transformed to the equation:

$$VMk(ijt) = VDk(ijt) - RESk(ijt) = a(ij).x(t) + b(ij).y(t) + c(ij).z(t) + d(ij)$$, where if

$$K(ij) = 1/\sqrt{A(ij)^2 + B(ij)^2 + C(ij)^2}$$, then

$a(ij) = A(ij).K(ij)$; $b(ij) = B(ij).K(ij)$;

$c(ij) = C(ij).K(ij)$; $d(ij) = D(ij).K(ij)$ and

$VMk(ijt) = VM(ijt).K(ij)$; $VDK(ijt) = VD(ijt).K(ij)$ and

$RESk(ijt) = RES(ijt).K(ij)$, where

VMk(ijt) is the measured ECG, amplitude of which was corrected by proper value of coefficient (K(ij); VDK(ijt) is the ECG of dominant dipolar component of equivalent source synthetized from VCG x,y,z ECGs for VCG spherical surface and RESk is RES corrected by the unit value of transfer coefficient. K(ij) can be interpreted as a relative expression of value of transfer coefficient of lead (ij).

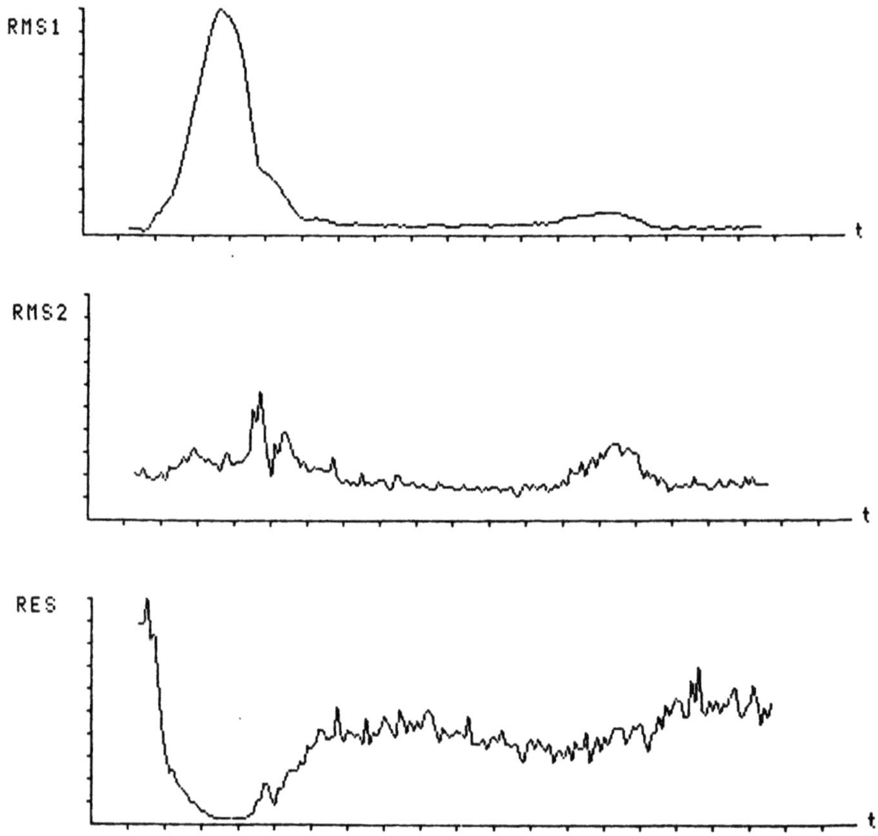

Fig. 1 - 3: Time sequence of RMS of dipolar component (Fig. 1), RMS of non-dipolar residue (Fig. 2) and ratio of non-dipolar residue within the Q-T interval (Fig. 3). Time step on the x axes: 20ms, the scale on the y axes: 90 uV, 20 uV and 2 uV respectively. The first peak on the RMS2 curve appeared in the 60th ms (11 uV), the second peak in the 74th ms (8 uV) from the onset of QRS.

The potential distribution of "non-dipolar residuum" on the unit transfer coefficient surface RESk(ijt) is obtained as a result of subtraction of BSPD corrected on the unit transfer coefficient surface and that created by the dominant dipolar component on the same surface.
This "non-dipolar residuum" both instantaneous (RES(t), RESk(t) and for QRS interval RES(QRS), RESk(QRS) was expressed as root mean square of potential (RMS(t), RMS(QRS) and correlation coefficient in regression

$R(t) = \sqrt{\text{Variance VD(ijt) / Variance VM(ijt)}}$ and

$R(QRS) = \sqrt{\text{Variance VD(ijt) / Variance VM(ijt)}}$

Results: The mean relative value of this "non-dipolar residuum" within the QRS interval in healthy subjects was found in level of 5% of whole signal. This expressed as RMS represents 5-10 uV. These values are comparable with results of multipole expansion, single value decomposition or conception of single moving dipole (Harumi et al).
Discussion: The amplitudes of ECGs VDk(ij) correspond to the normalized value of transfer coefficient and their orientation in space is the same as direction of original ECGs from the chest surface. This fact allows to visualize these normalized potential distributions on the surface having the same dimensions and angular distribution as original surface of visualisation of BSPD created by unrolled measured-off part of the chest surface.
The procedure described allows to unify (in the VCG system of axes) extracardiac factors influence on the BSPD properties. Procedure described does not require technically difficult and time consumpting lead points coordinates measurement, that could be, moreover, the source of significant errors in resulting values.

References:
(1) Drška, Z.: In: Abstracts of 13th Internat. Congress on Electrocardiology, Washington, 90 (1986)
(2) Harumi, K., H. Tsunakawa, S. Kanesaka, G. Nishiyama: In: Electrocardiographic Body Surface Mapping. Ed.: R. Th. van Dam, A. van Oosterom, Martinus Nijhof Publishers, Dordrecht et al, 283-288 (1986)

Modelling and simulation of the ventricular excitation and repolarization in relation to the heart mechanics

BENDEL,U.

Institute of Physiology, Berlin, GDR

Summary
On the base of a tube like model of the heart the electrical activity can be modeled and simulated by means of a computer program, so that the accompanying mechanical activity can be calculated. Thereby the connection of the two important activities of the heart - the electrical and the mechanical - becomes possible. The electrical activity can be grafically represented by means of the computer simulation program.

1. Introduction

The base of the complete activity of the heart for the function of the cardio-vascular system is the electrical activity of the heart (Fig. 1 shows the causal course). That is why big attention is paid to the electrical activity which consists of the excitation and the repolarization. The pronounced function of the heart as an organ is to realize the mechanical function of a pump. Therefore it is necessary not only to look at the single phenomena as a model approach but to view the complete relation, that means the connection between the electrics and the mechanics.

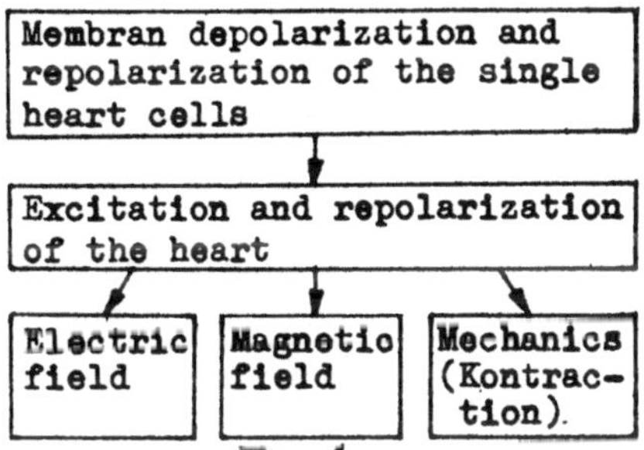

Fig. 1

2. Mathematical description of the heart chamber as a tube

Starting point for a simple mathematical description is the model of a piece of muscle (muscle segment)/1/,/2/. This mathematical model makes the description of the dynamics of the movement of the heart chamber possible and considers within this the electrical phenomena - the excitation and repolarization. For such a muscle segment the differential equations for the movement can be declared for the forces on the sides K_1, K_2 and the movements of the

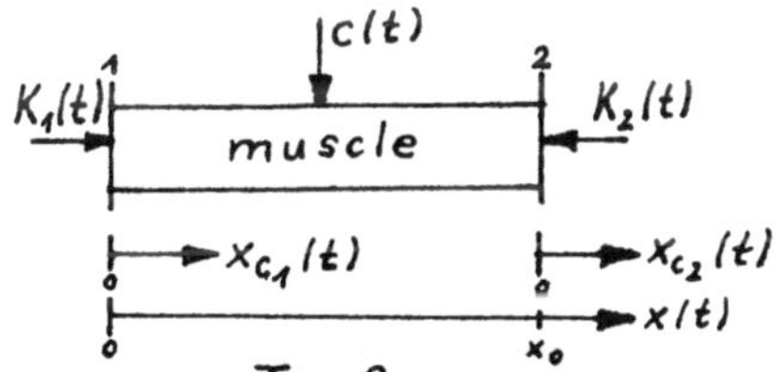

Fig. 2

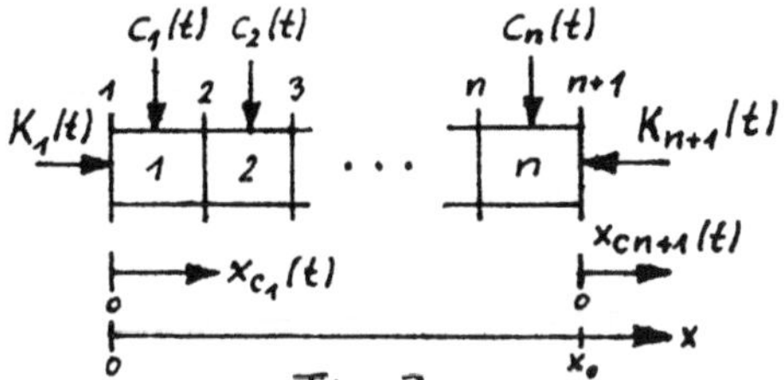

Fig. 3

sides x_{c1}, x_{c2} depending on the parameters of the muscle MP and the free intracellular Ca^{++}-ion concentration c(t) see Fig. 2

$$x_{c2} = f_1(x_{c1}, K_2, c, MP) \quad (1)$$
$$K_1 = f_2(x_{c1}, K_2, c, MP)$$

MP - parameters of the muscle

c - calcium quantity for the contraction, which will released by the depolarisation of the membran .

Even for several such segments put together one behind the other, which yield a long muscle, the differential equations for the movement can be declared (Fig. 3)

$$x_{cn+1} = f_3(x_{c1}, K_{n+1}, c_1, \ldots, c_n, MP_1, \ldots, MP_n) \quad (2)$$
$$K_1 = f_4(x_{c1}, K_{n+1}, c_1, \ldots, c_n, MP_1, \ldots, MP_n).$$

Putting such a muscle together to a ring form and considering instead of the ways and the forces the volumina (bloodflows i_1, i_2) and the pressures p_1, p_2 in connection with the flow resistances a simple model of the heart chamber hence follows (Fig. 4) /3/

$$i_2 = f_5(i_1, p_2, c_1, \ldots, c_n, MP_1, \ldots, MP_n) \quad (3)$$
$$p_1 = f_6(i_1, p_2, c_1, \ldots, c_n, MP_1, \ldots, MP_n).$$

It is possible to build up such a ring out of several layers. Furtheron several such rings can be put together to a complex heart chamber. A tube like heart chamber can therefore be constructed by an amount of rings (ri), layers (sc) and segments (se, sgm). Each segment possesses an input signal

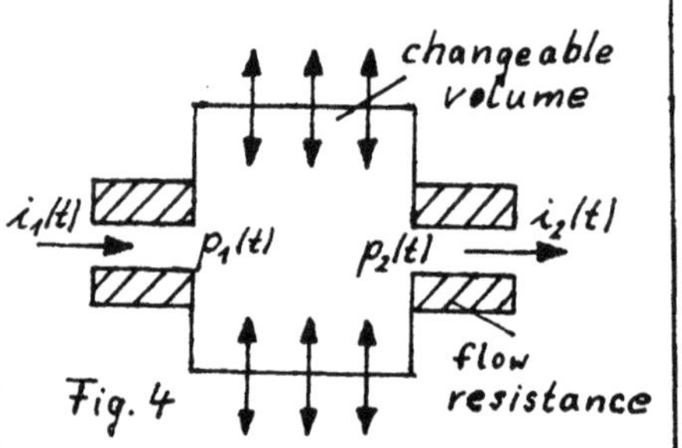

Fig. 4

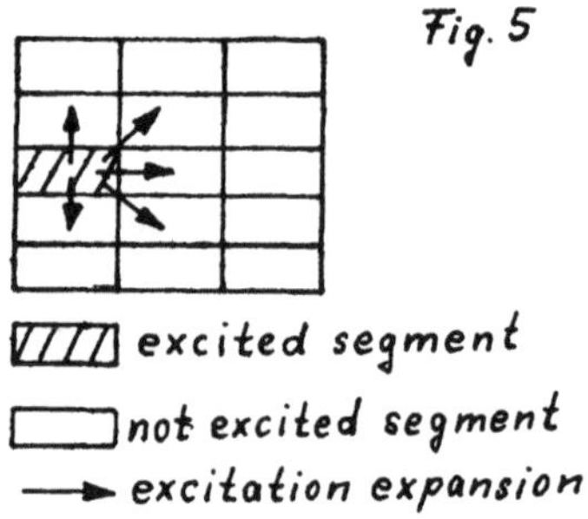

Fig. 5

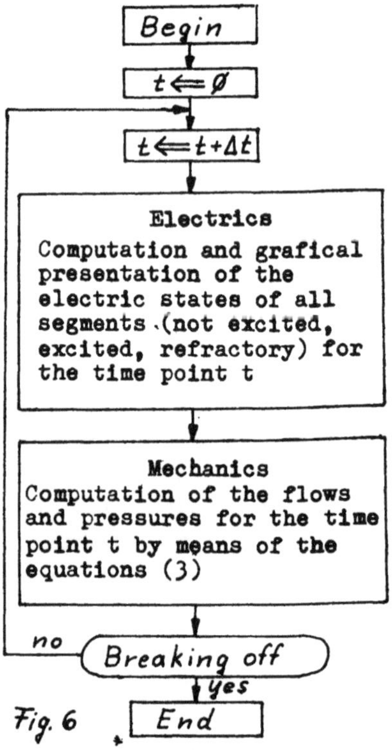

Fig. 6

c_i, which describes the free intracellular Ca^{++}-ion concentration and by this the electrical state of each single segment. By means of the submitted differential equ.(3) the flows i and pressures p of the heart chamber can be calculated depending on the $c_i(t)$ in their time course. The precondition however is the time pattern of the $c_i(t)$ (chronological excitation pattern of the single segments).

3. <u>Possible excitation of the segments of the tube like heart chamber</u>

The chronological pattern of the c_i that means the excitation (activation) and the repolarization has to be committed. The most simple case results in a neglection of the whole excitation conduction system and only to admit a depolarisation of neighbouring segments by an already excited segment (example Fig. 5 of a two dimensional expansion of the excitation). The characteristics of the single segments - electrical as well as mechanical - are enclosed in the muscle parameters MP_i, equ.(3). Hereby as well as by means of the assumed pattern of excitation c_i physiological and pathophysiological courses may be simulated. Therefore a starting point (center of excitation) must exist. In a second step, the conduction system can be simulated too, which brings the excitation on special pathways to the segments.

4. <u>Computer simulation of the excitation and repolarization</u>

By means of a relatively simple computer simulating program the explained conception can be realized (Fig. 6). The whole time course is divided into adjustable parts of time with the same length. In every part of time a complete

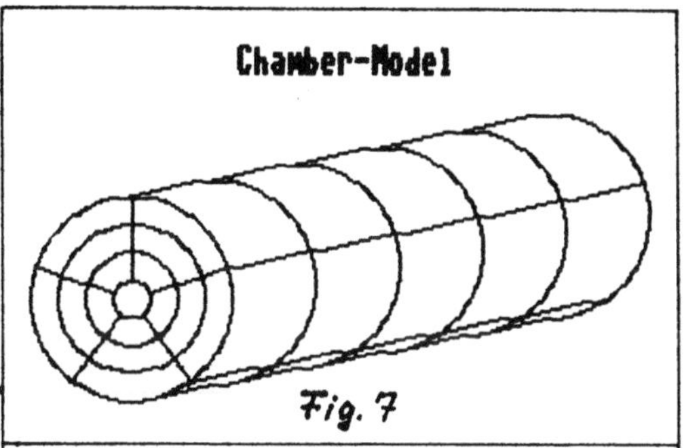

Fig. 7

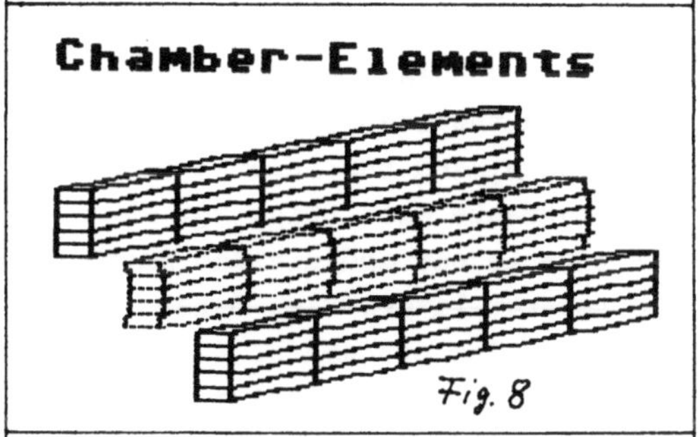

Fig. 8

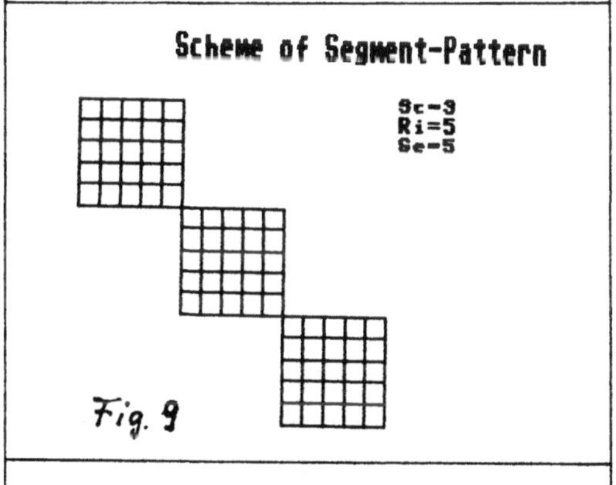

Fig. 9

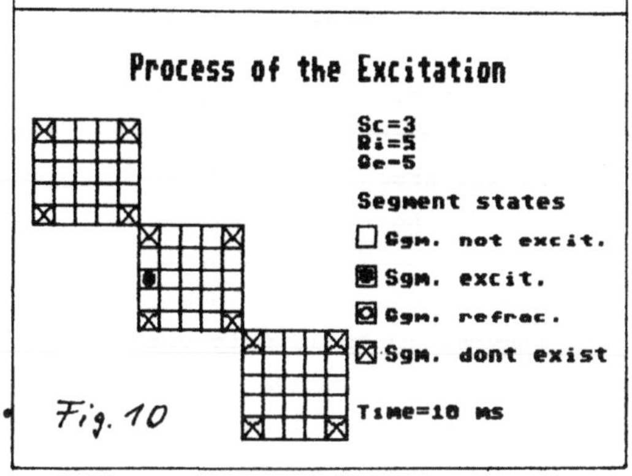

Fig. 10

computation of the electrical states of all segments is performed. Now it is possible to compute the solutions of the differential equ.(3) of the heart chamber for the blood flows and the pressure for every part of time by bigger efforts. Thereby the mechanical parameters can be computed step by step depending on the electrical state of the single segments of the heart chamber. However the base for this is the pattern of excitation and repolarization of the single segments of the heart chamber.

5. A simple example to illustrate the computer simulation

A tube is viewed, constructed of 5 rings and 3 layers, whereby the first and the last ring consist of 3 segments, and the inner 3 rings of 5 segments each (Fig. 7). When the tube is cut and divided into the seperat layers Fig. 8 is achieved. The pattern of the segments can be schematically presented as in Fig. 9. A choseable segment is the pace-maker segment (Fig. 10). Starting from this segment the excitation spreads till all segments are excited (Fig. 11, 12,13). Then the repolarization starts (Fig. 14,15,16) and afterwards the segments are excitable again (Fig. 17,18) and the process can start again. For this example the electrical parameters of all segments are assumed to be the same for ease. The time for the conductance of the excitation from one segment to the next is 20 ms. The excitation time is 250 ms and the repolarization time is 50 ms. The part of time for the computation is 10 ms. In the figures 10 to 18 only characteristical time points are choosen. The program is build up in such a

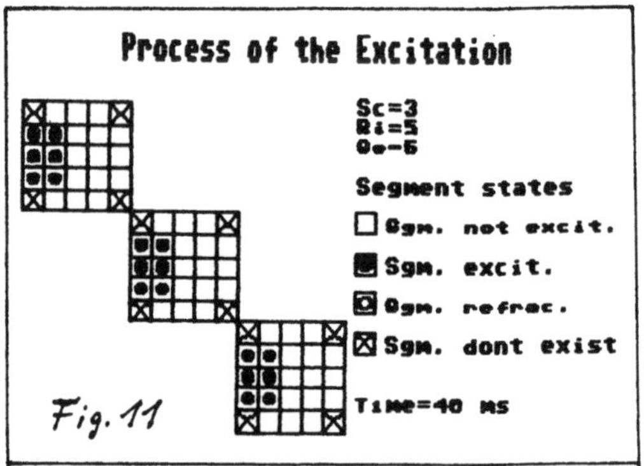

Fig. 11

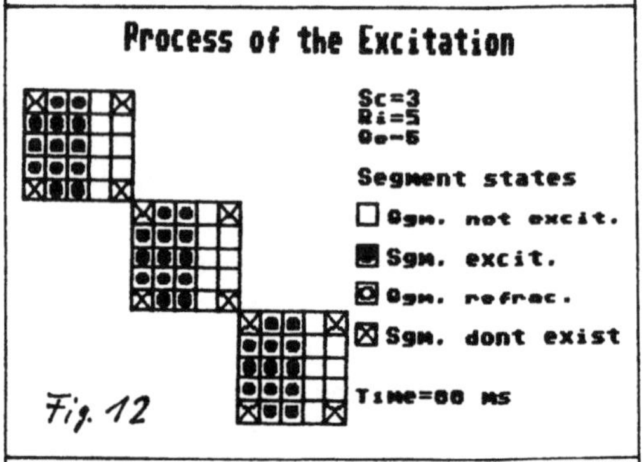

Fig. 12

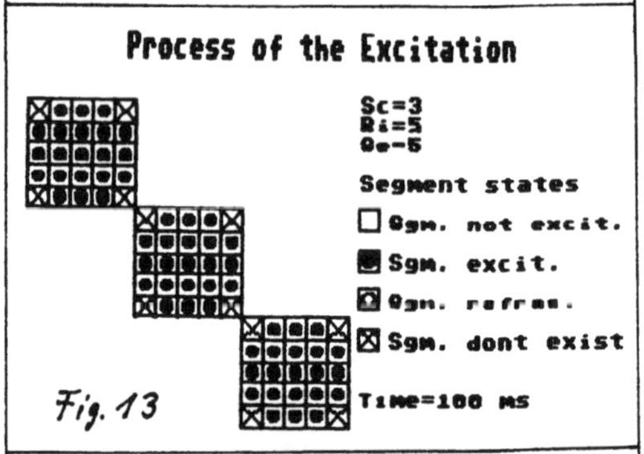

Fig. 13

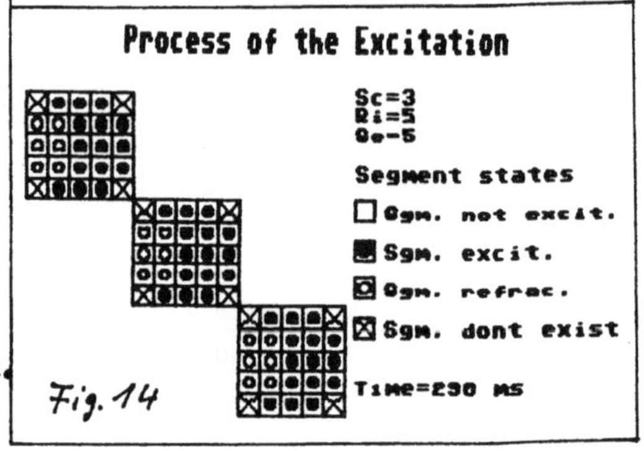

Fig. 14

way, that any values can be set for ri, se and sc. This is also considered in the graphical representation. The course of the program can be interrupted at any time points,in order to make a hardcopy on a graphic printer. With a colour graphic system the representation on the monitor can be composed of different colours.

The order of the differential equ. (3) increases with the amount of rings, layers and segments. Therefore a fast and an efficient computer is nessecary for the calculation of the solutions.

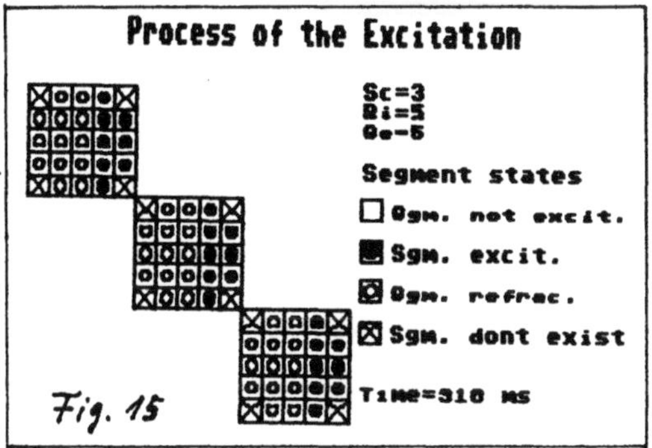

Fig. 15

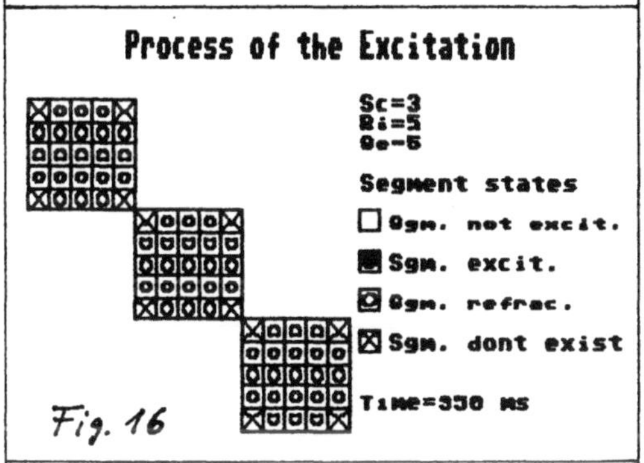

Fig. 16

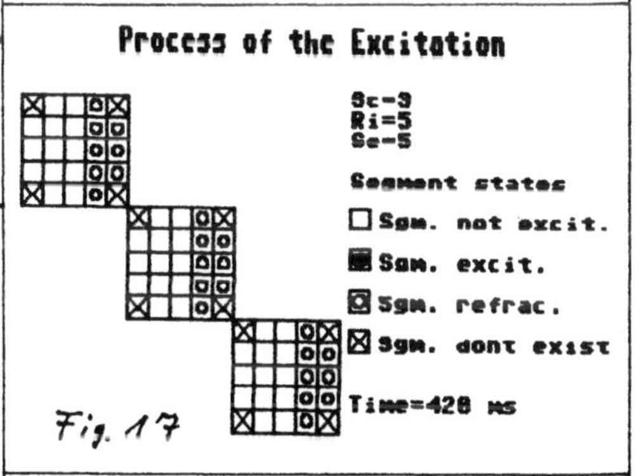

Fig. 17

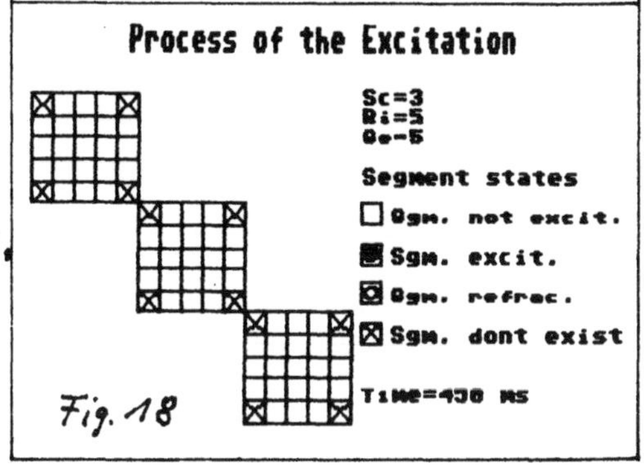

Fig. 18

6. <u>Extensions</u>

Two reasonable extensions are possible :

1.The consideration of the excitation conducting system.
The conduction of the excitation along the Hiss-bundles, the left and right bundle branches and the Purkinje fibers can be hereby simulated.

2.The composition of 4 tube like heart chambers to a complete heart. The simulation of the expansion of the excitation through the both atria, the passage through the AV-node and the excitation of the ventricles are hereby very realisticaly possible.

<u>References</u>

/1/Bendel,U.:Eine neue Systemtheorie der Muskelmechanik.studia biophysica 75(1979)H.1,S.31-40

/2/Bendel,U.:Habilitationsschrift 1987,Humboldt-Universitat Berlin

/3/Bendel,U.:Dynamisches Herzkammermodell auf der Grundlage des Modells eines gekrümmten Muskels. messen-steuern-regeln 24(1981)H.11, S.617-622

The auther thanks Mrs.Dr.K.P. Leiterer for her valuable help in translating this paper.

Dynamic Anisotropy of Atrioventricular Nodal Conduction? Computer Modelling Experiments

MAREK MALIK, DAVID WARD, A. JOHN CAMM

Department of Cardiological Sciences
St. George's Hospital Medical School
Cranmer Terrace, Tooting, London SW17 ORE, England

SUMMARY

The atrioventricular (AV) node is one of most complicated cardiac structures and the complexity of its function is very important from the clinical point of view. Several different physiological and pathophysiological hypotheses have been suggested in order to explain the AV nodal complex behaviour which is known from laboratory measurements and clinical observations. Most of these hypotheses explain the complexity of the nodal function as an integration result of complex behaviour of individual nodal cells and conduction fibres.

Special mathematical theory describing the function of conduction element networks and a complex computer model simulating the transmission of excitation within the cardiac tissues, have been employed to test the hypothesis that the complexity of the nodal structure itself may be responsible for its behaviour and that separated nodal cells and fibres may be considered to operate in a rather simple way.

Different network structures have been created using conduction elements which instantaneously change their state from resting to depolarized and vice versa. The computer simulation technique enables the functions of these networks to be evaluated. When considering a structure with different refractory periods of its elements and with anisotropic conduction, we were able to model different complicated phenomena of AV nodal function (1).

INTRODUCTION

AV nodal external behaviour, i.e. the function of the whole structure, such as the dependences of nodal conduction delay and repolarisation periods on the heart rate, can easily be recorded and measured in the clinical laboratory. Based on such laboratory investigations, different mathematical descriptions of AV nodal function have been reported (2-5). In spite of detailed knowledge of the external nodal behaviour, the internal functioning of the node, i.e. the properties and operations of its individual elements and fibres, is known only approximately. Laboratory studies enable separate nodal fibres to be examined; however, the interactions and mutual influence between intranodal cells are still not readily accessible by laboratory techniques. Hypotheses explaining internal nodal functions are therefore based mainly on logical speculations, and usually complex properties of individual cells are supposed. Most such hypothetical explanations employ the principle of decremental conduction, although different theories are also reported (6-8).

The aim of this paper is to present basic evidence that complicated AV nodal functions can be explained by supposing its individual elements to behave in a simple way in the context of a complex structure. To provide this evidence, we used a computer model of the cardiac conduction process which has been employed to simulate the behaviour of different hypothetical AV nodal images.

METHOD

The computer model used for this study has been documented in more detail elsewhere (9,10). It is not a fully realistic model which is capable of all aspects of the ECG generation process. However, simulation studies of the AV nodal properties require that images of not only AV nodal tissue but also of atrial and ventricular musculature, of the sinus node, etc., are incorporated in the model. In spite of this, the realization of these structures surrounding the AV node may be concise.

Fig. 1. Model organisation of heart images: S- sinus nodal element, A- atrial musculature, V- ventricular musculature, AVN- complex structure representing the AV node.

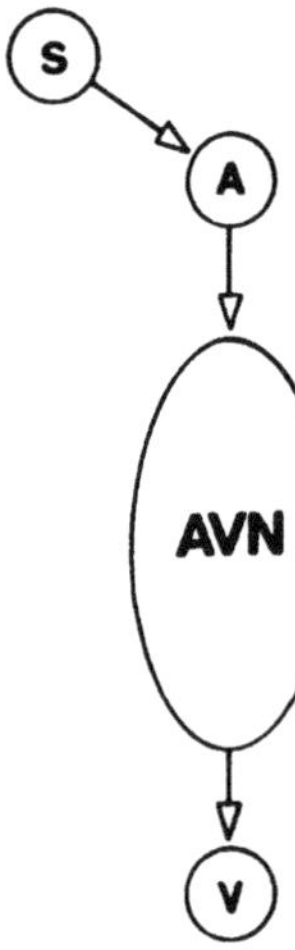

We have therefore experimented with a computer model enhancing the AV nodal structure and introducing only sigle elements to represent the sinus node, atria, and the ventricular myocardium (Fig. 1.).

All the elements used to create the artificial AV nodal model are treated in a simple way. The modelled node is composed of elements which transmit the excitation wavefront. The model distinguishes the depolarised and resting states for all elements and supposes the changes between them to be instantaneous. The excitation transmission speeds and repolarisation periods may differ for different elements.

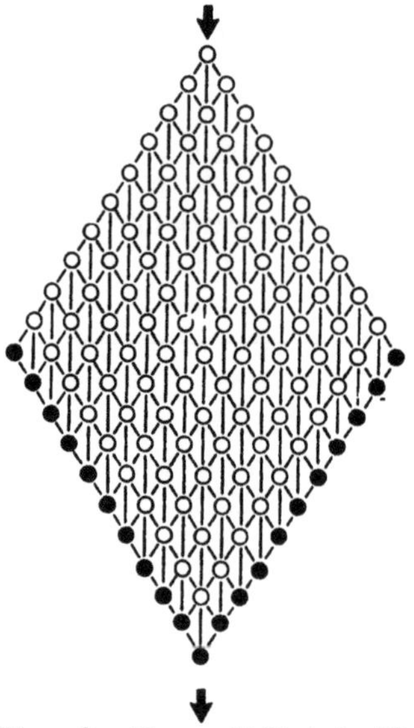

Fig. 2. The artificial AV nodal structure used in experiments in the first series. The open circles denote the elements with short repolarisation (250 ms), the solid circles denote the Rosenblueth layer having a prolonged repolarisation (450 ms). The conduction within the node is anisotropic: the delay between neighbouring elements parallel with the long axis has been set at 10 ms per connector, and 19 ms per connector in other directions. Retrograde conduction within the Rosenblueth layer is nearly instantaneous, the anterograde conduction within the layer has been varied.

Individual model elements are linked together using special connectors which transmit the excitation from one element to another. Depolarisation and resting states are not introduced for these connectors, but signal transmission delay is considered for them. Moreover, both uni- and bidirectional connection between two elements can be comprehended. In the case of a bidirectional link, the difference between anterograde and retrograde excitation speeds may be introduced.

Each computational experiment produces and exact time table of depolarisation and repolarisation events of all or of selected model elements. Using this tracing, the way in which the excitation radiates through the artificial AV node may be followed. For more 'realistic' display of results, a simulated single lead ECG record is also produced. The form of P (or P-Ta) waves and of QRS-T complexes is not generated by the model, but predefined approximate shapes are used. However, the timing of the generated ECG complexes, i.e. the appearance of P waves and QRS complexes, is exact and corresponds to the depolarisation events of atrial and ventricular musculature elements.

The results presented here were obtained using a new version of the model which was implemented on an IBM PC AT computer.

EXPERIMENTS AND RESULTS

Fig. 3. Experimental results of first series producing Wenckebach AV block. The anterograde conduction within the layer is heterogeneous: between 36 ms per connector at ventricular output point and 1 ms per connector at atrial border of the layer. The structure produces clinically relevant patterns of Wenckebach periods which include decremental shortening of RR intervals. Atrial coupling intervals: a - 445 ms, b - 435 ms, c - 425 ms, d - 415 ms.

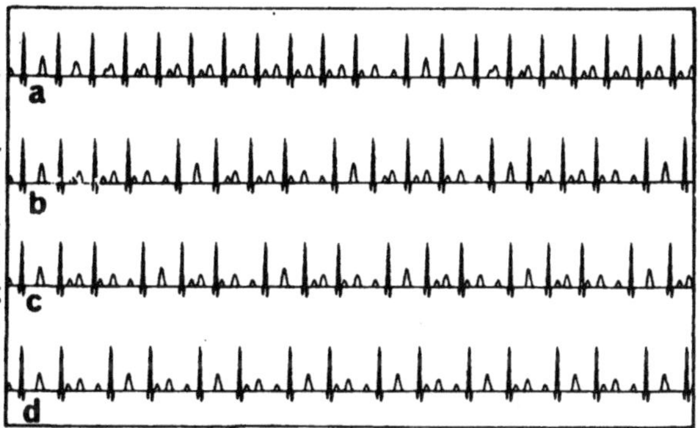

The first experimental series utilised an AV nodal structure based on the Rosenblueth hypothesis (11). Rosenblueth suggested (6,12) that the prolongation of the AV nodal conduction delay with shorter cycle length is not due to incremental delay exhibited by all nodal fibres, but that the excitation is delayed by a single special layer. This principle has been incorporated in a simple AV nodal model (Fig. 2.) having the form of a regular mesh and introducing conduction speed differences between pathways along and across the node. The ventricular border of the node represents Rosenblueth layer and its repolarisation period is prolonged. Retrograde conduction within the layer is nearly instantaneous, while the anterograde conduction properties of the layer were changed in the experiments. When introducing a sufficient difference between repolarisation intervals of the internal nodal elements and the Rosenblueth layer, 2nd degree AV block can be modelled and computer experiments reproduce Wenckebach periods. A constant anterograde delay causes the reproduced Wenckebach periods not to exhibit the shortening of successive RR intervals (13). To achieve such a decremental shortening of RR intervals during each period, a heterogeneous anisotropy within the layer was considered. When setting the anterograde conduction within the layer to be slowest near to the ventricular output, the structure simulates clinically relevant periods (Fig. 3.) but it does not reproduce a realistic VV/AA relationship (1). To improve the modelled VV/AA conduction plot, we considered an inverse ordering of the intra-level anterograde conduction heterogenity. However, this did not produce clinically relevant reproduction of Wenckebach periods (the modelled curve exhibits prolongation of successive RR intervals in each period).

According to the results of the previous series, the anisotropy and repolarisation interval differences between different layers can contribute to the complexity of the nodal function. We have therefore examined a more complicated nodal image (Fig. 4.). For some sinus node frequencies, this AV nodal image behaves satisfactorily while for other frequencies, the results do not resemble clinical records (Fig. 5). The exact tracing of computational experiments shows that the peculiar unrealistic rhythm models are due to collisions of modelled wavefronts at different internodal levels.

DISCUSSION

In spite of all important simplifications and restrictions of our computer model and of employed AV nodal structures, the experimental results provide evidence that the complexity of the AV nodal structure may itself be responsible for its complex behaviour.

In the first series of experiments, Wenckebach period reproduction was rather realistic although very simple elements were used to create the nodal model. However, the same nodal image could not reproduce the anterograde conduction curves suggesting that different anisotropical structures might be responsible for different aspects of AV

Fig. 5. The experimental results from second series. The sinus rate differs in the seven cases. The sinus nodal coupling intervals are: a - 350 ms, b - 320 ms, c - 310 ms, d - 315 ms, e - 280 ms, f - 300 ms, g - 215 ms.

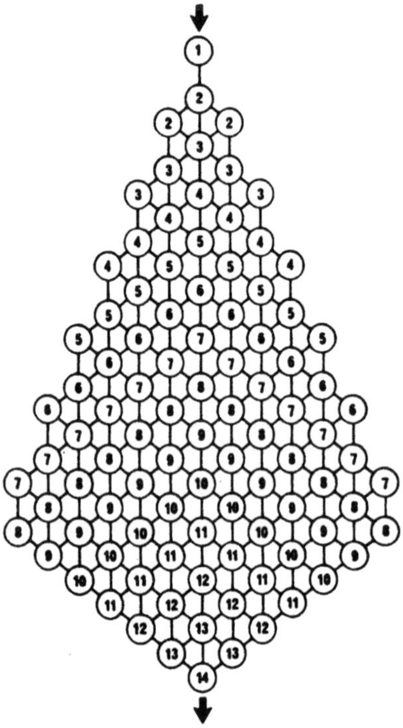

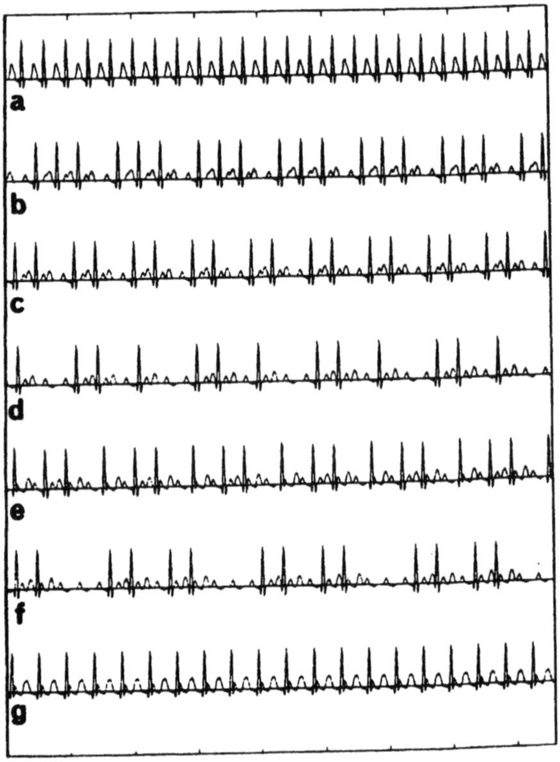

Fig. 4. The structure of the AV nodal image used in the second series of experiments. The node is composed of 14 layers with different properties. The elements denoted with same numbers have the same properties: the element (1) transmits the excitation most slowly (16 ms) and has the shortest repolarisation period (200 ms). For other layers, the conduction delay was shortened and repolarisation period prolonged to 3 ms and 330 ms of the element (14).

nodal function.

Results from the second series suggest that the complex nodal organisation may cause the wavefront of excitation to be delayed and blocked at different nodal levels. Though producing unrealistic results, the structure shows the importance of collisions of wavefronts invading and transversing the AV node.

(1) Malik M, Camm AJ: PACE (1988), in press
(2) Heethaar RM, van der Gon JJD, Meijler FL: Cardiovasc. Res. 7, 105 (1973)
(3) Heethaar RM, de vos Buchart RM, van der Gon JJD, et al: Cardiovasc. Res. 7, 542 (1973)
(4) Dorveaux L, Heddle W, Jones M, et al: Int. J. BioMed. Comput. 17, 227 (1985)
(5) Dorveaux L, Heddle W, Jones M, et al: PACE 8, 646 (1985)
(6) Rosenblueth A: Am. J. Physiol. 194, 491 (1958)
(7) Levy MN, Martin PJ, Zieske H, et al: Circ. Res. 36, 697 (1974)
(8) Young M-L, Wolff GS, Castelanos A, et al: Am. J. Cardiol. 57, 131 (1986)
(9) Malik M, Cochrane T., Davies DW, Camm AJ: Med. Biol. Eng. Comput. (1987), in press
(10) Malik M, Camm AJ: this proceedings
(11) Malik M, Ward D, Camm AJ: PACE (1987), submitted
(12) Rosenblueth A: Am. J. Physiol. 194, 495 (1958)
(13) Sandoe E, Bjarne S: Arrhythmia, Fachmed AG, St. Gallen, 1984

Instability of Multipole Model of Cardiogenerator Caused by Measurement Errors

PROCHOROV V.N., GAGIEV N.G., KUZNETSOV V.P., KARPUSHOV E.N.

Institute of biology
Komi branch of the Academy of Sciences of the USSR
Syktyvkar, USSR

SYMMARY

Real multipole components errors were investigated. Conclusion is made that geometrical parameters: a body shape and electrode localization must be measured with the accuracy of 2-3 cm.

INTRODUCTION

A multipole representation of the cardiac electric generator is one of the widely used approach to the solution of the so-called inverse problem in electrocardiology. However real methods of description of the excitation wave propagation through the myocard by means of the multipole components appear to be rather sensitive to relatively small errors of the components values. So the physiological interpretation of such calculation results used to be doubtful.

The multipole coefficients evaluation consists in the surface integration of measured potentials multiplied by the appropriate functions of co-ordinates of the body surface points. So the coefficients accuracy is determined by the errors of measurement of the potentials and the geometrical values. In addition, some variations may be caused by a priori valued parameters of a mathematical model for the body shape approximation. The problem of the relative role of the above factors is not quantitatively solved. So one has no apportunity to establish acceptable accuracy levels for the recording systems and the procedures of experiment.

INVESTIGATION RESULTS

In our investigation measurements have been performed with the multichannel measuring system developed in the Komi branch of the Academy of Sciences of the USSR. There were used 64 electrodes placed over the torso at 4 horizontal planes between the sternal notch and the umbilicus levels. Surface integrals have been calculated by the triangulation method. Side triangles were determined by electrodes co-ordinates. The upper part of the body was modelled by the cone surface with the height h_1, the part of the body below the umbilicus level was modelled by the cilinder with the height h_2. It should be noted that there are no mathematical arguments for choosing of h_1, h_2 values while the multipole components largly depend on this parameters.

The results of multipole errors investigations are presented in

TABLE 1. Relative errors (%) of multipole components caused by potentials and geometrical parameters measurement errors

	Factor 1	Factor 2	Factor 3	Factor 4	Factor 5	Factor 6
A10	15	1	1	1	5	0
A11	20	1	7	1	1	0
B11	10	7	5	5	1	0
A20	10	5	10	5	5	20
A21	25	20	15	20	7	20
B21	10	25	20	5	1	10
A22	5	1	1	1	1	10
B22	15	5	7	1	5	10
A30	30	10	10	10	35	25
A31	15	7	5	5	15	20
B31	25	20	20	20	1	10
A32	1	1	1	1	1	5
B32	1	5	10	5	1	5
A33	1	1	1	1	1	1
B33	1	1	1	1	1	3

Table 1. Strings of the table correspond to multipole components. It is used usual notation: A_{1i} , B_{1i} - dipole, A_{2i} , B_{2i} - quadrupole, A_{3i} , B_{3i} - octupole components. Columns correspond to investigated error factors. Factor 1 - measured potentials variations, caused by the errors in registration equipment, sample preprocessing and physiological variations of the heart activity during one hour of experiments. Factor 2 and 3 - variations of the h_1 and h_2 values. Factor 4 - errors of measurement of the distance between electrodes levels. Factor 5 - variations of angular and radial co-ordinates of electrodes. Factor 6 - multipoles center variations. All geometrical values were artificially variated in range of ± 2 sm.

The multipole errors are represented in relative form (in per cent). For the multipole of order n it was used as a unit the value:

$$U_n = \max_{t,i} |A_{ni}(t), B_{ni}(t)|,$$

t- time during QRS-interval.

Multipole components were calculated in the initial frame of references, then they were recalculated to the new one. The new frame of references was shifted by the vector $\mathbf{R}$ and its Z-axis was oriented along $\mathbf{D}$ -vector. $\mathbf{R}$ -vector was determined as the weighted mean of radius-vector of moving electrical center of the heart generator. $\mathbf{D}$ -vector was the weighted mean of dipole component $\vec{d}(t)$. The weights were proportional to $\|\vec{d}\|$.

Figure 1 shows the role of factor 1 for one of the normal volunteers, the relationship between dipole, quadrupole and octupole scales along Y-axis was 1 : 0.2 : 0.008.

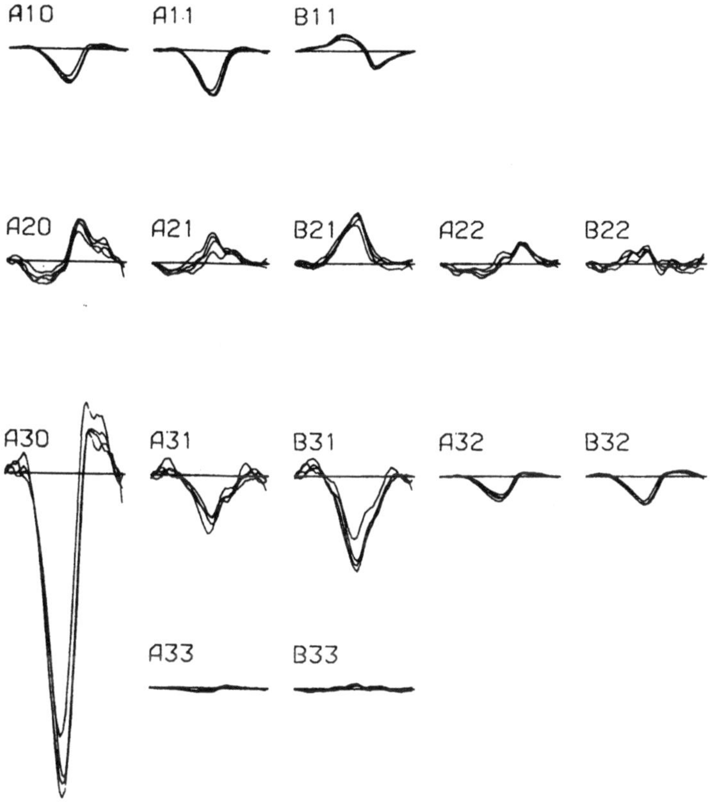

FIG. 1 REAL VARIATIONS OF MULTIPOLE COMPONENTS IN SINGLE SERIES OF FOUR MEASUREMENT OF NORMAL VOLUNTEER, REGISTRATIONS WERE REPEATED WITH TIME INTERVAL 15 MIN.

To illustrate the influence of multipole errors on maps of the heart electrical activity we used one of the possible approach for the mapping. Namely the potentials on sphere with radius R-have been calculated from evaluated multipole components. Then the instant maps have been integrated on time during QRS-interval. The procedure is analogous to the well known body surface time integral technique. Examples of such maps are presented on Fig.2. R-value was taken 7.5 cm, dipole, quadrupole and octupole components were used for potentials calculation, maps were constructed in above mentioned "own" frame of references. Three maps at the left column belong to one normal volunteer and reflect the influence of "Factor 1". Upper and middle maps at the right column belong to other normal men and the third one to LBBB-patient. The shaded area on maps is positive.

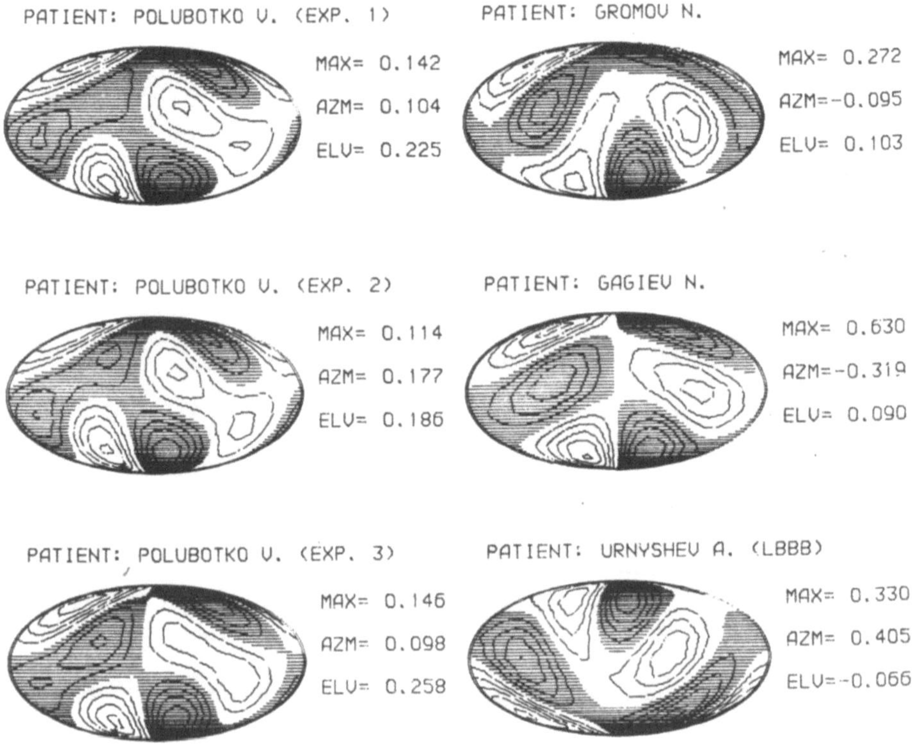

FIG.2 TIME INTEGRAL MAPS OF MULTIPOLES MODEL POTENTIAL ON SPHERE. MAX - MAXIMAL VALUE OF THE FUNCTION; AZM, ELV - AZIMUTH AND ELEVATION OF THE HEART ELECTRICAL AXIS.

CONCLUSION

Received data presented on Table 1 and Fig.1,2 show that real measurement errors of multipole components must be taken into account when a mapping procedure based on multipoles is been developed. The main conclusion is that in case of men heart investigation 2-3 cm errors of geometrical parameters:electrodes co-ordinates and mathematical modelling of a body shape may lead to the same multipole errors as ones caused by a physiological variability.

BODY SURFACE MAPPING - THEORY AND METHODS

Body Surface Isopotential Maps Properties after the Transfer Coefficient Unification

DRŠKA, Z., MÁLKOVÁ, A., VALOVÁ, D.

Institute of Physiological Regulations, Czechoslovak Academy of Sciences, FN Bulovka, pav. 11, 180 85 Prague 8, Czechoslovakia

Summary
Matrix of ECGs from the chest surface was corrected to the unit transfer coefficient surface (VCG spherical surface) using the method described elsewhere (Drška, Z.). In comparison with original body surface potential distribution (BSPD), the maps after correction exhibited elevation of amplitudes in general and tendency to the equilibrium of amplitudes of both positive and negative areas of distribution. Differences in position of potential peaks were observed during the whole QRS interval and additional potential peaks most frequently within the 20th to 50th ms of QRS interval appeared. These finding are in agreement with the presumption that the method of correction used, leads to the unification of extracardiac factors influence on the properties of BSPD and to the reduction of the smoothing influence of the thorax on the BSPD.

Introduction: The aim of this paper was to verify the character and significance of changes obtained in maps of isopotential lines within the QRS interval as a result of correction of BSPD to the unit transfer coefficient surface using the method described elsewhere.

Materials and methods: Matrix of unipolar ECGs was measured from the chest surface in horizontal, 18 cm wide zone, with its upper margin in the level of the jugulum. Seven silver-chlorid floating electrodes set was used for measurement in regular grid with the step of 3 cm in both vertical and horizontal directions. Orthonormal ECGs of Frank VCG system was also registered. These sequentional measurements were then synchronized using the QRS course of reference ECG lead. In this time the sampling frequency equal to 1000 Hz has been used. The data for visualization were interpolated using the cubic splines to the matrix of 64x256 points. Amplitudes were visualized in 256 gray levels and in 16 levels of pseudocolorisation. The procedure for transfer coefficient unification was applied to unify extracardiac factors influence on the BSPD (Drška, Z., Drška, Z. et al). This method consists of individual ECG amplitude correction to the unit VCG spherical surface, achieved by the normalization of the transfer coefficients corresponding to x,y,z VCG axes. These coefficients have been obtained by solution of 3 (x,y,z) linear equations system for every element of ECG matrix.

Measurementsfrom a group of healthy subjects (11) and subjects with ischemic heart disease (31) were studied. For technical reasons (i. e. sequentional measurements of ECGs) subjects with sinus rythm were included only.
Results: In comparison with the maps of original potential distributions from the chest surface, the corresponding maps after correction exhibited elevation of amplitudes in general. Significant tendency to the equilibrium of both positive and negative areas of distribution was found. Differences in position of potential peaks were observed during the whole QRS interval and aditional potential peaks most frequently within the 20th to 50th ms of the QRS interval appeared.
For example the map of BSPD in healthy subject (Fig. 1 up) after correction to the unit transfer coefficient surface (Fig. 1 bottom) exhibited the increase of the level of potentials generally in all distribution. The shift of positive peak from the left precordium to the left axillary area and the second positive peak in the left inferior part of the back appeared. Increased (5times) negative peak shifted from the upper to the middle part of the back to the right of the spine.
Similar situation can be observed in the maps of subject with old anterolateral myocardial infarction (Fig. 2). After transfer coefficient unification the level of potentials in negative area increased 3times and multiple peaks both positive and negative appeared.
In subject with old posterior myocardial infarction in the map after correction two negative potential peaks appeared in the inferior part of the back and in the right axillary area.

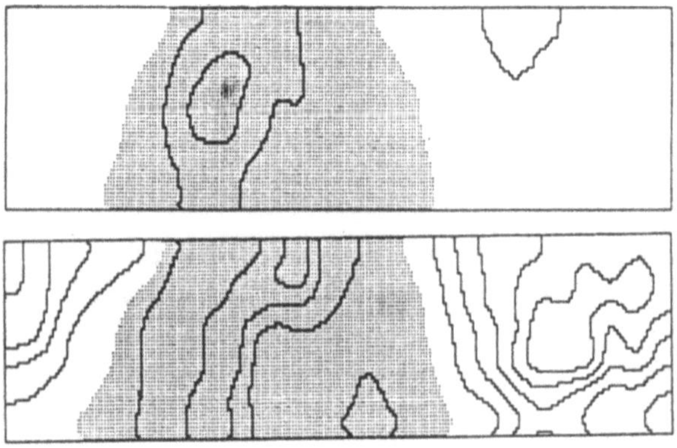

Fig. 1a: Isopotential map on the chest surface in a healthy subject (27), (20 ms before maximum vector of QRS, interval between isolines is 413 uV).
Fig. 1b: Isopotential map on the surface with unit transfer coefficient in the same subject and in the same instant of QRS.

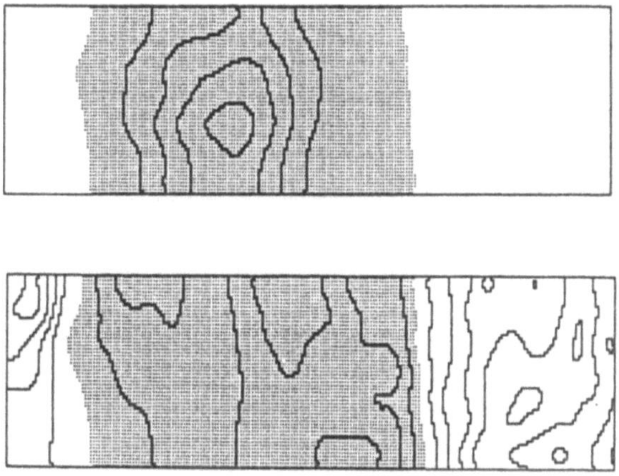

Fig. 2a: Isopotential map on the chest surface in the subject with old anterolateral myocardial infarction (65), in whom significant stenosis of the left coronary artery trunk was proved by angiography.(20ms before maximal vector of QRS, interval between isolines is 231 uV).
Fig. 2b: Corresponding isopotential map after correction of BSPD to the unit transfer coefficient surface.

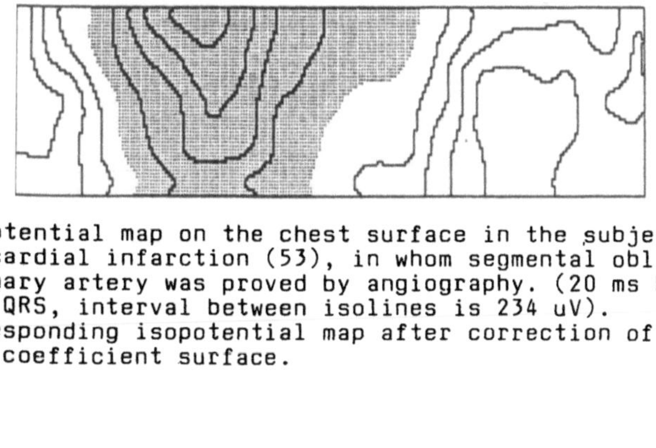

Fig. 3a: Isopotential map on the chest surface in the subject with old posterior myocardial infarction (53), in whom segmental obliteration of right coronary artery was proved by angiography. (20 ms before maximal vector of QRS, interval between isolines is 234 uV).
Fig. 3b: Corresponding isopotential map after correction of BSPD to the unit transfer coefficient surface.

Discussion: Described findings are in agreement with the presumption that the method of correction used, leads to the unification of extracardiac factors influence on the properties of BSPD and to the reduction of smoothing influence of the thorax on the BSPD (Rudy, Y.). These results also testify to reduction of non-dipolar residue within the IHD subjects in relation to healthy subjects (Tsunakawa, H. et al).

References:
(1) Drška, Z.: In: Abstracts of 13th Internat. Congr. on Electrocardiology, Washington, 90 (1986)
(2) Drška, Z., D. Valová, A. Málková: Proc. of 14th Internat. Congr. on Electrocardiology, Berlin (1987), in this issue
(3) Rudy, Y.: In: Electrocardiographic Body Surface Mapping. Ed: R. Th. van Dam, A. van Oosterom, Martinus Nijhoff Publishers, Dordrecht et al, 247-258 (1986)
(4) Tsunakawa, H., K. Hoshino, S. Kanesaka, K. Harumi, Y. Okamoto, Y. Teramachi, T. Mosha: Jpn. Heart J. 26, 319-334 (1985)

Electromagnetic field of heart contraction kinetics.
Electromagnetic kin etocardiography: theory and clinical application.

KRÁL V., KOČÍ M., HÖNIG J:

Institute of Physiological Regulations, Czechoslovak Academy of Sciences, FN Bulovka, pav. 11, 180 85 Prague 8, Czechoslovakia.

Summary.

Electromagnetic kinetocardiography (EM KCG) is a new noninvasive method, which in principle transforms heart walls movement into the secondary electromagnetic field (EMF) variations. The primary RF field evokes mainly on endocardial planes, the electrical charge layers. These sources change due to the heart motion and originate the secondary EMF distribution on the chest surface. We measure these EMF variations topographically and directly as a divergence of intensity $\vec{E}$. Processed isodivergence $\vec{E}$ maps and maps of their time differences demonstrate the dynamics of ventricular motion in a global view. The method was verified by angiocardiography and echocardiography on patients with ischemic heart disease. The results are in accordance with both comparative methods.

The method EM KCG depends on interactions of the primary EMF (13,56 MHz) with inhomogeneous intrathoracic medium. This field consists of a magnetic induction $\vec{B}_0(t)$ of the current loop (inductor) closing around the chest and of vortex field $\vec{E}_0(t)$ creating in conductive body medium Foucault currents $J_0(t)$. (Fig. 1.) These Primary currents traverse the surfaces separating myocardium and intracavitary blood. Because of the different conductivities (σ) and permittivities (ε), the sudden "voltage jumps" are created there. They can be explained by single layers of charges spread over endocardial surfaces of both ventricles. Because of the heart motion these layers form the time-space dependent multipolar sources of the secondary EMF. This field propagating on the body surface reflects the ventricular walls kinetics and is measured directly as divergence of $\vec{E}$ (div $\vec{E}$). The reason of the div $\vec{E}$ measurement is to differentiate multidipolar sources on endocardial planes of both ventricles. The discrimination ability of div $\vec{E}$ is demonstrated by a model experiment. Two dipoles d_1, d_2 were located in electrolytic model of thorax (Fig.2.). The surface distribution of the field of this dipoles was measured as a potential , intensity $\vec{E}$ and div $\vec{E}$. The topographic surface measurement of potential gives at most a simple dipolar distribution, so that the right and left ventricular sources could not be well distinguished in isopotential maps. The distribution of $\vec{E}$ shows two peaks of intensity referrend to particular dipoles. The distribution of div $\vec{E}$ differentiates the two dipoles by two separate sinks and sources best. The div $\vec{E}$ has physical significance of density of charge (ρ). May be defined mathematically according to the tensor of the second rank G_2. The sum of diagonal components of its symmetrical part is proportional to div E. It can be said, that the charge densities over the precordium image charge densities over the heart endocardial planes.

The secondary EMF is created in our case by two positive and two negative endocardial charge layers (see Fig. 1.). The polarity of these reverses of course each cycle of RF generator frequency. Detection enables us to measure secondary EMF only during one particular hemi-cycle of primary EMF frequency. Under such conditions we suppose negative charges on the right ventricular free wall and positive ones on the septal plane. The left ventricular septal plane is analogically negative and the residual endocardial surface positive. Measured distributions are converted to tensorial maps of isodivergence $\vec{E}$, which show in every one picture the state of motion of both ventricles and septum. Such movie maps (dynamic maps) give a characteristic panoramatic view of cardiac motion throughout systole and diastole.

The conception of isodivergence $\vec{E}$ maps and maps of their differences (time differences of div $\vec{E}$ relate to the current densities of flowing charges - div $\vec{J}$) is such that the number of isolines increases if the distances of ventricular parts relatively to the measuring points increases too. Synergic contraction manifests itself in isodivergence $\vec{E}$ maps at regions corresponding to different ventricular planes by characteristic distributions of polarities, which do not change its sign throughout all cardiac cycle (see Fig. 3a, b, c). The contrary polarity indicates always the paradoxical motion of corresponding ventricular walls. It occurs mostly in the left ventricular periapical area. If change outlasts the whole systolic phase it signifies dyskinesia. Polarity reverse appearing only in a part of the ejection phase may document a certain state of tardokinesia, hypokinesia or akinesia. These asynergias are always accompanied by lower amplitude of div $\vec{E}$. Similar paradoxical response is also found in the relaxation phase.

Clinical experiences in EM KCG were gained on more than 200 persons with normal and pathological myocardial contraction. Studying and comparing maps of isodivergence E with results on torso model and with results of ventriculokardiography (VG) and 2-D echocardiography (ECHO), we found in maps the areas where the ventricular segments with normal and abnormal kinetics are projected. We stated likewise the criteria as to the type and extension of contraction asynergias. The maps of healthy persons show full regularity as to the distribution of the right and left ventricle segments localisation.

Set of 110 persons with chronic coronary disease was compared as to the types of asynergia with VG and ECHO. The statistics of results concerns mainly the sensitivity of EM KCG method. The Tab. 1. compares groups after the anterior (MIA) and posterior (MIP) infarction to the type of contraction changes. The columns signify numbers of "false positivity" (+), equivalence (=) and "false negativity" (-), sensitivity (%) and sensitivity with a drift. In group MIA is one-sided drift in EM KCG to the "false positivity" (=). This unambiguous shift demonstrate higher sensitivity in differentiation of the type of asynergia. The sensitivity in group MIP shows on the contrary a drift of EM KCG to the more "false negativity" (=). These results refer to the fact, that the postero-inferior ventricular segments cannot be detected by EM KCG. We have informations only from neighbouring segments (inferior, lateral and basal) and from specially altered kinetics of the anterior and apical areas. The score of types of asynergia (normokinesia-1, hyperkinesia-2, hypokinesia -3, akinesia-4 and dyskinesia-5) shows correlation with a high significance in froup MIA and lower in group MIP (Tab. 2.).

The developed method is supported by many model experiments and by the theory explaining all phenomena in detail. The maps of isodivergence $\vec{E}$ display the kinetics of ventricular walls on the base of the movement of charge layers spread over the endocardial planes. In this respect EM KCG differs from the other methods dealing with a ventricular projections or cross-sections. The maps of isodivergence $\vec{J}$ present in global view the synchrony of contraction of different ventricular parts. This is the distinct advantage of EM KCG over the other methods, which cannot gain similar results in a single way.

Tab. 1.

Group MIA	VG - EM KCG (n=32)					ECHO - EM KCG (n=56)				
	+	=	-	%	=	+	=	-	%	=
Dyskinesia	7	17	-	100,0	100,0	11	24	-	96,0	96,6
Akinesia	1	1	-	12,5	100,0	4	0	1	0,0	91,7
Hypokinesia	5	1	-	50,0	100,0	3	5	1	50,0	90,0
Normokinesia	-	2	-	28,6	100,0	-	2	-	40,0	100,0

Group MIP	VG - EM KCG (n=36)					ECHO - EM KCG (n=46)				
	+	=	-	%	=	+	=	-	%	=
Dyskinesia	1	0	-	0,0	50,0	1	2	-	66,6	100,0
Akinesia	2	4	1	50,0	91,7	2	5	1	55,6	91,7
Hypokinesia	4	12	3	80,0	93,0	4	19	3	79,2	91,7
Normokinesia	-	3	2, 4	23,1	42,9	-	3	3, 3	21,4	42,8

Tab. 2.

MIA	VG (n=34)	ECHO (n=52)	MIP	VG (n=36)	ECHO n=46)
EM KCG	r=0,65^{+++}	r=0,75^{+++}	EM KCG	r=0,42$^{+(+)}$	r=0,56^{+++}
				p 0,001^{+++}	p 0,05^{+}

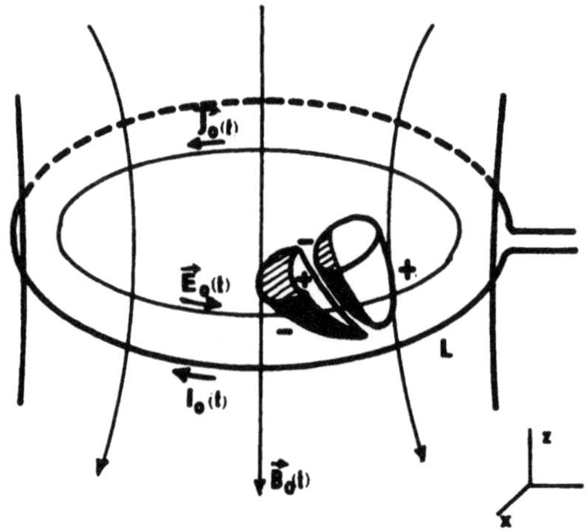

Fig. 1. Magnetic induction $\vec{B}_0(t)$ of one turn coil L fed by current $I_0(t)$ sets in the thorax current density $\vec{J}_0(t)$ and intensity $\vec{E}_0(t)$. Eddy currents flowing throgh the heart ventricles generat od endocardial surfaces the electrical charges because of different conductivities of blood and myocardium. These charge layers follow the motion of the heart walls and creates thus the secondary electromagnetic field of the heart motion.

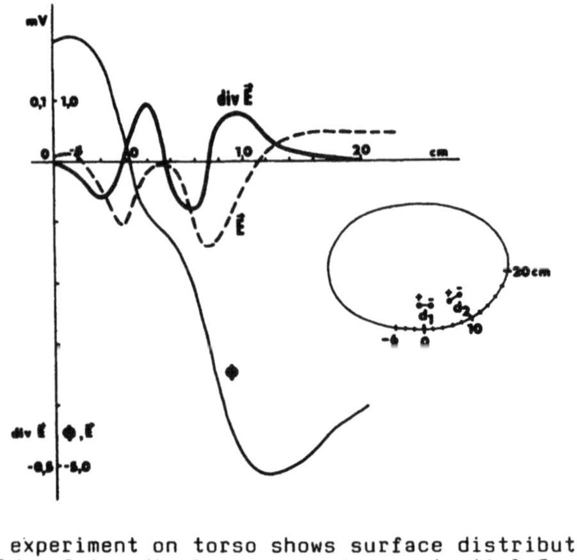

Fig. 2. Model experiment on torso shows surface distribution of the secondary fields of two dipoles measured as potential Φ, intensity E and divergence $\vec{E}$ (div $\vec{E}$). The distribution of potential Φ is that of one dipole only. Distribution of intensity $\vec{E}$ show two maxima corresponding to the locations of the two dipoles. The distribution of div $\vec{E}$ differentiate sources and sinks of the both dipoles. The space derivatives of potential thus enables to differentiate the multidipolar sources of the electric field.

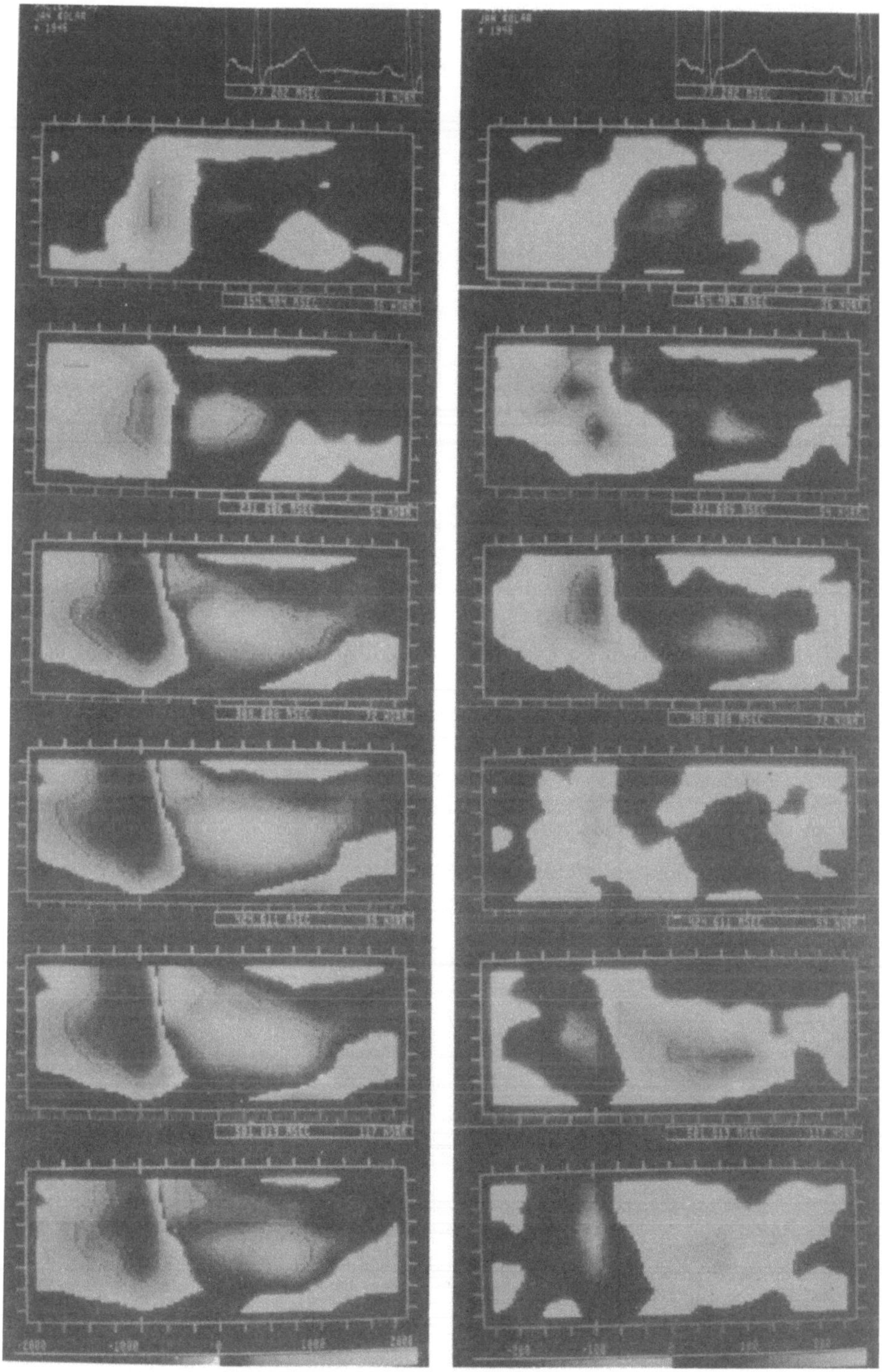

Fig. 3. Example of dynamic maps of isodivergences in 80 ms sequences of a healthy subject. On the left side are the maps of divergence $\vec{E}$ (div $\vec{E}$) and on the right one the maps of divergence of current density (div $\vec{J}$).

Data acquisition for ECG-mapping.

KRENZKE, GERHARD
Humboldt-Universitaet zu Berlin, Klinik Innere Medizin,
Schumannstr. 20-21, Berlin 1040, GDR

An ECG-mapping equipment with concentric mounted electrode-holders is described, which enables the measurement of the distance from the ECG-electrodes to the midpoint of the heart. This distance is used to calculate "corrected" ECG-maps.

There are some well known problems concerning ECG-mapping. The first is the different shape of the thorax, which makes it difficult on the one hand to find an electrode-holder universally suitible and on the other hand to obtain comparable maps from patient to patient. The variability of the thorax shape also influences the magnitudes of the ECG-map, as we know, so that we can say, that the ECG-map is partly a copy of the thorax shape. And therefore we should ask, if it is possible to consider the thorax shape. Another problem is the electrode contact, which depends on the electrode configuration, the contact medium and also the electrode pressure. These are of course not yet all problems of the ECG-data acquisition, but this selection of problems we tried to overcome with the development of a special ECG-data acquisition equipment for ECG-mapping.

A bicycle ergometer for lying position of the patient is completed with a car, which slides on two rails on both sides of the patients pad rest. This car carries two casings on which 75 electrode-holders are mounted. The upper part with 48 electrodes can be turned up. The lower part with 27 electrodes carries a hole plate on which the patient lies. The patient is placed between the two casings in such a way, that the midpoint of the equipment is identical with the midpoint of the heart. For this reason the equipment can be moved motor driven in three directions parallel to the body axises of the lying patient. The ECG-electrodes are movable in the electrode-holders. The direction of moving goes through the midpoint of the equipment. Therefore the possible positions of one ECG-electrode are, independent of the thorax shape and the patient, always placed on the same line, which has constant angles against the body axises. If we use the midpoint of the heart as the second virtual lead point, than we have a system of constant lead axises, which are independent of the patient. The electrode-holder consists of a cylinder and a piston on which the ECG-electrode is mounted. The piston is moved by airpressure respectively underpressure. The distance of the electrode from the midpoint of the equipment is measured electrically. The surface of the electrodes is gilded.We use usual electrode paste as contact medium.

As mentioned above the midpoint of the equipment is moved so, that it coincide with the midpoint of the heart. But where is the midpoint of the heart? At present we use the results of FRANK's investigations (*). According to these the midpoint is situated in the range of the 4.th ICS. In the horizontal plain its distance from the thorax midpoint is 0.094B and 0.148D respectively, where B is the thorax width and D the thorax depth. As virtual electrical midpoint of the heart we use the central terminal of WILSON.

The electronic equipment for data acquisition stores the ECGs on an analog tape. After converting this into a digital record the off-line processing is controlled by using a display terminal. By technical reason only three ECG-channels are recorded simultanously. Parallel to these three leads marking pulses are stored on the fourth track of the analog tape. The marking pulses are gained from the R-wave of one of the bipolar limb leads. The distance between two pulses serves as measure for the RR-distance. With a special algorithm a series of such 75 beats is selected that are most similar each other. This algorithm takes the first beat of the first lead and searches the best fitting beats in all other leads. The best fitting beats are those which have RR-distances of smallest deviation. So we get a set of 75 beats. In the same way we take the second beat of the first lead for the search program etc. The groups of beats are sorted according the mean square deviation. The typical beat in every group has a RR-distance which best suits the mean value of RR-distances of the whole group. This typical beat of the first group is represented on the screen. The symbol M marks the time point of the front side of the marking pulse. It is possible to alter the time window of the represented heart cycle as well as the amplitude scale. Than five ranges of amplitudes have to be determined. Every range get a symbol. At three free eligible cursor time points the amplitudes of the ECG-curves are measured, and according to the amplitude ranges every electrode point on the map get a symbol. Because of the three time points we also have three maps on one display picture (see figure). With the same follow up we can get a so-called "corrected" map. In this all amplitudes are multiplied by the squared distance of the ECG-electrode from the heart midpoint. If we use two cursor points, it is possible to determine the area under the ECG-curve between these two points with the normal ECGs as well as with the distance corrected ECGs. The last possibility is the representation of so-called "difference"-maps. For this purpose the FRANK-ECG is used. All electrodes for the FRANK lead system are implemented in the acquisition equipment too. The rotating vector calculated from the FRANK-ECG can be projected on all derivation lines, which are formed by the lines between the heart midpoint and the ECG-elctrodes. Between these virtual ECGs and the corrected ECGs the difference is calculated. The virtual ECGs serve

amplitude-map

	1	2	3	4	5	6	7	8	9	10	11	12	13	14	15	16
1			1	1	1					3	2	2	2	2		
2		1	1	1	1	2				3	3	2	2	2		
3	1	▪	▪	▪	1	2	3	3	3	3	3	3	2		2	2
4	2	1	▪	▪	1	2	3	4	3	3	3	3	3		2	2
5	2		▪	▪	2		4	4	4	3	3	3	3	3	2	2
6	2		1	1	3		4	4	4		3	3	3	3	2	2
			1	1	1					3	3	3	3	2		
		▪	▪	▪	▪	1				3	4	3	3	3		
	▪	▪	▪	▪	▪	1	4	5	4	4	4	3	3		1	1
T2	▪	▪	▪	▪	▪	2	5	5	5	4	4	3	3		1	1
	1		▪	▪	▪		5	5	5	4	4	4	3	3	1	1
	1		▪	▪	1		5	4	4		3	4	3	3	1	1
			2	2	2					3	3	3	3	3		
		1	1	1	1	2				4	4	3	3	3		
T3	1	1	1	▪	▪	2	5	5	5	4	4	3	3		2	1
	1	▪	▪	▪	▪	2	5	5	5	4	4	3	3		2	1
	1		▪	▪	1		5	5	5	4	3	3	3	3	1	1
	1		▪	▪	1		5	4	3		2	3	3	2	2	1

5)=+1000 µV
4)=+0500
3)= 0000
2)=-0500
1)=-1000
▪ <-1000

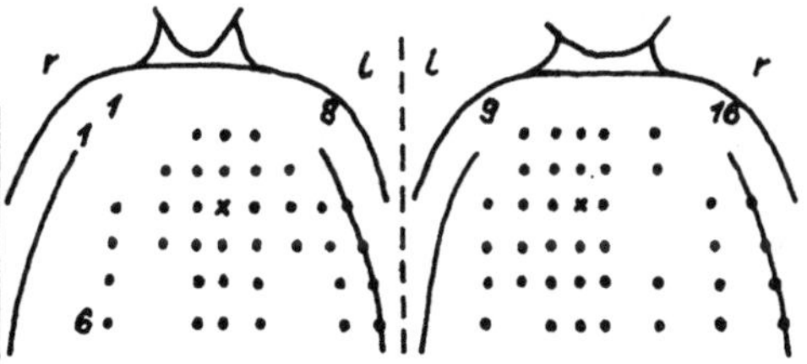

corrected amplitude-map

			2	2	2					3	2	2	2	2		
		1	1	2	2	2				3	3	2	2	2		
T1	▪	▪	▪	1	2	2	3	3	3	3	3	3	2		1	▪
	1	▪	▪	▪	1	2	3	3	3	3	3	3	3		1	1
	1		▪	▪	1		4	4	4	4	4	3	3	3	2	1
	2		▪	▪	3		5	5	5		4	4	4	3	2	2
			2	2	2					5	4	4	3	2		
		▪	▪	1	1	1				4	4	3	3	3		
	▪	▪	▪	▪	▪	1	4	4	4	5	4	3	3		▪	▪
T2	▪	▪	▪	▪	▪	2	5	5	5	5	5	4	4		▪	▪
	▪		▪	▪	▪		5	5	5	5	5	4	4	3	▪	▪
	▪		▪	▪	▪		5	5	5		4	5	4	3	▪	▪
			2	2	2					5	4	4	3	3		
		1	1	2	2	2				5	4	4	3	3		
T3	▪	▪	1	1	1	2	4	5	4	5	5	4	4		▪	▪
	▪	▪	▪	▪	▪	2	5	5	5	5	5	3	3		▪	▪
	▪		▪	▪	▪		5	5	5	4	4	3	3	3	▪	▪
	▪		▪	▪	▪		5	5	4		2	3	3	2	▪	▪

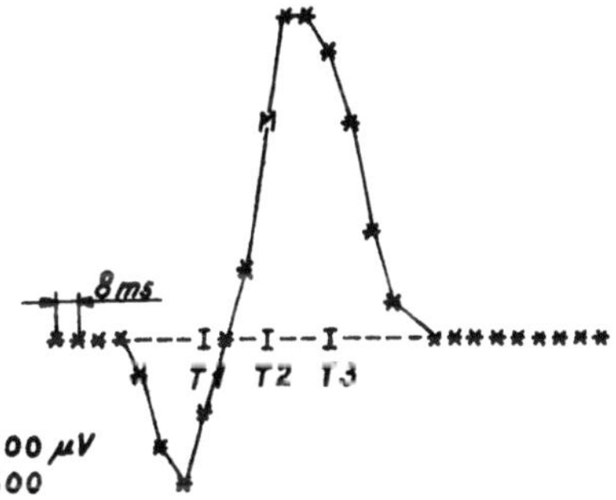

5)=+1000 µV
4)=+0500
3)= 0000
2)=-0500
1)=-1000
▪ <-1000

difference-map

			5	5	5					2	1	1	1	1		
		5	5	5	5	5				▪	▪	▪	1	1		
T1	2	1	3	5	5	4	4	4	2	1	▪	▪	▪		1	1
	2	▪	▪	▪	3	5	5	4	3	2	2	1	1		1	1
	2		▪	▪	3		5	5	5	2	2	2	1	1	3	3
	4		▪	▪	5		5	5	5		3	5	4	3	4	3
			5	5	5					3	3	3	1	1		
		5	5	5	5	4				▪	1	▪	1	1		
	1	2	5	5	4	4	5	5	2	2	1	▪	1		▪	▪
T2	▪	▪	▪	▪	1	5	5	5	5	4	3	1	1		▪	▪
	▪		▪	▪	▪		5	5	5	3	3	3	2	2	▪	▪
	▪		▪	▪	1		5	5	5		3	5	5	3	▪	▪
			5	5	3					3	3	3	2	2		
		5	5	3	3	1				2	2	1	2	2		
T3	3	4	5	5	2	2	4	4	2	4	3	2	3		1	2
	▪	▪	2	2	▪	2	5	5	5	4	3	2	2		▪	▪
	▪		▪	▪	▪		5	5	5	2	2	2	2	2	▪	▪
	▪		▪	▪	▪		5	5	4		▪	2	2	▪	▪	▪

Figure
Different methods of map analysis for the same patient with LVH, LBBB and anterior infarction.

5)=+0400 µV
4)=+0200
3)= 0000
2)=-0200
1)=-0400
▪ <-0400

as an expression of the mean potential distribution over the thorax surface in the sence, that this distribution is caused only by a dipol. Local disturbances of the dipol field are to be detected by this method.

Finally an example is to demonstrate the differences of the different methods of mapping analysis. We use the maps of a 53-year-old patient with ischaemic heart disease, left ventricular hypertrophy, incomplete left bundle branch block and anterior myocardial infarction (see figure). The uncorrected map shows at the time point T1, about 40ms after the beginning of QRS, activation in the lower part of the map beside the midaxillary line, marked with the 4. The undoubted activation of the inferior region at the time point T1 is better demonstrated in the corrected amplitude-map. We also see that a region of the lateral and posterior wall is activated (cipher 4). If the activation in the left chamber runs from the apex to the base the corrected map shows at the time points T2 (65ms) and T3 (90ms) higher potentials at the back positions of electrodes as the not corrected map. The LVH is better represented. The infarct region is especially shown in the difference map at the electrode points 5,3;5,4;6,3;6,4. Other negative values are in balance with positive values caused by hypertrophy. We hope that the combination of the demonstrated different methods of map analysis raises its contents.

(*) Frank, E.: An accurate clinically practical system for spatial vectorcardiography.
Circulation 13, 737-749 (1956)

System for clinical mapping and modelling the heart generator.

TYŠLER M., ROSÍK V., TURZOVÁ M.

Institute of Measurement and Measuring Technique, Electro-Physical Research Centre, Slovak Academy of Sciences, 842 19 Bratislava, Czechoslovakia.

Summary

Kardiomat system based on PDP-11 compatible personal computer with measuring subsystem expansible up to 64 channels enables to measure 24-lead ECG, standard 12-lead ECG or VCG. The amplifiers with bad electrode contact indication, controlled gain and selectable frequency response ensure good signal quality. The modular software includes packages for input of personal patient data, ECG measurements, body surface potential mapping, modelling the electric generator and the excitation of the heart. All results can be presented using color graphic display or graphic printer. Additional PDP-11 software for 12-lead ECG and VCG analysis can be run.

Introduction

The aim of the work was to develop a practical measuring and processing system for clinical electrocardiology which could make possible to use the classical computerized ECG and VCG classifications along with some new methods based on body surface potential mapping and, at the same time, to use the system for additional studies in electrocardiological research and clinic.

Material and methods

The hardware of the system consists of two basic parts: analog multichannel measuring unit and the microcomputer.

Electronic circuits of the measuring unit are segmented into several pluggable modules. This structure enables adjustment of the hardware to the demands of particular use.

The KZ-1 module implements standard limb leads I, II, III, aVR, aVL, aVF along with the signal of Wilson central terminal W. In addition, the module contains a circuitry for active neutralization through the right leg (N). The HZ-1 module picks up and processes signals from 8 chest leads. Use of several these modules enables to expand the system up to 64 channels (leads). Each measuring channel of the modules KZ-1 or HZ-1 contains an input buffer amplifier followed by a differential 3-OPA instrumentation amplifier in such way, that the resultant voltage gain is 1000. Modules also contain circuits for active shielding of the patient cables and for indication of bad electrode contact.

Signals from the KZ-1 and HZ-1 modules are fed to 16 channel controlled amplifier, sample/hold and multiplexer modules MP-1. The gain is digitally controlled in 4 steps. Outputs of all MP-1 modules are connected and fed to the A/D converter.

The measuring channels have input resistance 1000 M Ohm, discriminant factor (without active neutralisation) 100 dB and maximal frequency range 0.05-1000 Hz (-3 dB).

The microcomputer based on PDP-11 compatible 16-bit processor includes keyboard, color monitor (256x256 points, 8 colors), two floppy disc drives and a matrix printer with graphics. The measuring unit is connected with the microcomputer using laboratory interface card.

The device is designed as a mobile table, on which the display, keyboard and the printer are placed. All other modules are in two cabinets (computer unit and analog measuring unit) under the table.

The modular application software implemented in the device is running under RT-11 operating system. Severals levels of menu enable users to specify desired function area (program units). At this time the following programs are available:

ECG measurement programs enable to measure standard 12-lead ECG (2.5 s record, 2 ms sampling period), Frank VCG (10 s record, 2 ms sampling period) and 24-lead ECG for mapping (2.5 s record, 2 or 4 ms sampling period). The programs enable also input of the patient data, check of the measuring subsystem, graphical presentation of the measured signals and automatic or semiautomatic determination of the basic ECG time parameters. Measured data files are formatted corresponding to the ECG classification and mapping program requires.

Program for body surface potential mapping involves the computation of the 150-point body surface potential map frames in selected time instants of the cardiac cycle. The estimation of the 150 point map frames using 24 measured leads is based on the method reported by Barr et al. (1) and is described by the matrix equation

$$\mathbf{W} = \mathbf{H}\ \mathbf{V}$$

where $\mathbf{W}$ is the 150x1 vector of estimated potentials, $\mathbf{H}$ is the 150x24 transformation matrix, determined by the least square method using a large groupe of subject, and $\mathbf{V}$ is the 24x1 vector of potential, measured at 24 optimally selected leads.

Program for isointegral mapping performs the computation and mapping of the body surface potential integrals over selected time intervals $\langle T_1, T_2 \rangle$. Integral p_i of potential $u_i(t)$ at i-th chest surface site

$$p_i = \int_{T_2}^{T_1} u_i(t)\, dt \ , \qquad i = 1,2,\ldots 150$$

is computed by means of trapezoid rule.

Programs for graphical output provide the display or graphical printout of the measured ECG signals (in selected scales and time intervals) and of the resultant potential and integral map frames in several modes (single map frame or group of them, using isolines or color surfaces). All figures are supplemented with basic identification text and parameter description.

Other supportinng programs enable the print-out of the measurement protocol, computed parameters and map tables, storing the patient personal data in small data base and calibration and testing of the system.

Results

The first experience and tests of the device show that it could be an economical and practical solution for both research and clinical use.

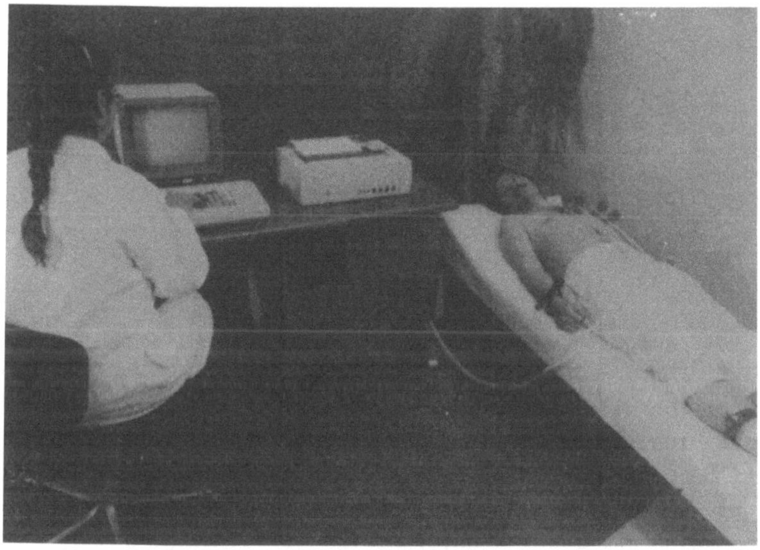

Fig. 1. Kardiomat system

Testing of the 24 lead mapping method on a group of subjects by means of comparing the total 150-point measurement maps and the maps estimated from 24 measured points gave the relative mean square error of 5.7 % and a correlation coefficient of 0.97 (average mean values for intervals, where rms signal $P > 0.1\ P_{max}$). The visual comparison showed good agreement for estimated and totally measured map frames.

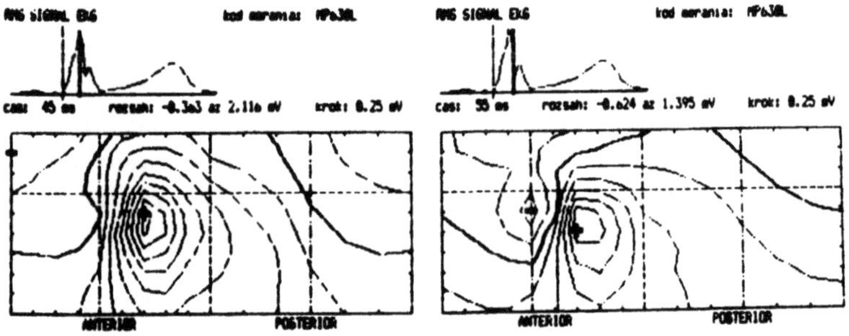

Fig. 2. Isopotential map frame samples for patient with myocardial infarction

Discussion and conclusions

The concept of KARDIOMAT device based on professional personal computer with the measuring unit specially designed for medical purposes and completed with appropriate application software makes the device a versatile tool for electrocardiological research and clinic. Using the same hardware, the other useful methods for patient examination or monitoring might be added according to the demands of the users. Software for modelling the electrical heart generator and heart surface excitation sequence, based on multipole model reported by Tyšler et al. (2), is under development. Implementation of Minnesota code and Pipberger program for ECG and VCG classification is expected. Possibility of using of Kardiomat system in magnetocardiographic research is also taken into consideration.

References

(1) Barr, R.C., Spach, M.S., Herman-Giddens, G.S.: IEEE Trans. biomed. Eng., BME-18, 125-138. (1971).

(2) Tyšler, M., Kužmová, J., Kneppo, P., Rosík, V., Kričfaluši, M.: Electrocardiology ´83. Proceedings of the 10th Intern. Congress on Electrocardiology, 160-163 (Excerpta Medica 1984).

How to image the differences between CEF-norm and actual condition of cardiac electric field using threedimensional isopotential maps without colour graphics ?

SLAVKOVSKÝ, P.; HULÍN, I.

Computing Centre, Slovak Academy of Sciences, Bratislava, Czechoslovakia
Medical School, Comenius University, Bratislava, Czechoslovakia

Mapping provides several types of maps which express the condition of cardiac electric field /CEF/. Isopotential, isointegral and isochronal maps express this condition in a form of surface. We describe the construction of these maps in our consideration with three possibilities of graphical representation of the surface: threedimensional, contour and character representation. One of the main problems in mapping is to make the CEF-norm /standard/ for values of these maps. CEF-norm will determine such parts of surface which express a normal condition of CEF and which must be represented graphically. We present the method of graphicall representation of parts of surface which are in or out of the CEF-norm for threedimensional isopotential maps with noncolour vector output.

1. Map classification with graphicall representation of maps

In our case mapping is based on following facts: 30 electrodes are placed on the chest of a person; the space surface is constructed from values of electrodes using interpolation method; the space surface is represented graphically. The space surface of CEF is represented by matrix of n x m values over the rectangular grid. This matrix is a numerical product of interpolation method. In our case the dimensions of matrix are: n=51, m=55. Using different methods for choosing of values of electrodes in one cardiac cycle the construction of three types of maps is possible. Isopotential map express the condition of CEF at a certain moment of one cardiac cycle i.e. for every electrode the value of electric potential at a certain moment is considered. Isointegral map express a quantity of electric potential produced by heart at a certain time interval $\langle t_1, t_2 \rangle$ i.e. for every electrode the value of definite integral at interval $\langle t_1, t_2 \rangle$ from values of electric potentials is considered. Isochronal map express course of a certain value of potential at time and at space i.e. for every electrode such time value from time interval $\langle t_1, t_2 \rangle$ is considered at which first time appears the considered value of electric potential. Each of defined maps provides specific information about the condition of CEF. These maps can be represented graphically in three ways: as a threedimensional map with perspective projection; as a contour map with contour lines; as a character map with character representation of values. Threedimensional map: The space surface, represented as matrix over the rectangular grid, is transformed to plane projection using perspective projection. The method of hidden line elimination is applied to obtain realistic resulting output. Contour map: It represents the space surface in a form of contours. Contour is a special set of points of surface which have the equal value of z-coordinate. The number of contours and their z-coordinates can be choosen arbitrary. Threedimensional and contour maps requires special devices for graphical output. Character map: The transformation of matrix values of surface into character matrix is the basic step for generating character map. The interval of values is divided into ranges and choosen characters are determined for every range. For every value of matrix the coresponding range of values and the character of this range is determined. Then the writting of character matrix is made using alphanumeric printer. The character representation does not require special devices for graphical output. Figure 1 provides example of isopotential map with threedimensional and contour representation in perspective view. The graphical outputs can be made using software products which were developed and implemented in Computing Centre of Slovak Academy of Sciences. The computing was carried out on the computer EC1045 and the graphical outputs on plotter DIGIGRAF.

2. CEF-norm and threedimensional isopotential maps /noncolour output/

We assume that the CEF-norm is known: for each time value of cardiac cycle for isopotential map it is determined with upper boundary matrix and bottom boundary matrix which represents the upper surface and the bottom surface of the CEF-norm /see Fig.3/. For arbitrary isopotential map only such parts of map are in the CEF-norm which are situated between upper boundary surface and bottom boundary surface. I.e. element a_{ij} of matrix $A=(a_{ij})$ of arbitrary isopotential map is in the CEF-norm when $a_{ij} \in \langle b_{ij}, u_{ij} \rangle$, where $B=(b_{ij})$ is the bottom boundary matrix and $U=(u_{ij})$ is the upper boundary matrix /i=1,2,...,51; j=1,2,...,55/. The element a_{ij} is over the CEF-norm if $a_{ij} > u_{ij}$ holds; element a_{ij} is under the CEF-norm if $a_{ij} < b_{ij}$ holds. This differences must be represented graphically. Using colour graphics devices we can determine: the first set of colours for parts of surface in the CEF-norm; the second set of colours for parts over the CEF-norm; the third set of colours for parts under the CEF-norm. The case of noncolour outputs is more complicated. Noncolour vector output on Figure 1 is represented with two types of edges: cross-edges which are parallel to yz plane and along-edges which are parallel to xz plane /x,y,z are coordinate axes, where y has the same direction as the longer side of surface and x has the same direction as the shorter side of surface/. Now we describe two principles for graphical representation of edges of surface which realize the differences between parts over, in or under the CEF-norm:
1. Only if both end-points of cross-edge are in or over the CEF-norm cross-edge is drawn; 2. Only if both end-points of along-edge are in or under the CEF-norm along-edge is drawn. In these way on the resulting

graphical output three types of region of surface are possible: 1. The over-region contains only cross-edges and represents part of surface over the CEF-norm; 2. The under-region contains only along-edges and represents part of surface under the CEF-norm; 3. The normal-region contains both types of edges and represents part of surface in the norm. We can see these regions on Figure 2 which contains threedimensional isopotential map with perpendicular projection of surface into the xy plane to better see the placing of regions on the surface. In this way we can obtain the noncolour vector output with parts of surface which are in, over or under the CEF-norm.

Nowadays two main problems in mapping are: 1. The construction of portable device based on personal computer with uniform number of electrodes, their uniform placing and with uniform interpolation method; 2. The construction of CEF-norm /standard/ for doing diagnosis. The solving of these problems will speed up the application of mapping.

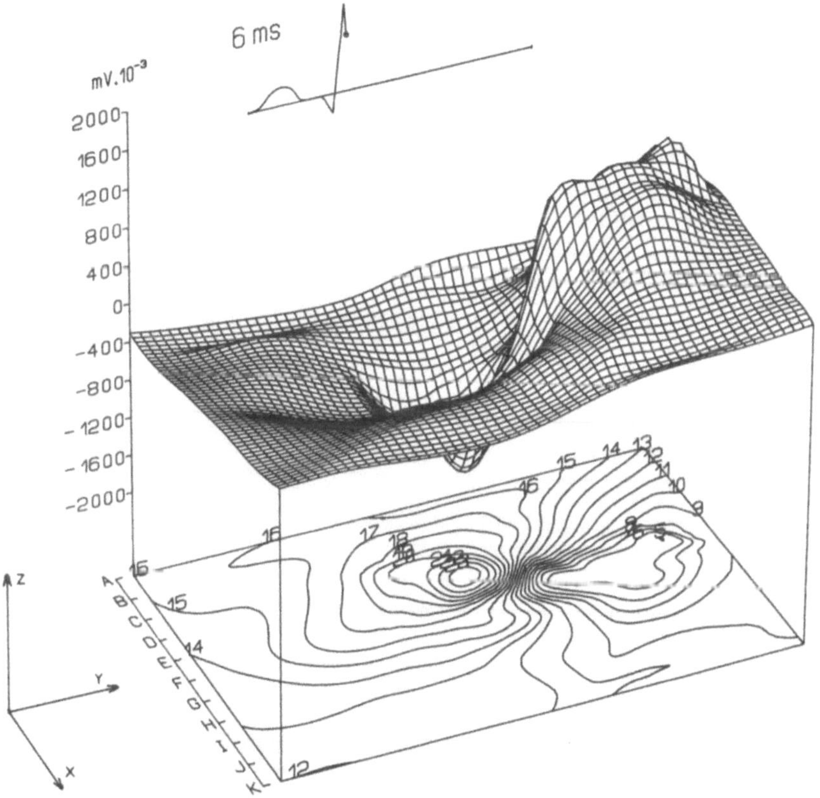

Figure 1 : Isopotential map at 6 milisecond with threedimensional and contour representation in perspective view .

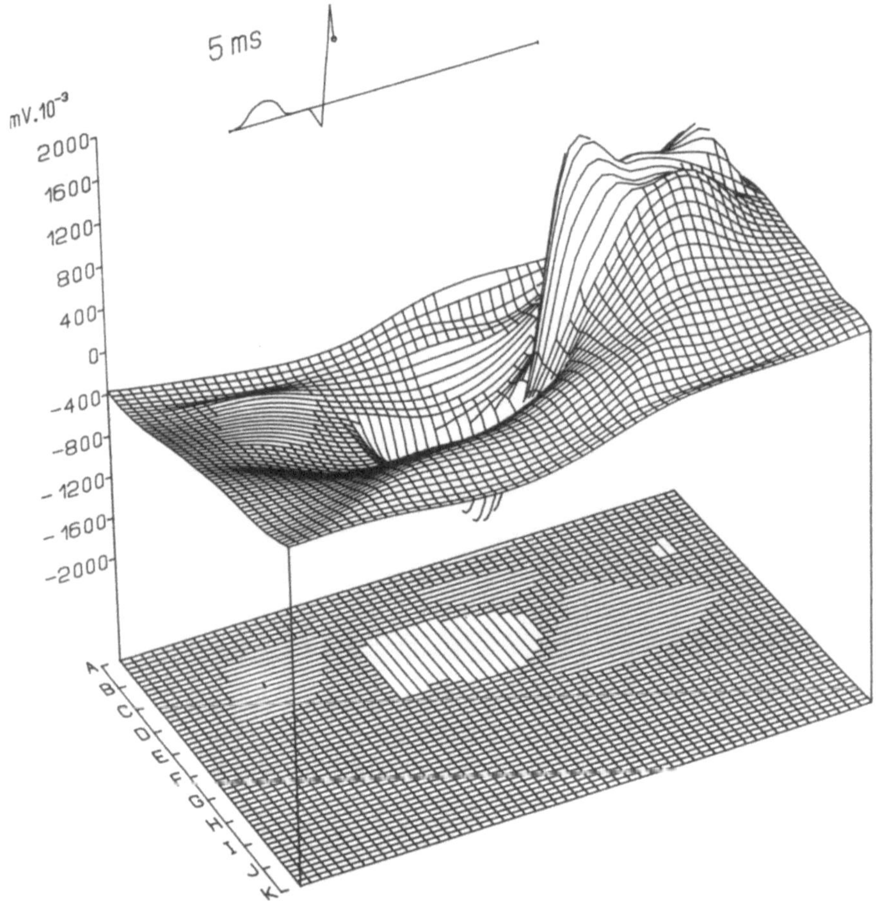

Figure 2 : Threedimensional isopotential map at 5 milisecond with perpendicular projection of surface into the xy plane and with regions of surface which are : in the CEF-norm, over the CEF-norm or under the CEF-norm .

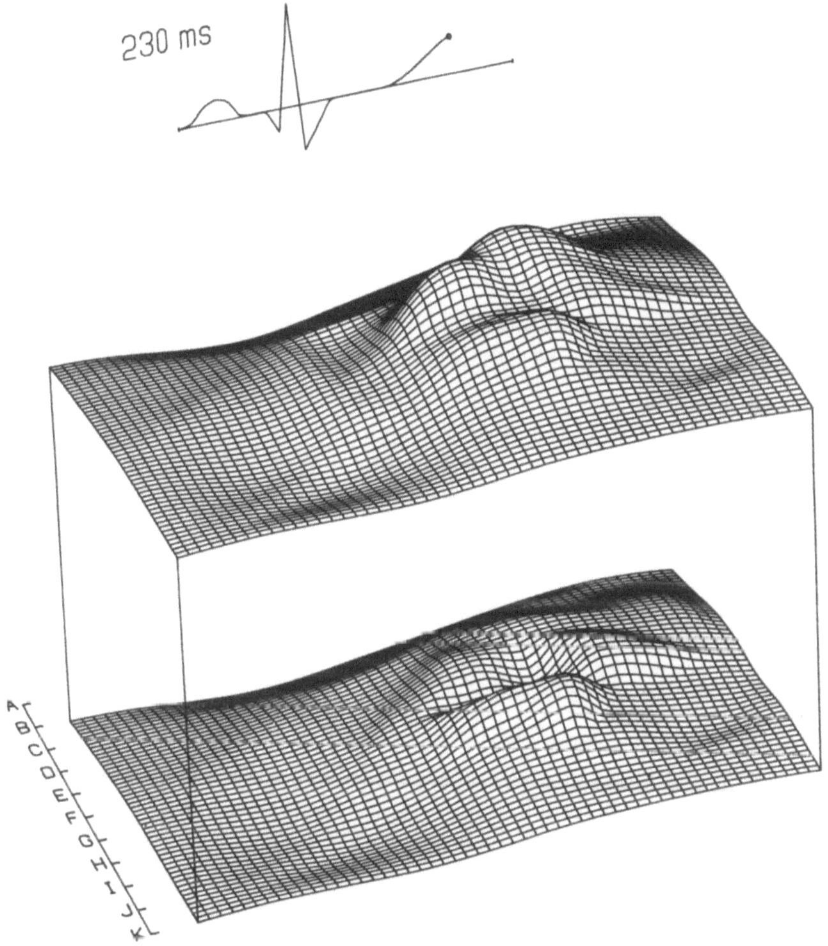

Figure 3 : The upper boundary surface and the bottom boundary surface of the CEF-norm for threedimensional isopotential map at 230 milisecond /the distance between both boundary surfaces is enlarged/ .

A BSPM Infrastructure: Product Description and Applications

Y.CHRISTOPHE, G.DE GEEST, P.DELMOITIE, E.NYSSEN, P.REYGAERT, A.PLETINCKX, I.SANSENS, P. DE MUYNCK, P.BLOCK, J.CORNELIS
Vrije Universiteit Brussel (VUB); Electronics dept. ETRO; Cardiovascular Research Unit HART
Pleinlaan 2 B-1050 Brussels
Belgium

Summary

This paper presents the hardware (acquisition, storage and display) and the software (data processing, data analysis, mathematical modeling) infrastructure for Body Surface Potential Mapping developed at our university. An overview of the features of both the acquisition equipment and the software will be given with emphasis on the user viewpoint.

A microprogrammable ECG data-logger designed in order to fulfil the many needs of an electrocardiographic research environment is presented. Its global architecture and the main specifications of each module are discussed.

A software package (running under UNIX 4.3BSD) has been designed on the basis of the same principles of modularity and versatility. This software can handle different types of maps (thoracic, hemi-thoracic, local,...) of various signals (XECG, high frequency activity,...); it supports comparative studies between measured maps and results from modeling studies, it generates body surface potential images and allows statistical data analysis.

Introduction

In the domain of multi-electrode data logging for biomedical signals, various system design strategies are possible (Delmoitie et al.):

1) a single processor for the acquisition control, the signal processing, the system supervision and the communication with the user
2) a custom hardware controlling the acquisition, microprogrammed and supervised by a general purpose workstation

The advantages of the first approach are a minimal amount of hardware and good acquisition versatility due to the full software control; the main drawback is the strongly limited data acquisition rate. The advantages of the second approach are a good acquisition versatility ensured by the microprogrammability of the controller, enhanced performances in data rate and sampling accuracy due to the decoupling of data processing and acquisition. Since the equipment is intended to be used in a clinical research environment in various applications involving biomedical signals with different amplitude and spectral characteristics (e.g. mapping of late potentials, ECG mapping during excercise, comparative studies between various biosignals,...),the main design aims are: high performance, good reconfigurability, modularity allowing the assembly of simplified versions for specific applications. Therefore design strategy 2 was choosen.

The software includes :

1) a package for the processing of BSPM's containing two main BSPM visualisation options:
   .the classical graphical display (isopotential lines)
   .a sequence of pseudo-coloured images which highlights the dynamic aspects of the evolution of the spatial potential distribution throughout the cardiac cycle
2) a package for mathematical modeling.

This software is running under the UNIX operating system on a VAX785 computer. It is possible to implement large fractions of this software on the acquisition equipment itself to constitute a powerful modular infrastructure for cardiological units, wanting to introduce BSPM's in their clinical or research activities.

Material and methods

A. The hardware (Christophe et al.):

The equipment for BSPM acquisition, storage, (processing), and display (figure 1) consists of four main parts

1) the data logger module (DLM)

2) the visualisation module

3) the workstation

4) the ECG signal conditioning block (SCB).

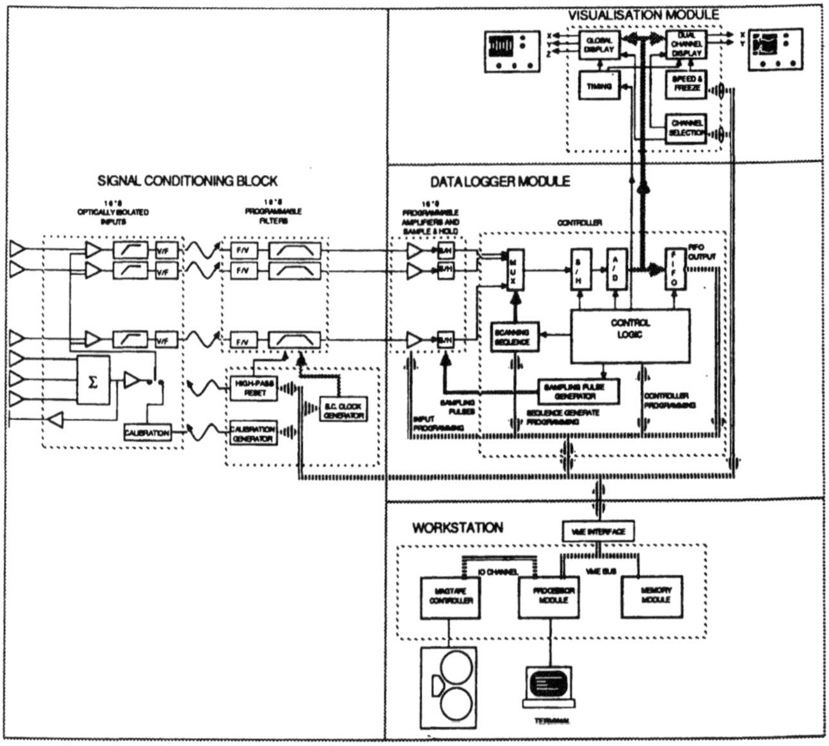

figure 1: Global overview of the acquisition equipment

1) The data logger module (DLM):

The DLM is a general purpose analog signal acquisition module primarily designed to be the intelligent slave of a versatile workstation based on a standard bussystem (VME). This approach allows configurability of the complete system on 2 levels:

- system configurability: Both on- and off-line data processing and storage can be realised by appropriate assembly of commercially available VME modules. The VME bus allows multiprocessing configurations.
- acquisition configurability: DLM settings may be programmed (number of input channels, and for each channel, gain and sampling frequency), and even external devices can be programmed through the DLM, for example the filter settings in the SCB, which is especially designed for ECG applications.

2) The visualisation module:

This module generates a graphical display of the incoming signals. In a global overview of the 128 input channels the instantaneous value of the amplitude is shown as a function of the channel number. This type of representation is suited to a fast and global control of the recordings. For a more detailed evaluation, a second graphical display is provided showing the incoming signal of two selectable input channels.

3) The signal conditioning block (SCB):

In order to improve the signal to noise ratio, especially during the recording of XECG's, Ag-AgCl electrodes with built in buffers (active electrodes) are appropriate. It is valuable in BSPM to attach the electrodes to velcro strips: it improves application speed, positioning accuracy and it reduces the probability of electrode misplacement while still allowing the use of different spatial sampling strategies on the thorax. The input pre-amplifiers are fairly classic: potentials are referenced to the Central Terminal of Wilson. A floating-patient circuit is obtained by isolation through optical fibers. The high cost of commercially available precision isolation amplifiers led us to design our own. The advantage of using long optical fibers is that the floating circuitry can be separated physically from the non-isolated equipment. The ECG filters have a low pass section with programmable cut off frequency, to allow a change in sampling mode without aliasing problems. Provisions are made for completely automatic calibration and diagnosis of the SCB and DLM steered by the workstation.

4)The workstation

The workstation may be any general purpose VME based microcomputer system. Its actual configuration is shown on figure 1. It is connected to a magtape unit providing mass storage facilities. Continuous storage of a 32 ksample/s data stream during a period of 10 minutes is possible. Memory modules in the workstation provide temporary buffering for higher rate data streams. The software for the communication with the operator and the programming of the sampling and visualisation parameters is an autonomous package, residing in the ROM memory of the workstation. It includes a menu-driven interface with the operator (setup of the acquisition and visualisation parameters, addition of comments to the recordings). The software provides a specific and protected environment for each user depending on the application domain and his qualification. All the information concerning the acquired signals including time pointers, acquisition settings and comments are stored together with the measurement data.

B.The software (De Geest et al.)

The software includes two packages:

1) a package for the processing of BSPM's
2) a package for modeling

1) Processing of BSPM's

ECG data coming from various equipments or research institutes are first converted to obtain a standardised storage of the signals (one mean or representative systole, pointers to relevant events on the acquired signals, identification data). The software package provides low pass or 50Hz notchfiltering and resampling at various frequencies. As the number of input signals and the sampling frequencies are arbitrary, the internal standard can handle various types of measurement data. The potential distribution is described by the values of the potentials on the vertices of a regular rectangular grid on which the electrode positions on the thorax are mapped. Since the electrode positions correspond to a subset of these vertices, the conversion of the measurement data to a description of the potential distribution requires some 2-D interpolation procedure. The 2 methods (Nyssen et al.) for this interpolation are based on a description of the electrode configuration and they take into account missing or faulty electrodes. Finally the software package includes programs to generate equipotential maps and potential images (Cornelis et al.), and it allows the creation of files for a statistical processing package.

2) Modeling

This software package includes the generation of triangulated surfaces and the design of a complete piecewise homogeneous, isotropic, non dispersive and linear electrical model of a volumeconductor. It implements a method for the solution of the forward potential problem (Lynn et al.): for an arbitrary source model the potential in internal points or points on the boundaries of homogeneous subregions are calculated. The software package also allows the computation of multipole moments of an arbitrary distribution of point sources and sinks generating the ECG signals. It implements a method for the inverse potential problem: the estimation of multipole moments from the ECG distribution (Geselowitz et al.).

Results

A summary of the specifications of the acquisition equipment is given in the following tables.

• DLM specifications	
Synchronous sampling	
MAX. NO. OF CHANNELS	128
NO. OF BITS AFTER ADC	12
MAX. DATA TROUGHPUT	256 ksamples/s
PER CHANNEL:	8 programmable gains
	choice out of 16 sampling frequencies

SCB specifications			
Active electrodes			
Floating input circuitry			
REFERENCE POTENTIAL	Wilson central terminal		
CMRR (50Hz)	with reinjection		≥100dB
	without reinjection		≥70dB
FILTER CHARACTERISTICS	low cut-off freq. f_{e1} (3dB point)		0.01 Hz
	high cut-off freq. f_{e2}		50-200 Hz
	fase linearity (f_{e1} to $0.9f_{e2}$)		>± 1%
	Amplitude characteristics	60dB point	$2.36f_{e2}$
		ripple in passband	<2%
LINEARITY	±0.5%		
SIGNAL-NOISE RATIO	±57dB		
GAIN	1000±5		

The software includes waveform recognition, generation of isopotential maps, synthesis of dynamic sequences of grey scale or pseudo-colour potential images on standard image processing equipment, a connection for generating input for statistical packages (e.g. BMDP). Moreover it allows mathematical modeling including forward and inverse solutions based on a multipolar heart model.The format of model generated maps is compatible with measured ones.The software developed for these studies is running under UNIX(4.3 BSD) on the VAX 785 infrastructure of the medical informatics dept. (MINF) and is available on request, as well as a documentation of the infrastructure.

Discussion and conclusions

We believe that the equipment and the portable program packages guarantee the feasibility of introducing the infrastructure in any technical research environment or clinical unit. The signal processing and analysis software is largely independent of the choice of the lead configuration (max 128 leads), and of the choice of the sampling frequencies (maximum total throughput 256kHz). The versatility of the acquisition settings (channel dependent gain, filtersetting, sampling frequency) allows a large range of applications.

The infrastructure is now used in studies involving normal male subjects, patients suffering from angina pectoris and CAD (demonstrated by coronary arteriography) with abnormal or normal 12-lead ECG. Several BSPM's were also recorded in patients with acute anterior, posterior inferior LVMI and RV involvement.

References

(1) P.Delmoitie, J.Cornelis, Y.Christophe, E.Nyssen, O.Steenhaut: 3-Tagung Elektronik - Technologie "Applikation mikro- und optoelektronischer Systemelemente", pp.19-25. Humboldt Universität, Berlin, DDR,(1985).

(2) Y.Christophe, J.Cornelis, G.De Geest, E.Nyssen, P.Delmoitie, P.Reygaert, P.Block: Advances in cardiology - Proc. 11th Internat. Congress on Electrocardiology, pp. 126-128. Centre de publications de l'université de Caen, France (1985).

(3) G. De Geest, J.Cornelis, E.Nyssen, Y.Christophe, P.Reygaert, P.Block: Computers in Cardiology, Boston, USA, (1986).

(4) E.Nyssen, J.Cornelis, M.Nyssen,Y.Christophe, L.Huyghens, and P.Block: Computers in Cardiology, Seatle, USA, (1982).

(5) J.Cornelis, E.Nyssen, M.Nyssen, Y.Christophe, P.Block, O.Steenhaut: SPIE 397, pp 288, 293,(1983).

(6) M.S.Lynn and W.P.Timlake: Publication 37.017, IBM Data Processing Division (Houston) (1978).

(7) D.B.Geselowitz: Proc.IRE, 48, pp. 75-79 (1960).

Spread of the atrial activation on the chest surface in healthy girls

POPPEROVÁ, E., HULÍN, I., SABOLOVÁ, K., MACO, M., TURZOVÁ, M., TYŠLER, M.

Department of Clinical Pathophysiology, School of Medicine, Comenius University, Bratislava, Czechoslovakia

Summary

Atrial activation sequences using ECG body surface isopotential mapping were studied in two groups of healthy girls in the age about 9 and 14 years. The oblique and vertical type of atrial activation patterns on the anterior chest have been recognized. The obtained results suggest suitability of the body surface mapping method in study the atrial activation developmental changes.

Introduction

The evolving techniques of ECG body surface mapping require development of adequate methods for their evaluation. In this respect we have studied ECG body surface isopotential maps generated during the atrial activation in pubertal age children. Our aim was to search for the physiological characteristisc of the atrial activation from the developmental point of wiev.

In our contribution we present some of our preliminary results obtained by studying the atrial activation in healthy pubertal girls.

Material and methods

Atrial activation sequences have been recorded and evaluated in two groups of healthy girls, consisting of nine and eight girls in age about 9 and 14 years, respectively. Their normal health condition was defined on the base of their medical history, general physical examination including 12-lead ECG and M-mode echocardiogram. The atrial activation potentials on the body surface have been recorded by electrocardiocoordinatorgraph EKKG-80 (Kneppo et al, 1979) in the proband sitting position while in apnea in expiration phase. A set of 19 electrodes is fixed on a cylindric frame which moves computer controlled along the chest in vertical direction. ECG signals are recorded in ten horizontal planes according to the spatial parameters of the chest. The sensed signals are being fed into the computer and subsequently processed.

The sequence of isopotential maps was plotted for each 10 ms with 50 μV steps between isopotential lines. The resulting atrial activation maps were evaluated at the P-wave peak and two 10 ms instances before and after it.

Results

The proband physical examination showed no significant differences between two age groups except, as it was expected, in the older girls significantly higher antropometric values and echocardiographic parameters have been found. Inspite of that, the observation of the atrial activation in body surface maps showed no significant difference in regard to the age difference of both groups. The detailed evaluation of the map parameters led to the similar results. The only significant difference has been obtained in the time interval between the P-wave onset and its peak, in average it was 52,6 ms and 40,4 ms in older and younger groups, respectively.

The map analysis showed that in both groups alike oblique and vertical types of atrial activation can be recognized in regard to the localization and migration of potential maxima and minima and the orientation of the zero potential line separating the fields of positive and negative potentials. In the first type (fig. 1) the activation is propagated on the anterior chest obliquely from upper right down to the left and the zero potential line tends to have the oblique direction from down-right up to the left.

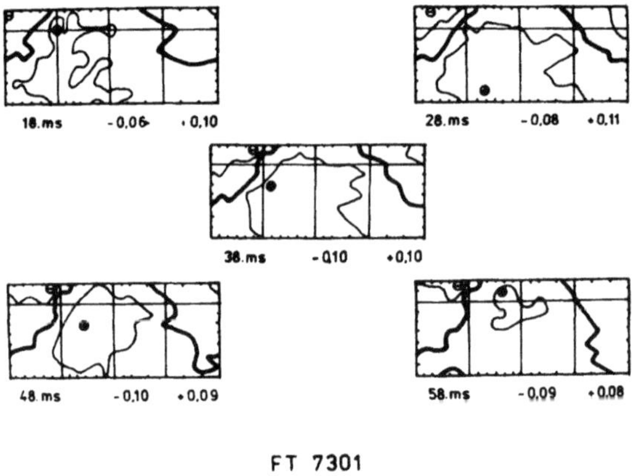

Fig. 1. The oblique type of atrial activation in healthy girl (FT 7301)

In the vertical type (fig. 2) the propagation is top-down and at or just next to the P-wave peak it turns to the left. In this type the zero potential line tends to be horizontal till the P-wave peak or just next to it and since then it takes form as in the oblique type. The oblique activation type was found in 6, while the vertical one in 11 cases regardless the age. During the activation spread on the anterior chest in both age groups the negative potential

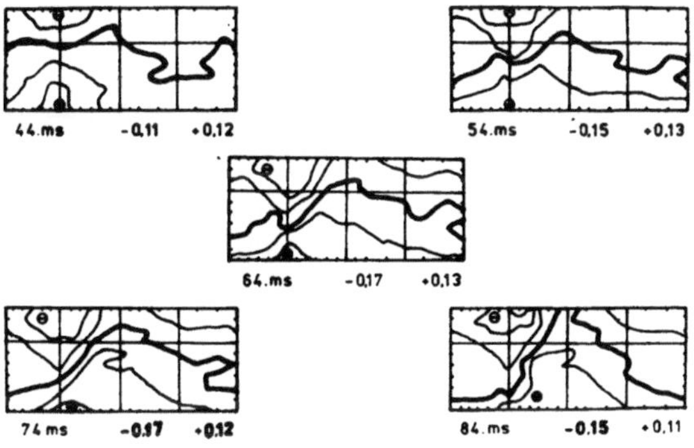

FT 7201

Fig. 2. The vertical type of atrial activation in healthy girl (FT 7201)

area has been extending on account of the positive potential area. We have also found that maps had dipolar character, however, in one 9 years old girl two potential maxima occured.

Discussion and conclusions

From the results of several authors who studied the atrial activation (Taccardi, 1966; Kawano et al, 1983; Stilli et al, 1983) it is possible to infer that this activation in healthy adult subjects is of the oblique type. We have found the oblique type of activation in our probands as well, however, the described vertical type was found in prevailing cases. This can be presumably ascribed to differing properties of the atrial activation in healthy children due to cardial and extracardial factors. The departure from dipolar body surface maps in one 9 years old girl could be due to the shorter distance between the heart and the chest. Similar results have been reported by Spach et al (1966) in ventricular activation study in children. However, for reliable results our study must be further extended. For this purpose we have already examined boys of the same age groups and the respective data are now under processing. We expect the obtained results will contribute to the elucidation of the atrial activation developmental characteristics in healthy children.

References

(1) Kneppo, P., V. Rosík and M. Tyšler: Progress in Electrocardiology, Pitman Medical Press, Glasgow, 212-214 (1979)

(2) Taccardi, B.: Circ. Res. 19, 865 - 878 (1966)

(3) Kawano, S., T. Sawanobori, and M. Hiraoka: J. Electrocardiol. 16, 151 - 160 (1983)

(4) Stilli, D., E. Musso, P. Barone, P. Ciarlini, A. Giuspini, E. Macchi, G. Regoliosi, and B. Taccardi: In Advances in Body Surface Potential Mapping, edited by K. Yamada, K. Harumi, T. Musha. Nagoya, The University Nagoya Press, 195 - 200 (1983)

(5) Spach, M.S., W.P. Silberberg, J.P. Boineau, R.C, Barr, E.C. Long, T.M. Gallie, J.B. Gabor, and A.G. Wallace: Am. Heart J. 72, 640 - 652 (1966)

Application of a bedside Microcomputer System for ECG Mapping after Myocardial Infarction

KNORRE,M.,KNORRE,H.,WIECHMANN,V.,ASSMANN,I.,KASSEL,P.and PORSTMANN,I.

Medical Academy of Erfurt, Nordhaeuser Str.74, 5010 Erfurt,GDR

1. Summary

A flexible microcomputer-based mapping system "MAP 100" for clinical and experimental conditions was developed. Special hardware and software permit the on-line data acquisition and analysis at the patients bedside. The results are represented on a colour graphic display and can be stored at floppy disk for further documentation and classification. First of all the mapping system is used for the praecordial ST-mapping after myocardial infarction. The estimation and alteration of ischemic area was observed of patients with anterior myocardial infarction. The coloured isopotential maps based on measured ST-levels from 35 ECG leads were compared with the CK-release and other clinical data.

2. Introduction

In general use the diagnosis of acute myocardial infarction and it's progress is founded mainly on the valuation of the CK-release and the electrocardiography. The method of multiple ECG registration and analysis gives additional information by using a higher number of electrodes than in conventional ECG leads and by calculating the distribution of electrical heart field. For cardiological diagnosis and monitoring an ECG mapping system can only gives advantages , if the method can be used with bedside data acquisition and analysis.

Therefore, we developed a mobile microcomputer mapping system which is applied at first in the Departement of Cardiology for estimation of ischemic area after acute myocardial infarction. The results and the variation of maps are compared with the course of the CK-release, with conventional ECG-leads and other clinical data.

3. Materials and methods

The flexibility of the microcomputer mapping system "MAP100" allows the connection of various electrode arrangements with a maximum of 100 electrodes. It's also possible to select the sampling rate (250Hz, 500Hz or 960Hz per channel), the signal resolution (8 or 10 bits) and the mode of map representation. This gives advantages in the experimental work.

The block diagramm of the "MAP 100" system is shown in figure 1. The analogue part consists of the arrangement of electrodes, the ECG amplifiers, the multiplexer and the high-speed AD-converters. The digitalized ECG signals are transfered to the digital part which has a Z 80 microcomputer as the central unit (CPU). This microcomputer interacts with an alphanumeric keyboard, with a floppy disk memory and a colour graphic display which has its own CPU and an additional 16 kByte memory.

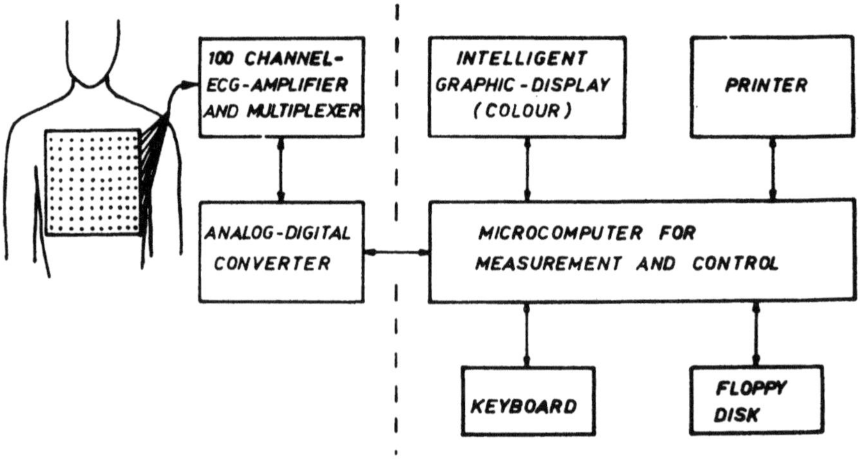

Figure 1: Blockdiagramm of "MAP100" system

At the beginning of data acquisition the user programm must be loaded by floppy disk and than the operator is guided through the procedure by the computer with "Yes" or "No" decisions.

For ST-mapping after myocardial infarction records from 35 praecordial sites are obtained. Fig.2 shows the placement of electrodes. To get a quick application and a good adjustment to the snape of thorax the 35 Ag/AgCl electrodes are assembled on a broad stretch bandage which has a flexible fastening and a sand bag is put on the praecordial thorax.The extremity leads RA, LL and LA are registrated additionally to form the Wilson-Central-Point for the unipolar EGC signals and to receive the Standard-II-lead as reference and for calculating the heart rate and RR-time interval. The Standard-II-lead and and all of unipolar surface leads are represented simultaneous on the display during the data acquisition for observing the quality of signals. About 20 seconds after interruption of recording the isopotential maps will be presented on the colour graphic display. For calculation of the ST-maps the ECG signals are sampled with 250 Hz per channel and the ST-levels are measured 100 ms

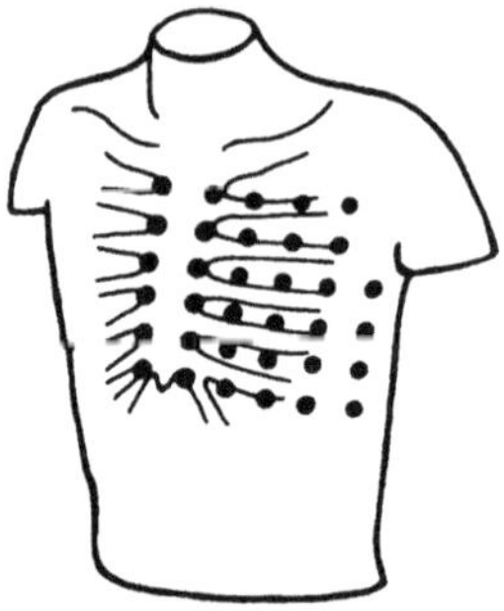

Fig.2:Electrodearrangement

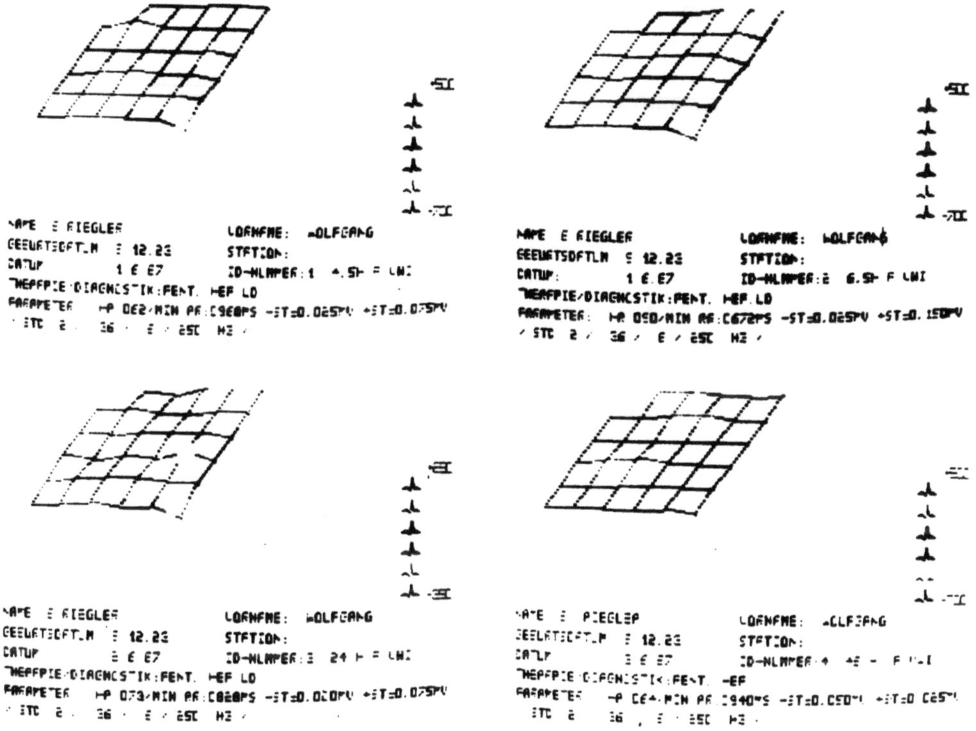

Figure 3:ST-maps of a 63 years old patient 4.5(a),6.5(b),24(c) and 48(d) hours after acute event

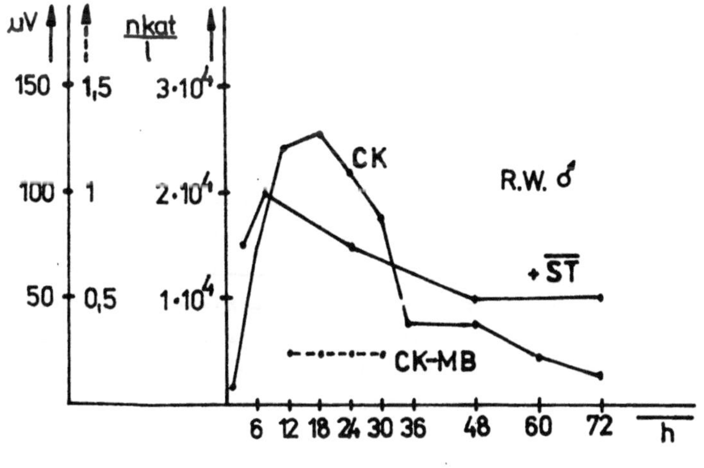

Figure 4: Course of CK-release and the mean ST-elevation of the same patient

after the maximum of R-wave. After correction according to the baseline shift the computer checks all ST-levels and automatically arranges the scale of colours for map construction. The maps can be displayed in 8 different colours and as 2- or 3-dimension pictures of coloured areas or coloured lines. The physician gets information about the mean ST-elevation and mean ST depression and about the number of surface leads which have ST-elevation or ST-depression.

In all patients with anterior myocardial infarction which were admitted to our coronary care unit within the first 6 hours after onset of pain was registrated a ST-map within the first hour of hospitalisation. Further measurements were carried out 6, 12, 24, 48 and 72 hours later. The displayed maps in regard of extent and distribution of the ST-elevations were compared with the CK-release, the therapeutic regime as well as the extent and place of coronary artery stenosis and the ejection fraction (angiographically) 1 to 3 months after the acute event.

4. Results

Up to now we have examined 12 patients with AMI. The inconvenience of the patients during the registration was small. In all patients we could record the maps in satisfactorily quality.

One example is shown in Figure 3. There are presented the ST-maps of a 63 years old man 4.5h, 6.5h, 24h and 48h after the acute event. The highest values of mean ST-segment elevation were present after 6 hours with a further decreasing till 72 hours. The maximum CK-release occured after 18 hours and after 60 hours normal values were reached. Comparing the course of mean ST-elevation and CK-release (Fig.4) we found out a large conformity. Till now the most of evaluated maps have correlated quite well with the other clinical data. However, significant differences between groups of patients with different medical managements have not yet be seen. Further measurements are nessecary, esp. the Q- and R-mapping for estimation of the infarct size.

5. Conclusions

Up to this day our results have shown, that the ST-segment mapping is a relatively suitable bedside method for estimation the extent of ischemia with only small trouble for the patient. In order to use the advantages of ECG mapping system for clinical practice the comparison of the maps with results of reference methods is nessecary. The ST-mapping after myocardial infarction with the "MAP 100" system gives us the first own experiences in the field of body surface mapping and will be the basis for enlargements of software for R- and Q- mapping to estimate the size of infarct too and for other clinical applications.

The Transfer Coefficient Unification Method for the Body Surface Potential Distribution Processing

DRŠKA, Z., VALOVÁ, D., MÁLKOVÁ, A.

Institute of Physiological Regulations, Czechoslovak Academy of Sciences, Bulovka, pav. 11, 180 85 Prague, Czechoslovakia

Summary

Studying the extracardiac factors influence on the heart electric field, the procedure enabled its unification influence on body surface potential distribution (BSPD) properties during the electrical systole was developed (Drška, Z.). This procedure does not require technically difficult and time consuming surface lead points coordinates measurement, which could be, moreover, the source of significant errors in resulting values.

Introduction: The differentiation of extracardiac factors influence on BSPD properties during the electrical systole seems to be for many years one of the basic problems of electrocardiology. A number of procedures solving the inverse problem for quasistationary field in volume conductor were developed (Forbes, A. D., Harumi, K. et al, Ruttkay-Nedecký, I. et al, Titomir, L. I.).

Materials and methods: The matrix of ECGs was synthetized from 3 orthonormal ECGs of Frank VCG system. Each matrix element was obtained by solution of 3 linear equations system using the least squares fit method. The relation between measured (VM(ijt)) and synthetized (VE(ijt)) ECGs can be expressed:

$$VM(ijt) = VE(ijt) + RES(ijt) - A(ij).x(t) + B(ij).y(t) + C(ij).z(t) + D(ij)$$

Following the multidipole as a equivalent source concept, ECGs synthetized from VCG orthonormal ECGs are interpreted as ECGs of dominant dipolar component of equivalent multidipole. Difference between measured and synthetized signals is interpreted as a sum of other dipolar equivalent source components ("non-dipolar residuum" - RES(ijt)).

By normalization of these coefficients corresponding to x,y,z VCG orthonormal ECG components for each element of ECG matrix (Drška, Z.) the extracardiac factors influence on the BSPD properties during electrical systole is possible to unify.

Using this normalization, where

$$K(ij) = 1/\sqrt{A(ij)^2 + B(ij)^2 + C(ij)^2},$$

the above mentioned equation is transformed to the equation:

$$VEk(ijt) = a(ij).x(t) + b(ij).y(t) + c(ij).z(t) + d(ij),$$ where

$a(ij) = A(ij).K(ij)$; $b(ij) = B(ij).K(ij)$;

$c(ij) = C(ij).K(ij)$; $d(ij) = D(ij).K(ij)$, where

VEk(ijt) is the ECG of dominant dipolar component of equivalent source synthetized from x,y,z VCG orthonormal ECGs. Its amplitude corresponds to the unit value of transfer coefficient. Above mentioned fact proves validity of following equation:

VMK(ijt) = VM(ijt).K(ij) = VEk(ijt) + RES(ijt)

Results: Achieved results are demonstrated on the isopotential map after extracardiac factors influence unification and on the resulting map of sum of higher degree dipolar components of equivalent multidipole in healthy subject.

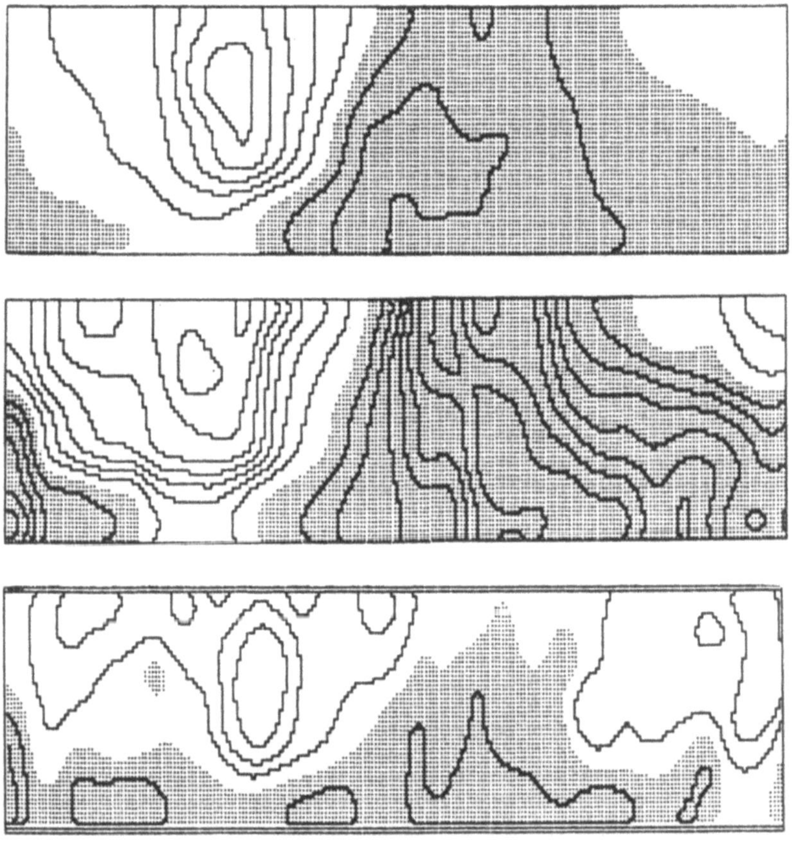

Fig. 1 - 3. Maps of isopotential lines of healthy subject from 50th ms of QRS: the map of measured BSPD on the chest surface (Fig. 1), the map of the same BSPD after its correction to the unit transfer coefficient surface (Fig. 2) and the map of resulting higher degree dipolar components sum (non-dipolar residuum) (Fig. 3). The isolines step is 230 uV in the first and the second map and 60 uV in the third map. Area of positive potential is shaded.

Discussion: Spatial orientation of corrected ECGs is identical with original ones from the body surface. This fact allows to visualize these corrected potential distributions on the surface that corresponds to original body surface isopotential maps projection plane, created by unrolled measured part of the chest surface. Used least squares fit method agrees with theoretically required total electroneutrality in potential field on equidistant surface.

Points in which the normalized ECGs are projected correspond to the end points of lead vectors in VCG system of axes. The radius vectors of these points have unit spatial amplitude. So, provided that Frank VCG system is orthonormal with sufficient precision, this spherical surface is concentric towards its origin point.

References:

(1) Drška, Z.: In: Abstracts of 13th Internat. Congr. on Electrocardiology, Washington, 90 (1986)
(2) Forbes, A. D.: Adv. Cardiol., 10, 199-208 (1974)
(3) Harumi, K. et al: In: Electrocardiographic Body Surface Mapping. Ed.: R. Th. van Dam, A. van Oosterom, Martinus Nijhof Publishers, Dordrecht et al, 283-288 (1986)
(4) Ruttkay-Nedecký, I. et al: Proc. of Conf, Biosignal 86, ČSVTS, DT Brno, 133-134 (1986)
(5) Titomir, L. I.: Avtomatičeskij analiz elektromagnitnovo polja serdca. Izdatelstvo Nauka, Moskva (1984)

Automatic QRS Onset Detection of BSPM by Spatial and Temporal Approach

GANG SUN, MS, CECIL W. THOMAS, PhD, RENNIE FRAENKEL, and JEROME LIEBMAN, MD

Biomedical Engineering Department
Case Western Reserve University
Cleveland, Ohio 44106, USA

SUMMARY: A new automatic algorithm, based on a spatial and temporal approach for detecting QRS onset in BSPM (Body Surface Potential Mapping) was developed. The new algorithm, along with three other algorithms (total energy, 3-lead and median), was tested in 73 normal and abnormal patients, and the results demonstrate the superior performance of the new algorithm. The new method is less sensitive to the noise, Ta of P wave, and the spatial location changes of QRS initial activation, and thus accurately detects the QRS onset.

INTRODUCTION: Recently developed BSPM techniques provide more information about the electrophysiological processes of human and animal hearts than in standard electrocardiography ECG or the orthogonal ECG (1,2,3). We find situations in which the BSPM data demonstrate events which are not evident in conventional ECG. Examples of such events are the right and left ventricular breakthrough, where the information lies in the spatial patterns and the relative timing of the events (1,3). These events are important, not just for their occurrence, but also for their timing after the QRS onset.

Previous techniques for determining the QRS onset basically utilized the one-dimensional ECG (4,5,6). In one dimensional ECG signals, the QRS onset can be defined as the point at which the signal changes from a constant level (zero slope) to a non-zero slope. A single lead or even a summation of multiple leads, may not detect onset correctly due to the effects of noise, artifact, and position variance of QRS initial activation of different patients and different diseases (4,5). We therefore developed a new QRS onset detection algorithm based on a spatial and temporal approach. Since the algorithm utilizes spatial and temporal information, it is invariant under location changes of QRS initial activation and less sensitive to the noise because the algorithm utilizes information in all three dimensions, i.e., spatial and temporal information.

MATERIAL and METHODS:

Data Acquisition and Preprocessing: see (1).

Patient Selection: Seventy three patients from age 5 to 43 with different cardiovascular diseases were included in this study, as listed in Table 1.

Table 1. Distribution of Selected Patients

Diseases	Number	Ages
Normal	30	20 - 43
Valvular AS	15	8 - 29
Other	28	5 - 30

QRS Onset Reference Selection: Two experienced investigators (RF and JL) determined the "reference onset time" for each patient by visual inspection of each patient's BSPM data.

Spatial and Temporal QRS Onset Detection Algorithm: By our observation, QRS initial activation begins with a small positive and/or a negative region, and then these regions grow larger and larger in both magnitude and region size. Movement of the maxima and minima within these expanding regions is minimal if at all. Our new algorithm takes advantage of this regional stability and first defines the QRS initial activation region. This step is critical because only that smaller region is used for the precise location of the QRS onset.

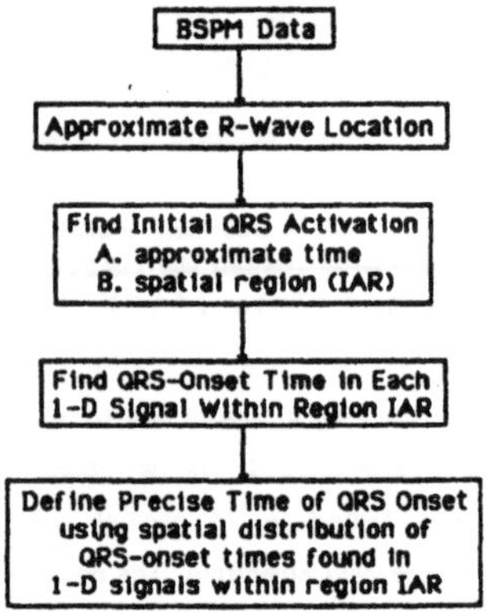

Figure 1. Flow chart of the spatial-temporal method for detecting QRS onset. (IAR - Initial Activation Region)

The algorithm (outlined in Figure 1) has three major steps:

Step #1: QRS initial activation region detection

1. Estimate the noise (NOISE) of the BSPM data by using a flat segment before the P-wave.
2. Find the total energy TE(i) of BSPM map verse time (i is the time index and the interval is 2 ms), i.e.:

$$TE(i) = \sum_{j=1}^{NE} p(j,i)^2$$

   where p(i,j) is the potential value of lead j at time i, and NE is the number of leads.
3. Find the maximum energy ME and its time MEL which is the approximate location of R-wave.
4. Find the trajectories of map maxima and minima, i.e., the locations of the maxima and the minima on the BSPM maps verses time, from MEL-49 to MEL, ie, over a total 100 ms.
5. Find the earliest segment (five consecutive maps) in which: a) the trajectory of the maxima and/or the trajectory of the minima does not change or only slightly changes, b) the potential increase along the trajectory exceeds a threshold, and c) the increase of region size exceeds a threshold.
6. Define the time of the middle map in the segment found in 5 as the approximate initial activation time (IAT) and the region of the fifth map in that segment as the initial activation region (IAR).

Step #2: Search backward from IAT for each lead j in IAR to find the ONSET of that lead. The ONSET in each lead is defined when the slope (time derivative)

$$2*p(ONSET,j) - (p(ONSET-1,j) + p(ONSET-2,j)) < NOISE/4$$

in a region of positive potentials, or when

$$(p(ONSET-1,j) + p(ONSET-2,j)) - 2*p(ONSET,j) < NOISE /4$$

in a region of negative potentials. This results in an activation onset timing map within the region IAR.

Step #3: Find the precise QRS onset time, which is defined as the time when at least two leads are at their onset time and at least two neighboring leads reach their onset time 2 to 4 ms later.

Other QRS Detection Methods:

For comparison, we used three other QRS detection algorithms on the same data. These methods are:

I. Total energy method:

1. Find the total energy TE(i) as defined in the spatial and temporal algorithm above.
2. Find the maximum energy ME and its time MEL.
3. Search TE(i) backward from MEL to find the time ME10L such that TE(ME10L) < 10 % of ME.

4. Search TE(I) backward from ME10L to find the time ONSET when:

$$2*TE(ONSET) - (TE(ONSET-1) + TE(ONSET-2)) < 0$$

Then the QRS onset is defined at the time ONSET.

II. 3-leads method (6):

1. Find the maximum energy ME of all three leads and its time MEL.
2. Search backward from MEL to find the time ME10L where the energy is less than 10 % of ME.
3. Search backward from ME10L for each of the three leads to find the ONSET in each lead j when

$$2*p(ONSET+2,j)+p(ONSET+1,j)-p(ONSET-1,j)-2*p(ONSET-2,j) < 10 \text{ mV} \quad \text{for } j=1,2,3$$

4. Define the QRS onset as the earliest ONSET of the three leads.

III. median method:

This is the same as the 3-lead method except: 1) use NE leads instead of 3 leads, and 2) the QRS onset is defined as the median of the NE individual onset times (instead of the earliest of the three leads).

RESULTS: As mentioned earlier, the QRS initial activation region detection in step #1 is very critical in this algorithm. The average and the standard deviation of the approximate QRS initial activation time IAT relative to the "reference onset time" are 6.3 ms and 4.1 ms respectively, and no IAT is earlier than the "reference onset time". The accurate QRS initial activation region detection thus provides a sound basis for the precise QRS onset detection.

The accuracy of the QRS onset detection among the four methods was compared to the standard (ie, the "reference onset time"). The results are summarized in Table 2, and the error distributions are shown in Figure 2.

Table 2. the mean and the standard deviation of the QRS onsets detected by the four method, relative to "reference onset time".

	Spatial-temporal	Total Energy	3-lead	Median
MEAN	-1.26 ms	0.84 ms	4.54 ms	7.78 ms
STD	2.1 ms	7.1 ms	11.0 ms	10.29 ms

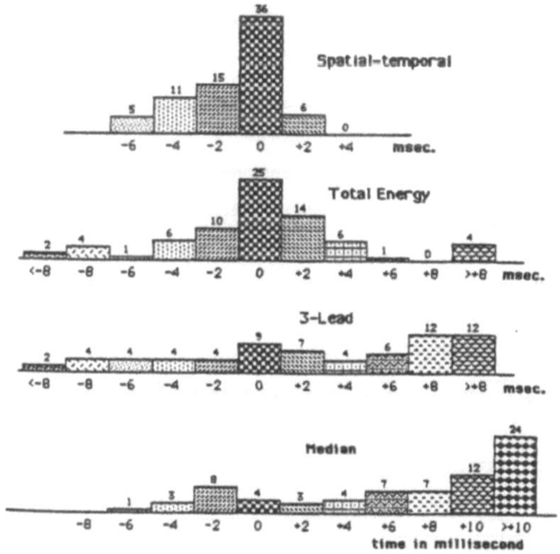

Figure 2. The error distribution of the QRS onsets detected by the four methods, relative to the "reference onset times". The negative error means that the detection is earlier than the "reference onset time".

The small mean, the small variance, and the narrow distribution of the results of the spatial and temporal method clearly demonstrate its superior performance compared with the other three methods.

DISCUSSION: The new method performs best as evidenced by the small mean error and the small variance in the onset values relative to the "reference onset times". In fact the computed onset values were mostly earlier than the "reference onset times", resulting in a negative mean difference. This negative mean was expected because the algorithm has more precision than is possible in a video display with only 31 levels (15 on positive side and 15 on negative side). In addition, the "smoothing" effect of the three dimension computation can better detect low-amplitude potentials in the presence of noise and artifact. The "total energy" method produced onset values with a small mean error, but the variance was excessive. The "median" and the "3-lead" methods performed poorly in both mean and variance.

The location of QRS initial activation varies from patient to patient and from disease to disease, and no fixed single or multiple lead set can detect correct QRS onset consistently (4,5). In addition, the Ta of the P-wave often temporally overlaps with the QRS initial activation. The "total energy" method integrates spatial energy including the energy of QRS initial activation energy, the energy of Ta of P wave, and the noise, resulting the relatively poor performance. Even without the noise, it still can not differentiate the QRS initial activation and the presence of the Ta of P wave. The "3-lead" method apparently lacks spatial information and has no information to reduce the effect of noise and artifact. Although the "median" method utilizes all 180 leads, it does not use the spatial information. In contrast, the new spatial and temporal approach combines the spatial and temporal information in the QRS initial activation process, so that it is insensitive to the position changes of QRS initial activation, and it ignores the Ta of P wave if it does not overlap with QRS initial activation spatially. In addition, the three dimensional processing reduces the effect of noise, resulting in more satisfactory performance.

The evaluation of these methods was done by using the "reference onset time" selected by two experienced investigators. The criteria of these two investigators in choosing the QRS onset time includes the spatial pattern changes of the maps in the QRS initial activation process, including the magnitudes. Although this selection is not absolutely correct, it is very close to the correct answer, since the experience enables the investigator to visually filter the noise by correlating the changes in consecutive maps near the initial QRS activation.

CONCLUSION: Both temporal and spatial information appears essential for QRS onset estimates for use in quantification of activation events. The new three-dimensional QRS onset detection algorithm is relatively insensitive to noise, artifact, position changes of QRS initial activation, and the Ta of P-wave, and thus it can accurately detect the QRS onset.

References

(1) Liebman, J, et al: J. Electrocardiol. 14, 249 - 260 (1981)
(2) Lux, RL: CRC Critical. Reviews in Biomed. Engr. 8, Issue 3, 253 - 279 (1982)
(3) Liebman, J, et al: J. Electrocardiol. 17, 329 - 346 (1984)
(4) Michael, D, et al: Circulation. 53, 447 - 451 (1976)
(5) Kenneth, L, et al: Circulation. 63, 933 - 937 (1981)
(6) Le, H.T, et al: IEEE Trans on Biomed. Engr. BME-32, 43 - 50 (1985)

Experimental Investigation of Cardiac Electric Field

ROSCHEVSKY M.P., BARABANOVA V.V., GAGIEV N.G., KALIBERDA N.M., KARPUSHOV E.N., KONDRASHOVA K.K., KUZNETZOV V.P., PROKHOROV V.N., ROSCHEVSKAYA I.M.

Institute of Biology
Komi Branch of the Academy of Sciences of the USSR
Syktyvkar, USSR

SUMMARY

To acquire a topographic and quantative description of epicardium electric activity, epi - cardial /body surface potential maps (ESM/BSM) were obtained with the use of multichannel computer-aided recording system wich had been reported of elsewhere. Two initial activation loci were discovered on the ventral part of ventricles in rat heart with normal activation sequence. Different BSM configurations were observed in Wystar (WY) rats, Wystar-Kyoto (WKY) rats with right ventricle hypertrophy and spontaneous hypertension Okāmoto rats (SHR).

INTRODUCTION

Multichannel computer-aided electrotopography techniques is widely used in comparative cardiology and biophysical simulation basic researches (1), so potential mapping is desi - dered to be rather appropriate in applied and clinical settings. Furthermore, ESM/BSM techniques is likely to provide a comprehensive analysis of cardiac regulation system and heart drugs pharmacodynamics.

METHODS

Rats were studied, a standard reference pattern in physiological, pharmacological, toxicological researches (2). Data were recorded simul-taneously, processed by computer, visua - lized as a series of ESM/BSM one every 1 msec with the use of 128-channel minicomputer-CAMAC system (designed by M.Roschevsky, V.Prokhorov, N.Gagiev, V.Kutnetsov, E.Karpushov). In order to reconstruct myocardial activation sequence that corresponds to BSM, an interactive computer programme was developed for numerical solution of so-called inverse problem of electrocardiology via evalvation of multipole coefficients (software by V.Kuznetsov).

RESULTS

Normotensive WV rats were sedates, anaesthetized, a midsternal incision on the chest enabled simultaneous recording of 64 epicardial electrograms shortly after 64-lead BSM were obtained (I.Roschevskava studies).

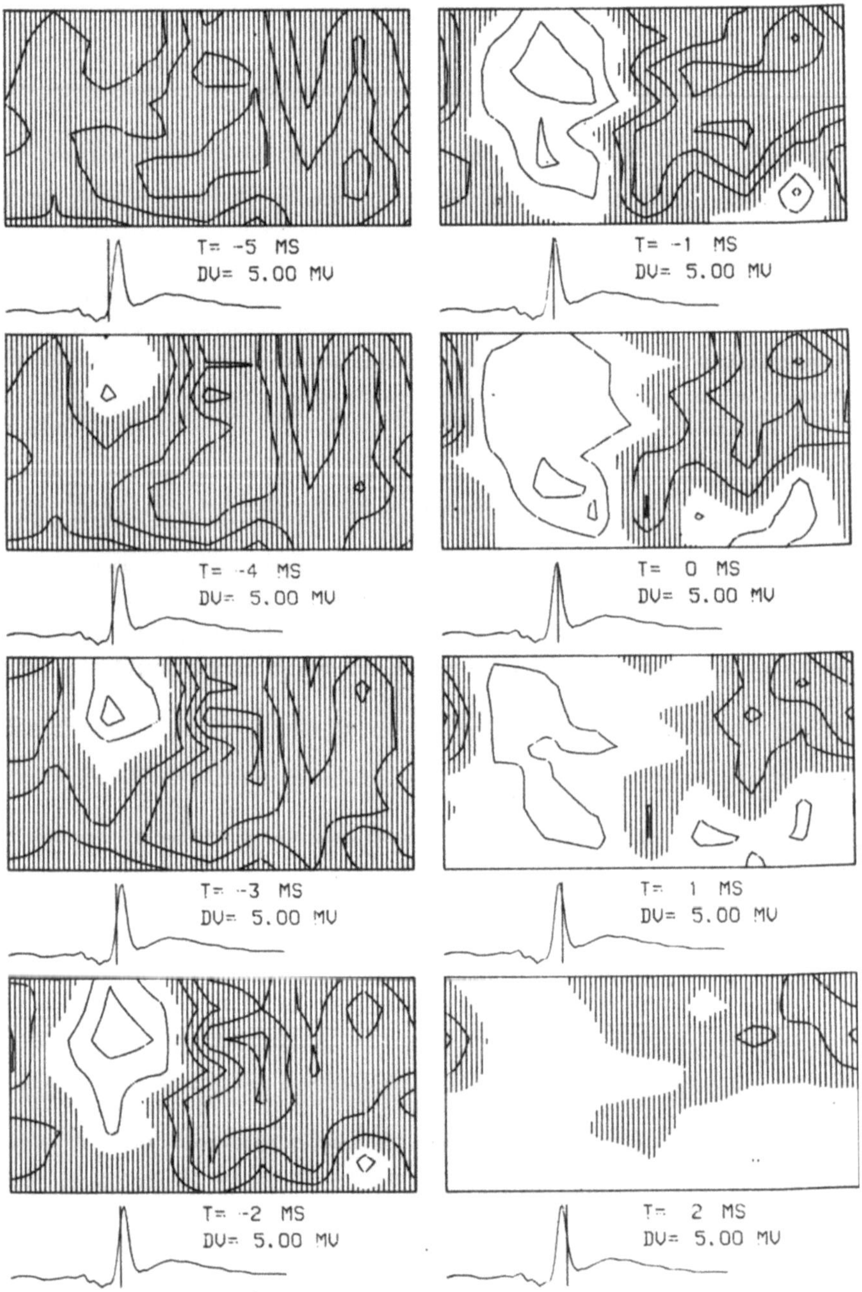

FIG. 1 EPICARDIAL SURFACE POTENTIAL MAPS IN WY PATTERN
64 - ELECTRODE ARRAY, 1000 HZ PER CHANNEL
(SHADED AREA - POSITIVE ONE)

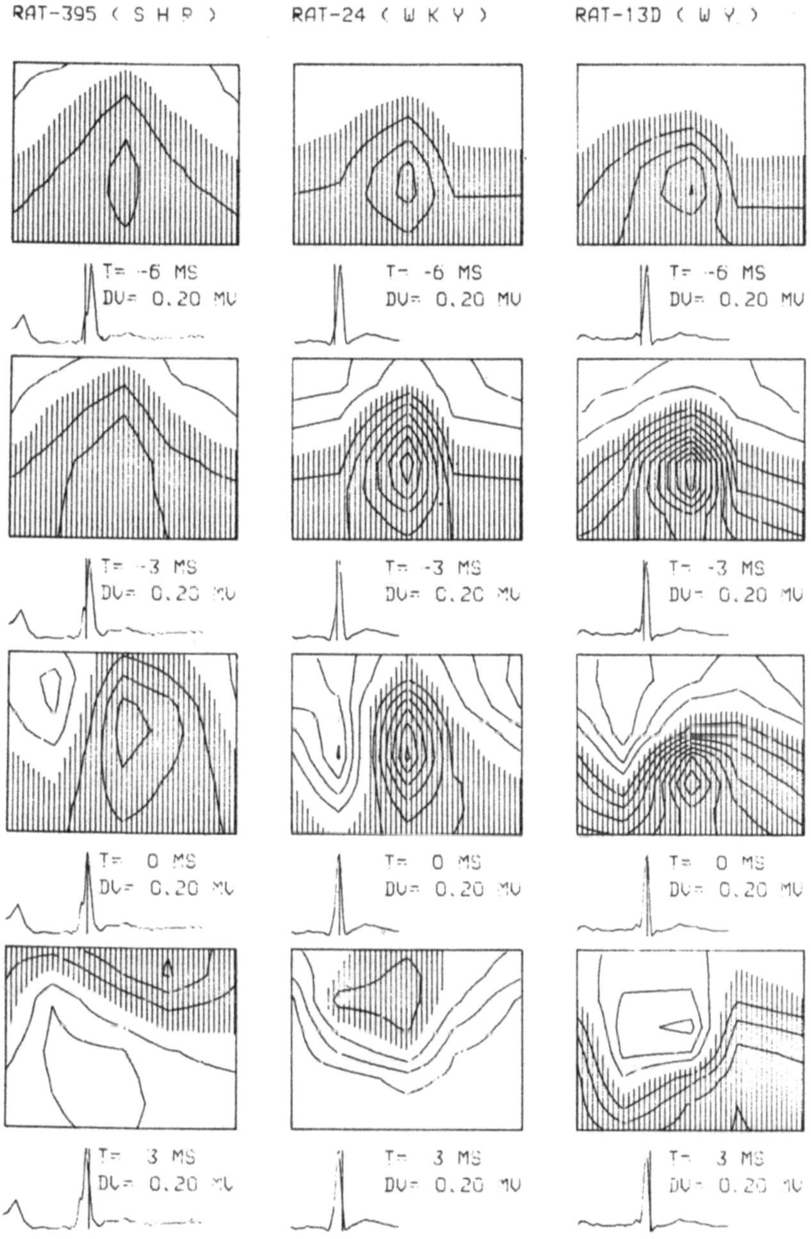

FIG. 2 BODY SURFACE POTENTIAL MAPS IN WY, WKY, SHR PATTERNS.
32 - LEAD ARRAY, 1000 HZ PER CHANNEL
(SHADED AREA - POSITIVE ONE)

Ventricular exitation occured to start on the right ventricular (RV) free wall and left ventricular (LV) apex, activation wavefront expanding along the septum into the LV free wall, its basal region and after all to LV base subepicardial surface. Activation wave co-vered subepicardial surface within 6-7 msec. Two initial activation loci were found on the ventral side of the ventricular subepicardial surface. Particular areas could be clearly recognized by visual inspection of ESM (Fig. 1).

BSM "images" were similar to ESM "origins",being a much more integrated, smoothed ones. Normal rat BSM possessed the only one potential minimum while ESM displayes two potential minima. Potential maximum reached its peak value 1,8-2,2 mV at 1-2 msec to R-wave peak, potential minimum - 1-2 mV and 1 msec from R-wave peak, respectively, i.e. potential extrema peak values could never be registered simultaneously. Potential extrema dipole vector changes its orientation up 30-40° during depolarization interval. Potential maximum traversed the mapping plane almost horizontally from the RV apex projection, ascending upward to the left at the end of the QRS interval. Potential minimum descended downward to the left at the angle of 60-80°, overlapping the RV projection.

BSM in normotensive WY rats, normotensive WKY rats with RV hypertrophy, spontaneous hypertension SHR rats were obtained with 32-lead array, placed evenly over the body (V.Barabanova, K.Kondrashova studies). Pattern maps were found to differ greatly in their topographic and quantative features (Fig. 2). Potential maximum in WY pattern migrated downward to the left toward the back at 5-6 msec from the onset of QRS. Potential maximum in WKY pattern moved upward to the right. Both potential extrema in SHR pattern decreased in voltage, potential minimum maintained its position, secondary potential extrema appeared during QRS interval.

CONCLUSION

We conclude that conparative analysis of epicardial and body surface maps would verify some of the inverse problem procedures and solutions. Significant differences in potential distribution patterns were observed, this information is considered to be useful for prospective applied and basic researches in comparative Cardiology.

REFERENCES

(1) Roschevsky M.P. Problems of Comparative Electrocardiology created by the Progress in Computer Mapping of the Cardioelectric Field: in "Models and Measurements of the Cardiac Electric Field".
E.Schubert ed., 131-134, (1982).

(2) The Rat Electrocardiogram in Pharmacology and Toxicology.
R.Budden, D.K.Detweiler, J.Zbinder eds., (1981).

BODY SURFACE MAPPING - CLINICAL APPLICATION

An analysis of multiple ECG leads in the patients with posterior myocardial infarction.

AMIROV R.Z., USHAKOV V.V.
The Central Scientific Research Institute of Health Resort and Physical Treatment.
The Kalinin Prospect 50, Moscow, USSR.

Summary.
In relation to location of myocardial infarction (MI) it is divided into the following types: local (16%), horizontal (40%), vertical (14%) and vertical-horizontal (30%). The first two types may be further subdivided into basal, central and diaphragmatic infarctions. As for a size, myocardial infarction may be presented as small, less than 10 leads (14%), medium-sized, up to 20 leads (38%), large, up to 30 leads (32%) and extensive, more than 30 leads (16%). In most patients with posterior myocardial infarction there are focal changes undetectable by 12-lead ECG. In all patients with myocardial distrophy there are focal changes on the posterior surface, which can't be detected in 12 leads.

Introduction. A number of studies has confirmed value of electrocardiotopic method for the diagnosis of myocardial infarction, of focal changes in particular, if they are absent on 12-lead ECG (1,2). Recent scientific papers have documented value of the diagnostic surface mapping.

Material and methods. One hundred forty six patients (127 men and 16 women) aged 36-80 years (8 patients under 40 years, 39 patients aged 41-50 years, 46 patients aged 51-60 years and 7 patients were over 70 years). 12-lead ECG reveals nonstable angina and compromised blood supply of the posterior left ventricular wall in 24 patients, myocardial distrophy in 8 and posterior myocardial infarction in 111 patients. All patients were hospitalized because of a severe pain syndrome (intensive chest pains ra iating to the left arm, left shoulder and so on).

Results. In the patients with ischemic heart disease seen as frequent angina attacks and compromised blood supply of the posterior left ventricular wall, IT reveals focal changes of an infarctional type in 19 (79.17%) patients. In remaining 5 patients of this group topography has confirmed the diagnosis of angina.

IT has revealed 2-24 (mean 10.95) leads containing an infarction-like type of ECG complexes. As for location these foci are distributed as follows: 8 patients have postero-basal myocardial infarction, three have postero-diaphragmatic MI, two topograms have revealed a postero-central focus irrespective of postero-basal and postero-diaphragmatic segments, in 6 patients this focus extends to the whole posterior wall: from a basal region to a diaphragmatic one.

The following case history is illustrative. Patient M. aged 52 years

Ischemic heart disease and hypertension had been present for 8 years. Two weeks before hospitalization her status was deteriorated,exertional angina attacks became more frequent, nearly constant dull pain was present in the intershoulder region. On february 25,1987 she exhibited a severe attack of chest pain accompanied with dizziness and syncope. The developing MI was suspected and an ambulance team delivered her in a poor status to the hospital. ECG registred a complete A-V block,ventricular contractions were 24-30/min.Resuscitativemeasures resulted in restoration of a sinus rhythm. There were no ECG signs of focal myocardial damages. A week later IT showed a small (3 leads) zero zone in the posterior wall on the electropositivity map (EPM)at the first electrode level. It corresponded to an area of QS waves on the electropositivity. A large area of the lowered potentials (21 leads) extended from a zero zone downward to the diaphragmatic area and horizontally to the anterior chest surface. The electronegativity map showed a zero area in three left inferior lateral leads. Here, there was a maximum of the electronegativity map (1.2mV). A maximal value of the electronegativity map was seen as S wave and was located at the second electrode level, to the right from the sternum. A zero zone and a zone of the lowered positive potential of the electropositivity map corresponded to an area of registration of negative and isoelectrical T wave, as well as a zone of ST segment elevated above an isoelectrical line. As reciprocation an area of ST segment lowered below an isoelectrical line was noted on the inferior anterolateral left chest surface. Thus, a topographic study helps to reveal posterior left ventricular myocardial infarction involving presumbly a posterobasal area.In the second group focal changes in the posterior left ventricular wall were noted in 8 (100%) patients with myocardial distrophy. They were fixed in 7-26 (mean 16.14)leads. As for localization of the damages, they were posterobasal and postero-diaphargmatic (three patients in each subgroup),postero central (1 patient) and vertically located focal changes (from a posterobasal to postero-diaphragmatic segment) (one patient). Comparison of the obtained results and clinico-laboratory data has allowed to make a diagnosis of MI. An analysis of IT in the patients of the third group, in whom there was evident MI of the posterior left ventricular wall according to 12-lead ECG,has helped to divide them into two subgroups: a)58 patients (52.25%) in whom ECG documented nonpenetrating myocardial infarction and IT revealed transmural damage and B) 53 (47.75%) patients, in whom both diagnoses coincided.IT revealed infarctional changes in the patients of the third group. Here, a zero zone on the electropositivity map and corresponding QS complexes on the electronegativity map covered 1-31 (mean 11) leads. Seventten patients had posterobasal MI. Eight patients had postero-diaphragmatic MI. A postero-central zone was affected in 2 patients. In 12 patients MI involved the whole posterior wall: from a basal to diaphragmatic area.

Nineteen patients had extensive MI, that is, a focus extended not only vertically, from the top to the bottom, but horizontally, involving the lateral and sometimes anterior left ventricular wall. During an analysis of the patients of group 3b we've revealed coincidence of the diagnosis of nonpenetrating MI in 27 patients and of transmural MI in 26 patients. The damaged area covered 4-29 (mean 14.42) and 7-49 (mean 29)leads. Extensive MI prevailed. Thus, a vertical (basal-diaphragmatic) variant was revealed in 9 patients and in 18 patients MI extended beyound the posterior left ventricular wall. Among local variants postero-diaphragmatic one was most commonly seen (in 14 patients), a postero-basal variant was noted on 10 topograms, a postero-central variant was diagnosed in 2 patients.
Conclusions.IT helps to reveal focal damages in the patients with clinical signs of unstable angina and compromised blood supply of the posterior left ventricular wall. in 79.17% of the patients of this group mapping of cardiac potentials from the whole chest surface has revealed infarctional changes.In the patients with myocardial distrophy of the posterior left ventricular wall there have been unrecognozed focal changes. Topographic analysis has revealed changes specific for MI, which are undetectable on standard ECG in 100% of the patients. Mapping of cardiac potentials has allowed to classify MI into variants and types in relation to quantitative estimation.

The legend.
Fig.1 Integral topogram taken in patient Ju. with posterior MI (see explanations in the text).

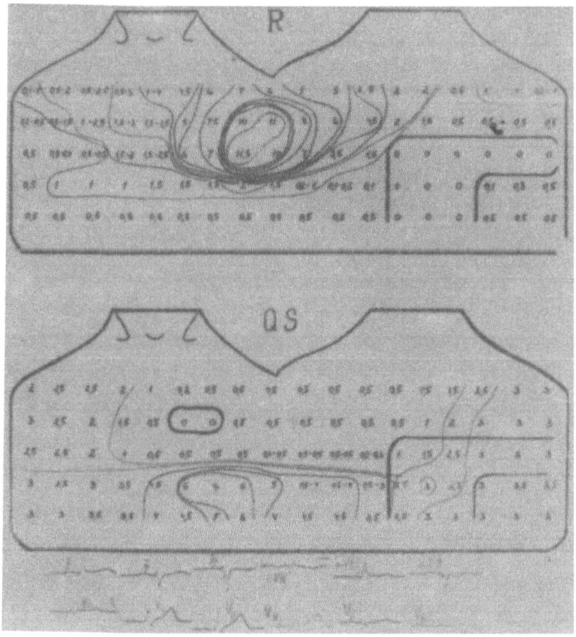

References.

(1) Amirov,R.Z: Electrocardiotopography. Moscow,(1965).

(2)Amirov, R.Z., Semenovitch, Z.G.: In: Adavances in electrocardiology. Ed. P.d'Alche, Universite de Caen,297-299, (1985).

RECOGNITION OF MYOCARDIAL ISCHEMIC AREAS BY COMPUTERIZED STRESS PRECORDIAL MAPPING

Gil,V.; Aleixo,A.; Andrade,M.J.; Seabra-Gomes,R.;
Almeida,F.; Especial,N.; Fernandes,J.(*)

HOSPITAL DE SANTA CRUZ-Servico de Cardiologia
Carnaxide-PORTUGAL

SUMMARY

Thirty seven individuals, 14 normals by clinical criteria and 23 patients, with CAD documented by cinecoronariography were studied by equilibrium radionuclide angiography and computerized 35-electrodes precordial mapping both at rest and after supine bycicle ergometer exercise. Correct identification of ischemic and non ischemis areas by stress mapping was made in 66.7% of cases with sensivity of 65%, specificity of 87.3% and predictive value of 94%. When consideringg only PTS out of medication, 73.8% correct identification was possible, with 75% sensivity, 80% specitivity and 92.3% predictive value. The area most often identified was the correspondent to RCA (82%). With exercise EF increased (75.7%) and RMSv decreased (78.4%). In some individuals, RMSv did, instead, increase with stress; in 60% of those, EF decreased with exercise.

INTRODUCTION

Coronary Artery Disease (CAD) continues to be a major cause of morbidity and mortality in developed countries. Its outcome depends mainly on the extent of coronary involvement and the degree of ventricular imparement (1).

During the last decades, efforts have been made to achieve reliable non invasive diagnostic methods appliable to its early diagnosis. Stress tests, either by bycicle ergometer or treadmill are among the most popular, because of its low cost, reproductiveness and hight sensitivity and specificity in diagnosing myocardial ischemia.

Several parameters of stress tests are known to be good indicators of prognosis. However, the information that they can provide concerning the extent of the ischemia and the degree of ventricular dysfunction is of relative value.

Other non invasive methods known to be superior for that purposes have the disadvantages of being too expensive or needing sophisticated equipment, like radionuclides.

In the last twenty years, body surface potencial mapping has been used to explore the electrical activity of the heart with more accuracy than the conventional ECG. However, only in recent years has the technique been completely used due to recent technologic developments, mainly in the field of microcomputers (2,3).

Stress computerized precordial mapping (SMAP) can improve the diagnostic accuracy of conventional stress tests and can provide important contribution concerning the site and extent of ischemia (4-8).

In the present study we used a computerized mapping system with 35 precordial electrodes , before and after supine ergometer bycicle exercise with the purpose of identifying ischemic areas and their relation to the diseased coronary arteries and to some parameters of ventricular dysfunction.

MATERIAL AND METHODS

We studied thirty seven individuals, 6 females (F) and 31 males (M), mean age 43.3 years, with computerized precordial mapping - MAPCARD system - and equilibrium radionuclide angiography (RNA) at rest and after supine bycicle ergometer exercise (SE). We considered two subgroups: A, 4 F and 10 M, mean age 32 years, clinically normals (N) and B, 23 patiens (PTS), 2 F and 21 M, mean age 53.9 years with documented coronary artery disease by conventional cinecoronariography (Sones or Judkins technique). 16 PTS had 3 vessel disease, 3 PTS 2 vessel disease and 4 PTS 1 vessel disease.

MAPCARD System (fig.1) (9,10) consists of: a versatile Data Acquisition System allowing simultaneous sampling of up to 36 channels at 250 Hz, 500 Hz or 1 kHz rates and 12 bit resolution; a personal computer, Sperry HT 500 with graphic capabilities with MAPAS (11), the apllication software; and printer and plotter facilities. We used a precordial network with 35 electrodes in a 5x7 matrix, 7 columns (1-7) of self-adhesive strips with 5 electrodes (A-E) at 3.5 cm inter-electrode distance. The strips are positioned over the chest with anatomical references: A1 over the second right intercostal space and strips 6 and 7 over anterior and left mid axillary line, respectively. Data collection was done at 500 Hz sampling rate.

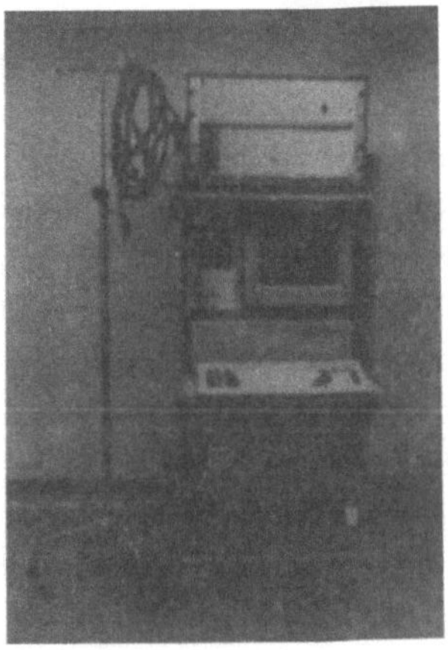

Fig.1 - MAPCARD system

The SMAP parameters considered were ST segment (80 msec after J point) isopotential maps in matrix areas corresponding to precordial projection of the three coronary arteries and its variation with stress (STv) and Root Mean Square amplitude variation (RMSv) with exercise.

The EXERCISE PROTOCOL adopted consisted on bycicle supine ergometer exercise with 2 minutes steps and 25 watts increments each stage. We performed an acquisition before and another immediately after maximum exercise defined by clinical criteria (anginal pain, ST depression, dyspnoea or fatigue).

RNA was performed after administration of 25 MCI of 99m Tc labeled "in vivo", using a Gamma Camera GE 400 T, with ECG gated 300 seconds acquisitions in LAO the "best septal" projection, before and after supine exercise (same protocol as for mapping). The image processing of equilibrium RNA including Ejection Fraction calculation was made according software of GE STAR system.

RESULTS

Mean Exercise Time (SEt) was greater in N (580.7±169.7 sec) than in PTS (430.4±133.1 sec) ($p<0.005$). In N, mean RMSv was 1413±357 mV in rest, and changed to 1221±484 mV with exercise; in PTS, mean RMSv was 1157±348 mV in rest and 1078± 377 mV with stress (fig.2). Mean EF% at rest was 63±10 in N and 57±10 in PTS and changed to 70±7 in N and 61±12 in PTS with

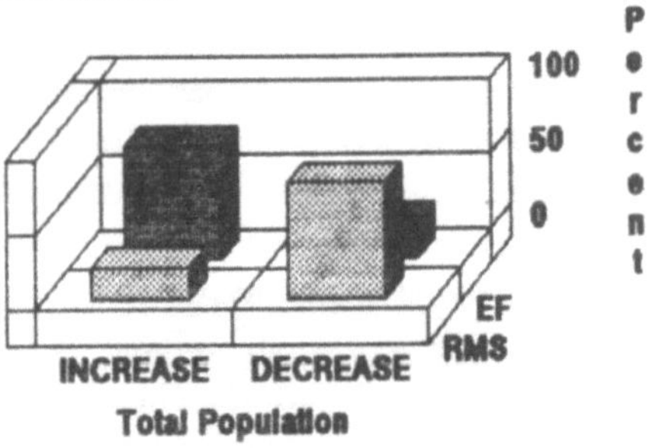

Fig.2 - Stress EF and RMSv variation

exercise (fig.2). Those differences were not statistically significant.

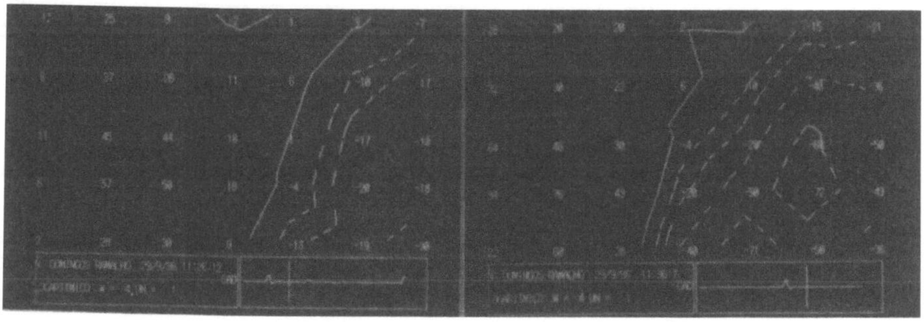

Fig.3 - Stress Equipotential Maps in a 3 vessel disease patient

In B group (69 areas, total), SMAP - STv correctly identified ischemic zones (fig.3) with a sensivity of 65%, specificity of 87.3% and a predictive value of 94%; when considering only PTS out of medication (42 areas), sensivity changed to 75%, specificity to 80% and predictive value to 92.3% (table 1).

TABLE 1

CORRECT IDENTIFICATION OF ISCHEMIC AREAS

ALL PATIENTS (69 areas)	
sensivity.........	65.0%
specificity.......	87.3%
predictive value..	94.0%
PATIENTS OUT OF MEDICATION (42 areas)	
sensivity.........	75.0%
specificity.......	80.0%
predictive value..	92.3%

In the majority of individuals, as in normals, with exercise EF increased (75.7%) and RMSv decreased (78.4%). In individuals (60%) in whom, on the contrary, RMSv increased with stress, EF decreased.

DISCUSSION AND CONCLUSIONS

In our series, correct identification of ischemic and non ischemic areas (as compared to the precordial projection of coronary arteries involved) was achieved in 46 of 69 areas (66.7%) of all PTS; considering only PTS out of medication, correct identification was made of 31 of 42 areas (73.8%) . The area more often correctly identified was the correspondent to the Right Coronary Artery (14 in 17, 82%). Left Circumflex and Anterior Descendent Arteries were identified respectively 61% (11 in 18) and 52% (12 in 23).

SMAP can also provide information about left ventricular dysfunction (12). In most individuals, with stress, EF increased and RMSv decreased. This was also the pattern observed in normals. In some individuals RMSv did, instead, increase with stress. In 60% of those, EF decreased with stress (against the general rule).

Our results confirm the possibility of identification of ischemic areas by this new non invasive method (4,7,8). Even when PTS were under anti anginal therapy it was possible to achieve correct identification in a significant number of cases.

In spite of the small number of cases studied, it seems likely that an association exists between EF% and RMSv variations with stress. This deserves further investigation.

In conclusion: 1 - SMAP is a reliable non invasive method in identifying ischemic areas in coronary patients. 2 - Stress RMSv and EF variations may be related.

BIBLIOGRAPHY

(1) - Vigilante,G., Weintraub,W., Klein,L., Schneider,R., Seelaus,P., Agarwal,J., and Helfant,R.:MEDICAL AND SURGICAL SURVIVAL IN CORONARY ARTERY DISEASE IN THE 1980'S. Am J Cardiol 58 , 926-931 (1986)

(2) - Yamada, K.: BODY SURFACE ISOPOTENTIAL MAP: past, present and future. Japanese Circulation Journal 45, 1-14 (1981)

(3) - Stilli,D., Musso,E., Macchi,E., Manca,C., Dei Cas,L., Vasini,P., and Taccardi,B.: BODY SURFACE POTENTIAL MAPPING IN ISCHEMIC PATIENTS WITH NORMAL RESTING ECG. Can J Cardio/Supplement A 107A-112A (1986)

(4) - Fox,K., Selwyn,A., Oakley,D., Shillingford,J.: RELATION BETWEEN THE PRECORDIAL PROJECTION OF S-T SEGMENT CHANGES AFTER EXERCISE AND CORONARY ANGIOGRAPHIC FINDINGS. Am J Cardiol 44, 1068-1075 (1979)

(5) - Essen,R., Hinsen,R., Spruss,K., Silny,J., Merx,W., Meyer-Erkelenz,J., Rau,G., and Effert,S.: AUTOMATED MAPPING OF ECG SURFACE POTENTIALS IN DETECTION OF ISCHEMIA DURING STRESS TEST. Computers in Cardiology, 41 (1980)

(6) - Miller III,W., Spach,M., Warren,R.: TOTAL BODY SURFACE POTENTIAL MAPPING DURING EXERCISE:QRS-T WAVE CHANGES IN NORMAL YOUNG ADULTS. Circulation 62,No3, 632-645 (1980)

(7) - Tavazzi,L., Guagliumi,G., Galli,M., Tosto,A., Imparato,A., Minuco,G.: CAN BODY SURFACE MAPPING IMPROVE THE DIAGNOSTIC POWER OF STANDARD ELECTROCARDIOGRAPHY IN EFFORT MYOCARDIAL ISCHEMIA? Can J Cardiol/Supplement A, 99A-106A (1986)

(8) - Farr,B., Vondenbusch,B., Silny,J., Rau,G., and Effert,S.: LOCALIZATION OF SIGNIFICANT CORONARY ARTERIAL NARROWINGS USING BODY SURFACE POTENTIAL MAPPING DURING EXERCISE STRESS TESTING.Am J Cardiol 59 ,528-560 (1987)

(9) - Especial,N., Almeida,F., Fernandes,J., Amado,J., Gil,V., Aleixo,A., Seabra-Gomes,R.: A PERSONAL COMPUTER-BASED SYSTEM FOR CARDIAC MAPPING.Computers in Cardiology, Boston, USA (1986)

(10) - Especial,N., Almeida,F., Fernandes,J., Aleixo,A., Suleman,A., Amado,J.: A MULTIPLE CHANNEL DATA ACQUISITION SYSTEM-AN APPLICATION IN CARDIOLOGY. In Eupsico 86, pp 1355-1358 North-Holland (1986)

(11) - Almeida,F., Especial,N., Fernandes,J., Amado,J., Aleixo,A., Gil,V., Seabra-Gomes,R.: MAPAS - AN INTEGRATED SOFTWARE PACKAGE FOR CARDIAC MAPPING. Accepted for presentation in Miami Technicon'87, Florida, USA, October 28-30 (1987)

(12) - Aleixo, A., Gil,V., Adao,M., Real,T., Seabra-Gomes,R., Especial,N., Almeida,F., Fernandes, J., Amado,J.: NON INVASIVE ASSESSMENT OF LEFT VENTRICULAR DYSFUNCTION THROUGH COMPUTERIZED BODY SURFACE POTENTIAL MAPPING. In 13th International Congress on Electrocardiology, Abstracts pp 37, Washington DC, USA (1986)

(*) F. Almeida, N. Especial are at LABORATORIO NACIONAL DE ENGENHARIA E TECNOLOGIA INDUSTRIAL - DEE, J. Fernandes is at INESC.

Electrocardiographic isopotential exercise and oesophageal stimulation maps in the diagnosis of myocardial ischaemia

JANOTA M., BYTEŠNÍK J., LEXA J., STUPKA J.

Institute for Clinical and Experimental Medicine, Vídeňská 800, P.O.B.10, 140 00 Prague 4, Czechoslovakia

Summary. Ecg mapping of Q, R, S and the ST segment with 56 praecordial leads was performed using the Cardiomap-1, a microcomputer system at rest, during exercise and atrial oesophageal stimulation. Exercise mapping was performed in 115, and oesophageal stimulation in 33 men. The exercise led to a typical increase in ST depression during mapping in patients with ischaemic heart disease (IHD). Oesophageal atrial stimulation evaluated by isopotential mapping was successfully used as an intervention test. In patients with IHD, stimulation ST maps of the left praecordium led to characteristic ischaemic changes as did the exercise test.

Introduction. In the diagnosis of myocardial ischaemia, 12-lead ecg is used not only at rest, but also during exercise, pharmacological intervention or during oesophageal atrial stimulation. Atrial stimulation evaluated by 12-lead ecg yielded results equally good as did the exercise test (1). ST mapping appears to be a new alternative examination helpful in myocardial ischaemia detection (2). The aim of our study was to use oesophageal atrial stimulation as an intervention technique evaluated by isopotential ST maps and to determine if it is as good as exercise ST maps.

Material and methods. A group of 115 subjects (45 controls and 70 patients with IHD) were examined by exercise mapping. Both stimulation and exercise mapping were performed in another 33 subjects (11 controls and 22 patients with IHD). All patients were examined clinically, by resting and exercise ecg and, most of them by coronary arteriography. The diagnosis of IHD is based on standard clinical criteria and the finding of a significant stenosis on coronary arteries.

Isopotential maps were obtained from a Cardiomap-1 microcomputer with a special praecordial multielectrode comprising 56 leads. It enables us to obtain maps of the Q, R, S wave amplitudes and of the ST segment 70 ms after the peak of the S wave. It evaluates automatically the sums of maximal values and areas of ST denivelations and of the Q wave. The examinations are carried out at rest, during exercise and during oesophageal stimulation. 3-minute exercise stages of 1W/kg and 1.5W/kg were used (3, 4). Atrial stimulation was stimulation using a bipolar Vygon electrode induced 40 cm from lips. A stimulator of our own design generates impulses of 2 ms and 10 ms width. As a rule, stimulation is performed at 1-minute intervals gradually with frequencies of 100, 120 and 140 with every stage examined twice.

Results. The values of ST elevation and ST depression sums before and after stimulation in controls just as in patients with IHD are given in Tab.1. While the sums of ST elevations decreased in both groups, the sums of ST depressions were significantly higher only in patients with IHD. This was regarded as a special sign of myocardial ischaemia.

Tab.1. Heart rate, sums of ST elevations and ST depressions at rest without stimulation and with stimulation in controls and in patients with ischaemic heart disease (IHD)

		HR/min		ST elevation mm		ST depression mm	
		$\bar{x}$	SD	$\bar{x}$	SE	$\bar{x}$	SE
	rest	71.3	3.9	28.3	8.3	3.2	1.6
controls	stimulation	145.5	5.4	15.7	6.5	7.6	1.8
	p <	0.001		0.05		n	
	rest	75.4	2.6	27.9	4.6	7.3	2.1
IHD	stimulation	142.7	2.2	12.6	4.4	46.2	3.8
	p <	0.05		0.05		0.05	

Fig.1 shows the results of rest and exercise mapping in controls and in patients with IHD. In controls during exercise, the sums of ST elevations increased, and ST depressions were without a significant change, and R waves decreased. In patients with IHD during exercise, the sums of ST elevation decreased and the sums of ST depression increased, R waves decreased as did in controls.

CHANGES OF ST ELEVATION + DEPRESSION + R WAVE IN EXERCISE MAPS

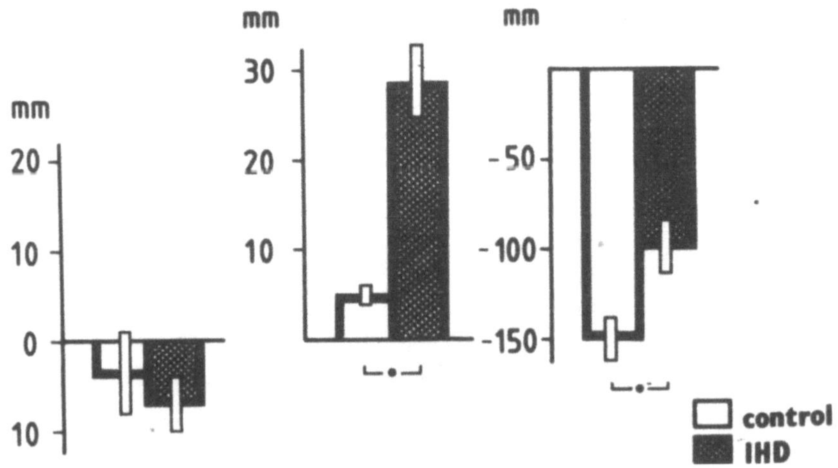

Discussion. The ideal aim of exercise ecg mapping is an accurate diagnosis of IHD, assessment of the extent of myocardial ischaemia and determination of the distribution of coronary artery involvement. The typical increase in postexercise ST depression sums and areas is recommended as a helpful and conclusive sign of myocardial ischaemia. We succeeded with this method in evaluating the dynamics of the disease, at follow-up just as in assessing the therapy (surgery, coronary angioplasty, etc.). More precious results of ST mapping can be obtained from the mean values of two or three measurements. This is not possible during the exercise test but it is possible at rest as well as during stimulation. This is one of the advantages of the stimulation method, another one being that the stimulation frequency reaches higher values than maximal exercise heart rate in IHD patients.

To conclude, atrial oesophageal stimulation evaluated by isopotential mapping was successfully used as an intervention test. In patients with IHD, stimulation ST maps led to characteristic ischaemic changes in maps in the left praecordium of the same type as those appearing during the exercise test. The authors believe that the oesophageal stimulation mapping test can provide more information than 12-lead stimulation ecg and can be used in some indications instead of exercise ST mapping, especially so in cases in which it is not possible to use the exercise test.

References: 1) Janota M. et al.: Prakt.lékař, 33, in press (1987), 2) Janota et al.: Noninvasive Cardiology Proc. 4th European Conf.Mechanocardiography, Budapest, 301-303 (1985), 3) Janota M. et al.: Vnitřní lék., 31, 8, 736-743 (1985), 4) Janota M. et al.: Xth World Cong.Cardiology, Washington, 14-19 September (1986) abstract.

Usefulness of the QRST integral maps to detect vulnerability to malignant arrhythmias in patients with old myocardial infarction.

BERTONI T., BREGHI M.L., MARCONI M., BONIFACCIO G., and DE AMBROGGI L.

Istituto di Scienze Medico-Chirurgiche, University of Milan, Italy.

INTRODUCTION

Malignant ventricular arrhythmias are the main cause of sudden death in patients with ischemic heart disease. Although different electrophysiologic mechanisms can be responsible for the initiation of the arrhythmias, an approach to the prediction of ventricular arrhythmias could be confined to the recognition of a cardiac condition of vulnerability to the various arrhythmogenic agents.

Evidence for the relation between vulnerability to arrhythmias and disparities of ventricular recovery times has been provided by experimental studies (1,2). Abildskov et al. proposed that local repolarization disparities can be detected at the body surface from the analysis of QRST integral distribution (3). Specifically, the non-dipolar components of QRST integral distribution were considered an index of repolarization disparity (4).

The aim of our investigation was to detect signs of repolarization disparities in patients with an old myocardial infarction (MI) and to correlate them with the occurence of sustained ventricular tachycardias (VT).

METHODS

Study population: Body surface maps (BSM) were obtained from 73 patients (age 51 ± 10 years) who had had an acute MI 1 to 82 months before the study, and from 30 healthy controls (age 36 ± 10). On the basis of the standard ECG, 38 patients showed a Q-wave infarction of the inferior wall, 22 of the anterior wall and the remaining 13 patients had a non-Q wave MI.

All MI patients were followed-up for a period of at least 18 months; 11 out of 73 patients had one or more documented episodes of VT before BSM recording or during the follow-up period, while the other 62 patients remained asymptomatic for arrhythmias.

BSM recordings: The system of BSM recording has been described in previous papers (5). Briefly, 140 ECG were recorded from the entire chest surface and converted in a digital format with a sampling rate of 500 Hz per channel. At each lead point the potential-time integral relating to the entire QRST interval was calculated as an algebraic sum of all instantaneous potentials multiplied by the sampling interval (2 msec). The times of QRS onset and of T wave offset were determined by careful examination of the instantaneous potential maps. The maps of the integral values (QRST I-maps) were displayed on a format reproducing the chest surface.

Eigenvector analysis: In order to detect and quantitate non-dipolar components of QRST I-maps, we applied the principal component analysis proposed by Lux et al. (6). In this kind of analysis each individual map is represented as a weighted sum of a limited number of fundamental patterns (eigenvectors), common to both control subjects and patients, ordered according to their decreasing importance. Previous investigations (4,5) demonstrated that the first 3 eigenvectors generally have a dipolar distribution, while eigenvectors beyond the 3rd are multipolar. Thus the cumulative contribution of the eigenvectors beyond the third to an individual map, expressed as percent contribution of the total map content, will be considered as "non-dipolar" content of that map.

Statistical analysis: Data are presented as mean ± standard deviation. Comparisons of sample mean values of different groups were made by means of Wilcoxon test for unpaired data.

RESULTS

QRST I-maps: In all subjects of the control group, the QRST I-maps showed a bipolar distribution of the integral values, with a maximum in the left mammary region and a minimum in the upper sternal-right clavicular area. The mean I-map of the group is illustrated in Fig. 1.

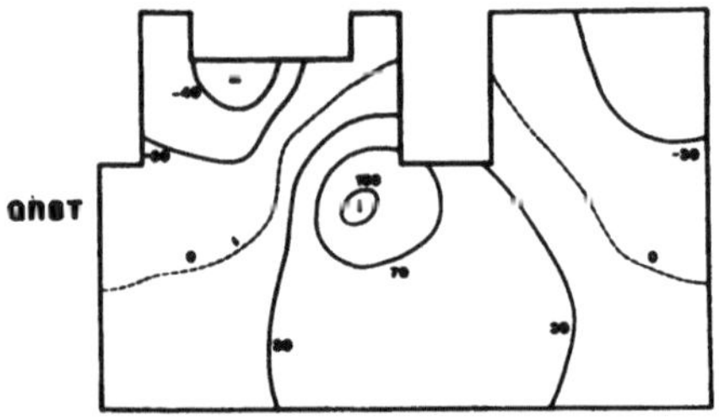

Fig. 1: Schema illustrating the anterior (left part) and posterior (right part) chest surface explored. Mean QRST I-map obtained from the control group. Values of the isointegral lines are expressed in μV•sec.

In the great majority of MI patients the QRST I-maps were bipolar with a different location of the negative and positive values, according to the site of the infarct (Fig. 2). Only in 7 patients (5 without and 2 with VT) there was a clear multipolar distribution of the values (Fig. 3).

Eigenvector analysis: Only the first 9 eigenvectors were considered since each eigenvector beyon the ninth accounted for a very small proportion of the total information content of the maps obtained in our study population. The spatial distribution of the first 6 eigenvectors

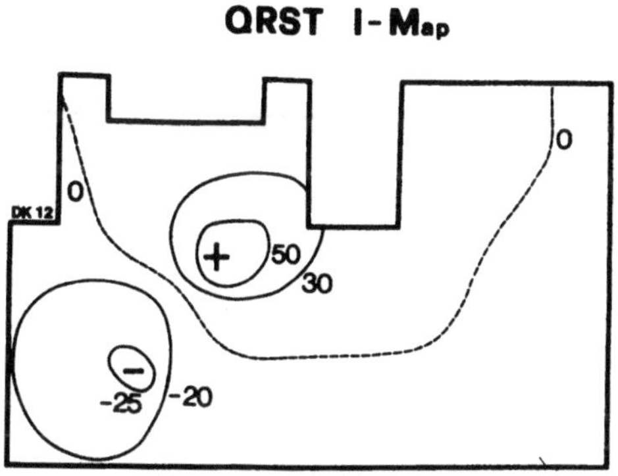

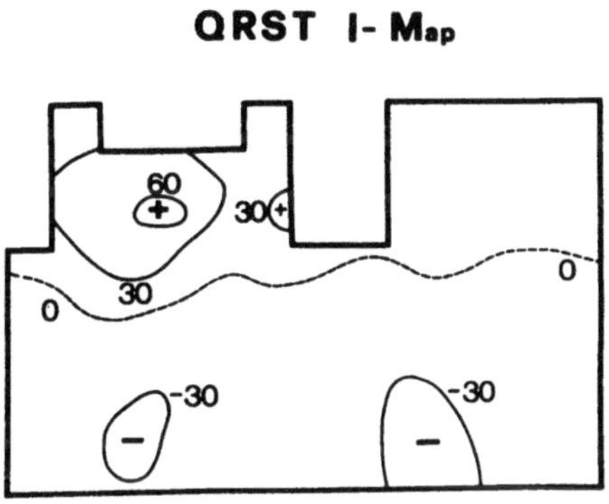

Fig. 2: QRST I-map from a patient with inferior MI without VT.

Fig. 3: QRST I-map from a patient with inferior MI and recurrent VT.

is illustrated in Fig. 4: the eigenvectors beyond the 3rd show a complex multipeak distribution. The cumulative contribution to each individual map of all eigenvectors beyond the 3rd, i.e. the non-dipolar content, is shown in Fig. 5.

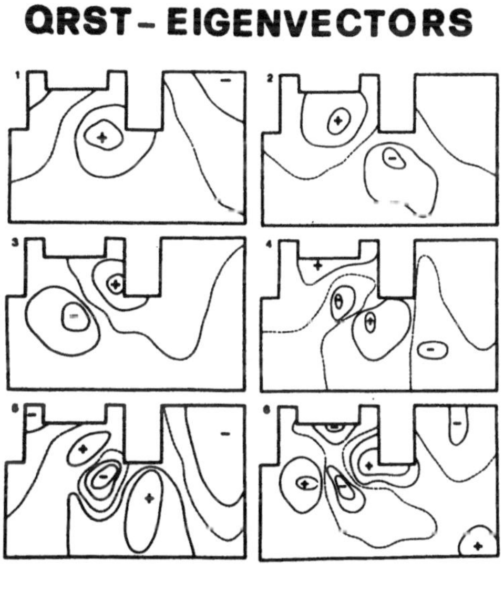

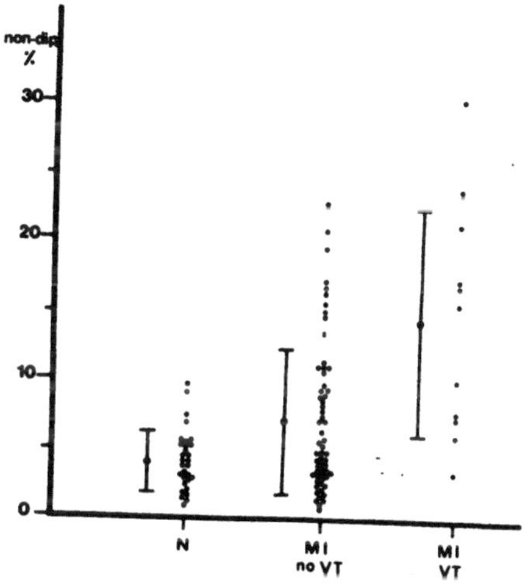

Fig. 4: Spatial distribution of the first 6 eigenvectors (1 to 6) derived from QRST I-maps of our entire study population.

Fig. 5: percentage of non-dipolar content of QRST I-maps in control subjects (N), in MI patients without VT and in MI patients with VT. Mean values and 1 SD are indicated for the 3 groups.

On average, the contribution of non-dipolar components to the individual QRST I-maps was significantly greater in MI patients than in controls (8.3 ± 6.4 % vs 4.1 ± 2.2 %, $p<0.001$) and, among MI patients, in those with VT (7.2 + 5,3 % vs 14.6 + 8.5 %, $p<0.001$). Considering the three

subsets of MI, i.e. anterior, inferior and non Q-wave, the non-dipolar content was slightly higher in anterior than in inferior MI (11.0 ± 6.6 % vs 8.2 ± 6.6 %, p: NS). In non Q-wave MI the non-dipolar content was similar (3.9 ± 1.8 %) to that of the control group.
An abnormally high non-dipolar content (exceeding mean value + 1 SD of the control group) was found in 4 out of 30 control subjects (13 %), in 28 out of 62 patients without VT (45 %) and in 9 out of 11 patients with VT (82 %).

DISCUSSION

Previous investigations have shown abnormalities of QRST integral maps which were related to the occurrence of life-threatening arrhythmias in patients with ischemic heart disease and with long QT syndrome (4,5,7).
In our study population, a clearcut multipolar distribution of the QRST integrals, which is likely related to a markedly disparate repolarization, was infrequently observed in both patients with and without recurrent VT. Thus the simple inspection of the QRST I-maps seems not to be useful in predicting the development of ventricular arrhythmias. On the other hand, by applying the eigenvector analysis we were able to detect and quantitate a high non-dipolar content in many QRST I-maps showing an apparent bipolar distribution.
In our MI patients the presence of a high non-dipolar content in the QRST I-maps was a sensitive index for the occurence of VT (82 %), but not a specific one. However, it cannot be excluded that in some of the patients without VT the high non-dipolar content of QRST I-maps might truly indicate a cardiac state of vulnerability, even though those patients never experienced episodes of VT. In fact, the non-dipolar content should not be equated with the actual occurence of arrhythmias, which still requires an appropriate trigger for initiating.
In conclusion, the high non-dipolar content of the QRST I-maps in patients with VT suggests the presence of local disparities in recovery duration and it might be considered an useful, noninvasive marker of susceptibility to malignant arrhythmias.

REFERENCES

1) Han J., Millet D., Chizzonitti G., Moe G.K.: Am. Heart J. 71, 481-487 (1966).
2) Han J., Garcia Dejalon P.D., Moe G.K.: Circ. Res. 18, 18-25 (1966).
3) Abildskov J.A., Burgess M.J., Urie P.M., Lux R.L., Wyatt R.: Circ. Res. 40, 3-7 (1977).
4) Abildskov J.A., Green L.S., Lux R.L.: in Zipes D.P., Jalife J. eds, Grune Stratton, 495-499 (1985).
5) De Ambroggi L., Bertoni T., Locati E., Stramba-Badiale M., Schwartz P.J.: Circulation 74, 1334-1345 (1986).
6) Lux R.L., Evans A.K., Burgess M.J., Wyatt R.F., Abildskov J.A.: Circ. Res. 49, 186-196 (1981).
7) Gardner M.J., Montague T.J., Armstrong C.S., Horacek B.M., Smith E.R.: Circulation 73, 684-692 (1986).

Nondipolarity of QRST area map and the ventricular arrhythmias following myocardial infarction

KENICHI HARUMI, HIROSHI TSUNAKAWA, GENYO NISHIYAMA, SHIGERU KANESAKA

Division of Cardiology, Showa University Fujigaoka Hospital,
1-30 Fujigaoka, Midori-ku, Yokohama 227, Japan

Summary

Nondipolarity of QRST area map was quantitatively studied by residue in relation to susceptivity for ventricular arrhythmias following myocardial infarction. (1) The residue of MI was lower in QRS area map and higher in ST.T and QRST area maps than that of normal subjects. (2) The residue of QRST area map in 12 patients with VT during the chronic phase was higher (34.5±10.3%) than no VT group (22.7±6.7%) and group of VT only during the acute phase (21.2±7.5%). (3) The QRST area residue exceeding 25% (mean + 2 SD of normal subjects) appeared to be a reliable index for the detection of VT during the chronic phase of MI. (4) The root mean square ratio of ST/QRST was 1.24±0.84 in anterior infarction and 0.51±0.33 in inferior infarction. These results suggest that the determination of the nondipolarity of QRST area map may be clinically relavant to detect substrate for VT during the chronic phase of MI. However, the site of infarction must be considered since the QRST area was influenced more intensely by ST segment deviation in anterior infarction.

Introduction

The QRST area map has been shown to predict the susceptivity for ventricular arrhythmias since it reflects the disparity of ventricular recovery properties.[1)2)3)] However, the detection of nondipolar component of the QRST area as a marker of increased disparity of repolarization has not been fully studied in patients with myocardial infarction (MI). In order to clarify further the clinical value of the area map, the nondipolarity of isointegral map quantitatively studied in relation to ventricular arrhythmias following MI.

Method

The subjects of this study were 27 normal adults and 55 patients with acute MI who were followed at least for 9 months. The patients with the history of previous infarction were not included. The patients were divided into groups A,B and C based on the feature of ventricular tachycardia(VT) following MI, determined by the continuous ECG monitoring during the acute phase (within 10 days from the onset) and by

Holter and exercise ECGs at the time of the convalescent and post hospital phases of MI. Group A consisted of 30 patients without VT throughout the study. Thirteen patients of group B developed VT only during the acute phase and 12 patients of group C showed VT during the chronic phase with and without VT during the acute phase.

Body surface mapping was recorded at the time of discharge, 40 days after the onset of infarction in the average. The body surface potentials were recorded from 64 points on the anterior chest and the time integral area of QRS, ST.T and QRST was calculated for each lead as a algebraic sum of the all potentials from the onset to the offset, multiplied by time interval, then displayed as isointegral map. Each intergral map was examined by means of dipole analysis as shown on the right lower panel of figure 1. This technique allows us to quantitate the nondipolar component included in the surface potentials, in addition to the localization of the optimal dipole .

In order to describe the nondipolarity, the term "residue" was introduced by equation 2. The root mean square ratio of ST/QRST was also determined to represent the relative magnitude of ST segment deviation to the QRST area.

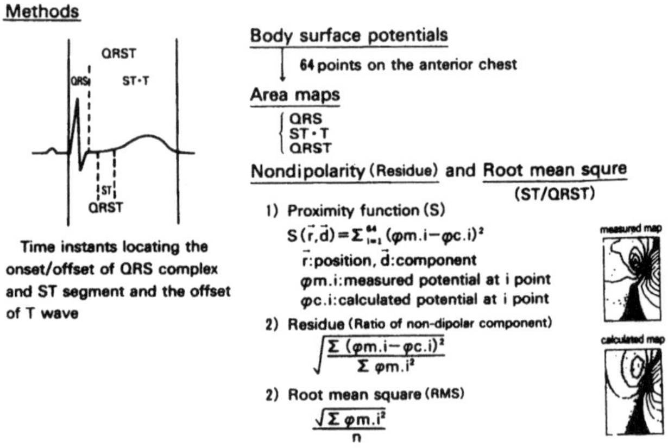

Fig.1

Results

Figure 2 shows the mean residue values of QRS, ST.T and QRST area maps in 27 normal subjects and 55 patients with MI. The residue in the cases of MI was significantly lower in QRS area and higher in ST.T and QRST area maps than that normal subjects. Killip score was 1.5±0.7, 1.7±1.0 and 2.1±0.7 and the left ventricular ejection fraction was 55±14, 53±16 and 37±15 in the groups A, B and C, respectively. There was no significant difference between three groups in their age, the percentage of anterior MI and the number of involved coronary artery.

The QRST area maps were then examined by the residue in relation to VT following MI. The mean residue of QRST area map in group C (43.5±10.3 %) was significantly higher than that of both groups A (22.7±6.7%) and B (21.2±7.5%). However, when the site of infarction was considered, overlapping of the residue value increased between three groups for anterior infarction and the separation of group C from other two groups was less clear in anterior infarction than in inferior infarction as shown in figure 3. This might have resulted from the higher residue value even in groups A and B in the anterior infarction. We arbitrarily defined the residue exceeding 25% (mean + 2 SD of normal subjects) as abnormally high non-dipolar contribution to the QRST area. It was obtained in 24 of 55 patients with higher prevalence in group C as shown on table 1. Further the clear differentiation of group C from other two groups was shown in inferior infarction.

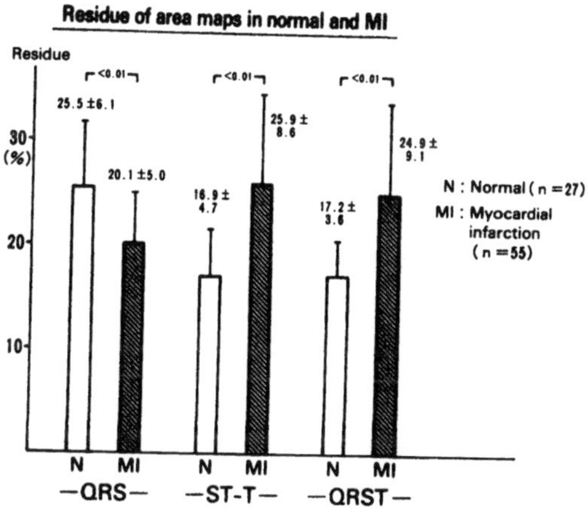

Fig.2

Discussion

There has been increasing interest to detect substrate for life threatening arrhythmias by means of noninvasive techniques. One of the most important electrophysiologic abnormalities for the development of such arrhythmias is an increased disparity in the recovery properties of ventricular muscle.[5] This nonuniform repolarization has been thought to be reflected on the QRST area.[1] More recently, the significance of the higher nondipolarity of the QRST area as a marker of increased nonuniform recovery was clearly shown in patients with malignant ventricular arrhythmias based on the multipolar potential distribution by visual interpretation of the map[2] and in patients with long QT syndrome assessed by higher contribution of the nondipolar eigenvectors.[3]

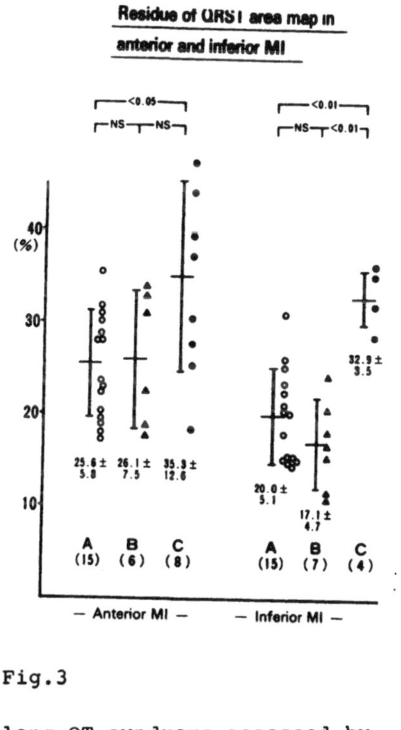

Fig.3

In this report, the nondipolarity of isointegral maps was quantitatively studied by residue in relation to susceptivity for VT following MI. Our previous studies on the clinical application to the residue using the equivalent dipole method have suggested that the nondipolar component has been successfuly estimated and could be applied to clinical use.[6) 7)] The results of this study demonstrated that although some overlapping of the residue value was noted between three groups in anterior infarction, the patients with VT during the chronic phase of MI could be predicted by the nondipolar QRST area map.

While the nondipolarity of the ratio QRST area depends primarily on the ventricular repolarization properties, other factors might influence the QRST area. Among several factors studied in this report, the magnitude of the ST segment deviation must be taken into consideration since the QRST area was more intensely influenced by the ST segment deviation in anterior infarction even more than one month after the onset of infarction.

Comparison of Residue of QRST area map

Myocardial Infarction (n=55)

	A	B	C*
Residue ≥ 25	10	3	11
<25	20	10	1

*P <0.01 compared with group A and B

Anterior MI (n=29)

	A	B	C
Residue ≥ 25	7	3	7
<25	8	3	1

NS

Inferior MI (n=26)

	A	B	C*
Residue ≥ 25	3	0	4
<25	12	7	0

*P <0.01 compared with group A and B

Table 1.

References

1) Urie,P.M.,et al: Circ.Res. 42, 350 - 358 (1978)
2) Gordner,M.J., et al: Circ. 73, 684 - 692 (1986)
3) Ambroggi,L.D., et al: Circ. 74, 1334 - 1345 (1986)
4) Okamoto, Y., et al: Jpn. Heart J. 23, 293 - 304 (1982)
5) Han ,J., and Moe,G.K.: Circ.Res. 14, 44 - 60 (1964)
6) Tsunakawa,H., et al: Jpn.Heart J. 26, 319 - 334 (1985)
7) Tsunakawa,H., et al: JACC, to be published.

Characteristic Features of the Cardioelectric Fields Mapped in Patients with Essential and Renal Hypertension

KNYAZEVA T.A., TITOVA G.A.

The Central Institute of Health Resorts and Physical Treatment
50 Kalinin Avenue, Moscow, USSR

Summary - Quantitative criteria for three degrees of the pronounced left ventricular hypertrophy (LVH) are devised. The LVH differential diagnostic features of essential (EH) and renal hypertensions (RH) are found, which are of particular importance in detecting the aetiology and stage of the disease. Greater informative value of the 90-lead integral cardiotopography (ICTG) is revealed as compared with the standard 12-lead ECG in the LVH diagnostics and dynamics.

Introduction - The study is aimed at finding the LVH characteristic features by quantitative criteria mapped in EH an RH patients using ICTG techniques.

Material and Methods - All in all 60 patients with arterial hypertension and with the LVH clinical and roentgenological signs have been investigated. 25 patients suffered from EH (second stage) and 35 were RH patients investigated 8-14 days after reconstructive operations on renal arteries. The patients were grouped according to the disease period (from 5 to 10 years), the blood pressure level (160-180/100-120 mm Hg) are age (30-50). The ICTG maps were drawn using 90 chest unipolar leads arranged on 5 horizontal levels uniformly all over the thorax (1). The following ICTG quantitative values were analysed: R, the total value of all R waves (Mv); ratios Rmax / Smax and $\frac{R}{QS}$; the area of the zero zone R (n R_o). ECG was taken in 12 standard leads, evaluated by the classic signs of the left ventricular hypertrophy. The LVH degree was determined in accord with the criteria devised by Knyazeva T.A. and Titova G.A. (2): These criteria are given in Table 1.

Results - ICTG resulted in detecting LVH in 100 % of the patients, while ECG detected LVH signs only in 57 %. In RH cases the third degree (dg) of LVH was detected in 66 % of the patients and the second degree in 34 %, while in EH cases the third degree was not detected in any patient, the second degree was detected in 68 % and the first degree in 32 %. The characteristic feature of LVH in RH cases is the presence of zero zones (R_o) on the right-hand side of the electropositivity map: for the second degree in 10-25 leads and for the third degree in more than 25 leads. There were no zero zones in EH patients with the first degree of LVH, while in those with the second degree zero zones were revealed in insignificant number (up to 10 leads). See Figure 1:

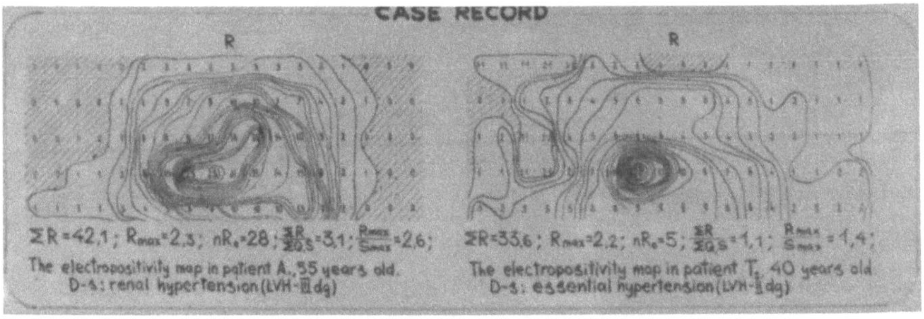

Discussions and Conclusions - The elaboration of quantitative criteria for the pronounced LVH makes it possible to create an objective LVH classification, which is of primary significance for specifying a stage of hypertension and even its aetiology, i.e. it can serve as one of the differential diagnostic criteria for evaluating EH and RH. The importance of the devised diagnostic criterion lies in the fact that the disease period does not always correlate with LVH signs in standard 12 leads (3) and R in ICTG (in contrast to ECG) makes it possible to take into account a shift of a maximum zone of positive potentials tothe left and downwards which is ordinarily the case in LVH. The appearance of zero zones (R_o) on the right-hand side of the electropositivity map is evaluated as a break in the dipole circular movement, which is caused by a considerable increase of R wave on the opposite (left-hand) side of the electropositivity map. It is confirmed by a gradual decrease of R wave with its follow-up disappearance (R_o). The area of a zero zone increases in proportion to the LVH degree, which is particularly evident in RH cases. Due to a gradual decrease of R till its disappearance the LVH cartogram differs from a sharp disappearance of R wave ("downfall syndrome") in transmural myocardial lesions.

Classification of the left ventricular hypertrophies
/according to the quantitative value of the degree/

	ΣR (mv)	$\frac{R_{max}}{S_{max}}$ and $\frac{\Sigma R}{\Sigma Q,S}$	nR_o (the number of leads)
norm	<25,0	0,7-1,2	is absent or <5
moderately pronounced (I degree)	25,0-30,0	<1,5	RH- <10 (EH-is absent)
cleary pronounced (II degree)	30,0-35,0	1,5-2,0	RH-10-25 (EH-<10)
strongly pronounced (III degree)	>35,0	>2,0	RH- >25 (EH-)

Therefore:

1) ICTG makes it possible to find specific differential diagnostic features of LVH in RH cases in contrast to EH: strongly pronounced values of hypertrophy (R 35.0; Rmax/Smax and R/ QS 2.0) and a large area of zero zones on the right-hand side of the electropositivity map.

2) Quantitative criteria of pronounced LVH are devised, thus making it possible to evaluate in a objective manner the degree of hypertrophy.

3) The specific feature of zero zones (n R_0) in LVH cases is that they appear due to a gradual decrease in the value of R wave in contrast to its sharp disappearance ("downfall syndrome") in focal myocardial lesions

References.

1) Amirov R.Z. Integral Topogramms of Cardiac Potentials. Nauka, Moscow (1973).

2) Knyazeva T.A., Titova G.A. Cardiology, 6, (pp. 91-92, (1986).

3) Shkhvatsabaya I.K. Proceedings of the Third All-Russian Cardiological Congress, pp. 187-188. Sverdlovsk (1985).

USE OF COMPUTER SYSTEMS TO DEVELOP NOVEL APPROACHES TO ELECTROCARDIOGRAPHIC ANALYSIS

A.V.Sobolev, G.V.Ryabykina, F.U.Gadzhaeva, Z.Z.Dorofeyeva, T.A.Sakhnova

Our study over many years to increase a diagnostic value of electrocardiographic and vectorcardiographic techniques by using computer systems [1,2] has prompted us to look for new criteria for evaluating curves produced in combined types of cardiac abnormalities. The McFee-Parungao system vectorcardiograms (VCG) and natural maps of 35 precordial leads ECG performed by the Maroko method were the major object of the study. The material was as follows: ECG signals from a patient were amplified, synchronized and recorded on an analog magnetograph. From the magnetograph the signal was entered into the computer storage through an analog-to-number converter. The input curves were displayed on the screen on which the physician marked the coordinates of the wave limits which were entered into the storage on the ECG with a vertical cursor. With this method, a total bank comprising VCGs and ECGs recorded in patients with a clinical diagnosis verified by various methods was formed. The bank is being constantly supplied. At present there are over 1,000 ECGs and VCGs in the bank.

The present studies proceeded along three interrelated lines: 1) nonconventional computer visualization of VCG; 2) determination of diagnostically valuable ECG and VCG parameters and 3) search for leads that are most informative in diagnostic criteria for cardiac abnormalities. Some results will be presented.

Spatial vector P loop imaging. We made an attempt to elucidate which parameters of a spatial P loop form were diagnostically significant for atrial enlargement. The imaging analysis of the loops projected to the routine planes has shown that they show a great polymorphism and inscribed traectories are very complicated both in normal and enlarged atria. We visualized the P loop projected to plane II when the loop approached its spatial position with best approximation. The analysis of the P loop projected to plane II simplified and became diagnostically valuable when the angle of view was correctly chosen (Fig. 1). Basis vectors W_1 and W_2 were so selected that the projection of P loop started and ended in the left half-plane and ran the origin of coordinates counterclockwise. Normally, P loops fall into two main types: those of type A are stretching along the vector W_1 direction, those of type B are stretching along the vector W_2 direction. The analysis of our material (33 and 32 cases with an isolated enlargement in the left and right atria, respectively) has shown that all loops are of type A in cases of right atrial enlargement and of type B in those of left atrial enlargement, and the loops shown a highly significant difference from normal with regard to oncreases in their respective diameters. Atrial enlargement is established on the basis of increase not only in loop diameter Dp, but in its area.

Role of middle QRS loop vectors in the diagnosis of ventricular hypertrophy [3]. While enlargement in either ventricle shifts the middle vector towards the enlarged portion, the position of the middle vector is diagnostically important to determine the type of one-sided hypertrophy. Synchronous enlargement in the both ventricles produces specific changes in the position of the middle vector in space. These changes are mostly reflected in the horizontal plane projection. The analysis of the middle QRS loop vectors in 81 healthy

P_{xyz}LOOP - PLANE Π

RIGHT ATRIAL ENLARGMENT

LEFT ATRIAL ENLARGMENT

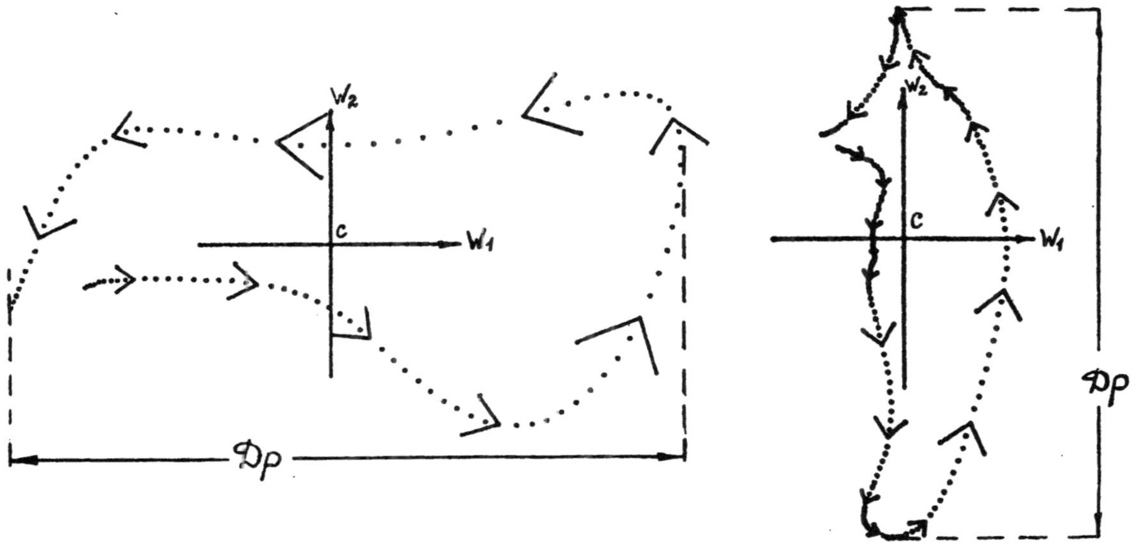

VARIANT A CONSIDERABLE ENLARGMENT $D_p(W_I)$

VARIANT B CONSIDERABLE ENLARGMENT $D_p(W_2)$

Fig.I VARIANTS OF P_{XYZ} WAVE IN PROJECTION ON "Π"PLANE.

subjects, 125 patients with left ventricular hypertrophy (LVH), 44 patients with right ventricular hypertrophy (RVH) and 80 patients with both ventricular hypertrophy (BVH) showed the following: according to the position of the middle vector, hypertrophy was found in 75 of 80 cases in BVH group, BVH being in 36 cases (Fig. 2). At the same time signs of combined hypertrophy were not detected by 12 leads ECG.

Search for leads most informative in the diagnosis of ventricular hypertrophy 4 . 35 precordial leads ECG were studied for value in the diagnosis of various types of ventricular enlargement. Different S and R wave sums were analysed in pairs (similarly to the method Sokolov and Lyon had developed for particular pairs of the precordial leads) to diagnose LVH in 88 patients with arterial hypertension and 71 healthy subjects. S waves from 1-4 lead columns and R waves from 4-7 columns were summands. For each of 400 sums formed in such a fashion we estimated percentage of cases with LVH when their values exceeded the higher control threshold $M_N + 2\sigma_N$. The sums for which the percentage was maximum were regarded as being most diagnostically significant. Such were $S_{32} + R_{14}$ and $S_{30} + R_{19}$. Their simultaneous use enabled the method sensitivity to be increased to 1.5-fold the routine ones. The much greater (63% versus 37% by the Sokolov-Lyon criteria) increase was reached in the diagnostically most complicated group involved 49 patients with moderate hypertrophized left ventricular myocardial mass (ranging from 160 to 200 g). Application of the similar sums of S and R wave areas allowed the diagnostic sensitivity to be increased up to 71% in this subgroup at 93 specificity.

Likewise, there are sums that are of most importance in the diagnosis of LVH in 57 patients with right ventricular enlargement. They simultaneous use of amplitude sums such as $R_8 + S_{12}$ and $R_{15} + S_{20}$

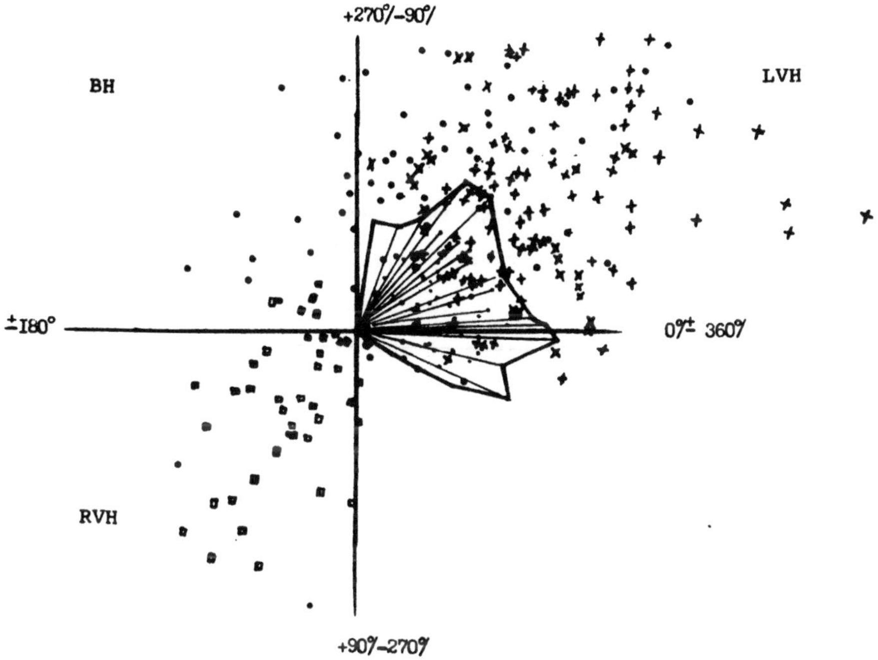

Fig.II Concentration Areas of L_{xyz} Mean Vectors Location

Areas of Mean Vectors in Norm Limited by Boundary Line.

Signes: X-LVH, -RVH, -BH

made it possible to attain 100% sensitivity in our samples (by the Sokolov-Lyon criteria, the sensitivity was 87.9%) at invariable specificity of 94.4%.

The results of studying the maps in BVH turned out to be the most interesting. Traditionally, cases with BVH were regarded as satisfying the criteria for diagnosing isolated types of both LVH and RVH. The analysis sensitivity in this case is minor. Different approach were applied to select diagnostic criteria for BVH. After distinguishing BVH cases from the normal ones, they were compared with ECG parameters in one-sided hypertrophy. The same groups of healthy subjects, patients with LVH and RVH, and 136 cases with BVH were analysed. The greatest variations were found between BVH and LVH while transforming S waves which appeared larger in size in the third vertical column, they are virtually equal in the first column in these two groups. Hence, the ratio of S wave amplitude and area in the third vertical column to S waves of the first vertical column should be used as a distinguishing feature of BVH and LVH. The distinction of BVH from RVH is regarded as to a greater extent being true for Rwave size and area in the leads of the seventh vertical column are lower than those in the BVH group, in the leads of the first vertical column they are higher. We chose the ratio of R waves in the seventh vertical column to R waves in the first vertical column to discriminate BVH from RVH.

Fig. 3 shows the most informative indices of differences found in BVH, RVH, and LVH, whose application produces 72.8% diagnostic sensitivity for BVH at 90.4% specificity. Application of the Sokolov-Lyon indices in the same group showed 9.6% sensitivity for BVH detection at 94.0% specificity.

The change-over of the above analytic methods to 6 precordial

ECG-35 MEAN INDICES USED TO DISTINGUISH BH FROM ISOLATED FORMS OF RVH AND LVH

ECG-35 INDICES	BH n = 136		LVH 160 gr. < MMLV < 200 gr. n = 27		LVH MMLV ≥ 200 gr. n = 12		RVH n = 57	
	M	σ	M	σ	M	σ	M	σ
AMPLITUDES RATIO								
a) TO DISTINGUISH FROM LVH								
R_{14}/R_1			5.5	3.8	7.0	3.4	0.5	0.6
								M+2σ =1.7
S_{25}/S_{27}	6.7	10.1	7.3	8.2	13.6	7.2	1.8	0.7
								M+2σ =3.2
b) TO DISTINGUISH FROM RVH								
$\frac{S_{10} + S_{17} + S_{24}}{S_1 + S_8 + S_{15}}$	2.8	3.2	0.9	0.4	1.0	0.3	5.1	7.1
			M + 2σ =1.7					
R_{27}/R_{17}	6.6	9.3	2.1	1.6	4.0	2.9	0.9	0.9
			M + 2σ =5.3					
AREAS RATIO								
a) TO DISTINGUISH FROM LVH								
R_{14}/R_1			9.9	10.3	16.4	18.9	0.3	0.4
								M+2σ =1.1
S_{25}/S_{27}	18.7	67.6	7.9	12.0	19.8	21.3	1.6	0.6
								M+2σ =2.8
b) TO DISTINGUISH FROM RVH								
$\frac{S_{10} + S_{17} + S_{24}}{S_1 + S_8 + S_{15}}$	3.4	4.8	0.7	0.3	0.8	0.3	7.9	17.1
			M + 2σ =1.3					
R_{27}/R_{17}	14.3	33.5	2.7	2.9	6.0	5.3	1.0	1.5
			M + 2σ =8.5					

leads V_1-V_6 proved to be highly effective. 55.9% (versus 9.6%) sensitivity of the method was observed at 95.8% specificity.

Thus, application of computer systems have been demonstrated to be feasible in developing novel approaches to the analysis of electrocardiograms.

REFERENCIES

1. Common standards for quantitative electrocardiography. CSE 5th Progress Report, 1985, Leuven. Ref. N CSE 85-12-05.
2. Pipberger, H.V., McCaughan, D., Littmann, D., Pipberger, H.A. et al. Clinical application of a second generation electrocardiographic computer program- Am.J.Cardiol., 1975, v. 35, p. 597.
3. Sobolev A.V., Ryabykina G.V., Krotovskaya T.A., Sergakova L.M., Kivaeva G.M. Informative value of different precordial ECG leads for the diagnosis of left ventricular hypertrophy. Kardiologiya, 1986, v. 26, No. 11, p. 23 (In Russian).
4. Gadzhaeva F.U., Sobolev A.V., Dorofeyeva Z.Z., Serchakova L.M., Dyakonova E.G., Markovskaya T.S., Randmaa I.L. Integral parameters of automatically reproduced spatial QRS loop in the diagnosis of myocardial hypertrophy. Kardiologiya, 1986, v. 26, No. 11, p. 18.

Specific features of the integral cardiac topograms in the patients with myocarditis.

R.Z.Amirov, Z.I.Semenovitch
The Central Scientific Research Institute of Health Resort and Physical Treatment.
The Kalinin Prospect 50, Moscow, USSR.

Summary.
A study of the cardiac electrical field by means of integral topography has allowed to reveal focal changes in 100 examined patients. In the patients with myocarditis focal changes are projected beyond the limits of 12-lead ECG:in the basal areas and over the right and posterior cardiac surface and they are similar to that ones seen in the patients with myocardial infarction. In these patients integral topograms have zero zones on the electropositivity maps of QS waves and on the opposite side there are zero zones on the electronegativity maps. In a number of patients there is a disbalance of cardiac potentials during QRS period.

Introduction. It is known, that in the patients with infective-allergic myocarditis ECG changes are basically limited by changes of T wave and ST interval. For the sake of the detailed investigation into the electrical cardiac field and development of new diagnostic indices in the patients with myocarditis we've studied multiple leads from the whole chest surface.

Material and methods. One hundred patients aged 23-49 years with infective-allergic myocarditis existing from 3 months to 5 years have been examined. Myocarditis had developed 7-14 days after infective disease (influenza, tonsillitis, pneumonia). In 75 patients this process had been latent and in 25 postmyocarditis cardiosclerosis had been diagnosed. Main signs of the disease were as follows: cardialgia, signs of the developing heart failure in 76%, cardiac rhythm disorders - extrasystolic arrhytmia- in 24%. Integral topography,registration of 90 chest leads and construction of the maps of distribution of the potentials during QRS period, ST interval and T wave maximum have been applied.

Results.In all patient integral topography has revealed myocardial changes covering an area of 1-10 leads and a sum of the potentials of QS waves 23.6-135mV on the electropositivity map. Focal changes are mainly projected onto the basal regions of the heart. In 42% of cases there are basal focal changes in the anterior and posterior wall, in 19% - in the posterior wall, in 18% - ther is a combined damage of the anterior,lateral and posterior wall and in 9% - the anterior and lateral wall is affected.

In addition,25% of the patients there is multifocal myocardial damage.

On the electronegativity maps there are zero zones (without Q-S waves) having an opposite projection in comparison to QS wave.

In 11 (12%) patients a zero zone on the electronegativity map corresponds to a value of QS wave, in 43 (48%) a zero zone is by 39% less, than QS zone. In 33% a zero zone is by 50% larger, than QS zone and only in two patients (2%) a zero zone is totally absent. A zero zone is, as a rule, projected onto the opposite pole along a diagonal from the right to the left or from the left to the right in relation to QS zone.

Alongside with it, there is a disbalance to a side of elevation of R_{max} and decrease of S_{max}.

All metioned changes are not and can'be revealed by 12-lead ECG. Integral topography and ECG have revealed changes in the electrical activity of the myocardium in 50 patients following treatment with carbonaceous baths.

All patients are distributed into 4 groups in relation to an extent of focal myocardial changes.

Group I includes the patients with a small affected area covering 1-10 leads.

Group II includes the patients with a middle-sized affected area covering 11-20 leads.

Group III includes the patients with a large affected area covering 31-40 leads.

Group IY includes the patients with an extensive affected area covering 31-40 leads.

In the patients of group I a zone of focal changes prevails in 4 leads. In the patients of group II (17%) a zone of focal changes covers 19 leads, of the third group (27%) this zone cavers 22 leads. In the patients of group IY teher is extensive myocardial damage. Physical treatment with carbonaceous baths has resulted in positive changes in the bioelectrical activity of the myocardium in the patients of group II, which are seen as a sum of the potentials in the zone of focal changes reduced by 18%, that is, from 55.2 ± 7.6 to 45 ± 7.02 ($p < 0.001$).

In relation to a degree of circulatory insufficiency a volume of the reparative processes in the myocardium has been changed following physical treatment with carbonaceous baths. Thus, in the patients without signs of circulatory insufficiency and with a zone of focal changes covering 10-20 leads there is a statistically confident reduction of the affected zone from 18.0 ± 1.0 to 11.0 ± 0.7 ($p < 0.05$) and of a sum of QS potentials from 79.60 ± 9.0 to 45.5 ± 2.0 ($p < 0.05$). As for $\frac{R}{Q,S}$ sum a disbalance is confidently increased from 1.27 ± 0.07 to 1.41 ± 0.06 ($p < 0.01$), which confirms marked reparative processes in the myocardium. While in the patients of the same group with circulatory insufficiency of stage I-2 there is favourable hemodynamic rearrangement confirming the elevated myocardial contratile function and lowered tonus of peripheral vessels according to the data of the tetrapolar chest rheography. In this category of patients focal myocardial changes are a sum of potentials, which is not essentially changed according to topographic data, just as in the patients receiving "placebo" treatment. Alongside with it in several patients ECG reveals insignificant changes seen as an elevated T wave amplitude and reduced extrasystoles. Integral topography has allowed to reveal presence and localization of focal changes, their extension and to calculate a sum of QS waves, $\frac{R}{QS}$ max disbalance and to examine favourable changes in these indices influenced by physical treatment with carbonaceous baths.

Conclusions:

1. A focal nature and degree of the myocardial damage has been revealed in the patients with myocarditis.
2. A zero zone is present on the electronegativity map in the area opposite to a zone of QS waves.
3. A disbalance of a disbalance of the maximum and sum of R and QS waves has been revealed.
4. Favourable changes in these indices in the patients with myocarditis influenced by treatment with carbonaceous baths have been followed up.

Legends.

Fig.I Integral topogram and ECG of patient P. with myocarditis. QS wave area covers 20 leads, a zone of the zero negative potentials covers 13 leads in the upper chest surface.

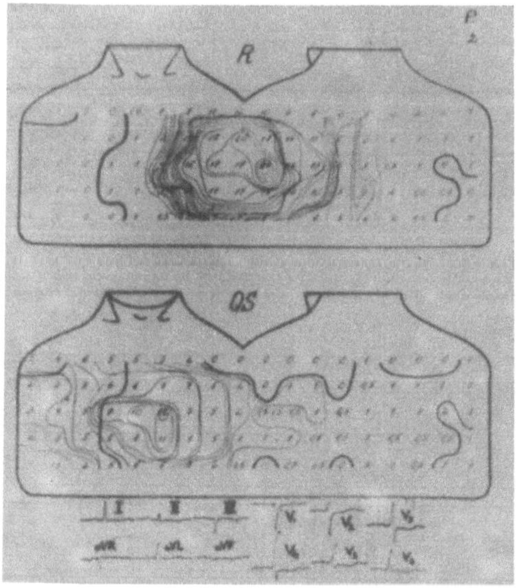

Fig. 2 Patient Zh. with myocarditis, a QS zone covers 19 leads, a zero zone of negative potentials covers 10 leads and is located in the posterio upper and lower chest surface.

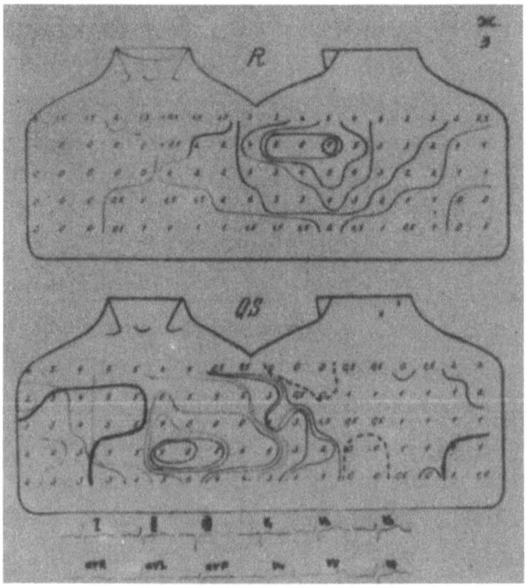

Estimation of the dipolar content of total body surface potential distribution in WPW syndrome.

BACHÁROVÁ,L., FILIPOVÁ,S., CAGÁŇ,S.
Medical Bionics Research Institute, Jedľova 6, Bratislava, Faculty of Medicine, Comenius University, Bratislava,Czechoslovakia

Summary.

In 7 patients with Wolf-Parkinson-White syndrome the body surface potential distribution was recorded from 30 unipolar leads by the modified method of Lux et al. along with physically corrected orthogonal ECGs (Frank lead system). Orthogonal waveforms served for chronocardiotopographic presentation of ventricular depolarization sequence on a spherical image surface with the aid of Titomir's mathematical model (DECARTO system). In this way the dipolar content of the body surface distribution was compared with uncorrected total information. Special interest was paid to the initial pre-excitatory ventricular activation, to the period of fusion of preexcitation with regular ventricular activation, as well as to the period of normal ventricular activation after the termination of preexcitation. With these two kinds of topographic presentation of ventricular activation the pathways of maximum positivity, the time function of maximum and minimum potential values, the temporo-spatial evolution of positivity areas, as well as the estimation of localisation of preexcitation on hand of 20-30 ms delta vectors were compared. This comparison allowed to evaluate the diagnostic value of non-dipolar body surface information in localising the origin of the preexcitation wave.

Introduction.

Preexcitation is a natural model for detection and study of two simultaneously present fronts of myocardial activation. The aim of this study was a comparison of body surface information obtained by ECG mapping with the dipolar information presented by dipolar electrocardiotopography (DECARTO system).

Material and methods.

Seven patients with WPW pattern were examined. In all patients body surface potential distribution were recorded by 30 leads (modified lead system according to Lux et al. 1979), as well as orthogonal physically corrected Frank electrocardiograms. Frank ECG signals were processed by Titomir's mathematical model (Titomir and Ruttkay-Nedecký, 1987) and presented in the form of activated areas on the spherical image surface as chronocardiotopograms (DECARTO system.)

Following comparable forms of presentation of BSPM and DECARTO system are presented:

(1) maps at selected instants of QRS:

- isopotential instantaneous maps,
- areas of activated points on the spherical image surface.

(2) magnitudes of potential extrema as a function of time:

- time function of the magnitude of body surface potential maximum and minima,
- time function of spatial vector magnitude.

(3) trajectories of minima:

- trajectory of minima on the body surface maps,
- trajectory of the mirror image of the spatial vector end-points.

(4) vectors connecting minima-maxima at selected instants of QRS:

- vector connecting minimum to maximum on BSPMs,
- connections of the spatial vector end-point with its mirror image on the spherical image surface.

Results:

Results of individual comparisons of BSPMs and DECARTO maps obtained in the same subject are illustrated on hand of a typical case. Patient J.J.,21 years old, male, with the accessory pathway location in the anterior septum, determined by the analysis of the body surface potential maps (Benson et al.1982, Iwa et al.1980) is presented on fig. 1-4.

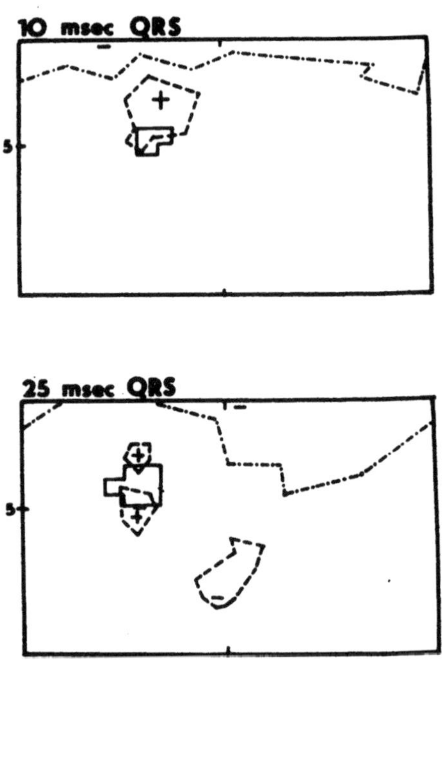

Fig.1. Comparison of body surface potential distribution (dot-dash line = zero line, dash line = positive and negative isopotential lines) and DECARTO areas of activated points (solid line). In 10 ms QRS (period of pure preexcitation) the body surface potential maximum is located on the left upper anterior surface of the chest. The DECARTO activation area is dislocated slightly downward. Max. = 0.224 mV, Min. = -0.054 mV, V_{10} = 0.081. In 25 ms QRS (fusion of preexcitation and normal activation) two maxima are located on the anterior surface of the chest, DECARTO activated area is located between two maxima. Max.1 = 0.947 mV, Min.1 = -0.121 mV, Max.2 = 0.841 mV, MIN.2 = -0.021 mV, V_{20} = 0.210 mV, V_{30} = 0.763 mV.

Fig.2. Comparison of time functions of magnitudes of potential extrema. Solid line = spatial vector magnitude. Dash line = preexcitation minimum. Dot line = normal activation minimum. Dot-dash line = BSPM maximum.

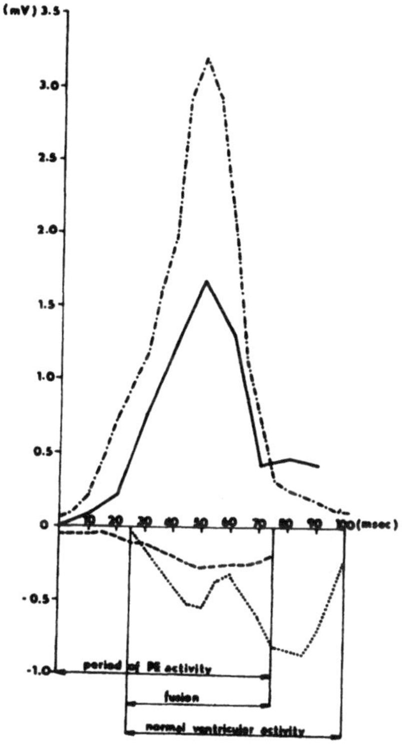

Fig.3. Comparison of trajectories of minima. Preexcitation minimum (dot line) was moving in a limited area high on left precordium, at the level of the 2nd intercostal space. Normal activation minimum (dash line) appeared in 20 ms of QRS on the left anterolateral abdominal surface, moving farther slightly upward anteriorly, and then from the 25 ms rotating posteriorly on the dorsal surface and from the 45 ms to 100 ms moving throug the anterior right chest surface to the middle of precordium. Mirror images of the end-points of QRS vectors (solid line) up to 50 ms are located posteriorly in the upper middle part, thereafter from 60 to 90 ms they follow pathway of normal BSPM minimum.

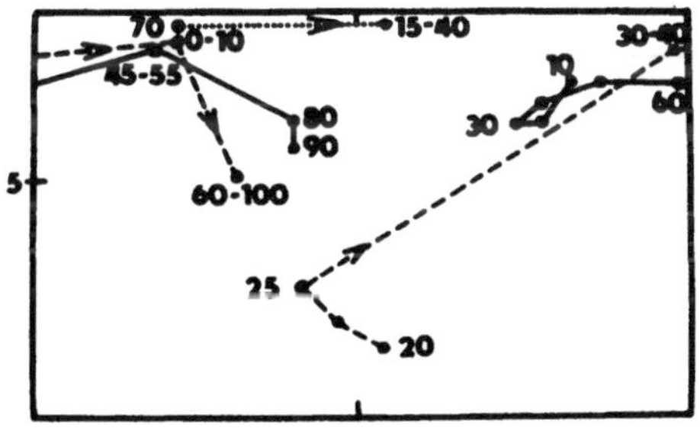

Fig.4. Comparison of the orientation of vectors connecting minima - maxima. BSPM - in 10 ms QRS (dot-dash line) and in 25 ms QRS (dot line) the orientations were from the upper pole anteriorly slightly downward to the midsternal area. Spatial vectors in 10 ms (solid line) and in 25 ms (dash line) were oriented from dorsal upper pole anteriorly to the middle. Both of presented methods (BSPM and DECART) have a qualitatively similar orientation of vectors connecting minima - maxima.

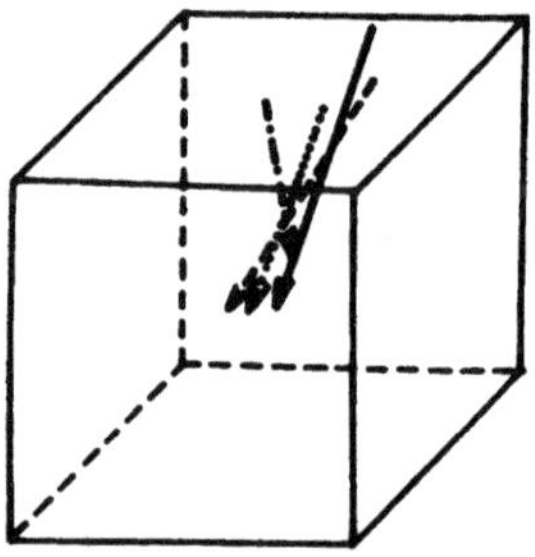

Discussion and conclusion:

In WPW two activation processes were distinquishable by the BSPM and by presentation of time functions of surface potential minima - period of preexcitation via accessory pathway and myocardial activation via normal conductivity system. The location of preexcitation was determined by BSPM.

DECARTO chronotopocardiograms enable to present the dipolar information in a qualitatively similar form to BSPM.

In WPW patients with accessory pathways located in the anterior septum or anterior left ventricle wall, the differences between data obtained by BSPM and DECARTO respectively, axis maps, were relatively small. The trajectory of the mirror image of the spatial vector end-point was distingtly irregular in the region representing the focus of preexcitation as determined by the analysis of BSPM.

With location of the accessory pathway in the posterior bazal ventricular wall the trajectory of spatial vector end-point was distingtly curled. The connections of minima-maxima during the period of preexcitation and during the fusion were oriented differently.

In conclusion, it is felt that that above demonstrated methods of non-invasive electrocardiographic analysis of WPW patients may contributed to the approximate localisation od preexcitation in the ventricle.

References.

1. Lux,R.L., Burgess,M.J. Wyatt,R.S., Evans,A.K., Vincent,G.N., Abildskov,J.A.: Circulation 59, 356-363 (1979).
2. Titomir,L.I., Ruttkay-Nedecký,I.: International J Biomed Comp 20, 275-282 (1987).
3. Benson,S.W.Jr., Sterba,R., Gallagher,J.J., Walston,A.,II.,Spach,M.S.: Circulation 65, 1259-1268 (1982).
4. Iwa,T.W., Kawasuji,M., Misaki,T., Iwase,T., Magara,T.: J Thorax Cardiovasc Surg 80, 271-279 (1980).

M A G N E T O C A R D I O G R A P H Y

High resolution magnetocardiography

NOWAK, H. (1), ALBRECHT, G. (1), BURGHOFF, M. (1), HEINKE, M. (2), KIRSCH, G. (3), VOLKMANN, H. (2), ZACH, H.-G (1)

(1) PTI Jena, Academy of Sciences of the GDR, Helmholtzweg 4, Jena, 6900, GDR
(2) FSU Jena, Dep. of Medicine, Div. of Cardiology, Karl-Marx-Allee, Jena, 6902, GDR
(3) FSU Jena, Sektion Physik, Helmholtzweg 5, Jena, 6900, GDR

Summary

High resolution magnetocardiography is used for the identification of signals of the conduction system e. g. His-Purkinje system or late field magnetocardiography.
The measurement technique, used by the biomagnetic group in Jena, will be briefly described. Latest results of measurements with patients (WPW syndrome, ventricular tachycardia) will be presented and discussed.

Introduction

Investigations on the electric and magnetic activity of the heart are current topics in cardiology research, and scientists are looking for more or new information about the human heart. There exist a lot of diagnostic methods and devices for heart investigation but both a well-established theory and a complete model are unknown. For that reason slightly unconventional methods as biomagnetic investigations are employed in basic research on the heart structure, on cardiac current distribution or on the conduction system of the heart.
The myocardial magnetic activity generates one of the strongest biomagnetic fields in the body and is caused by the same current distributions that generate the electric potentials in the biological volume conductor.
Since 1963 researchers have been studied the phenomena of the magnetic field of the heart, hoping that the magnetocardiogram (MCG) might provide diagnostic information about cardiac activity not present or visible in the electrocardiogram.
For this purpose, high-resolution magnetocardiography (HR MCG) is used for the identification of signals of the conduction system (1) HR MCG seems to be promissing for the localization of sources, one of the advantages of the magnetic technique(2).

Methods

The magnetocardiographic measurements were carried out in an unshielded room of the biomagnetic laboratory in Jena. The equipment consists of a dc thin film SQUID UJ 111 with integrated input transformer (3) and a second order gradiometer with 28 mm in diameter and a baselength of 50 mm. The input sensitivity of the system is 20 fT $Hz^{-1/2}$ for white noise. This is sufficient for high-resolution magnetocardiography when signal averaging is employed. The method is discribed more in detail in (4).

Results

A non-invasive recording of late potentials with QRS triggered averaging in the ST-segment in a patient with ventricular tachycardia is shown in Fig. 1. All curves are recordings of the V1V6 lead, where (a) is a reference lead, (b) is a HR ECG with late potentials after 100 averagings and 30 Hz high-pass filtering and (c) after 60 Hz high-pass filtering.

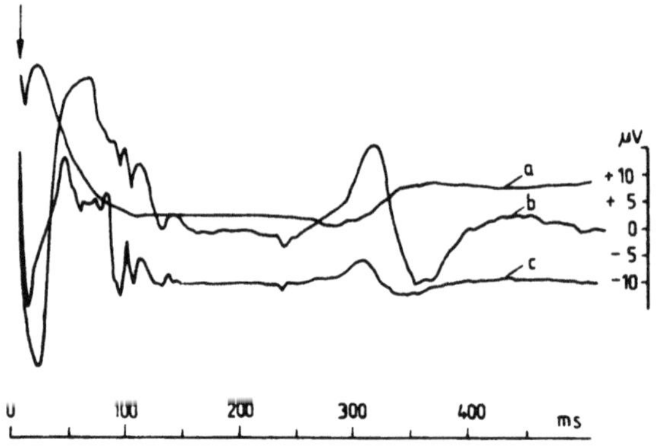

Fig. 1 . Late potentials in the ST-segment on a patient with ventricular tachycardia.

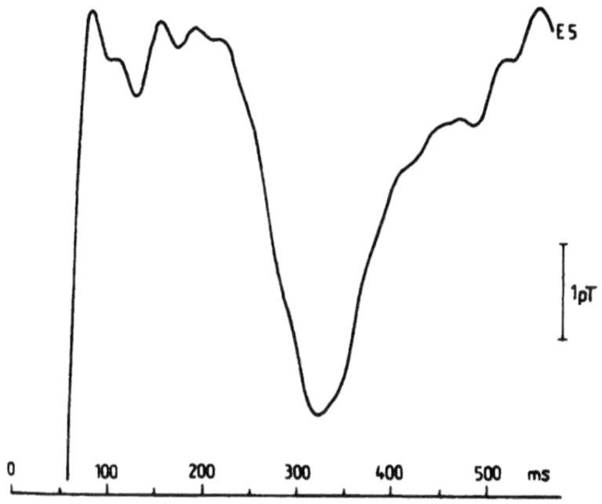

Fig. 2 . HR MCG recording (recording position E5) on the same patient as in Fig. 1.

In Fig. 2 a HR MCG of the same patient is shown for position E 5 of the Saarinen grid (5).
Both in the HR ECG and the HR MCG are signals evident which are contrasted with normal ST-segment. These signals are due to late excitations of the heart and represent late potentials and late fields, respectively. Altogether we carried out such investigations with 25 patients with episodes of ventricular tachycardia. Both HR MCG and HR ECG recordings were performed during sinus rhythm.

Conclusions

Finally we want to remark that the biomagnetic research can essentially be improved by multichannel systems. It will be possible to look at simultaneous magnetic events at different points because it is strongly suspect that some interesting information are going to emerge.
In accordance with other biomagnetic groups we think that this new field of research and the application of superconducting devices shall become important for cardiomagnetic studies.

References

(1) Nowak, H., G. Albrecht, M. Burghoff, W. Haberkorn and H.-G. Zach, Functional localization: A challenge for biomagnetism, (1987), in press

(2) Erne, G.N., H.-D. Hahlbohm, J. Korsukewitz and H.P. Lehmann, Biomagnetism, Applications and Theory, Pergamon Press, New York, 148 - 152 (1985)

(3) Berthel, K.-H., G. Albrecht, G. Kirsch, H. Nowak, W. Vodel and H.-G. Zach, Proceedings of the 4th Czechoslovakian Symposium on Weak Superconductivity, Smolenice, 53 - 63 (1986)

(4) Albrecht, G., K.-H. Berthel, M. Burghoff, G. Kirsch, W. Haberkorn, H. Nowak, H. Volkmann, M. Heinke, H.-G. Zach, Proceedings of the 6th Int. Conf. on Biomagnetism, Tokio (Aug. 1987), in press

(5) Saarinen, M., P. Siltanen, P.J. Karp and T. E. Katila, Ann. Clin. Res. 10, 1 - 43 (1978)

The Influence Of Inhomogeneities On ECG And MCG Mapping *)

CH. EICHTINGER, P. WACH, E. TELSA, S. SCHUY

Institute of Biomedical Engineering, Technical University of Graz
Inffeldgasse 18, A-8010 Graz, Austria

Summary

The influence of the inhomogeneities on ECG and MCG body surface maps was studied using a physical thorax model. The field distributions of a dipole source were measured with and without inhomogenieties and compared with calculated distributions based on a simple model with an analytical solution. Although the boundaries induce large changes in the local values, the patterns still reflect the underlaying current dipole source very well. We found that the MCG maps are closer to a dipolar pattern than the ECG maps.

Introduction

Initial studies of the MCG forward problem using torso models with high symmetry lead to the conviction that the magnetic field component normal to the frontal plane is less affected by the inhomogeneities than the electric potential measured on the body surface. Numerical studies and investigations using physical models based on realistic geometries (Horacek 1973, Hosaka et.al. 1976, Cuffin and Geselowitz 1977, Peters et.al. 1983) however showed that MCG is affected by the inhomogeneities as much as ECG. These studies considered mainly the changes in the local values. Horacek et.al. (1987) pointed out that in spite of large changes in local values the MCG maps of a current dipole very well reflect the underlying source even in the presence of boundaries.

The purpose of this study is to compare the deviation of electric potential and magnetic isofield maps of a current dipole from the dipolar pattern induced by the inhomogeneities. A quantitative criterium for these deviations is given.

*) supported by FWF - project nr. 5491

Method

The model used was a plexiglas tank with realistic torso shape. This tank has been filled with saline solution with a conductivity of 2mS/cm to simulate the average body conductivity. A lung model could be inserted into the tank to represent the internal inhomogeneities reducing the conductivity to about one third in this region. The dipole source has been formed by two small brass spheres seperated 18mm from each other. The dipole was fed by a current at a frequency of 1kHz with an amplitude of 0.1A through a twisted pair of wires. Due to the high current and frequency used the magnetic field outside the tank could be measured by an induction coil magnetometer. The electric potential was measured by silver electrodes built into front wall of the thorax. The 36 measuring positions for both ECG and MCG agreed with the rectangular standard grid of Saarinen. Only the magnetic field component normal to the frontal plane was measured. Both electric and magnetic signals were bandpass filtered to eliminate interference at line frequency.

The dipole has been located in the anterior part of the myocardium pointing downwards to the left leg and forward.

Mappings were taken from the model both with and without lungs. In addition dipolar maps have been calculated using the infinite homogeneous volume conductor as thorax model.

Results

Figure 1 shows the calculated, figure 2 and 3 the measured maps from the homogeneous and the inhomogeneous thorax model. The field distributions from the thorax model are very similar to the calculated patterns although the electric potential is somewhat more affected by the boundaries.

To get a measure for the differences which discribes the deviation from the dipolar pattern we scaled the calculated values by a constant factor in order to reach the least squares fit to the measured values. The standard deviation of the remaining differences of the 36 positions is then a quantitative criterium for the distortion of the dipolar shape.

The scaling factors were 0.61 (hom. magn.), 0.70 (inhom. magn.), 1.1 (elec. hom.), and 1.4 (elec. inhom.). The standard deviations of the remaining differences after scaling are 5% (magn. hom.), 7% (magn. inhom.), 11% (elec. hom.), and 12% (elec. inhom.) of the difference between maximal and minimal value in the particular map.

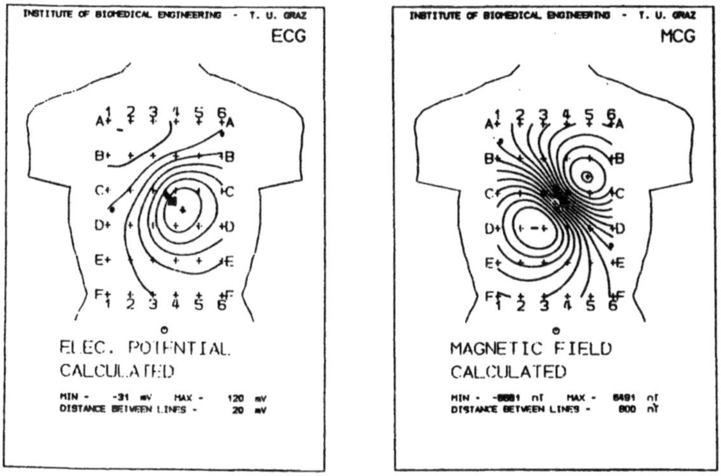

Figure 1: Calculated field distributions of a dipole source

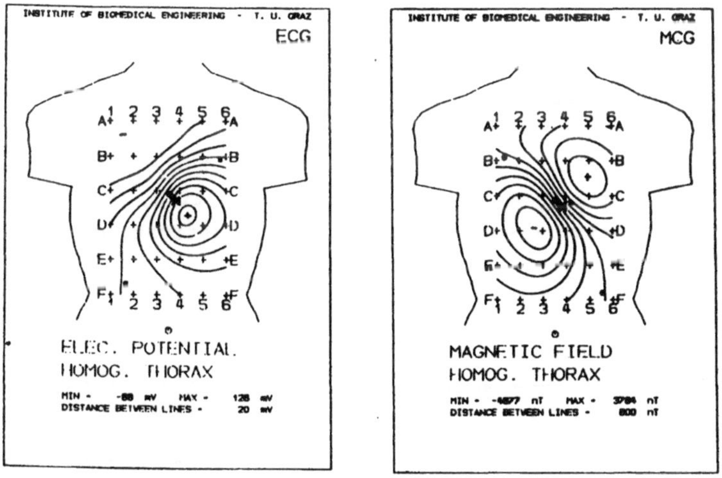

Figure 2: Electric potential and magnetic field of a dipol in the homogeneous thorax model

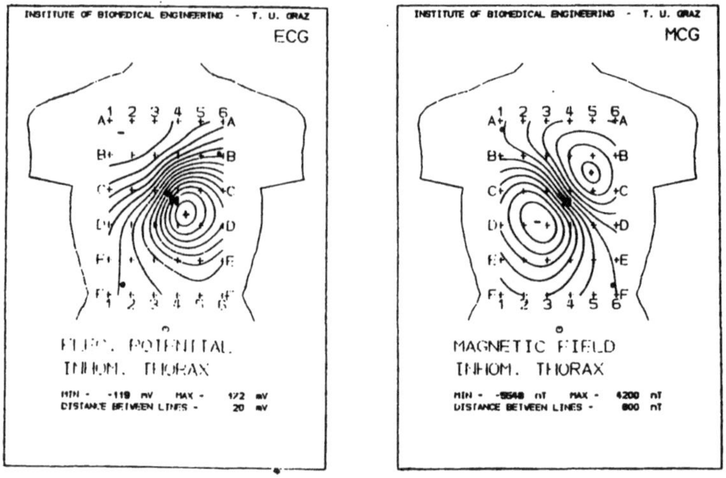

Figure 3: Electric potential and magnetic field of a dipole in the inhomogeneous thorax model

Discussion

The magnetic field appeares to be less affected by the inhomogeneities in our investigation than the electric potential. The MCG maps are closer to dipolar patterns than the ECG maps. This could result in a more accurate source localisation when using the magnetic data.
Nevertheless one has to take into account that these results are based on a special assumption of geometry, dipole position, and dipole direction. To get more general information, further investigations are needed.

References

(1) Horacek, B.M.: IEEE Trans. Magn. MAG-9, 440-44 (1973)
(2) Hosaka, H., D. Cohen, B.N. Cuffin, B.M. Horacek: J.Electrocardiol. 9, 418-25 (1976)
(3) Cuffin, B.N., D.B. Geselowitz: IEEE Trans.Biomed.Eng. BME-24, 242-52 (1977)
(4) Peters, M.J., M.J.M. Swennenhius, A. van Oosterom, J.J. Wevers-Henke: Nuovo Cimento 2D, 324-39 (1983)
(5) Horacek, B.M., C. Purcell, R. Lamothe, R. Merritt, C. Kafer, S. Periyalwar, S. Dey, L.J. Leon, G. Stroink: Physics in Medicine and Biology 32, 121-24 (1987)

On basic models for magnetocardiographic studies

W. HABERKORN, G. ALBRECHT and N. LANGHOFF

ZWG, Academy of Sciences of the GDR, Rudower Chaussee 6,
Berlin, 1199, GDR

Summary

The cardiac sources are represented by multiple current dipoles, a linear source, and planar current dipole layers. For the volume conductor the elementary shape of the conducting half-space is considered. Based on these models, the complete external magnetic fields are determined analytically. Furthermore, the effect of magnetic dipoles arising from circulating currents is discussed.

Introduction

The aim of magnetocardiographic studies is to obtain information about the clinical condition of the heart from the extracorporeal magnetic field. For the quantitative analysis of magnetocardiograms the physical description of the heart and the thorax is needed. Note that the source localization can be performed only on the basis of appropriate models. The purpose of the present study is to consider basic models and to determine the corresponding magnetic fields analytically. The field sources are represented by elementary current dipole models (1). For the thorax the model of the conducting half-space (2) is chosen.
Frequently in magnetocardiographic studies, only the field component normal to the volume conductor is considered. The present analysis includes the complete external field distributions.

Methods

The starting point is the expression for the magnetic field produced by a current source in a bounded volume conductor (3).

If the source is represented by multiple current dipoles, then

$$\vec{B}(\vec{r}) = \frac{\mu_0}{4\pi} \sum_n \frac{\vec{p}_n \times (\vec{r} - \vec{r}_n)}{|\vec{r} - \vec{r}_n|^3} + \frac{\mu_0}{4\pi} \sum_l \int_{F_l} (\sigma_i^l - \sigma_o^l) U(\vec{r}\,') \frac{(\vec{r} - \vec{r}\,')}{|\vec{r} - \vec{r}\,'|^3} \times d\vec{f}_l' \tag{1}$$

The first contribution is the field of the source directly, where $\vec{p}_n$ are the moments of the current dipoles located at $\vec{r}_n$. In the second term which describes the effect of the volume conductor σ_i^l and σ_o^l are the conductivities on the inside and outside of the surface F_l between regions of different conductivity, and U is the corresponding electric potential. For the elementary shape of the homogeneous conducting half-space $z < 0$ the second term of Eq. (1) contributes nothing to the component of the magnetic field normal to the surface $z = 0$ (2). This component resulting from the first term of Eq. (1) alone can be written as

$$B_z(\vec{r}) = \frac{\mu_0}{4\pi} \sum_n \frac{(y - y_n) p_{nx} - (x - x_n) p_{ny}}{|\vec{r} - \vec{r}_n|^3} \ . \tag{2}$$

Furthermore, at a point outside the half-space the magnetic field is irrotational and can be expressed as the negative gradient of the magnetic scalar potential Ψ . Starting from the normal component of the magnetic field, this potential can be determined by an appropriate integration procedure.

Results

The method suggested above is used to derive analytically the magnetic scalar potential for basic models of cardiac sources. Considering the case of discrete current dipoles, we obtain for Ψ the solution

$$\Psi(\vec{r}) = \frac{\mu_0}{4\pi} \sum_n \frac{(y - y_n) p_{nx} - (x - x_n) p_{ny}}{(x - x_n)^2 + (y - y_n)^2} \left(1 - \frac{z - z_n}{|\vec{r} - \vec{r}_n|} \right) \ . \tag{3}$$

It can be seen that components of the current dipoles oriented normal to the surface do not provide contributions.
The next basic model is a linear source (1) which lies in the $y = 0$ plane and is parallel to the x axis. For a uniform distribution of current dipoles pointing in the x direction, the magnetic scalar potential is found to be

$$\Psi(\vec{r}) = \frac{\mu_0 q}{4\pi} \sum_{\sigma = \pm} \left\{ \sigma \arctan \frac{(x - \sigma l)(z + d)}{y[(x - \sigma l)^2 + y^2 + (z + d)^2]^{1/2}} - \sigma \arctan \frac{x - \sigma l}{y} \right\} , \tag{4}$$

where q is the constant dipole density, d is the distance of the line from the x axis, and $\pm$ l are the dimensions of the line along the x axis.

Another source model is a planar sheet of uniformly distributed current dipoles which are perpendicular to the layer (1). Considering the rectangular shaped sheet which lies in the x = 0 plane, we obtain the expression

$$\Psi(\vec{r}) = \frac{\mu_0 \tau}{4\pi} \sum_{\sigma=\pm} \Big\{ (z+d+\sigma b)\,\mathrm{arsinh}\frac{z+d+\sigma b}{[x^2+(y+\sigma a)^2]^{1/2}} - [x^2+(y+\sigma a)^2+(z+d+\sigma b)^2]^{1/2} \tag{5}$$

$$-(z+d-\sigma b)\,\mathrm{arsinh}\frac{z+d-\sigma b}{[x^2+(y+\sigma a)^2]^{1/2}} + [x^2+(y+\sigma a)^2+(z+d-\sigma b)^2]^{1/2}$$

$$+\sigma b \ln[x^2+(y+\sigma a)^2] \Big\} ,$$

where τ is the constant dipole density, d is the distance of the layer center from the surface of the volume conductor, and 2 a, 2 b are the width and the height of the layer, respectively.

Discussion

The expressions for the magnetic scalar potential presented above yield also if the medium of the half-space consists of flat slabs of uniform conductivity lying parallel to the surface. The corresponding magnetic fields follow by taking the negative gradient

$$\vec{B}(\vec{r}) = -\nabla \Psi(\vec{r}) \,. \tag{6}$$

Note that the complete field distributions are needed for the analysis of magnetocardiographic measurements with multichannel systems which detect not only the normal, but also the tangential field components.

Furthermore, the results of this study provide the means to investigate the effects of extended sources and to determine the boundary conditions for representing a generator by a single current dipole. A more detailed analysis is presented for the linear source model embedded in the conducting half-space. For x = 0, the positions of the extrema of the magnetic field component normal to the surface are found to be

$$y = \pm \frac{1}{2}[(z+d)^2+l^2]^{1/2} \left\{ \left[\frac{9(z+d)^2+l^2}{(z+d)^2+l^2} \right]^{1/2} - 1 \right\}^{1/2} \tag{7}$$

The comparison with the result for a single current dipole shows the effect of the source dimension. In addition, the expansion of Ψ with respect to the length of the source is considered. The first-order term agrees with the expression for a single current dipole (2). For the next higher order contribution we obtain the result

$$\Psi^{(3)}(\vec{r}) = \frac{\mu_0}{4\pi}\frac{l^3 q y}{x^2+y^2}\left\{\frac{y^2-3x^2}{3(x^2+y^2)}\left[\frac{z+d}{N^{1/2}}\left(\frac{1}{N}+\frac{2}{x^2+y^2}\right)-\frac{2}{x^2+y^2}\right] - \frac{(z+d)x^2}{N^{5/2}}\right\}, \quad N = x^2+y^2+(z+d)^2 . \qquad (8)$$

It can be seen that the first deviations from the behaviour of a single current dipole are proportional to l^3.

Furthermore, the situation of magnetic dipoles located in the half-space is considered. It is assumed that the dipoles arise from circulating currents. If such currents exist, they do not provide contributions to the electrocardiogram (4). The effect of the magnetic dipoles having the moments $\vec{m}_n$ is represented by the potential

$$\Psi(\vec{r}) = \frac{1}{4\pi}\sum_n \frac{\vec{m}_n(\vec{r}-\vec{r}_n)}{|\vec{r}-\vec{r}_n|^3}, \quad \vec{m}_n = \mu_0 I_n \int_{F_n} d\vec{f}_n , \qquad (9)$$

where F_n is an area enclosed by the corresponding circulating current I_n.

Finally, we remark that similar considerations can also be made for the case that the field sources are located in the spherical volume conductor.

References

(1) Haberkorn, W., and G. Albrecht: this volume

(2) Cuffin, B.N., and D. Cohen: IEEE Trans. Biomed. Eng. BME-24, 372 - 381 (1977)

(3) Geselowitz, D.B.: IEEE Trans. Magn. MAG-6, 346 - 347 (1970)

(4) Wikswo, Jr., J.P., and J.P. Barach: J. theor. Biol. 95, 721 - 729 (1982)

The DC SQUID SYSTEM 3 - a new tool for investigations of magnetic activities of the heart

VODEL, W.; KOCH, H.; ORTMANN, W.

Department of Physics of the Friedrich Schiller University Jena, Max-Wien-Platz 1, Jena, 6900, G.D.R.

Summary

In this paper we present a new dc SQUID system, recently developed and produced in a small series by the Department of Physics of Friedrich Schiller University Jena/GDR. The high sensitivity of this device allows to study biomagnetic phenomena of the human body as indicators of physiological conditions. One of the most interesting and intense magnetic fields normally emitted from the human organism are those from the heart.

Introduction

The superconducting quantum interference device (commonly known by the acronym SQUID) is the most sensitive magnetic flux detector known today. It has often been referred to as a cryogenic or superconducting magnetometer, and indeed the measurement of extremely small magnetic fields is one of its most important applications. Important new methods can now be employed in medical research and clinical diagnostics, especially in the modern field of biomagnetism of the human body.
Electrical measurements of physiological potentials are well established in clinical diagnostics. Analogous measurement of physiological magnetic fields, however, are relatively unknown to researchers and clinicians. These measurements are providing to be of considerable significance and the subject of a great amount of current research.

Material and methods

The basic components in DC SQUID SYSTEM 3 are as follows:
- **DC SQUID sensor**: As magnetic field sensor in the constructed measurement system serves a multiloop thin film SQUID (1) on the basis of $Nb-NbO_x-Pb$ Josephson tunnel junctions with dimensions of 2.6 x 2.6 μm^2 shunted by stripes of Ag/In with a resistivity between 1 and 3 Ohms at the working temperature (4.2 K, boiling point of liquid helium). Tightly coupled to the SQUID loop is a thin film input coil with twice 18 turns providing an input inductance of 0.8 µH. The coupling factor between input coil and SQUID loop obtains 0.8. Both the SQUID

loop and the input coil are made in a gradiometric configuration in order to cancel uniform background fields. The overall size of the complete SQUID sensor is only 3×5 mm^2. Typical values are a critical current of about 30 µA, a SQUID inductance of 50 pH, and a input current sensitivity of 0.38 $\mu A/\emptyset_o$ ($\emptyset_o = 2.07 \times 10^{-15}$ Vs, magnetic flux quantum). To reduce the influence of ambient magnetic fields all SQUIDs are enclosed in a leaden capsule with dimensions of $24 \times 11.5 \times 5 mm^3$.

- **Low noise preamplifier**: It includes the matching transformer and a low noise amplifier. The input transformer matches the dc SQUID sensor to the noise minimum impedance of the amplifier. The overall amplification is about 4×10^4. Amplifier and SQUID sensor are shielded against static fields and rf-radiation.
- **SQUID-controller**: This electronic unit includes the circuitry that simplifies operation and significantly improves performance when working in noisy magnetic environments. A special notch filter with high performance is enclosed which is automatically synchronized with the line frequency. It attenuates the line frequency part in the signal and its harmonics up to the 31st.
- **Power supply**: This seperate unit includes in addition to the normal operation mode the possibility to supply the SQUID-controller from a battery set.

The magnetic signal is transferred to the input coil of the SQUID sensor by means of a superconducting flux transformer forming a symmetrical 2nd order gradiometer (2) developed at the Physikalisch Technisches Institut Jena of the Academy of Sciences of the GDR. The baselength of the gradiometer (i.e. the distance between the pick-up coil and the middle compensating coil) is 50 mm and the diameter of the one-turn pick-up coil amounts to 26 mm. Three superconducting adjustable discs are used to compensate the imbalance resulting from inaccuracy of manufacturing by the factor 10^5 (3).

Results

The noise properties of the SQUID sensors were measured using a HP 3582 A spectrum analyzer at the Dep. of Physics of the Helsinki University of Technology.*) For an optimal choise of current and flux bias point, a white flux noise spectral density of 1×10^{-5} $\emptyset_o/Hz^{1/2}$ was observed above 0.02 Hz. This corresponds to an effective current noise in the input coil of 3.8 $pA/Hz^{1/2}$, and an effective energy sensitivity of 5×10^{-30} J/Hz. No 1/f noise component was observed. The noise limited magnetic sensitivity of the complete equipment (with connected gradiometer) is about 60 $fT/Hz^{1/2}$ in our unshielded laboratory and 20 $fT/Hz^{1/2}$ during "quite" neight hours.

*) The authors are very grateful to Prof. T. Katila and J. Nenonen for their continous and helpful support to resolve the noise measurements.

Discussion and conclusions

The achived sensitivity of the constructed measurement equipment of 20 - 60 $fT/Hz^{1/2}$ and the obtained results (4) indicates that high quality magnetocardiograms can be measured in a laboratory or a hospital environment without the need for expensive magnetic shielding. Beyond it the described dc-SQUID system is also suitable for high resolution magnetocardiography e.g. PQ segment, His-Purkinje (HP) system, and ST segment studies. Because of the better local resolution of the magnetic measurement method (compared to electrocardiography) it seems possible that high-resolution magnetocardiography could be used in the near future to help in diagnostic of myocardial deseases.

References

(1) Berthel, K.H. et al.; Proceedings of the 4th Czechoslowak Symposium of Weak Superconductivity, Smolenice, April, 1986

(2) Nowak, H. et al.; Functional localisation: A challenge for biomagnetism; in press

(3) Haberkorn, W. et al.; Feingerätetechnik 31, H. 12, pp. 547- 548, 1982

(4) Nowak, H. et al.; Proc. of the 14th Intern. Congress on Electrocardiology, Berlin, August 17 - 20, 1987

Electromagnetic kinetocardiography.
Measurement technique, hardware and software.

KOČÍ M., HÖNIG, J., KRÁL V.

Institute of Physiological Regulations, Czechoslovak Academy of Sciences, FN Bulovka, pav. 11, 180 85 Prague 8, Czechoslovakia.

Summary.

The paper deals with technical details concerning electromagnetic kinetocardiography (EM KCG), while physical principles and clinical results are published in another paper. Technique of primary electromagnetic field EMF generation, secondary EMF measurement and computer aided data evaluation are described in more details. Some of resulting maps of isodivergence $\vec{E}$ are shown.

Generation of the primary EMF.

The induction loop is tightened around the chest of patient at the level of heart ventricles (Fig. 1.). The loop inductance with tuning capacity creates resonant circuit tunable to the frequency of 13,56 MHz crystal controlled power generator. Resonant current $I_0(t)$ in the loop is about 0,5A and sets magnetic induction of about $1,5.10^{-6}$T. Varying magnetic flux generates in conductive chest medium eddy currents with the density of 19 A/m^2 near surface. Output power of generator is manually controlled up to 3 W.

Measurement of the secondary EMF.

Topographic measurement of the secondary EMF is carried out by a special multielectrode probe. The probe is constructed to sum by the analog way the diagonal components of tensor G_2. The output is proportional to the divergence of intensity $\vec{E}$. The probe consists of 23 idependently adjustable electrodes in order to reach good electrical contacts with the irregular chest surface. The electrode configuration forms in fact the base for the Poisson´s equation. The probe has 7 channels allowing simultaneous measurement of div $\vec{E}$ at 7 measuring points. The probe is attached to the loop but may be loosely shifted along to perform successive measurement in 2cm steps. All measurements form a standard matrix of 7 x 15 measuring points, which enclose precordial area 14 x 30 cm. One standard ECG lead is recorded simultaneously in order to synchronise all measurements of div E.

Equipment for EM KCG.

Analog RF signals detected and preamplified by probe reguire aditional amplification to fit the consecutive processing. Differential AC coupled low frequency ymplifiers are used in 7 channel arrangement. Amplifier gains are controlled manually. Every amplifier is calibrated by AC signal 50Hz 1 mV peak to peak. The probe and the ECG amplifiers are galvanically separated from the other electronics.

Computer aided data evaluation.

The informations from all measurements are synthetised in isoline maps. This task can be executed on any computer, so our aim was to develope a programme that could be easily modified for particular target machine. Data processing can be divided to two phases.

1. Data asquisition and preprocessing.

As a results of 2 years experiences with EM KCG recording, we can describe today´s "standard" method. Data are recorded sequentially in 15 probe positions with sampling interval 4 msec, record length in each probe position is 1500 samples. Each record contains 3-6 systoles from which only the best one is stored. The selection is carried out automatically. The criterion is the minimal baseline drift. The next step is the baseline level subtraction and the time normalization to minimize the unwanted influence of heart rate changes. The resulting record has 256 samples for each point on chest surface. The position of two subsequent R points on ECG is the 40th and the 240th sample respectively.

We developed the "skeleton" program, to which only 3 modules must be added for any computer:

- A/D converter driver, which is totally hardware dependent
- graphics with procedures-draw point, vector and character
- I/O disc operations, which may be operating system dependent.

2. Data evaluation.

This phase includes the display of resultant EM KCG time courses or maps on graphic display or printer in order to determine the diagnosis and the patient´s file menagement.

Many procedures for two-dimensional arrays presentation were developed in our computer laboratory for EM KCG, standard ECG mapping and brain mapping. The library includes the procedures for different modes of black and white and color display, some examples see Fig 3.-6. This maps can be displayed as a movie pictures on a screen or can be printed out. Fast algorithms for map interpolation and isolines detection were specially designed for small machines, so the system may run even on 8-bit CPU´s.

Today two versions of software are in practical use. The first runs on PDP 11/34A under the RSX-11M operating system, the second on Kontron Cardio 2000 under the CP/M operating system. The first is written in Pascal, the second in Fortran (Microsoft F80) both with a small portion of code in assembly language. In contrast to widely used PDP the Cardio 2000 is not well known and it needs a special comment. This computer is delivered as an additional image processing unit of the ATL ultrasound imaging system. It consist of special array processor for image processing and the host Z80 based CPU. For EM KCG the simple A/D unit was added. Because EM KCG method can be a good complement to cardiological investigation and Cardio 2000 computers can be found in many echo laboratories, we belive, that our Cardio 2000 software can be very important for future clinical applications.

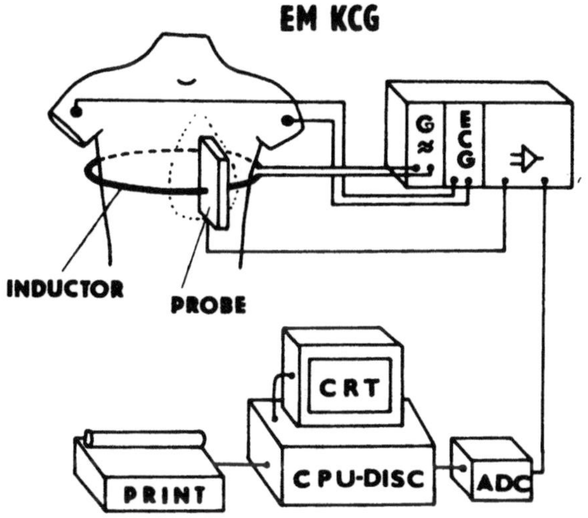

Fig. 1. Diagram of Electromagnetic Kinetocardiography equipment with a computer service.

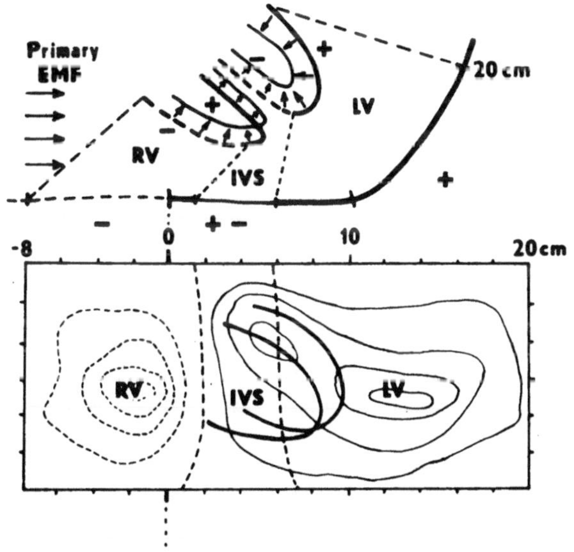

Fig. 2. Endocardial charge layers motion and its projection on the thorax surface represented for a certain instant by isodivergence E map. RV is right ventricle, IVS interventricular septum and LV left ventricle.

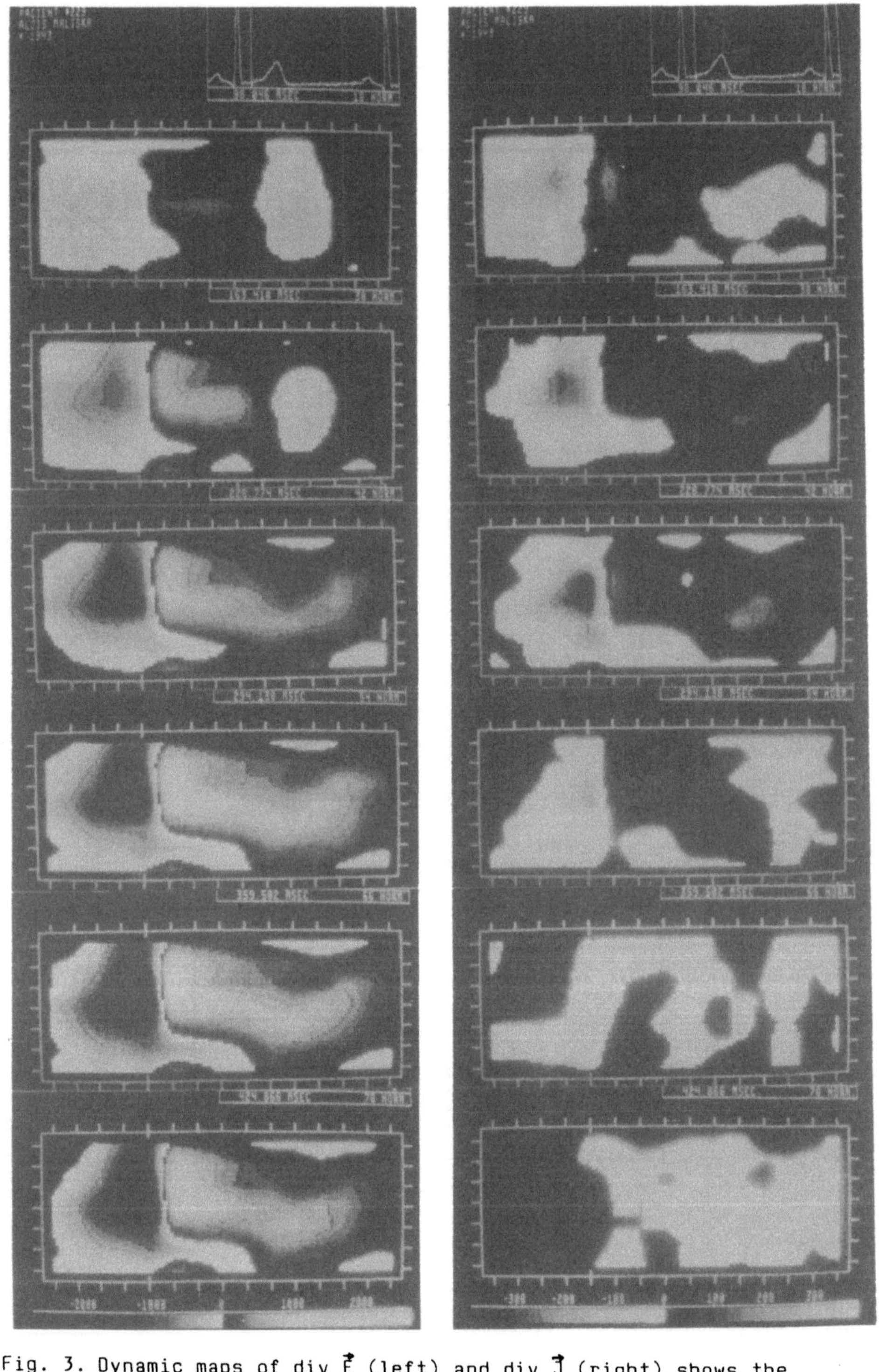

Fig. 3. Dynamic maps of div $\vec{E}$ (left) and div $\vec{J}$ (right) shows the inferio-septal dyskinesia after myocardial infarction.

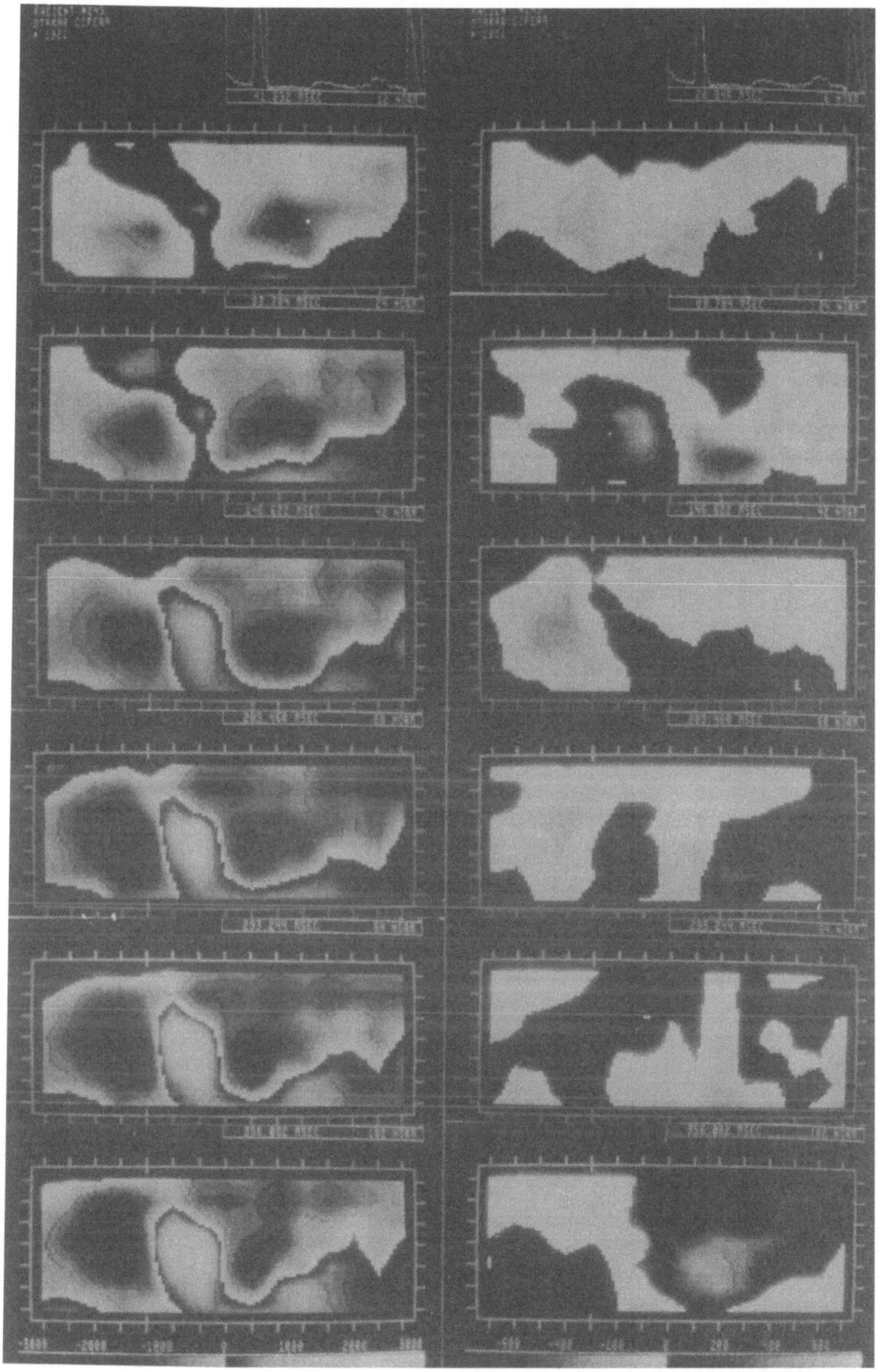

Fig. 4. Dynamic maps of div $\vec{E}$ (left) and div $\vec{J}$ (right) shows the antero-apical dyskinesia after myocardial infarction.

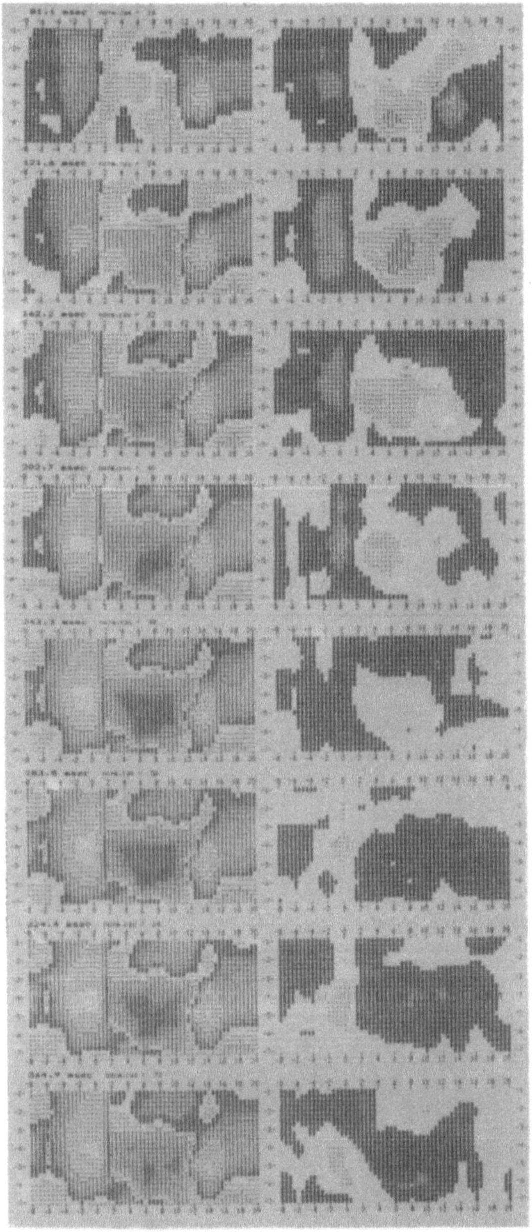

Fig.5. Printed maps of div $\vec{E}$ and div $\vec{J}$ display apico-lateral dyskinesia.

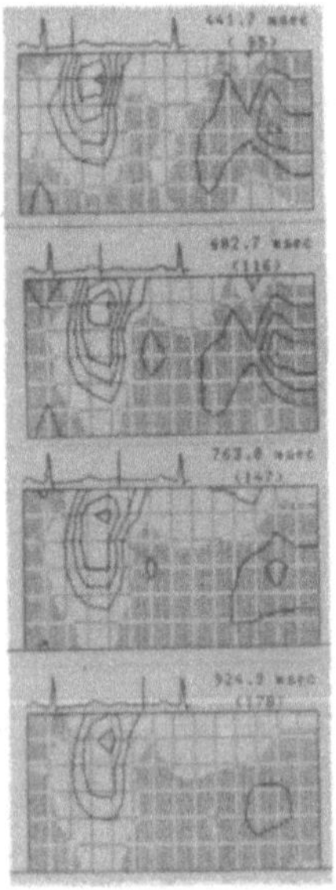

Fig.6. Example of another type of printed div $\vec{E}$ maps.

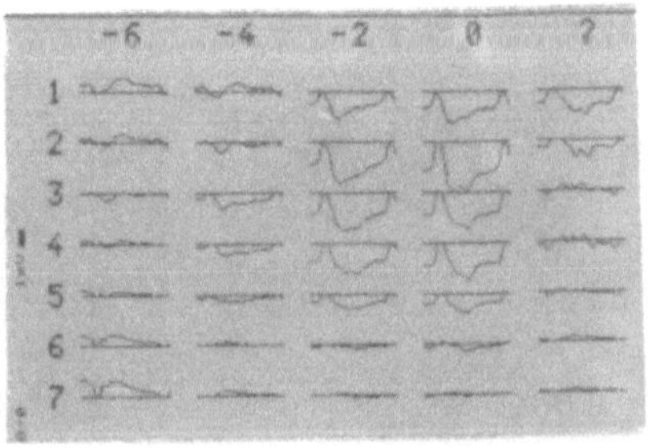

Fig.7. Some printed time courses of div $\vec{E}$.

V E C T O R C A R D I O G R A P H Y

THE RELATIONSHIP BETWEEN THE 12-LEAD STANDARD ECG AND THE XYZ VECTOR LEADS

Uijen* G.J.H., Oosterom** A. van, Dam* R.Th. van

* Department of Cardiology, University of Nijmegen

** Laboratory of Medical Physics and Biophysics

University of Nijmegen

P.O. Box 9101 6500 HB Nijmegen, The Netherlands

Summary

Different transfer matrices for synthesizing the 12-lead Standard ECG from observed XYZ vector lead signals have been analyzed. The analysis entailed the computation of both the RMS and the MAXABS errors between simulated and observed signals for all individual subjects in a population, as well as the mean values of these errors, $\overline{\text{RMS}}$ and $\overline{\text{MAXABS}}$. The matrices considered were:

M1, derived by us using statistical techniques,

M2, derived by Dower, based on Frank's image surface,

M3, a more recent version of M2, also published by Dower.

Explicit forms of these matrices are tabulated. For M1 we found $\overline{\text{RMS}}$ = 145 µV (largest individual value: 300 µV), $\overline{\text{MAXABS}}$ = 757 µV (largest individual value 2168 µV !). For M2 and M3 the corresponding errors were even larger. A similar analysis has been carried out on a transformation matrix M4, which we derived for synthesizing the signals of the XYZ vector leads from observed 12 lead ECG's. For M4 we found $\overline{\text{RMS}}$ = 52 µV (largest individual value: 91 µV) and $\overline{\text{MAXABS}}$ = 163 µV (largest individual value 373 µV). It is concluded that neither the XYZ → 12-lead transfer, nor the 12-lead → XYZ transfer is acceptable as a standard routine.

Introduction

The synthesis of the 12-lead Standard ECG (ECG) from recorded XYZ leads in Frank's vector cardiogram (VCG) has been advocated by Dower [1,2,3,4]. The motives for such a procedure are

1) the possibility of applying diagnostic computer packages to recorded VCG signals,

2) the storage of VCG rather than ECG data requires less space.

Ever since this procedure was suggested we have doubted its validity. In our data base a sufficiently large number of well documented cases have now been collected to allow us to easily test Dower's claims. The results of this test are reported in this paper. In addition we have used another method for deriving such a transfer matrix (M1), based on a statistical (least squares) technique. Dower has published several transfer matrices, all assumingly based on Frank's image surface. We will consider an earlier version (M2) and a later version (M3).

Intuitively, the expansion of the three XYZ signals to the larger number of 12 in the ECG cannot be error free. It would be error free if the cardiac electrical activity could be entirely represented by a single dipole but, as is well known, this is not the case.

The converse procedure, synthesizing the XYZ signals from the larger data set of the (twelve) observed ECG signals, does not seem to be hampered by the same theoretical difficulty. Here the crucial question is: does the sampling of the three dimensional volume conductor as performed by the lead system of the ECG allow a sufficient recovery of all three vector components. In particular, the Z-lead might pose a problem. We have tested this procedure by using the same data base. The resulting transfer matrix will be denoted M4.

The quality of matrices M1 to M4 has been analyzed by computing the values of the RMS and the MAXABS errors between actual and synthesized data for all subjects and for all four matrices considered.

Materials and methods

Single beat ECG signals in N = 106 subjects (54 normals; 52 chronic infarctions) have been collected using a 64-lead BSM system [5]. These 64 leads have both the nine electrodes of the ECG and the seven electrodes of the Frank VCG system as subsets. The signals were sampled at 500 samples per second. The voltage position reference was Wilson's Central Terminal. The QRS interval (length 100 ms) was documented by storing all T = 50 samples (QRS data), the subsequent interval of 400 ms (STT data) was documented by storing T = 50 samples at 8 ms intervals. The three XYZ signals were obtained by appropriately weighting the signals recorded at the seven Frank leads. After sampling the ECG of subject n the data are represented by a matrix $E^{(n)}$ of dimension (12,T); the VCG of the same subject by matrix $V^{(n)}$ of dimension (3,T). Similarly the ECG's of all N subjects studied are represented by matrix E of dimension (12,NT) and their VCG's by a matrix V of dimension (3,NT).

Transfer matrix M1

The synthesized ECG data, denoted by $\tilde{E}$ is computed as a linear combination of the data contained in the VCG by

$$\tilde{E} = M1\ V,$$

with M1 the associated transfer matrix. This matrix is computed by requiring the norm between the estimated $\tilde{E}$ and the observed E data to be minimal. The well known solution to this least squares estimation problem is

$$M1 = E\ V^t\ (V\ V^t)^{-1} \qquad (1)$$

in which t denotes the transpose-, and -1 denotes the inverse of a matrix.

In this expression $E\ V^t$ (dimension (12,3)) is proportional to the cross covariance between the ECG and the VCG signals. This transfer matrix M1 (derived from the entire data set) is used to synthesize the ECG data of individual n : $\tilde{E}^{(n)}$ from the observed VCG data $V^{(n)}$ of that same individual by

$$\tilde{E}^{(n)} = M1\ V^{(n)}. \qquad (2)$$

Transfer matrices M2 and M3

These have been taken from the work of Dower [1] and [2] respectively.

Transfer matrix M4

The synthesized VCG $\tilde{V}$ is computed as a linear combination of the data contained in E by

$$\tilde{V} = M4\ E\ ,$$

with M4 the associated transfer matrix. Similar to the procedure described for deriving M1, this matrix M4 is computed as the solution to a linear estimation problem. Consequently, it may seem as if

$$M4 = V\ E^t\ (E\ E^t)^{-1}$$

were the required solution. However, since the ECG contains at most eight linearly independent signals this computation must be carried out by using the subset E_8 containing the data from the six precordial leads and any two limb leads rather than the redundant data set E. Accordingly we have

$$M4 = V\ E_8{}^t\ (E_8 E_8{}^t)^{-1}\ . \qquad (3)$$

This matrix M4 (derived from the entire data set) is used to synthesize the VCG data of individual $\tilde{V}^{(n)}$ from observed ECG data $E^{(n)}$ of that same individual through

$$\tilde{V}^{(n)} = M4\ E^{(n)}\ . \qquad (4)$$

Error analysis

The quality of the synthesis is analysed by comparing synthesized and recorded signals at all time instants and in all leads considered. For the VCG → ECG synthesis this leads to an error matrix $\varepsilon^{(n)} = \tilde{E}^{(n)} - E^{(n)}$, for which two norms are used:

$$RMS_n \triangleq \{ \frac{1}{LT} \sum_{\ell=1}^{L} \sum_{t=1}^{T} (e_{\ell t}^{(n)})^2 \}^{1/2}\ , \qquad (5)$$

and $$MAXABS_n \triangleq \max_{\substack{\ell=1,L \\ t=1,T}} e_{\ell t}^{(n)}\ . \qquad (6)$$

L is the number of leads considered.
In the analysis of matrices M1 to M3 L=12; in the analysis of M4 L = 3.

Results

The various transfer matrices considered are listed in tables 1 to 4. Matrices M1 and M4 are based (Eqns. 1 and 3) on the data of the QRS interval.

Table 1: transfer matrix M1 derived from QRS data using Eqn. 1 and applied to Eqn. 4.
Table 2: Dower's transfer matrix specified in [1].
Table 3: Dower's transfer matrix specified in [2].

weights for resulting standard leads	Table 1 (vector leads) X	Y	Z	Table 2 X	Y	Z	Table 3 X	Y	Z
I	0.79	-0.24	0.08	1.05	-0.28	0.19	0.632	-0.235	0.059
II	0.24	1.05	-0.01	0.37	1.45	-0.14	0.235	1.066	-0.132
III	-0.56	1.29	-0.09	-0.68	1.73	-0.33	-0.397	1.301	-0.191
aVR	-0.51	-0.41	-0.03	-0.71	-0.59	-0.03	-0.434	-0.415	0.037
aVL	0.67	-0.77	0.08	0.87	-1.01	0.26	0.515	-0.768	0.125
aVF	-0.16	1.17	-0.05	-0.15	1.59	-0.24	-0.081	1.184	-0.162
V1	-0.52	-0.06	-1.04	-0.65	-0.67	-1.06	-0.515	0.157	-0.917
V2	-0.15	-0.35	-1.76	0.06	-0.86	-1.58	0.044	0.164	-1.387
V3	0.69	0.38	-1.16	0.99	-0.42	-1.50	0.882	0.098	-1.277
V4	1.34	0.68	-0.49	1.67	-0.13	-0.84	1.213	0.127	-0.601
V5	1.09	0.64	0.01	1.53	-0.06	-0.14	1.125	0.127	-0.086
V6	0.65	0.52	0.23	1.10	-0.06	0.33	0.831	0.076	0.230

Table 4
Transfer matrix M4; derived from QRS data using Eqn. 3 and applied in Eqn. 4.

	VR	VL	V_1	V_2	V_3	V_4	V_5	V_6
X	-0.52	0.82	-0.01	0.04	0.05	0.05	0.07	0.37
Y	-1.53	-1.09	0.03	-0.02	-0.02	0.03	-0.07	0.08
Z	0.43	-0.01	-0.26	-0.28	-0.14	0.04	-0.15	0.34

The 106 error measures RMS_n (Eqn. 5), resulting from the application of matrices M1, M2 and M3 to recorded VCG data are presented in Fig. 1 in the form of histograms. The mean values and standard deviations are also indicated. The left panels represent the errors observed over the QRS interval; the right panels those observed over the STT interval. In Fig. 2 the $MAXABS_n$ (Eqn. 6) values are presented in the same manner.
In Fig. 3 the synthesized ECG's resulting from the application of M1 are shown superimposed on the waveforms of the simultaneously recorded actual signals. For this (worst case) RMS_n = 300 µV; $MAXABS_n$ = 2168 µV.

Figure 4 depicts the corresponding results which were observed in the application of (Dower's) M3. For this (the same) subject we found RMS_n = 451 µV, $MAXABS_n$ = 2920 µV.

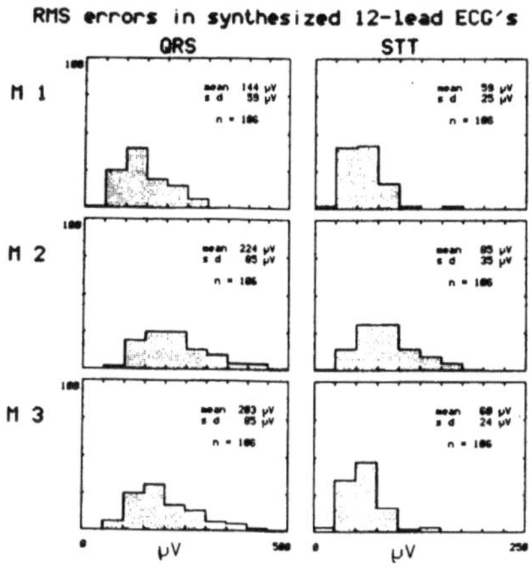

Figure 1
Histograms of RMS_i error values resulting from the use of transfer matrices M1, M2, M3 in Eqn. 2 for all 106 subjects.
Left panels: QRS interval; right panels: STT interval.

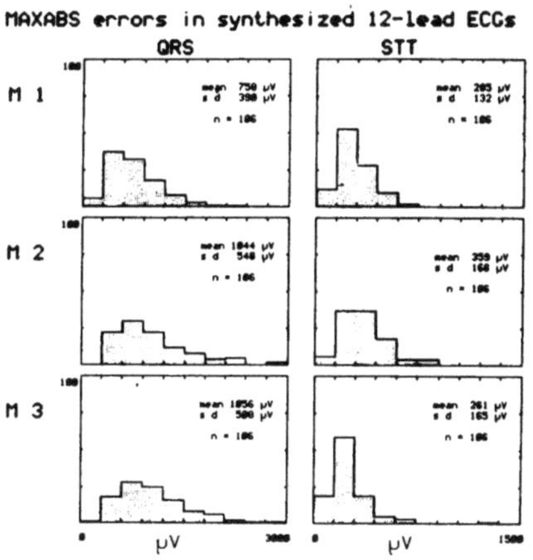

Figure 2
Histograms of $MAXABS_i$ error values; remaining legends as n Fig. 1.

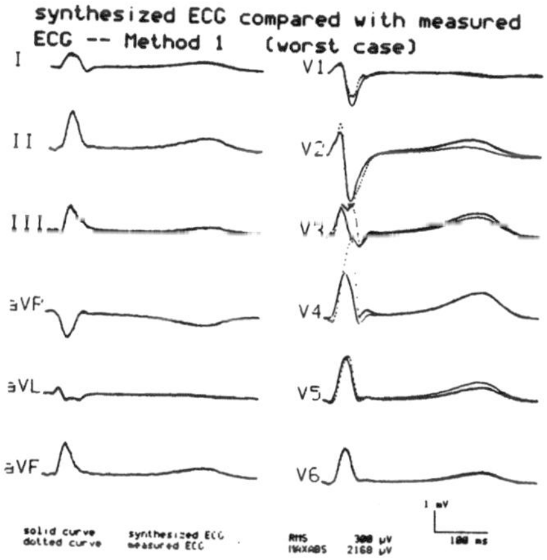

Figure 3
Synthesized (solid lines) Standard ECG waveforms resulting from the application of M1 to the VCG of an individual, superimposed on the ECG waveforms (dashed lines) recorded in the same individual; worst case; errors as indicated.

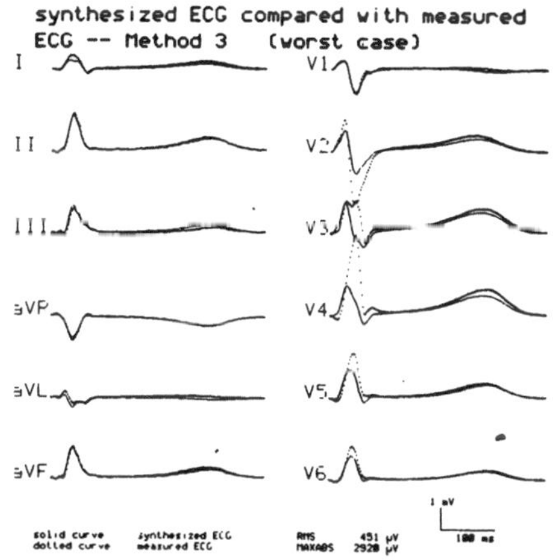

Figure 4
As in Fig. 3, but for a different transfer matrix: M3.

In a similar way the results of the ECG → VCG procedure (Eqn. 4) is presented. Figure 5 shows the histograms of the RMS and the MAXABS errors; Fig. 6 depicts both the synthesized and the observed XYZ lead signals, both for the worse case (RMS = error 91 μV; MAXABS error = 373 μV) and best case (RMS = 19 μV; MAXABS = 60 μV).

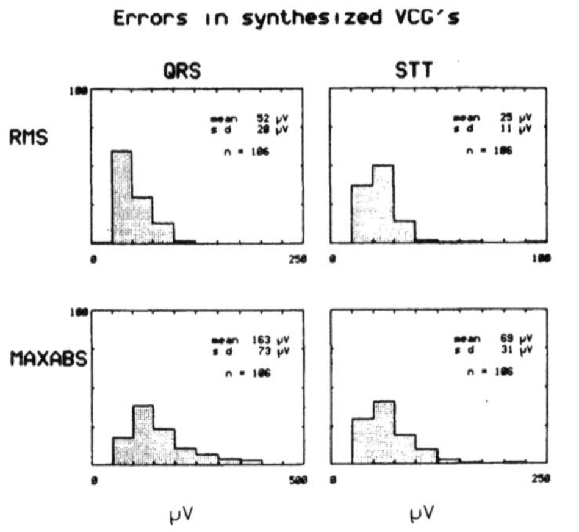

Figure 5
Histograms of errors resulting from the use of transfer matrix M4 (Eqn. 3) in Eqn. 4 for all 106 subjects.
Upper panels: RMS errors; lower panels: MAXABS errors. Left panels QRS interval, right panels STT interval.

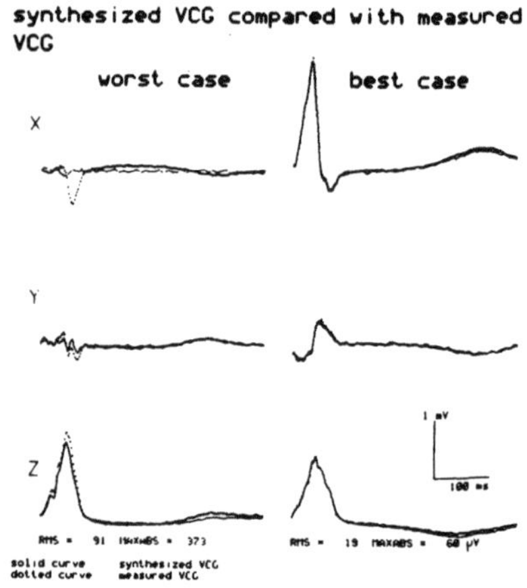

Figure 6
Synthesized VCG (solid lines) resulting from the application of M4 to the ECG of an individual, superimposed on the VCG waveforms (dashed lines) recorded in the same individual; left panel: worst case; right panel: best case; errors as indicated.

Discussion

The transfer matrices M2 and M3, taken from the work of Dower, clearly give rise to very large errors in individual cases, and this in spite of the fact that a relatively homogeneous (sober) data base was used in our test including just two diagnostic categories.

In his evaluation of the procedure Dower used the indirect test of running both the original and the synthesized signals through a commercially available computer package for the automatic interpretation of ECG's. The observed diagnostic accuracies were found to be of about the same quality.

There is some confusion about the exact specification of Dower's second transfer matrix (our M3), the specification of which does not seem to match its hardware realization as presented in Fig. 1 of [2].

There have been several other studies investigating the relationship between ECG and VCG waveforms.

Zywietz et al. [6] used transfer matrices derived from the lead vector concept and from an inhomogeneous torso model. A correspondence measure was documented being the maximum amplitude ratios within the P, Q, R, S and T waves. Considerable discrepancies between synthesized and recorded waveforms were demonstrated. No explicit versions of the transfer matrices used were documented.

Wolf et al. [7] used statistically derived matrices (similar to our M1 and M4) and Dower's M2. Their analysis was based on correlation coefficients for individual leads, amplitude differences in Q, R and S waves and on a comparison of the diagnostic interpretation produced by a computer package for ECG interpretation. They found that the diagnostic accuracy of the procedure implied in our matrix M4 was acceptable; but that the procedure implied in matrices like M1 to M3 are not acceptable. No explicit forms of the transfer matrices used were presented.

Our work supports the main conclusions of Zywietz et al. [6] and of Wolf [7] and is at odds with Dowers conclusions. Our transfer matrix M1 seems to behave somewhat better than Dower's M2 and M3 but not sufficiently so to advocate its use in any way at all. The procedure implied in M4 seems to work slightly better again than the procedure implied in matrix M1 (M2, M3) but large individual errors will be encountered when such procedure is used in a large population. We do not believe that these matters would improve sufficiently if a time variant transfer matrix, as proposed by Zywietz et al. [6] and Tuinstra et al. [8] were used.

The main conclusion of our work is that neither for the purpose of automatic ECG interpretation, nor for the purpose of data reduction in general the vector cardiogram is an appropriate intermediary.

Far more appropriate means of data reduction are available [9,10,11].

References

1. Dower G.E.: J. Cardiol. 1, 101-116 (1968)
2. Dower G.E. and H.M. Machado: Progress in Electrocardiology, 264-271 (Pitman Medical, Tunbridge Wells, 1979)
3. Dower G.E. and H.B. Machado: J. Cardiol. 12, 249-261 (1979)
4. Dower G.E.: J. Cardiol. 17, 189-192 (1984)
5. Heringa A., G.J.H. Uijen and R.Th. van Dam: Electrocardiology '84. Amsterdam, Excerpta Medica (1982), 297-301.
6. Zywietz C., H. Abel, H.P. Mock and B. Rosenbach: Adv. Cardiol. 16, 82-86 (Karger, Basel, 1976)
7. Wolf H.R., P.M. Rautaharju, V.C. Unite and J. Stevast: Adv. Cardiol. 16, 87-97 (Karger, Basel, 1976)
8. Tuinstra C.L. and M. Visser: Adv. Cardiol., 21, 198 (Karger, Bassel, 1978)
9. Lux R.L., A.K. Evans, M.J. Burgess, R.F. Wyatt and J.A. Abildskov: Circ. Res. 49, 186-196 (1981)
10. Evans A.K., R.L. Lux, M.J. Burgess, R.F. Wyatt and J.A. Abildskov: Circ. Res., 49, 197-208 (1981)
11. Uijen G.J.H., A. Heringa and A. van Oosterom: IEEE Trans. Biomed. Eng., BME-21, 706-714 (1984)

Planarity of the spatial QRS loop. Comparative analysis in normals, infarcts, ventricular hypertrophies and intraventricular conduction defects.

ARNAUD P., MORLET D., RUBEL P.

INSERM U 121, Hôpital Cardio-vasculaire, 69394 Lyon Cedex 03, France.

SUMMARY : An original planarity index computed by the Lyon VCG program has been tested in normal and abnormal populations (1435 subjects). Providing information about any kind of loop distortions, it showed a relative independence from other VCG parameters, and a good stability. Lowered in abnormal tracings, especially in BBBs, it proved to be a useful tool for the normal-abnormal discrimination.

INTRODUCTION : An almost perfect planarity of the spatial QRS loop is known as a characteristic of normal hearts (1, 2, 3). Since 1972 the Lyon VCG program (4) has routinely computed an original planarity index (5) as follows :

METHOD : The spatial area between two consecutive vectors is defined as a vector dS_i (Fig. 1). The geometrical area vector (GAV) is computed as the sum of dS_i vectors over the whole loop. The GAV magnitude equals the total QRS area if the loop's planarity is absolutely perfect. It decreases in the case of poor planarity because dS_i vector directions fluctuate. So we compute the relative magnitude of GAV expressed as a percentage of the total QRS area (GAV%).

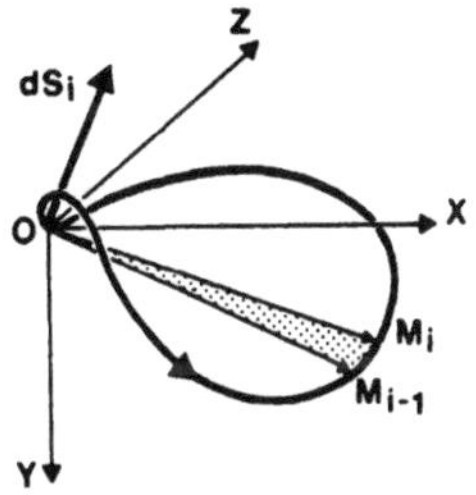

$$GAV\% = \frac{|\Sigma\, dS_i|}{\Sigma\, |dS_i|}$$

This index provides an indirect assessment of the presence of distorted segments lying outside the preferential plane of the loop. The larger and more distal these segments, the lower the GAV%. Moreover, the GAV% may be lessened if a part of the loop is concave (even if the concavity is located in the preferential plane) or if the entire loop shows a figure of eight, or if it is relatively narrow as compared with a rounded loop (see below correlation between GAV% and QRS area).

The stability of GAV% was tested in a preliminary study in three different populations recorded with the Lyon system : 1. For 87 in-patients recorded twice at ten minutes interval without moving the electrodes, the absolute difference of GAV% values was calculated : mean = 2.4, 96% range = 0-7. 2. For 267 young normal subjects, recorded twice at a time interval varying from 1 to 11 months, we obtained : mean difference = 2.7, 96% range = 0-9. 3. For 8 young normal subjects, each recorded 23 to 26 times during a 24 hour period, the electrodes being attached in the same place, the standard deviation of GAV% computed for each subject was respectively : 1.0, 1.1, 1.5, 1.6, 1.9, 1.9, 2.1 and 3.7, the mean values of GAV% ranging from 79% to 96%.

POPULATIONS : The study was performed on 1435 subjects recorded with the Lyon system (4) using the Frank leads. Eleven groups were investigated :

YN : young normals : 267 healthy male subjects, 17 to 26 years old (mean=20).

WP : working population : 214 male subjects, 22 to 62 years old (mean=38), without any history of cardiovascular disease and with a normal, visually controlled, VCG.

HT : heart transplantation : 98 patients, 15 to 67 years old (mean=47) recorded during the ambulatory follow-up more than two months after surgery.

Adult populations with pathological diagnoses according to clinical data and usual investigations, and to ECG and VCG criteria (the latter from the Lyon program (6)) :

RVH : right ventricular hypertrophy : 57 patients ; the degree of RVH according to VCG criteria was moderate (28% of the cases), medium (47%) and severe (25%).

LVH (m) : moderate left ventricular hypertrophy : 130 patients.

LVH (s) : severe or medium left ventricular hypertrophy : 188 patients (respectively 45% and 55%).

IMI : inferior or postero-inferior myocardial infarction : 110 patients.

AMI : anterior or antero-septal or antero-lateral myocardial infarction : 98 patients.

RBBB : complete right bundle branch block : 82 patients - either pure RBBB (20 cases) or associated with RVH (22 cases) or with LVH or biventricular hypertrophy (22 cases), or consecutive to open heart surgery (18 cases).

RBBB + LAFB : complete right bundle branch block associated with left anterior fascicular block : 36 patients - a ventricular hypertrophy could be associated. In 3 cases the RBBB originated from surgery.

LBBB : complete left bundle branch block : 155 patients - either pure LBBB or associated with an LVH or a coronary disease.

Table 1 : Smallest, largest, mean values, standard-deviations and 96% range of GAV% in 11 populations.

Population	N	min - max values	mean value	standard - deviation	96% min - max values
NP	214	66 - 97	88.8	5.6	71 - 96
YN	267	35 - 97	87.2	8.0	65 - 96
HT	98	47 - 98	87.8	10.2	50 - 97
RVH	57	32 - 96	82.2	11.6	43 - 95
LVH(m)	130	15 - 97	82.0	14.7	37 - 96
LVH(s)	188	8 - 97	76.3	19.7	23 - 96
IMI	110	33 - 96	82.0	12.6	40 - 96
AMI	98	10 - 89	60.7	21.3	16 - 88
RBBB+LAFB	36	30 - 89	68.5	15.8	35 - 89
RBBB	82	6 - 92	54.9	20.6	18 - 86
LBBB	155	3 - 91	48.6	21.1	11 - 86

RESULTS : Table 1 shows the GAV% values in the 11 populations. YN, NP and HT mean values are not significantly different ($p<0.01$). Discarding the HT group whose normality is debatable, we then regrouped YN and NP in order to perform pairwise t-tests of group means (Table 2).
The choice of an optimal threshold value of GAV% aimed at discriminating between normal and abnormal tracings is of interest. We tested several values between 75% and 84%. The value leading to the optimal balance between sensitivity and specificity in discriminating between each abnormal group and YN+NP was 80%. Moreover, this value concords with our daily experience. With such a threshold value, GAV% alone gave the following results :- YN+NP : 89.6% classified as normals (GAV% > 80%)-in other groups the percentage of cases classified as abnormal (GAV% < 80%) was respectively : AMI : 78.6%, LBBB : 91.0%, RBBB : 86.6%, and together LBBB, RBBB and RBBB + LAFB : 86.8%. Concerning the other groups i.e. RVH, LVH and IMI, no discrimination was found.

Table 2 : Pairwise t-tests of group means with the Bonferroni significance level (+++ : 1%, ++ : 5%, NS : non significant)

	RVH	LVH(m)	LVH(s)	IMI	AMI	RBBB +LAFB	RBBB	LBBB
YN+NP	NS	+++	+++	+++	+++	+++	+++	+++
RVH		NS	NS	NS	+++	+++	+++	+++
LVH(m)			++	NS	+++	+++	+++	+++
LVH(s)				NS	+++	NS	+++	+++
IMI					+++	+++	+++	+++
AMI						NS	NS	+++
RBBB+LAFB							+++	+++
RBBB								NS

Table 3 : Percentage of tracings correctly classified at the 11 first steps of discriminant analysis.

Step	Variable entered	normal	abnormal	total
1	EL MAXV	78.6%	69.3%	72.6%
2	GAV%	86.7%	70.6%	76.4%
3	LAI A	89.2%	73.6%	79.2%
4	LAS MV	89.4%	73.6%	79.3%
5	M MAXV	90.2%	73.9%	79.8%
6	AZ GAV	91.3%	74.4%	80.5%
7	D MAX HAV	92.1%	75.4%	81.4%
8	QRS DUR	90.0%	77.3%	81.9%
9	RA A	89.4%	78.0%	82.1%
10	LP D	90.9%	78.2%	82.7%
11	D C N	90.6%	79.0%	83.2%

Another aim was to appreciate the relative power of GAV% for normal-abnormal discrimination as compared with other VCG parameters. A stepwise discriminant analysis (BMDP package) was performed between normal population (YN + WP) and abnormal population (all other groups) with GAV% and 25 spatial QRS parameters. These parameters were selected from the Lyon program as being the more efficient ones for the diagnoses concerned. Table 3 displays the ranking of the 11 parameters entered first : GAV% was entered at the second step, after elevation of the maximum vector (EL MAXV). At this step 76.4% of the whole population were correctly classified. The sensitivity was 70.6% and the specificity was 86.7%. The parameters entered next were : relative area in the left anterior inferior octant (LAI A), relative magnitude of the left anterior superior maximal vector (LAS MV), magnitude of the maximum vector (M MAXV), azimuth of GAV (AZ GAV), time delay between maximum vector and half-area vector (D MAX HAV), QRS duration (QRS DUR), relative area in the right anterior quadrant (RA A), octantal duration in the left posterior quadrant (LP D), number of direction changes (more than 90°) in the course of the spatial loop (D C N). At this eleventh step 83.2% of cases were correctly classified. No improvement was obtained when introducing the other 15 parameters.

On the other hand, we investigated the correlations between GAV% and 10 parameters representative of the main QRS features for the normals (YN + WP), for each of the pathological groups and for all the latter together. We observed a poor negative correlation ($r = -0.30$, $p < 0.001$) with the number of direction changes for the whole population. The correlation was better between GAV% and QRS duration ($r = 0.52$, $p < 0.001$) for the whole population due to the presence of bundle branch blocks, but inside each group no significant correlation was observed. The correlations were not significant with QRS maximal magnitude and very poor with total QRS area, except for LVH (m) ($r = 0.43$, $p < 0.001$) for RBBB ($r = 0.38$) and for IMI ($r = 0.38$). But we must point out that the partial correlations between GAV% and QRS area after discarding the linear effects of QRS magnitude were $r = 0.40$ for the YN + WP group and $r = 0.34$ for LBBB. This means that disregarding the maximal QRS vector magnitude, a narrower loop, corresponding to a smaller QRS area, may lead to a lower GAV% value. Such a feature is usual in LBBB (5).

DISCUSSION : Several kinds of planarity index have been published (7,8). The GAV% index computed by the Lyon program is different : it takes into account the global planarity of the loop and in addition it is affected by the presence of concave or distorted segments and by the more or less narrow shape of the loop.

A quasi experimental circumstance was afforded by 6 of our patients who suffered RBBB consecutive to open heart surgery with right ventriculotomy. In 5 cases the post-operative GAV% value was - 11 to - 37 (mean = -23) lower by comparison with the pre-operative one. Paradoxically, an increased GAV% (+27) was observed in the 6th patient due to a particular evolution of the loop.

GAV% remained stable when calculated several times for the same subject.
The scatter of GAV% values was smaller in the normal by comparison with abnormal populations (SD up to 21).

Mean values were significantly different ($p < 0.01$) in normal population (YN + NP) and in the other groups except RVH. In LVH, cases with severe hypertrophy had lower GAV% values than moderate ones (mean 76 versus 82). In myocardial infarction, since both anterior and inferior infarcts had different mean values from normals, the former had significantly lower values than inferior infarcts (mean 61 versus 82). As expected the smallest values were due to intra-ventricular conduction defects (9). Mean values were 49 in LBBB and 55 in RBBB (N.S. difference). The RBBB values were not significantly different when a right or left ventricular hypertrophy was in association. In the case of LAFB associated with RBBB the values were significantly higher (mean = 69 versus 55, $p < 0.01$). If this result is to be corroborated in more homogeneous and larger populations, the following interpretation could be suggested : in the pure RBBB, a late anterior right activity develops outside the preferential plane at the QRS end. This explains a low GAV% value. If a LAFB appears, the main (leftward) part of the loop moves up and back and its orientation becomes opposite to the terminal anterior displacement of QRS. So we can suppose that these two parts of QRS tending to be inscribed in neighbouring planes, cause the GAV% value to be higher.

Finally, the more interesting point to be discussed is the diagnostic value of GAV%. A threshold value of 80% seemed to be optimal for the normal-abnormal discrimination. It gave a specificity level of 89.6%.
When compared with other VCG parameters by means of stepwise linear discriminant analysis between normals and abnormals, GAV% was found to be entered at the second step and to allow 76.4% of tracings to be correctly classified. But this rank is questionable, various parameters having a multimodal distribution because of the inhomogeneity of the populations.
Moreover, correlations with other parameters demonstrated that GAV% was a relatively independent one. Thus it may be supposed to provide a new diagnostic information and to be a useful tool for the detection of any activation disorder either in normals or in heart diseases.

Acknowlegment : We are grateful to M. Th. Rameaux for providing technical assistance.

References

1 - Schellong, F. : Grundzuge einer Klinischen Vektordiagraphie des Herzens, Springer -Berlin, (1939).
2 - Rochet, J., and M.M. Vastesaeger : Arch. intern. Physiol. 49, 113, (1939).
3 - Sulzer, R., and P.W. Duchosal : Helv. Physiol. Acta 4 : 285, (1946).
4 - Arnaud P., and P. Rubel : in : Trends in computer-processed Electrocardiograms, J.H. Van Bemmel and J.L. Willems eds, North-Holland, 175, (1977).
5 - Roland, J.G., P. Rubel , M.C. Forlini , P. Arnaud : in : New Frontiers of Electrocardiology, de Padua F. ed., Research studies press, 214, (1981).
6 - Arnaud P. : in : Electrocardiographic body surface mapping, Van Dam R. Th. and Van Oosterom A. eds., Martinus Nijhoff publ. 225, (1986).
7 - Hiraoka, M., S. Kawano , T. Sowanobori , S. Kokusho : Jpn- Heart J. 23, 39, (1982).
8 - Mossard J.M., J. Baruthio , S. Voegtlin , J. Chambron , A. Sacrez , R. Voegtlin : Arch. Mal. Coeur, 8, 887, (1984).
9 - Arnaud P., P. Rubel : in : 5e Colloque de Vectocardiographie et Electrocardiographie Quantitative, Marseille, Abstract p. 1,(1983).

This work was supported in part by DRET under Grant N°84/144.

New routine VCG-analysis with high diagnostic power in LVH and RVH

ESPERER, MARIA; BEIN, GEORG

Universitätskinderklinik, Kaiserin Auguste Victoria Haus
Heubnerweg 6, D-1000 Berlin 19

A new simple method of VCG-analysis was developed to allow differential diagnosis of isolated aortic and pulmonary stenosis and to estimate the severity of right and left ventricular pressure overload.

The purpose of this study was first to find out reasons of the diagnostic deficiency in common VCG-analysis. Secondly we looked for new simple VCG-criteria more sensitive than those usually used.

The VCG of 25 children with aortic stenosis and those of 30 patients with pulmonary stenosis, aged 2 to 15 years, were explored with special interest for the loop's circumference in the transverse plane. VCG with RBBB had been excluded. Eight, partly not yet described loop types were defined to be specific for LVH or RVH, respectively (fig. 1). Criteria that depend on the enlargement of right directed vectors failed in diagnosing type B and E of RVH and even showed false positive results concerning type C of LVH. On the other hand it was impossible to identify LVH-type C using VCG-criteria recording enlarged left directed vectors. Erroneously LVH was suggested applying such criteria to RVH-type B.

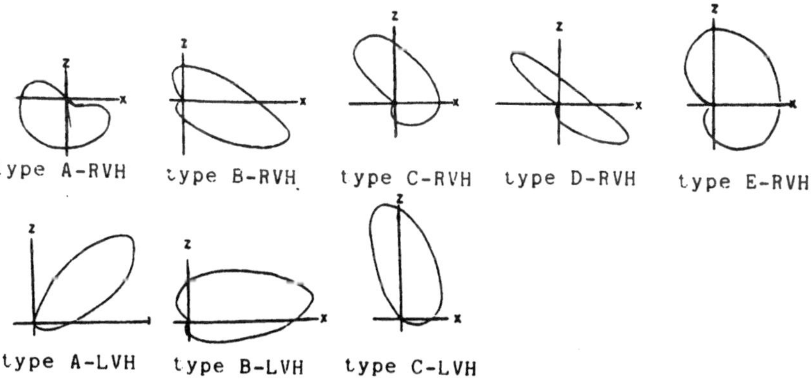

Fig.1: QRS-loop types of right and left ventricular pressure overload

Regarding the quadrant distribution of the loops' circumference as highly informative we measured the length of the 4 loop segments in each quadrant of the transverse plane. For simplifying this procedure we printed a scale of graticules with 1cm (≙1 mV) subdivisions in a circular array on a transparent foil which was put on the original VCG prints. Thus the quadrant number N (equalling the number of sudivisions cut by the vector loop in each quadrant) and the maximal amplitude M of each quadrant rapidly were determined (fig. 2).

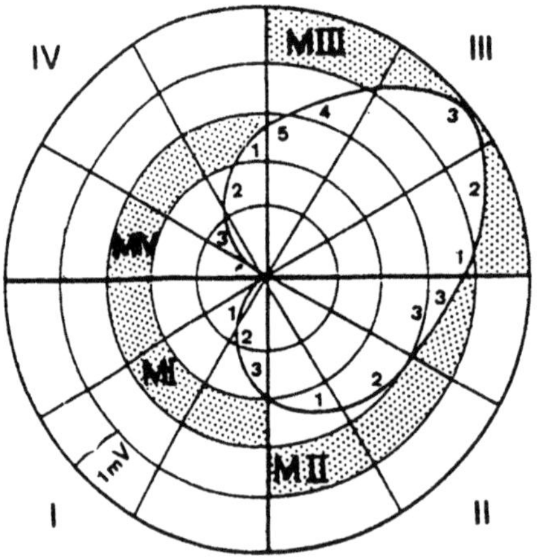

NI = 3
NII = 3
NIII = 5
NIV = 3

MI = 3 mV
MII = 4 mV
MIII = 5 mV
MIV = 3 mV

Fig.2: Determination of quadrant numbers N and maximal amplitudes M.

We found highly significant differences of the quadrant number NI, NIII and NIV between the two patient groups (fig. 3). The maximal amplitudes of the third quadrant (MIII) differed also highly significantly. By multiplication of N and M we got a further variable, the so-called "corrected area" CA of each quadrant. (In contrast to the real area it increased in case of hypertrophy-specific figure of eight or elongation of the loop.) As expected, there were highly significant differences of CAI and CAIII between both groups.

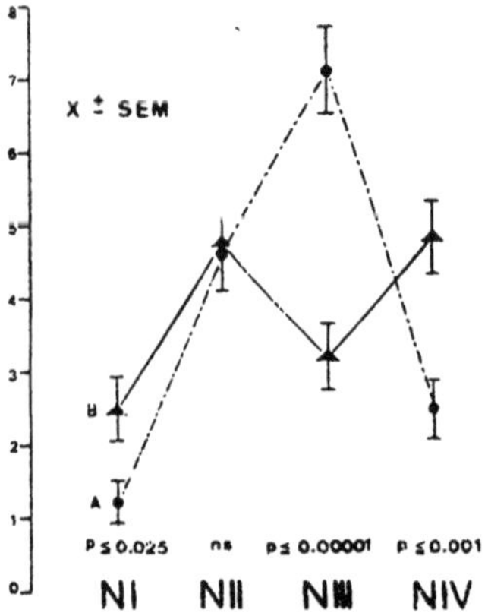

Fig.3: Quadrant numbers of the LVH (A)- and RVH-group (B).

In order to identify each described loop type we calculated hypertrophy specific criteria on the basis of N and M, which reflected best the different quadrant topography of the loops (tab. 1).

Table 1: List of 7 RVH- and 4 LVH-criteria.
The value below each variable is defined either as the upper or as the lower limit of the 95%-tolerance range of the corresponding variable of the reference group (p 0.025).

RVH-criteria							LVH-criteria			
Nright/Nleft	Nant	MII-MIII (mV)	NIV	NIII-NIV	NIV/MIV (mV^{-1})	$\sum\Delta M$ (mV)	CAright-CAleft (mV)	CAIII-CAI (mV)	Mant-Mpost (mV)	CApost-CAI (mV)
>1	≥13	≥1	≥8	≤-5	≥2	≤4	≤-50	≥39	≤-6	≥67

Type A of RVH was easily recognized by using the quotient Nright/Nleft (Nright/Nleft = (NI+NIV)/(NII+NIII) >1). This criterion, however, could not be applied to type B-RVH with its considerable left directed vectors. A high anterior quadrant number (Nant = NI+NII ≥13) or the difference MII-MIII (≥1mV) classified this RVH-loop type and allowed clear discrimination from the similar loop type B of LVH. Type C-RVH could be identified either by NIV ≥ 8 or, in case of only relative enlargement of posteriorly oriented right forces, by the difference NIII-NIV (≤-5). If both criteria failed, type C-RVH nonetheless could be recognized by using the quotient NIV/MIV (≥2mV^{-1}), because a relative small MIV was related to this loop type. Furthermore the otherwise impossible differentiation between the similar loop types C-LVH and C-RVH was made by using the two latter criteria, which were negative in case of loop type C-LVH. Type D-RVH, the double-tipped transitional form between mild (type B) and moderate (type C) severity, was found out by using one of the criteria applied to type B or C. None of these variables, however, was applicable to type E of RVH with its homogeneous distribution of circumference among the 4 quadrants. Thus we calculated the sum of the differences of the 4 maximal amplitudes (each >3mV) and got the result ($\sum\Delta M = |MI-MII| + |MII-MIII| + |MIII-MIV| + |MIV-MI| \leq 4$) small enough to identify this loop type.

Type A-LVH could be diagnosed, if the difference between left and right corrected area (CAright - CAleft = (CAI+CAIV) - (CAII+CAIII)) was less than -50mV. In some cases of posterior loop rotation with consecutive underrepresentation of the second quadrant, where left forces were not large enough, the variable CAIII-CAI (≥39mV) proved to be of diagnostic value. The first criterion (CAright - CAleft) was positive in type B-LVH with loop elongation into the left quadrants II and III.

The difference between the posterior and right anterior corrected area (CApost - CAI = (CAIII+CAIV) - CAI $\geq$67mV) revealed type C-LVH. The difference between the anterior and posterior maximal amplitudes (Mant - Mpost = (MI+MII) - (MIII+MIV) $\leq$-6mV) discovered an only relative enlargement of the posterior forces.

Even type B-RVH showed positive results in the first, type C-RVH in the last two LVH-criteria. But the first-step-using of the RVH-criteria proved RVH-loop characteristics and avoided diagnostic errors.

The sensitivity of this new method of VCG-analysis was 83% (LVH) and 89% (RVH), respectively. A differential diagnosis between both groups was possible in 96%.

In order to establish criteria that reflect severity of the underlying hypertrophy it is necessary to register any of the possibly enlarged vector forces regardless of their direction. RVH-loops prefer quadrant I (type A), II (type B) and IV (type C), neglecting the third one. Therefore we calculated the variable RG (right gain) = CAI+CAII+CAIV--CAIII, that correlates with the RVPSP: $r=0.68$, $p\leq0.001$ (fig. 4, left). In case of LVH-loops which prefer the quadrants II (type B), III (type A) and IV (type C), neglecting the first one, we created the parameter LG (left gain) = CAII+CAIII+CAIV-CAI. Instead of the absolute values of N we used here the relative quadrant numbers N%. Fig. 4 (right) demonstrates the correlation with the LVPSP: $r=0.78$, $p\leq0.001$.

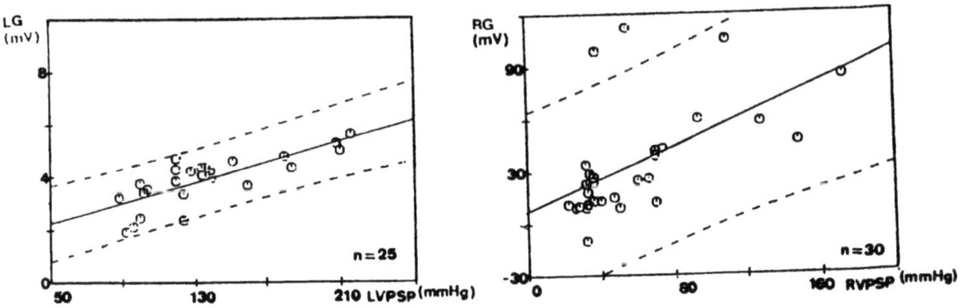

Fig.4: Correlations of vectorcardiographic variables with hemodynamic data determined by heart catheterization. RG = right gain, LG = left gain, RVPSP = right ventricular peak systolic pressure, LVPSP = left ventricular peak systolic pressure.

With special regard to the various loop shapes this new method of analysis can be applied to all loop types of RVH and LVH, respectively. Furthermore it allows the cumbersome differential diagnosis between similar loop types of contrary ventricular hypertrophy, which usually is more difficult than distinguishing them from normal vectorcardiograms. Altogether this method decodes well the information of VCG and being easily practicable it should be qualified for routine use in the assessment of congenital valvular heart disease.

Vectorcardiographic identification of anteroapical infarction

ITO,S.; TAMURA,M.; MAEDA,T.; NAKAGAWA,M.; HARA,M.; TAKAKURA,T.;SAIKAWA,T.
department of medicine I, medical college of oita, japan

Summary

Electrocardiographic (ECG) and vectorcardiographic (VCG) identification of myocardial infarction (MI) involving the LV apex still remains controversial. We try to clarify the VCG criteria of anteroapical (AAp) MI that involves the LV apex on left ventriculogram (LVG), Tl-201 Scintigram (SCG) and 2-D echocardiogram (2-D). The subjects constitute 18 patients (pts), mean age of 57 ± 10 years, with acute MI. The ECG V4 showed poor r, qR, qRs or QS. Wall motion abnormalities and perfusion defect were noted on LVG and SCG at AAp areas. On VCG, we classified our pts into 3 groups according to the pattern of the horizontal plane (HP) QRS loop such as a 8-F pattern with CW rotation of the afferent limb 3, CW rotation of the efferent limb 11, and miscellaneous group with minimal QRS change or normal 4. Frontal plane (FP) max QRS vector is widely distributed in the range between -86 and + 224°. Initial CW rotation of the QRS loop in the FP and sagittal plane (SP) is noted in only 10/18(55.6%). Miscellaneous group showed 'bite" formation in the initial and efferent limb with initial superior force, and also marked posterior deviation of the max QRS vector in the HP.

Introduction

The sensitivity and specificity of the ECG and VCG to accurately detect MI of the anteroseptal, anterolateral, lateral, diaphragmatic or inferior, posterior LV walls are very high [1), 2)]. However, their identification of MI involving the apical segments might be relatively less capable and still controversial [3) - 11)].

Because of the lack of optimal ECG and VCG criteria for the detection of apical MI, we try to clarify the anterior MI that involves the LV apex, which has proven to have asynergy on LVG.

Materials and methods

The subjects constitute 18 patients, mean age of 57 ± 10 years, 17 men and 1 woman, who have documented episode of acute MI. The ECG of all pts met the criteria of acute MI. The ECG V4 showed rS, qR, qRs or QS, and no abnormal Q waves are noted in leads II, III, and aVF. LVG performed 1 month after the onset of acute MI showed asynergy of the AAp and lower part of the septal wall.

Results

Table 1 shows the list of all pts in the next conditions : 1) ECG V4 and aVF, 2) LVG asynergy, 3) the severity of coronary arteries, 4) SCG, and 5) ejection fraction (EF) on 2-D. All pts showed defect or hypoperfusion on SCG, except 3 pts with higher EF on 2-D with only reduced contractility on LVG. Fig. 1 shows the HP VCG of all pts classified according to the degree of asynergy in the apical segments. 5 pts showed reduced, 8 none, 3 dyskinetic, and 2 aneurysmal contractility respectively.

Fig. 1 The horizontal plane VCG of all patients classified according to the degree of asynergy in the apical segments.

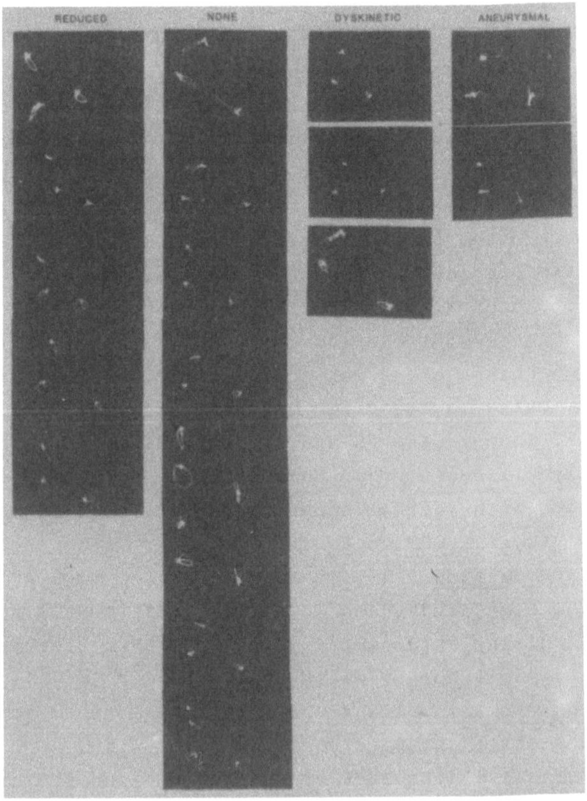

Dr. Young et al already classified VCG in asynergy of the AAp areas into 7 groups [2]. Our pts fit only 3 patterns such as type C with a 8-F pattern with CW in the afferent limb, type D with CW in the efferent limb, and miscellaneous group. The most established quantitative criteria for diagnosing antero-septal or localized anterior infarction and antero-lateral infarction are : 1) A posterior location of the 0.02 second vector and 2) A duration of initial rightward forces greater than 0.022 second. The application of these 2 criteria to our pts showed that none fulfilled both simultaneously, 16/18 (88.9%) only 1, none 2 and 2/18 (11.8%) fulfilled neither criteria.

The angle of the FP max QRS vector is widely distributed in the range between -86 and + 224°. Dr. Hugenholtz stated that the observation of initial CW rotation in association with the max QRS vector in the range between + 270 and + 20° in the FP constitutes one of the most reliable signs of of AAp infarction [1]. Our pts fit these criteria in only 14/18 (77.8%). He also stated that CW rotation in the SP occurs when the anterior as well as the apex is involved. Again, only 10/18 (55.6%) in our pts showed initial CW rotation in the FP and SP.

4 cases designated as miscellaneous group should be mentioned further. 2 cases have a small "bite" of their efferent limbs with initial q waves in the FP and SP. The third case showed marked abnormal posterior deviation of the max QRS vector in the HP (-90°) with left anterior hemiblock. The fourth case also has bites of its initial and efferent limb with q

Table 1 The list of all patients

Name	Age	Sex	ECG in V4	q in aVF	LVG '83	'86	CAG '86	'87	'88	Grade	Defect or hypoperfusion in TSG	EF in UCG
M.K.	61	M	qR	-	red	red	50	90		SVD	+	61
T.H.	38	M	rS	+	red	red		75	100	SVD	+	64
A.Z.	64	M	rS	-	red	red	90		75	TVD	-	65
A.M.	47	M	rS	+	red	red	90	75		SVD	-	73
T.T.	53	M	qR	+	red	red	90			DVD	-	86
M.K.	62	M	QS	-	non	non		90	75	TVD	+	42
S.H.	60	M	QS	-	non	non	75	90		SVD	+	46
K.T.	64	M	QS	+	non	non		75		SVD	+	50
T.S.	80	F	QS	-	non	non		100		TVD	+	50
U.M.	58	M	QS	-	non	non	75			SVD	+	51
M.H.	57	M	QS	+	non	non		75		SVD	+	56
T.M.	32	M	qR	-	non	non		90	50	TVD	+	62
M.M.	70	M	rS	+	non	non		90	99	SVD	+	67
A.S.	44	M	QS	+	dys	non		100		SVD	+	29
T.M.	54	M	QS	-	dys	red		100		TVD	+	34
K.H.	60	M	QS	-	dys	a/e	99			DVD	+	39
H.S.	63	M	qRS	-	ane	non		100		SVD	+	28
K.Y.	71	M	QS	+	ane	non		99		SVD	+	38

Fig. 2 The horizontal plane VCG of 4 patients designated as miscellaneous group.

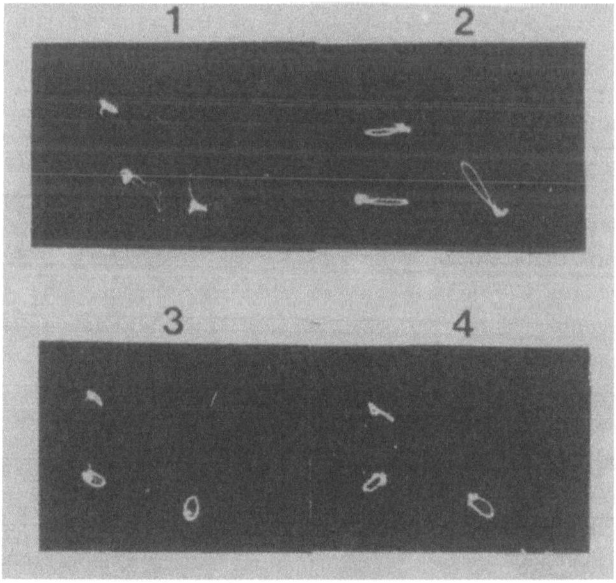

waves in the HP and SP (Fig. 2).

Discussion

Dr. Port and associates proposed that the VCG criteria for identificati-on of AAp infarction are ; 1) in the H^D, both efferent and afferent limbs of the QRS loop are mostly or completely CW, and 2) if the max H^D amplitude is $\geqq$1.8 mV, then the earliest posterior force must be to the right of the point of origin [3]. Our 18 pts met these criteria in only 7/18 (39.8%).

Dr. Surawicz mentioned about apical infarction that it is acceptable term in describing infarction and that this term has merrit because often inferior infarction slightly overlaps the apex and manifests its-elf in Q waves in leads V3 or V4 as well as in II, III and aVF [5]. He also stated that the term may be misleading because it has been used in the past to describe massive circumferential involvement of the entire apex [5]. On the contrary, Dr. Selvester stated that inferior infarcts don't involve the apex circumferentially as do anterior infarcts [6]. The results in this study appears to support the latter concept.

Conclusions

When the VCG shows one or more of the following criteria, anterior infarction with apical segment involvement is highly suspected :

1) CW rotation of at least the early part of the efferent limb and/or the early part of the afferent limb associated with posterior locati-on of the 0.02 second vector.
2) "bite" formation in the efferent limb with initial superior force.
3) Marked abnormal posterior location of the max or half-area vector associated with abnormal posterior location of the 0.02 sec. vector.

References

(1) Hugenholtz,P.G.,C.E. Forkner et al : Circulation 24 : 825-850 (1961)
(2) Young,E., P.F. Cohn et al : Circulation 51 : 467-476 (1975)
(3) Port,S., A.D. Fortune et al : J. Electrocardiol. 13 : 245-252 (1080)
(4) Rothfeld,B., J.L. Fleg et al : Am. J. Cardiol. 53 : 715-717,(1984)
(5) Surawicz,B., H.Uhley et al : Am. J. Cardiol. 41 : 130-145 (1978)
(6) Selvester,R.H., J.C. Solomon, J.L. Gillespie : Circulation 38 : 684-690 (1968)
(7) Starr,J.W., G.S. Wagner et al : Circulation 53 : 229-234 (1976)
(8) Phillips,H.R., J.W. Starr et al : Circulation 53 : 235-240 (1976)
(9) Savage,R.M., G.S. Wagner et al : Circulation 55 : 279-285 (1977)
(10) Seino,Y., H.M. Staniloff et al : Am. J. Cardiol. 52 : 37-42 (1983)
(11) Roark,S.F., R.E. Ideker et al : Am. J. Cardiol. 51 : 382-389 (1983)

Normal areas of Frank VCG instantaneous vector end-points-comparison with the VA program evaluation.

BACHÁROVÁ,L., MELOTOVÁ,J., POPÍK,P.
Medical Bionics Research Institute, Jedľová 6, 833 08 Bratislava, Czechoslovakia

Summary.

Physically corrected orthogonal Frank lead system electrocardiograms were processed in a group of 482 unselected subjects as well as in a group of 448 patients with cardiac pathology by the VA (Pipberger) program of automated ECG evaluation, implemented on a SM 4-20 minicomputer. The group of subjectes with normal results was defined by lack of abnormal diagnostic statements in the print-out of the Pipberger program. In this group of subjects parameters of instantaneous QRS vectors at 10 ms time intervals from the beginning of QRS were written out and used for construction of spatial vector end-points projected onto the horizontal and left sagittal planes. Only in 34.1 % of ECG evaluated as normals by the VA program in the group of unselected subjects and in 11.2% in the group of cardiac patients,respectively, were found to have all instantaneous QRS vector end-points within normal reference areas obtained by nonparametrical procedure on a probability level of 0.95 in another group of 123 healthy subjects. This results underline the problem of bordeline abnormality of vectorcardiographic parameters which remains unappearent if the classification is made only by exclusion of pathological teatutes or by classifying the subject as fitting into normal reference parameters or not.

Introduction.

The problem of separating normal ECGs from pathological ones and the classification of pathological ECGs is a problem of diagnostic decision making in automated ECG analysis. The aim of this study was to assess ECG records evaluated as normals by the VA program by means of reference areas for normal location of instantaneous planar vector end-points.

Material and methods:

Two groups of ECG record were examined. 1)group of 482 unselected subjects examined for screening purpose aged from 20 to 71 years, average age 38.9 yrs (236 males, 246 females).2) Group of 448 patients aged from 7 to 82 yrs, average age 47,8 yrs. (245 males, 203 females) with cardiac pathology or complaints suggesting heart disease, referred for electrocardiographic investigation by cardiologist.

Orthogonal physically corrected Frank ECGs were recorded by a three-channel electrocardiograph Chirastar 32 U (Chirana, Czechoslovakia) and evaluated on-line by VA program (Pipberger 1975) implemented on the Czechoslovak minicomputer SM 4-20 (Melotová et al.1975). Only ECGs with absence of any pathologic diagnosis of QRS with VA program were considered.

Values of x, y, z coordinates of instantaneous vectors in 10 ms time intervals from 10 to 60 ms QRS were taken from the intermediate processing of the Pipberger program and used for construction of spatial vector end-points projected onto the horizontal and left sagittal planes.

Locations of instantaneous vector endpoints were evaluated with respect to reference areas for the planar projections. Reference areas of planar vector end-points (horizontal and left sagittal planes) were constructed nonparametrically on the probability level p = 0.95 according to Ruttkay-Nedecký (1982) in a group of 123 healthy subjects (Bachárová and Melotová, 1986) fig.1 and fig.2.

Fig. 1. Reference areas of instantaneous planar vector end-points (horizontal plane) for 10 to 80 ms of QRS in form of polygons.

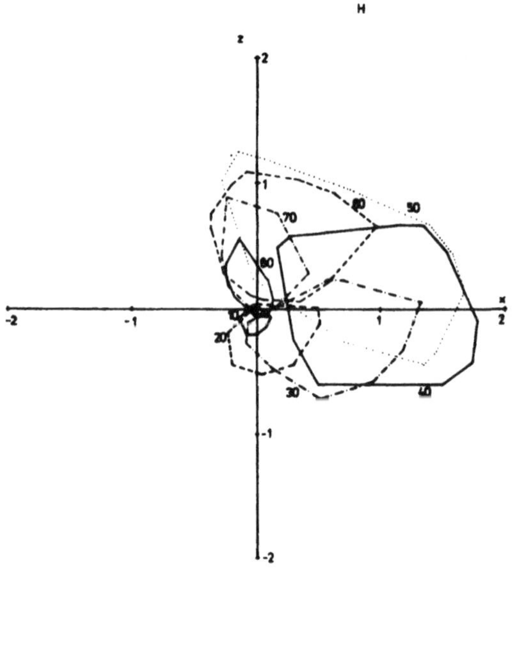

Results:

In the group of 482 unselected subjectes 370 ECG records were assessed as normal by the VA program. From these 126 records (=34.1%) had the 10 to 60 ms instantaneous vector end-points within the normal references areas. Probability of abnormally located vectors for 10 ms time intervals of QRS is indicated in the table 1. Average probability of abnormally located planar vector endpoints for this group was p=0.24.

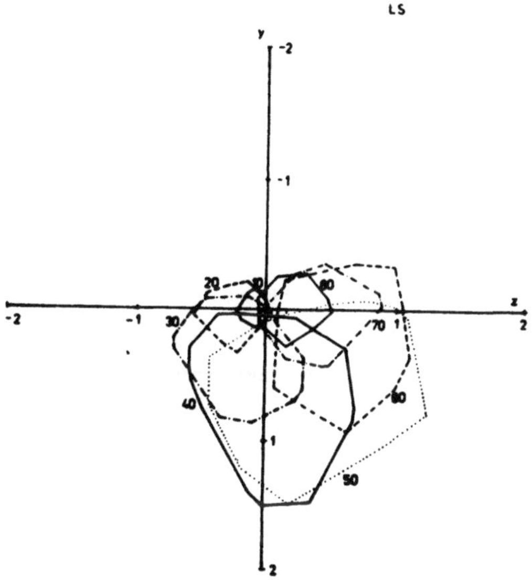

Fig. 2. Reference areas of instantaneous planar vector endpoints (left sagittal plane) for 10 to 80 ms QRS in form of polygons.

Table 1. Probability of abnormally located instantaneous vector endpoints from 10 ms to 60 ms QRS in the group of unselected subjects.

ms of QRS	p
10	0.33
20	0.18
30	0.19
40	0.24
50	0.27
60	0.22

Table 2. Probability of abnormally located instantaneous vector endpoints from 10 ms to 60 ms QRS in the group of cardiac patients.

ms of QRS	p
10	0.49
20	0.32
30	0.42
40	0.48
50	0.51
60	0.46

In the group of 448 cardiac patients 134 ECG records were evaluated as normal according to VA program. From these 134 records only 15 records (= 11.2%) had all observed instantaneous vector endpoints located within normal reference areas. Probability of abnormally located vector for 10 ms time intervals of QRS is indicated in table 2. Average probability of abnormally located planar vector endpoints for group of cardiac patents was p = 0.45.

Discussion and conclusion.

The algorithm of Pipberger' VA program was based on the estimation of the posterior probability that an individual with observational multidimensional vector falls in a given diagnostic category (Cornfiel et al.1973). Posterior probability of any pathological category less than 10 % was supressed in the print-out. It follows that the conclusion that a given QRS pattern belongs to norm is given by exclusion of patterns belonging to a pathological category.

In contrast, the assesment of normal ECG patterns on the basis of instantaneous vector end-points localisation within the polygons of norm defined the normal pattern positively on a 95 % probability level.

Two extreme categories were separated by the above mentioned procedure - the category of pathological ECGs and the category of normal ECGs. Between these two extremes there is a set of records with abnormally located instantaneous vector end-points, which are out of the norm, but don' t belong to a typical or suspected pathological VCG pattern. This undefined intermediary set comprised 65.9 % of ECG records determined as normal by the VA program in the group of unselected subjects and even 88.8 % in the group of cardiac patients. The probability of occurence of abnormally located vectors increased from 20 ms QRS to 50 ms QRS, in 60 ms QES it slightly decreased. Relatively high probability of abnormal location was found in 10 ms QRS in the group of unselected subjects as well as in cardiac patients. These results underline the problem of bordeline abnormality of vectorcardiographic parameters which remains unapperent if the classification is made only by exclusion of pathological teatutes or by classifying the subjects as fitting into normal referenoo paramcters or not.

References.

1. Pipberger,H.W.:Automated ECG Analysis System, VA Res. Center for Cardiovascular Data Processing. Washington, Vet.Adm.Hosp.,105,(1975)
2. Melotová,J.,Ruttkay-Nedecký,I.,Smolák,L.,Bachárová,L.,Mokráň,L.,: Automated System of Screening Vectorcardiography (in Slovak). Research Institute of Medical Bionics, Bratislava, 50, (1975)
3. Ruttkay-Nedecký,I.:BLL 59, 682-690 (1973)
4. Bachárová,L.,Melotová,J.: BLL 86, 603-611 (1986)
5. Cornfield,J.,Dunn,R.A.,Batchlor,Ch.D.,Pipberger,H.V.: Comp.Biomed.Res.,6, 97-120 (1973)

Shape of the QRS loop and the stability of transformation coefficients between two different VCG lead systems

V. SZATHMÁRY, L.A. POPOV, O.V. BAUM, Š. ŠAJBAN, I. RUTTKAY-NEDECKÝ
Inst. of Normal and Pathol. Physiology, Slovak Acad. Sci., Sienkiewiczova 1, 81371 Bratislava, ČSSR; Inst. of Biological Physics, Acad. Sci. USSR, SU 142292 Pushchino, USSR

Summary

The mutual transformation coefficients for cardiosignals recorded by two different corrected orthogonal lead systems (Frank, McFee-Parungao) computed by one of the standard methods as well as using regularization methods lack stability. This instability may be caused by degeneration of the system of linear equations necessary for the calculation of transformation coefficients. This in turn may be due to the fact that the heart vector end points are usually distributed on one plane during ventricular depolarization. This has led to the suggestion of a new method for the determination of transformation coefficients. The x and z components of one lead system are expressed as a function of the same two components of the other lead system, while y components linearly depend on x and z components in their own lead systems. Relatively stable coefficients were obtained with this method in a group of healthy subjects, using the Frank and McFee-Parungao lead systems.

Introduction

Practical vectorcardiography still lacks agreement on standard use of a defined lead system. Owing to this, determination of appropriate transformation relationships seems to be the only way of comparing and calculating electrocardiosignals recorded using different lead systems.

The aim of the present work was to develop a method for mutual transformation of electrocardiosignals which, in the framework of the computation algorithm, would eliminate procedures leading to instability of the solution to the system of linear equations and/or to instability of the determined coefficients of mutual transformation [1][2].

Transformation of electrocardiosignals means transformation of electrocardiosignals measured using one electrocardiographic lead system to values of electrocardiosignals which would be measured from the same person and during the same interval but using another (different) VCG lead system.

Theory and Methods

The analysis of characteristics of transformation coefficients determined by the standard method [3] has shown an indirect relationship between the stability of these coefficients upon the administration of low-level random noise and planarity of spatial QRS loop. In other words, the use of parameters of planar QRS loop results in singularity of the linear equation system matrix used to determine transformation coefficients, and thus in instability of solution. The proposed method for the determination of transformation coefficients is based on the assumption that the spatial QRS loop is planar. It arises from the above assumption that transformation may be performed for this loop so as the two axes of the new orthogonal system lie in the loop plane. Such a reference coordinate system was introduced by directing axis y along the loop polar vector, by directing axis x along the maximal heart vector, and by directing axis z perpendicular to the new axis x and y. Denoting time courses of voltage components x, y and z measured simultaneously using two different lead systems $U1_x(t)$, $U1_y(t)$, $U1_z(t)$ and $U2_x(t)$, $U2_y(t)$, $U2_z(t)$ respectively, the transformation of vectorcardiogram components from the original to the reference coordinate system is given by the following system of equations:

$$\begin{aligned} Ui_{xR}(t) &= Ci(1,1).Ui_x(t) + Ci(1,2).Ui_y(t) + Ci(1,3).Ui_z(t) \\ Ui_{yR}(t) &= Ci(2,1).Ui_x(t) + Ci(2,2).Ui_y(t) + Ci(2,3).Ui_z(t) \\ Ui_{zR}(t) &= Ci(3,1).Ui_x(t) + Ci(3,2).Ui_y(t) + Ci(3,3).Ui_z(t) \end{aligned} \quad (1)$$

where $i = 1$ or 2 and denotes the respective lead system, $Ci(j,k)$ stands for $j,k = 1,2,3$ and denotes reference transformation coefficients. With planar loop, $Ui_{yR}(t) = 0$, or $Ui_{yR}(t) \ll Ui_{xR}(t)$, and/or $Ui_{zR}(t)$ when end points of cardiac vectors lie near the reference plane. Introducing the condition of planarity into the system of transformation equations allows to express one of the original voltage components in terms of linear combination of the two other voltage components. Chosing component y as being linearly dependent, we obtain for each lead system

$$Ui_y(t) = -\frac{Ci(2,1)}{Ci(2,2)}.Ui_x(t) - \frac{Ci(2,3)}{Ci(2,2)}.Ui_z(t) \quad (2)$$

Employing relationship (2), the transformation equations between two different lead systems may be written as

$$\begin{aligned} Ui_x(t) &= Kj(1,1).Uj_x(t) + Kj(1,2).Uj_z(t) \\ Ui_z(t) &= Kj(2,1).Uj_x(t) + Kj(2,2).Uj_z(t) \\ Ui_y(t) &= Ai(1).Ui_x(t) + Ai(2).Ui_z(t) \end{aligned} \quad (3)$$

where $Kj(m,n)$ for $m,n = 1,2$ are transformation coefficients, $Ai(m)$ for $m = 1,2$ are the same coefficients as in relationship (2). When reconstructing vectorcardiogram components in the first system from those in the other system, $i = 1$ and $j = 2$, while $i = 2$ and $j = 1$ for inverse reconstruction.

The quality of the transformation method based on the system of equations (3) was tested by comparing it with the standard method as used by H.C.Burger et al. [3]. The standard method uses following transformation equations:

$$\begin{aligned} Ui_x(t) &= Lj(1,1).Uj_x(t) + Lj(1,2).Uj_y(t) + Lj(1,3).Uj_z(t) \\ Ui_y(t) &= Lj(2,1).Uj_x(t) + Lj(2,2).Uj_y(t) + Lj(2,3).Uj_z(t) \\ Ui_z(t) &= Lj(3,1).Uj_x(t) + Lj(3,2).Uj_y(t) + Lj(3,3).Uj_z(t) \end{aligned} \quad (4)$$

where $Lj(m,n)$ are transformation coefficients for $m,n = 1,2,3$. With both methods, the respective transformation coefficients were determined for vectorcardiogram components by the method of least quadratic deviations applied to the respective transformation equations. Stability of transformation coefficients was evaluated by estimating the variability upon the administration of random noise to input VCG components. Standard de-

VCG study of the S-T segment changes in pts with MI treated or not with i.v. Streptokinase.

PALMIERI M., GOTTI G., ZILIO G., CATTARINI G., MORATTI P.

Servizio di Cardiologia e CCU - Ospedale Provinciale - Monfalcone - Italy

Summary

In order to study the S-T modification during the acute phase of the MI treated or not with i.v. Streptokinase (SK: 1.500.000 I.U.), 62 consecutively admitted pts, 50 men and 12 women, aged 45-82 (mean 60.2), underwent a VCG recording within 4 hours after onset of symptoms, subsequently repeated every 6 hours for 48 hours, and then every 12 hours up to the discharge of the pt from CCU to a sub-intensive area (50-100 hrs). At the same time, blood samples were drawn until a total CPK release curve was obtained. VCG vector differences, with regard to spatial amplitude, S-T max(mV), S-T vector shifting (mV) and its planar deviation were plotted as a function of time. In 35 SK pts, with respect to 27 non-SK pts, the followings were noted:

1) The S-T showed an important voltage reduction during the whole period of observation in all treated pts.
2) In all cases important planar shifting of S-T vectors are recorded especially when reciprocal changes in diametrically opposed areas occur, or associated ischemic areas are present.
3) Also the T wave demonstrates a reduction of voltage after SK, even if no definitive considerations could be made with regard to its morphology.
4) Although the early onset and peak of CPK in SK-pts, no correlation has been found in this group between S-T max absolute values and CPK release curve.

So the S-T segment is almost always reduced after SK and is not a reliable parameter for monitoring the acute phase of MI, when the diagnosis of infarcted area extension or expansion is concerned.

Introduction

Spatial VCG has been proved to be an important diagnostic and prognostic procedure for monitoring the depolarization phase during the acute stage of the MI, in order to verify the extent of the ischemic lesion and to have a morphologic and a semi-quantitative evaluation of the area at risk for necrosis(1,2,3,4,5,6) For this purpose, this study has been carried out firstly, to check the repolarization phase during the acute stage of MI and to compare the VCG data in pts receiving or not i.v. streptokinase, in order to confirm the effect of this fibrinolytic on the infarcted area and on the S-T segment. Secondly, to correlate these data with the total CPK release curves, being this marker a reliable one for the appreciation of the infarcted area extension (3).

Material and methods

62 pts, 50 men and 12 women, aged 45-82 (mean 60.2) consecutively admitted in the CCU within 4 hours after the onset of symptoms of MI, underwent a VCG recording, subsequently repeated every 6 hours for 48 hours, and then every 12 hours up to the discharge of pts from CCU to sub-intensive area(50-100 hrs). At the same time, blood samples were drawn until a complete total CPK release curve was obtained(see Table 1). The admission of the pts to the study fulfilled the following criteria:

1) No history of previous MI;

2) Admission within 4 hours after onset of symptoms;

3) Absence of intraventricular conduction disturbances(IVCDs) prior or subsequent to MI;

4) Cardiac symptoms lasting 30 m' or more, with elevation of S-T segment = 1 mm in leads I,II,III,aVL,aVF, or = 2 mm from V_1 through V_6;

5) Non pericardial friction rubs during the clinical course.

Table 1

COHORT OF PATIENTS

TOTAL N.62		MEN: 50	WOMEN: 12
AGED 45-85 (MEAN 60.2)			
MI SITE	N.	SK	NON-SK
INFERIOR	36	20	16
ANTERIOR	26	15	11
TOTAL	62	35	27

STREPTOKINASE 1.500.000 I.U. I.V.
WITHIN 4 HRS AFTER ONSET OF SYMPTOMS

No pts had i.m. injections, DC shock or major troubles of plasma electrolytes.

Data analysis

For the analysis of our data we have chosen the following method. The repolarization phase has been investigated with the following measurements: 1) Spatial amplitude of S-T vector, with S-T vector Max (mV);2) mean change during time of S-T vector (mV);3) planar deviation of S-T in H,F,LS planes. Spatial amplitude of S-T vector has been checked with the formula: S-T (mV) = $X^2 + Y^2 + Z^2$. The registration of S-T at the admission has been chosen as reference, and the following recordings have been subtracted from this in order to obtain the so called "vector difference". Then we have made some confrontations between the spatial parameters and the cardiac enzymes of total CPK release curves, in order to check the variations of these parameters during the therapeutic interventions with the fibrinolytic treatment.

Results

PLANAR ORIENTATION AND DIFFERENCES OF S-T VECTORS REPORTED AS MEAN. INFERIOR MI: S-T vectors are mostly directed downward,forward and to the right in F(+90°,+170°)and LS(+46°,+168°)planes. In the H plane two subgroups of pts are recognized according to the angular displacement of S-T vectors:group A,with SK and non-SK pts presenting posterior and right shift of the vectors(+82°,+165°);and group B,in which an anterior vectorial shift is present(-62°,-150°).Mostly of the pts in group A showed an S-T depression in the precordial leads of the standard ECG,so that the posterior shifting of S-T vectors could be seen as a reciprocal change in a diametrically opposed area.ANTERIOR MI: in the H(-50°,-125°)and in LS(+65°, 135°)planes the orientation of the S-T vectors is forward,as espected for the MI site.In the F plane other to groups of pts are individualized according to the upward-left(-35°,-65°)or downward and right(+105°,+145°)direction of their S-T vectors.The angular displacement resulting in downward shift is mainly present in pts with an important S-T depression in leads II,III,aVF of the ECG,irrespective of the treatment received.

S-T VECTOR VARIATIONS IN AMPLITUDE DURING THE TIME FROM ADMISSION OF PTS UP TO THE 60th HOUR.VCG RECORDING EVERY 6 HRS FOR 48 HRS AND THEN EVERY 12 HRS UP TO THE 60th HR.As can be seen in Table 2,the S-T vector amplitude in treated pts with SK is constantly lower with respect to that of the other group, irrespective of the site of the MI.

Table 2 - ST AMPLITUDE (mV)

HOURS		10	20	30	40	60
ANTERIOR MI	SK	0.20	0.14	0.20	0.17	0.12
	NON-SK	0.28	0.22	0.25	0.20	0.13
INFERIOR MI	SK	0.18	0.11	0.14	0.13	0.10
	NON-SK	0.35	0.22	0.25	0.17	0.13

COMPARISON BETWEEN S-T VECTOR VARIATIONS IN AMPLITUDE AND CPK VALUES IN THE ACUTE STAGE OF MI. The comparison of the S-T Max in absolute values with those of total CPK release curve demonstrates that in non-SK pts a close correlation exsists between S-T Max and CPK samples during the time of observation, with a high correlation coefficient (r=0.5), whereas in SK pts there is no correlation at all in the two parameters.

Table 3 - VCG AND CPK VARIATIONS WITH RESPECT TO MI SITE.

SITE	ANTERIOR MI		INFERIOR MI		TOTAL (n=62)	
SK TREATMENT	yes(n=15)	no(n=11)	yes(n=20)	no(n=16)	yes(n=35)	no(n=27)
S-T V.Max (mV)	0.20 (0.14/0.27)	0.428 (0.18/0.7)	0.224 (0.07/0.5)	0.34 (0.14/0.56)	0.20 (0.07/0.7)	0.375 (0.14/0.7)
MEAN TIME OF PEAK APPEARANCE	12.7(4/22)	17.14(3/72)	10.2(2/35)	20.6(1/66)	15.82(4/70)	19.65(1/72)
CPK Max (IU/lt)	3934 (1519/7197)	1731 (306/3024)	1736 (980/2556)	1722 (377/3008)	3006 (377/7197)	1733 (306/3800)
MEAN RELEASE TIME HOURS	15.2 (9/24)	33.7 (13/48)	16.14 (8/35)	24 (16/39)	15.35 (8/35)	27.5 (13/48)

The Table 3 is inclusive of the S-T mean vector amplitude and mean CPK values plotted with the time and MI site, in SK and non-SK pts. It shows that in the first group the S-T mean voltage remains always lower during the observation period with respect of the same parameter in the other group, as previously explained ; whereas the mean CPK peak values of the SK pts appear earlier and higher. However, the CPK curve is followed by a faster drop in the next hours, so that the area outlined by the curve is obviously reduced with the time, the other curve being longer and higher the followings days. Moreover, in both S-T vectors curves a nearly constant finding is represented by a second increase starting about the 25th hour up to the 45th with a plateau for about 20 hours. The interpretation of this finding is reported in the discussion. On the T wave, it can be said that large variations intra-group is the rule when the observation is made on its orientation , voltage and morphology. There is a faster planar modification of T after SK, a consistent reduction of T vectors plotted with time in SK pts and a prevalence of the oval-roundish shape during the acute phase of MI.

Discussion and conclusions

Considering the data obtained in our study on the repolarization phase in the acute stage of MI, the following remarks can be made. SK and non-SK pts do not demonstrate significant differences in the plane orientation of S-T vectors during the first hours of observation. The predictable angular displacements are widely distributed intra-and intergroup, and even if some interest is raised in the presence of posterior shifting of S-T vectors mean differences in the H plane in pts with inferior MI, and the partial inferior position of S-T forces in the anterior MI, these shiftins may be due to reciprocal changes of S-T vectors in a diametrically opposed area or to an associated ischemic zone, rather than to any difference created by the different pharmaceutical intervention. On the other hand a nearly constant finding has been the recording of a lower S-T vector amplitude in SK pts, in the whole period of observation. The importance of this finding must be pointed out for the interpretation of the VCG data in various clinical settings following the acute stage of MI. Even if the mechanism of this finding has not been sufficiently explained as yet (recanalization of coronary vessels or improvement of repolarization with another mechanism?) its importance may arise in the differential diagnosis of MI complications as infarcted area extension, expansion or pericardial reaction to a transmural MI(7,8). Furthermore, in our cases it must be pointed out the increase of S-T vector amplitude from the nearly 25th hour for 15-20 hours in both groups of pts. Considering that pts presenting friction rubs due to pericardial reaction did not meet the criteria to enter the study,than this increase in vector amplitude may represent either the silent reaction of pericardium in the infarcted zone or the VCG signs of extension or expansion in the same zone.In fact,only in few cases the real presence of a MI extension could be demonstrated by the coexistence of a higher shifting of CPK values in agreement with the first findings,while MI expansion was only suspected when a consonant increase of the enzymatic curve was not present in the meantime. For the orientation of T wave,in SK pts there have been only minor modifications with respect to the pts of the other group.Also T wave demonstrates a voltage reduction after SK,even though no definitive considerations could be drawn with respect to its morphology.The presence of earlier and higher total CPK values in the first hours of MI are compatible with a favourable course of MI in our pts,perhaps for a reperfusion of vessels in the infarcted area.Unfortunately these events have not been demonstrated by a coronary artery angiography,but the clear improvement in clinical conditions along with the reduction of S-T vectors amplitude as results in the VCG findings,and the enzymatic behaviour all together play an important role to admit the existence of an infarcted area reduction and a hemodynamic improvement in the clinical course.Under this point of view our data seem in accordance with those reported in the literature(9,10,11,12).Summarizing the data obtained in our study,we can say: 1)the S-T showed an important voltage reduction during the whole period of observation in all treated pts.2) in all cases,important planar shiftings of S-T vectors are recorded,especially when reciprocal changes in diametrically opposed areas occur,or associated ischemic areas are present . 3)Also the T wave demonstrates a reduction of voltage after SK,even if no definitive considerations could be made with regard to its morphology. 4)Although the early onset and peak of CPK in SK pts,no correlation has been found in this group between S-T Max absolute values and CPK release curve.So the S-T segment is almost always reduced after SK and is not a reliable parameter for monitoring the acute phase of MI,when the diagnosis of infarcted area extension or expansion is concerned.

References

(1) Sederholm,M.,P.Grøttum,L.Erhardt,J.Kjekshus: Circulation, 68, 1006-1011 (1983)

(2) Colle,J.P.,G.Le Goff,E.Aouizerate,J.Bonnet,J.Ohayon,P.Besse,H.Bricaud:Arch.Mal.Coeur,79,292-300(1986)

(3) Bleifeld,W.,D.Mathey,P.Hanrath,H.Buss,S.Effert: Circulation, 55, 303-311 (1977)

(4) Wikswo,J.P.Jr.,S.C.Gundersen,W.Murphy,A.K.Dawson,R.F.Smith: Circul.Research, 49, 1055-1062 (1981)

(5) Kronenberg,M.W.,M.Hodges,T.Akiyama,D.L.Roberts,D.A.Ehrich,Th.L.Biddle,P.Nyu.Circulation,54,756-761(1976)

(6) Wickline,S.A.,J.J.McNamara: Circulation, 57, 910-920 (1978)

(7) Hutchins,G.M.,B.H.Bulkley: Am.J.Cardiol., 41, 1127-1132 (1978)

(8) Piccolo,E.,P.Delise,G.Zuin,A.Bonso,S.Romano,V.Ricciardiello,D.Fisher,F.Tani,C.Forleo,V.Portulano,L.Tini Brunozzi,L.Meniconi: G.Ital.Cardiol., 17, 57-62 (1987)

(9) Ganz,W.,I.Geft,J.Maddhi,D.Bermann,Y.Charuzzy,P.K.Shah,H.J.C.Swan: J.A.C.C., 1,1247-1252 (1983)

(10) Rentrop,P.,H.Blanke,K.R.Karsch,H.Kaiser,H.Kostering,K.Veitz: Circulation 63, 307-311 (1981)

(11) Blanke,H.,D.Von Hardenberg,M.Cohen,H.Kaiser,K.R.Karsch,J.Holt,H.Jr.Smith,P.Rentrop: J.A.C.C., 3, 657-661 (1984)

(12) Grøttum,P.,J.K.Kjekshus: J. Electrocardiol. 19, 337-346 (1986)

D E V E L O P M E N T A L

E L E C T R O C A R D I O L O G Y

Experimental Simulation of the Postnatal Decrease of Pulmonary Vascular Resistance: Effect on the ECG

DELLAS, S., EIFRIG, Th., SCHWARTZE, H.

Institute of Pathological Physiology, Karl Marx University, Leipzig, GDR

Summary

The QRS period of humans' and other mammalians' ECG undergoes a rightward shift during the first 3 days of life which could not be explained from growth effects. During the same period the heart rate (HR) increases. The decrease of pulmonary vascular resistance (PVR) normally occuring during this early life span had been produced pharmacologically in newborn guinea pigs. The changes of the excitation spread caused by the acute decreased PVR are the same as in uninfluenced growing guinea pigs during the first days of life. Accordingly, the changes of the QRS complex, of uninfluenced growing guinea pigs must be evoked by the same mechanism: a left ventricular volume loading caused by the decreasing PVR.

Introduction

The excitation spreading period of humans' and other mammalians' ECG undergoes a typical shift during the first 3 days of life and the HR increases. These changes could be caused by a left ventricular volume loading as a result of the decreasing PVR; the main decrease of PVR in a lot of mammalian species develops at the same period as the changes of the ECG. The aim of our study was the experimental simulation of the process of the early postnatal decrease of PVR.

Material and methods

11 two-days-old guinea pigs were narcotized i.p. by o.15 mg Etomidate (Radenarkon$^{(R)}$, VEB Jenapharm, GDR) per 1oo g body weight, and additionally by a subcutaneous injection of o.5% Lidocainhydrochloride (Xylocitin$^{(R)}$, VEB Jenapharm, GDR) at the jugular region. An intravenous infusion of 1o µm/kg/min prostaglandin E_2 (PGE_2, Minprostin$^{(R)}$, Upjohn GmbH, FRG) was applied via the vena jugularis. ECGs were recorded with the Frank lead system before, during and after the infusion of PGE_2. Treatment of the signals was off-line and resulted in analog-digital converting of the QRS complex and computation of horizontal and frontal vector loops and the HR from the RR intervals.

Results

During the infusion of PGE_2 significant alterations of the VCG occured in 6 of the 11 cases (paired match t-test, $\alpha = 0.05$), exclusively in form of a rightward shift of parts of the QRS loop. In 5 animals this extensive rightward shift resulted in a reversion of the vector loop type; the 6th case showed a rightward directed VCG already before starting the infusion. The remaining 5 of the 11 cases showed no significant alterations of the QRS loop, as will be discussed later.

In Fig. 1 the averaged time normalized horizontal vector loops of all 11 animals before and during the PGE_2-infusion are presented. The rightward shift of the mean QRS loop during the infusion becomes obvious. For comparison Fig. 2 shows averaged time normalized horizontal vector loops of 12 uninfluenced growing guinea pigs. The left part of the 2nd day loop is considerably cut off, the portion in the right front increased.

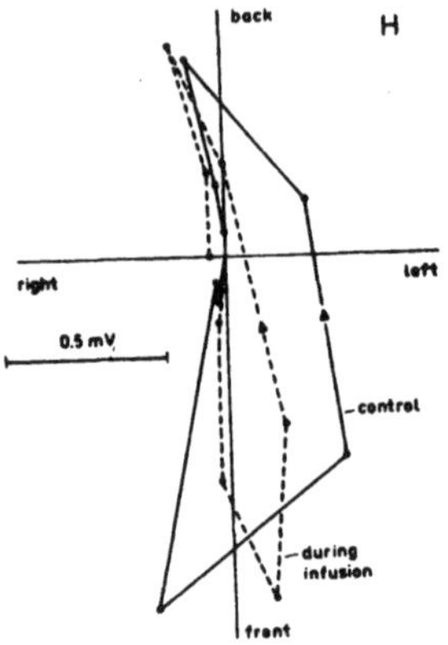

Fig. 1. Averaged time normalized horizontal vector loops before and during infusion of PGE_2.

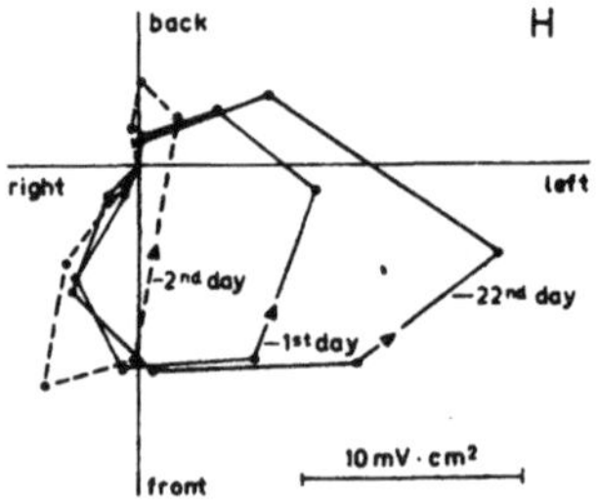

Fig. 2. Averaged time normalized horizontal vector loops of 12 uninfluenced growing guinea pigs (reproduced by permission from Joel 1984).

The averaged HR was found to be 44 bpm higher during the PGE_2-infusion than before (t-test, $\alpha = 0.05$). However, HR increase could not be seen in each particular animal (Fig. 3). But, if a change of the positional type of the QRS loop occured the HR increase was obligatory. In uninfluenced growing guinea pigs the averaged HR also exceeds significantly the initial value by 25 bpm at the age of two days while no significant change can be proved at the following days (Fig. 3).

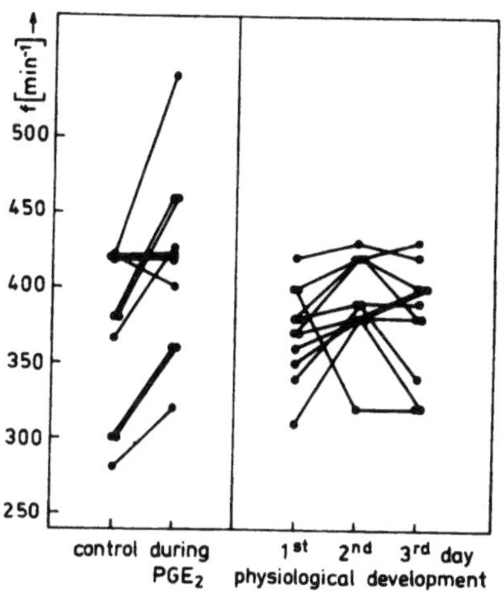

Fig. 3. Left panel: HR of 11 guinea pigs before and during the infusion of PGE_2; Right panel: Increase of HR of uninfluenced growing guinea pigs during the first days of life (by permission from Joel 1984).

After having finished the infusion the VCG changes and HR increases showed a retrograde tendency, but they did not vanish completely within 15 minutes.

Discussion

Early rapid alterations of the VCG start shortly after birth and take place during the transitional circulation period. In newborn guinea pigs and human newborns, functional closure of the fetal shunts is finished within the first day of life (Moss et al. 1963, Dellas 1985). The most important event of the following newborn period is the decrease of the PVR. The most rapid decrease of PVR in humans and in guinea pigs occurs during the first 2-3 days of life (Emmanouilides et al. 1964, Strittmatter-Bolleter 197o).
Acute decrease of the postnatally high PVR can be produced in guinea pigs by i.v. infusion of PGE_2 (Okpako 1972). No side effects are to be expected on the systemic circulation and the ductus arteriosus (Piper et al. 197o, Coceani et al. 1978).
A significant pharmacologically produced decrease of PVR is only possible in cases with high initial PVR. Because the natural decrease of PVR begins immediately after birth, in 4 of the 11 two-days-old guinea pigs neither VCG alterations nor HR increase could be found during the PGE_2 infusion. The remaining animals showed both, alterations of the VCG and of the HR strictly corresponding to adequate changes of similar direction and magnitude in uninfluenced animals within the first

3 days of life (Joel 1984).
Decreasing PVR causes a decrease of arterial pressure and an increase of venous pressure in the pulmonary circulation with corresponding changes of systolic pressure of the right heart and enddiastolic pressure of the left heart. Increased left ventricular enddiastolic pressure reflexly increases HR (Thorén, Lundin 1983) and produces alterations of the VCG (Millard et al. 1978), in turn being responsible for the outlined acute directional changes to the right of the newborns' ECG.

References

(1) Joel, A.: Diss. A, Med. Fak. Karl Marx University, Leipzig 1984

(2) Moss, A.J., G. Emmanouilides, E.R. Duffie: Pediatrics 32, 25-30 (1963)

(3) Dellas, S.: Diss. A, Med. Fak. Karl Marx University, Leipzig 1985

(4) Emmanouilides, G.C., A.J. Moss, E.R. Duffie Jr., F.H. Adams: J. Pediat. 65, 327-333 (1964)

(5) Strittmatter-Bolleter, E.: Med. Diss., Zürich 1970

(6) Okpako, D.T.: J. Pharm. Pharmacol. 24, 40-46 (1972)

(7) Piper, P.J., J.R. Vane, J.H. Wyllie: Nature 225, 600-604 (1970)

(8) Coceani, F., P.M. Olley, I. Bishai, E. Bodach, E.P. White: in Coceani and Olley, Adv. Prostagland. Thrombox. Res. 4, 325-333 (1978)

(9) Thorén, P., S. Lundin: in Ganten and Pfaff, Current topics in neuroendocrinology 3, 32-61 (1983)

(10) Millard, R.W., B.C. Hodgkin, C.V. Nelson: Am. J. Physiol. 235, H182-H187 (1978).

Conception and results of neonatal electrocardiographic screening

SPARR, K.-D.; MOCKE, D.
Children's clinic of the Military Medical Academy, Bad Saarow, GDR

Summary: The purpose of this study was to detect congenital heart failures, cardiomyopathies and conduction disturbances which can already be of haemodynamic importance in the neonatal period or infancy, and to make statements on the normal development of neonatal electrocardiogram. 3500 newborns have been included in ECG screening on their fifth day of life since October 1980. Conventional leads by EINTHOVEN, GOLDBERGER and WILSON as well as orthogonal FRANK leads were used. - Electrocardiograms not showing normal pattern were demonstrated in 15 % of the total group of newborns. It was evident that a pathological QRS vector occurred in approximately 15 % of electrocardiograms, being mainly in the range between 180° and -60°. This was documented by a negative elevation in FRANK ECG. Time, amplitude and heart rate values known from literature could be confirmed to a large extent. - A positive T wave was seen in 2,8 % of the cases in right precordial leads. - The diagnosis of a WOLFF-PARKINSON-WHITE syndrome was made in 9 cases.

Introduction: The purpose of our investigatiens was to contribute to an early detection of congenital angiocardiopathies including neonatal disorders of impulse formation and conduction and possibly to make a statement on the effects of fetal hypoxias on specific myocardium by introducing screening electrocardiography in neonatal period. - Similar investigations were made by study groups around Southall (1976, 1981) and Jones (1979).

Material and methods: About 3500 neonates have been included in our ECG screening on their fifth day of life since October 1980. - Both conventional leads and orthogonal leads by FRANK were used. Interpreting the results it has to be taken into account that short-time ECG leads, which recorded 100-150 cardiac cycles, were evaluated with priority. - 51.2 per cent of the newborn infants were males and 48.8 per cent females. The average birth weight was 3265 g. Only four per cent of the children weighed less than 2500 g. 3.6 per cent were preterm infants. - Only in 7.8 per cent of the neonates Apgar score at 5 minutes was less than 8. - Approximately 20 per cent of all newborns included in screening were moved to children's clinic for a variety of reasons. Respiratory adaptation disorders occurred in 9.5 per cent of the cases. - A vitium cordis was suspected in 2.5 per cent of the newborn infants. In 44 per cent of these suspect cases the diagnosis proved true in further course. - One part of statistical data, which could be expected as representative and identical, is related to an analysis of findings in 1005 children.

Results: Neonates with ECG findings requiring a check-up and with pathological ones, respectively, had clinical and electrocardiographical control examinations at monthly intervals up to the completed first year of life. - While in the first month of life still 31 per cent were asked to come to a check-up examination, there were only 6 per cent in the 6th month of life and 3.5 per cent of the initial group in the 12th month of life. - While 99.8 per cent of all newborn infants were included in neonatal ECG screening, 90 - 95 per cent came to check-up examinations. - Direction deviations of QRS not corresponding to age on the fifth day of life were the cause of most findings requiring a check-up. - Approximately 15 per cent of all newborns showed an angular range from more than 180° to -60°. - While in the third month of life QRS direction was in physiological range again in 80 per cent of the children, it was unchanged out of normal range corresponding to age in 20 per cent. This patient group showed typical ECG patterns indicating a hemiblocking. In about 70 per cent the pattern corresponded to a left anterior hemiblock. - Even though functional peculiarities in the infrabifurcal conduction system depending on maturation are probable for such processes in the neonatal period (Mücke 1987), as to stable atypical QRS integral vectors it is not possible to decide with certainty, whether changes caused by hypoxia are aetiologically concerned or a primary genetically determined impulse conduction anomaly is present. - Repolarisation disorders in the form of positive T waves in right precordial leads were observed in 2.8 per cent of the cases. - Still approximately 20 per cent of this group turned out to be "non-responders" in the fourth week of life, i.e. positive T waves remained in right precordial leads without clinical signs of a cardiac disease. - It has to be mentioned, however, that T can become negative also in absence of a cardiopathy at a later date. - Children with delayed decrease in pressure in the pulmonary vascular system are possibly concerned here. Mean heart rate was 130 ± 17 beats/minute in the whole group. The range was between 65 and 180. A higher heart rate was observed with lower birth weight. - A sinus arrhythmia could be demonstrated in almost all electrocardiograms. - Abrupt rate changes were partly diagnosed. In about 2 per cent of them one could think of sinuatrial blocks. - These and minor arrhythmias could be confirmed both by longtime leads and cardiospirograms. - Bradycardia phases rarely lasted longer than 30 seconds. - Our studies could confirm the known time values for P and QRS duration. - The PQ interval was not dependent on heart rate, while a negative correlation was found between the QT interval and the heart rate. - Recording short-time ECG leads 9 WPW syndromes were diagnosed in our study. This corresponds to an incidence of 1:400. Taking into account also the intermittently occurring or[1] WPW syndromes, incidences published so far and found in our study would be exceeded. - This aspect and the fact that a WPW syndrome can be the aetiological basis of the development of tachycardic dysrhythmias in neonates, but in fetuses too, require therefore a consequent supervision of these children. - In 2 cases of WPW syndromes we diagnosed supraventricular tachycardias occurred in the postnatal period.

[1] "concealed"

Discussion and conclusions: To sum up it can be said:

1. that mainly maturation processes of the cardiac conduction system are a cause of an atypical direction of ventricular conduction, but disorders caused by hypoxia or congenital impulse conduction anomalies come into consideration in approximately 20 per cent. The left anterior fascicle is probably affected in 70 per cent of all cases here.
2. that early detection of congenital angiocardiopathies by an ECG screening is of importance only inasmuch as it must concern clinical pictures which can be identified by repolarisation disorders, signs of hypertrophy, direction deviations and other ECG characteristics. In addition to hypoplastic right heart syndromes recirculation vitia being of special haemodynamic importance are first of all concerned.
3. that as far as disorders of impulse formation and conduction can be recorded with short-time leads, a definitive statement can be made about these disorders.
4. that more importance has to be attributed to pre-excitation syndromes in the neonatal period and early infancy. An incidence of the WPW syndrome of 1:400 is probably to be expected.
   Since haemodynamically important cardiac arrhythmias can develop, an ECG screening in neonatal period may well be justified.

References:

(1) Southall, D. P., D. G. Vulliamy, M. J. Davies, R. H. Anderson, E. A. Shinebourne, A. M. Johnson: Brit. med. J. 2, 615 - 618 (1976).

(2) Southall, D. P., A. M. Johnson, E. A. Shinebourne, P. G. B. Johnston, D. G. Vulliamy: Pediatrie 68, 58 - 66 (1981).

(3) Mücke, D.: Kinderärztl. Praxis 55, 227 - 232 (1987).

(4) Mücke, D.: Kinderärztl. Praxis 55, 321 - 328 (1987).

Some aspects of the body surface mapping and echocardiographic findings in healthy children

MICHALÍK, D., HULÍN, I., MAŠURA, J., MACO, M., TYŠLER, M., TURZOVÁ, M.

Department of Clinical Pathophysiology, Medical School, Comenius University, Bratislava, Czechoslovakia

Summary
Two groups of healthy children aged 9 and 14 years were studied. The somatic and echocardiographic parameters in both groups were related to the body surface potential maps (BSPM) constructed from potentials recorded by 190 electrodes on the torso surface. Qualitative evaluation of BSPM showed no relation to the age and heart mass. The multifactorial analysis including somatic, echocardiographic parameters and cardiac electric events suggested the complex influence of the cardial and extracardial factors.

Introduction
Body surface potential mapping provides better electrophysiologic information about cardiac events than standard 12-lead electrocardiogram. It is known that body surface potential pattern distributions in ventricular activation are similar in both sexes. On average, however, QRS potentials are slightly higher in the male subjects of each age group, probably due to larger heart size (Green et al, 1985). The aim of our work was to search for the possible relations between morphological and electrophysiological cardiac parameters in both sexes during prepubertal and pubertal period.

Material and methods
Two groups of healthy children in age about 9 and 14 years were studied. All children were considered to be normal on the base of medical history, physical examination, 12-lead electrocardiogram and M-mode echocardiogram (ATL 51 D and EMG 666 B computer). After taking a set of needed somatometric parameters the electrophysiological examination was performed on the subject in sitting position. The electrocardio-coordinator EKKG-80 (Kneppo et al, 1979) was used for this purpose. ECG signals were recorded according to the torso geometry by 19 electrodes in ten levels (190 points), from the axilae to the navel. The sampling rate during QRS complex was 250 per second. The ventricular activation was analysed qualitatively and quantitatively.

Results
Both age groups of children differed significantly in some somatic parameters. The mean value of body weight was 32,4 and 52,4 kg, body

height was 139 cm and 166 cm and chest circumference (CC) was 64 and 77 cm, respectively. The CC to weight ratio was 2,0 and 1,5 respectively. The echocardiographic examination showed that the mean interventricular septum thickness in the first group was 7,1 mm and in the second one was 8,6 mm, the left ventricular posterior wall was 5,8 and 7,7 mm, left ventricular diastolic diameter was 39,6 mm and 44,2 mm respectively. Left ventricular end-systolic volume, calculated from echocardiographic values was 15,5 ml and 22,4 ml, left ventricular diastolic volume was 63,3 and 87,2 ml, stroke volume was 47,8 and 67,6 ml, respectively. The heart mass calculated according to the Devereux and Reichek (1977) formula was in the first group 87,8 g and in the second one 142,5 g (the difference was 62 %). The qualitative comparison of body surface isopotential maps in both groups showed no essential pattern difference. The QRS total root-mean-square (RMS) potential was considered as an important quantitative BSPM parameter. It represents the cardiac electric field total intensity. The average total RMS potential value in the younger group was 6,689 mV and in the other one was 7,246 mV, but the difference was non-significant. The multifactorial analysis of some somatic, echocardiographic and electric parameters showed:

1. the subjects with high total RMS potential (above 7000 mV), heart mass value (above 120 g) had the low CC/weight ratio (under 1,6)
2. the subjects with low total RMS potential and heart mass value had the high CC/weight ratio
3. the combination of mentioned factors in the rest of subjects was very variable.

This multifactorial analysis re-devided the most of our probands into two dominant groups. In the first one the total RMS value was significantly higher (8,214 mV) than in the second one (5311 mV), as well as the heart mass value which was 155 g and 76,8 g respectlively.

Discussion and conclusions

Liebman et al. (1981) presented the qualitative observation of the QRS BSPM in 40 normal children. Their results concerning the localisation and migration of the potential maxima, minima and zero potential line are the same as ours. Potential pattern distribution in our children did not change in regard to the age as it was described by Green et al. (1985). The multifactorial analysis showed that cardiac electric events are in better relation to the combination of somatic and echocardiographic parameters than to the age. Because of the small number of examined subjects the definite conclusion of this phenomenon requires to extend the number of followed children.

References

(1) Green, L.S., R.L. Lux, C.W. Haws, R.R. Williams, S.C. Hunt, and M.J. Burgess: Circulation 71, 244 - 253 (1985)

(2) Kneppo, P., V. Rosík, and M. Tyšler: In Progress in Electrocardiology, Pitman Medical Press, Glasgow, 212 - 214 (1979)

(3) Devereux, R.B., and N. Reichek: Circulation 55, 614 - 618 (1977)
(4) Liebman, J., C.W. Thomas, Y. Rudy, and R. Plonsey: J. Electrocardiology 14, 249 - 260 (1981).

FRANK ECG of adolescents

Jacobi, S.; Mücke, D.
Women's[1] clinic of the Military Medical Academy, Bad Saarow, GDR

Summary: Normal ranges for time, amplitude and angular values of ECG were obtained in 200 adolescents between 15 and 18 years of age. EINTHOVEN, GOLDBERGER and WILSON (V_1 - V_6) as well as FRANK leads were used. Our studies were of screening nature. The results showed that body height has the greatest influence on ECG. The so-called physiological incomplete right bundle branch block has been relatively often found in the conventional ECG in 39 %. Regardless of this finding, similar morphological changes occurred in 13,5 % also in FRANK lead -z. By comparing our results with those given in literature effects of centenary acceleration on our own results could be demonstrated.

Introduction: The main purpose of the present study was to obtain valid and up-to-date electrocardiographic normal values for adolescents in the GDR. At the same time investigations were carried out to gain experience in using electrocardiography as a screening method. A comparison of our results with data of other authors given in literature 20-25 years ago was to allow statements about the acceleration process on normal ranges of electrocardiographic parameters.

Material and methods: Electrocardiograms (ECG) were recorded with the conventional lead systems by EINTHOVEN, GOLDBERGER and WILSON as well as the corrected orthogonal FRANK leads (x, y, -z) in 258 healthy probands 15 to 18 years old. All ECG were visually interpreted. A 6-channel electrocardiograph was used. The normal value group consisted of 90 male and 110 female adolescents. These 200 adolescents were subdivided into 4 groups of 50 probands each according to their age of birth. Body height, weight and chest circumference were measured and parameters required for comprehensive ECG description obtained in each adolescent.

Results and discussion: Detailed calculations of the correlation between body height, weight and chest circumference as well as age on the one hand and time as well as amplitude values of the corrected orthogonal FRANK leads on the other hand were made to study the influence of somatic parameters and age on electrocardiographic values. 92 different correlations were studied in this way. It was found that according to the number of significant correlation coefficients body heigh had the strongest influence on adolescent ECG. Less frequently electrocardiographic parameters were influenced by chest circumference, body weight and age. Nevertheless, establishing normal values related to body heightin adolescents is not considered as effective. Values obtained in especially small or very tall individuals of a given age group should rather compared with normal values of adjacent age groups. Relatively few significant electrocardiographic age differences were obtained in this study. They were mainly related to the group of 18-year-old adolescents differing already somatically.

[1] and Children's

In considering the rather slight differences in means in the age groups, however, the evident dispersions have to be taken into account (fig. 1.). In this figure dispersion of R, S and T amplitudes in FRANK lead y is shown in the 4 age groups.

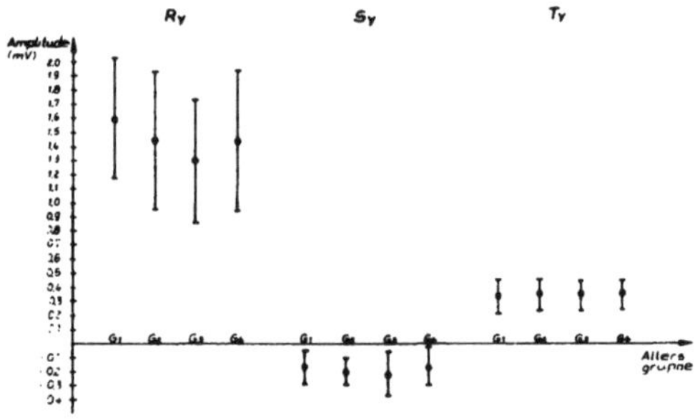

Fig.1. Dispersion of R, S and T amplitudes (lead y) in the 4 age groups
This great dispersion clearly indicates the influence of puberty. Correlation studies concerning the dependence of P-Q and Q-T intervals on heart rate showed no significant effects of heart rate on the P-Q interval, but indicated the known close relation between heart rate and Q-T interval. The limits of elevation and azimuth for P, QRS and T vectors in the 4 age groups are seen in figure 2:

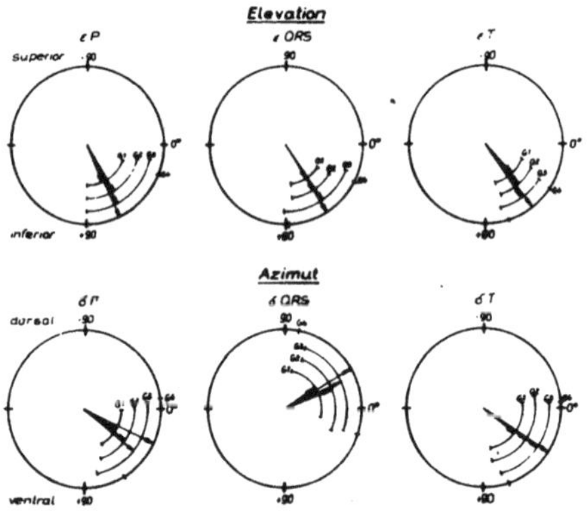

Fig. 2. Limits of elevation and azimuth in the 4 age groups
Since the normal values obtained for elevation and azimuth of the maximum instantaneous vectors and mean integral vectors resulting from plane integration differed only slightly, limits for mean integral vectors are not given in this figure. Simultaneous calculation of maximum instantaneous and mean integral vectors will lead to additional information mainly for the evaluation of pathological ECGs showing a deformation of P, QRS and T. Figure 3 shows essential features of the QRS complex in FRANK leads x, y and -z. The ventricular complex showed very different configurations in adolescents. This QRS configuration of x and y leads, however, was dominant in all 4 age groups

(fig. 3.). The predominant majority of ventricular complexes in lead -z was characterized by deep S waves. None of the 200 probands studied had a Q wave in lead -z. Consequently, a Q wave in lead -z has to be considered as an indication of pathological changes in heart.

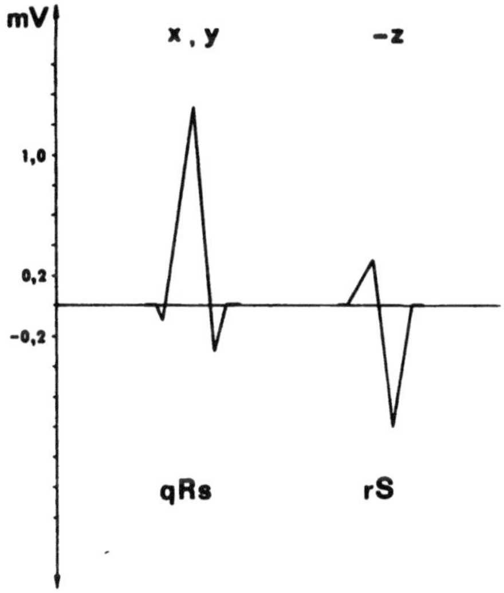

Fig. 3. Essential features of QRS in FRANK

The so-called physiological incomplete right bundle branch block (PIRBBB) was more frequently observed in conventional leads in adolescents we studied than in literature. Taking into account the criteria for the exclusion of a pathological incomplete right bundle branch block, a constant or intermittond occurrence of a second R wave in V_1 and/or V_2 could be established in the total normal value group in 39 %. Prevalence found in literature is varies between 2 and 26 % (1, 2, 4). The high prevalence of this so-called PIRBBB found in our study could be explained by school, competitive and leisure-time-sport activities of most adolescents and possibly by the effects of centenary acceleration. Morphologically equivalent configuration changes of QRS complex could also be observed in FRANK lead -z. In lead -z a second R wave constantly or intermittently occurred in 13,5 %. Since these configuration changes occurred, however, also indopendontly of the changes in conventional ECG mentioned above, FRANK ECG can't be considered as an indicator differentiating pathological changes from physiological ones. The influence of centenary acceleration is to be studied by comparing somatic and selected electrocardiographic parameters with those given in literature 20-25 years ago. Means for body height and weight were evidently higher in 200 adolescents of the present study examined in 1981 and 1982 than in pupils of 12-year schools of the same age studied by MARCUSSON in 1956-1958. There has been an increase in body height of 5-6 cm in male and 4-5 cm in female adolescents over 25 years. Alterations were observed also in body weight. There has been an increase of 3-5 kg in male and 3-4 kg in female probands over this period (3). In comparing our results with means of Q, R, S and T amplitudes of conventional ECGs in healthy young male and female adults, which were published by SIMONSON in 1961, an evident increase in almost all mean amplitude values was seen in adolescents examined in the present study (5). Evaluating these comparisons the influence of the acceleration process can be assumed. A total of 258 persons were examined in the present study. 200 of them were included to obtain normal values. The majority of all 258 probands were pupils of a 12-year school. Electrocardiography as part of this study was used as a screening method in pupils. Conventional ECGs could be recorded in 188 of 196 pupils, that means 96 % were included. Using conventional evaluation methods we determined the figures of ECGs interpreted as "normal", "abnormal" or "pathological". After a further anamnestic and clinical examination of adolescents with a conventional ECG requiring a check-up there were 40 abnormal and pathological, respectively, ECG findings in 36 adolescents. These abnormal findings are essentially classified:

1. disorders of impulse formation in and below the sinoatrial node in 15 adolescents,
2. a LOWN-GANONG-LEVINE syndrome in 8 persons,
3. a first-degree atrioventricular block in 1 proband,
4. a left anterior hemiblock is suspected in 5 adolescents, which was combined with a complete right bundle branch block without evident signs of hypertrophy in 2 cases,
5. a complete right bundle branch block in 1 proband,
6. a hypervoltage without further signs of a hypertrophy in 3 pupils,
7. a Q-T syndrome is suspected in a 16-year-old girl.

Conclusions: On the basic of a comparison of our own results with data given in literature 20-25 years ago the influence of the centenary acceleration process can be assumed. In comparison with corresponding data given in literature the so-called PIRBBB was more frequently - in 39 per cent - observed in conventional leads in healthy adolescents we examined. This prevalence could be explained by the great number of adolsecents regulary going in for sports. Without overestimating electrocardiography as a screening method, this study shows that abnormal findings have to be reckoned with in the population.

References:

(1) Kuppardt, H., et al: Ärztl. Jugendk. 62, 415-423 (1971).
(2) Lichtman, J., et al: Arch. internal Med. 132, 763-770 (1973).
(3) Marcusson, H.: Das Wachstum von Kindern und Jugendlichen in der Deutschen Demonkratischen Republik. Berlin 1961.
(4) Reindell, H.; and H. Klepzig: Die neuzeitlichen Brustwand- und Extremitäten-Ableitungen in der Praxis. Stuttgart 1958.
(5) Simonson, E.: Differentation between normal and abnormal in eleccardiography. St. Louis 1961.

Prevalence and clinical relevance of different physiological variants of right ventricular conduction in infancy, childhood and adolescence

PFEIFER, H. J.; MÜCKE, D.
Children's clinic of the Military Medical Academy, Bad Saarow, GDR

__Summary:__ Prevalence and clinical relevance of morphologically different physiological variants of right ventricular conduction shall be commented on in infancy, childhood and adolescence. A total of 1102 ECG leads in 571 male and 531 female healthy children and adolescents 1 month to 19 years old were evaluated for this study. EINTHOVEN, GOLDBERGER and WILSON (V_1 - V_6) as well as FRANK leads were recorded on a 6-channel electrocardiograph under the same lead conditions and visually interpreted. In analyzing ECGs, a classification into 6 morphologically different groups of physiological right ventricular conduction was chosen at random. Prevalence found in the various groups classified according to sex (girls: 41 - 81 per cent; boys: 35 - 88 per cent) and age (39 % in infancy; 81 % in puberty) is interpreted and compared with heterogeneous results given in literature.

__Introduction:__ Prevalence and clinical relevance of morphologically different variants of right ventricular conduction (RVC) shall be discussed with special regard to the so-called physiological incomplete right bundle branch block (PIRBBB) in infancy, childhood and adolescence.

__Material and methods:__ A total of 1102 ECG leads in 571 male and 531 female healthy children and adolescents one month to 19 years old was evaluated for this study. - The 23 chosen age groups with female and male probands and the total number are seen in the table 1. - Due to

Table 1. Age groups of the study

group No	age	Σ	♂	♀	group No	age	Σ	♂	♀
1	2 - 3 m	51	26	25	13	8 y	49	26	23
2	4 - 6 m	46	30	16	14	9 y	51	29	22
3	7 - 9 m	50	28	22	15	10 y	51	23	28
4	10 - 12 m	49	24	25	16	11 y	45	27	18
5	13 - 18 m	50	24	26	17	12 y	42	23	19
6	19 - 24 m	47	23	24	18	13 y	45	23	22
7	2 y	41	22	19	19	14 y	45	23	22
8	3 y	46	24	22	20	15 y	50	25	25
9	4 y	47	30	17	21	16 y	50	21	29
10	5 y	47	24	23	22	17 y	50	18	32
11	6 y	50	28	22	23	18 y	50	26	24
12	7 y	50	24	26	months = m ; years = y				

the very marked cardiovascular changes, especially in the first year of life, age groups were formed here, covering a period of three months each. The second year of life was subdivided into two periods: from 13 to 18 months and from 19 to 24 months. - After the age of two, grouping was made by years. - EINTHOVEN, GOLDBERGER, WILSON leads (V_1 - V_6) as well as the corrected orthogonal leads by FRANK (x, y, -z) were recorded on a 6-channel electrocardiograph under the same following lead conditions: Proband in lying position; FRANK electrodes A, I, C, E and M at the level of the fourth intercostal space, WILSON electrodes for V_1 and V_2 in the fourth intercostal space on the right and left parasternally and according to existing convention, respectively, synchronous leads from V_1 to V_6 also at a paper speed of 100 mm/sec. - All leads were visually interpreted. - Interpreting the electrocardiograms, a random division into 6 morphologically different variants of physiological RVC was chosen (fig. 1.):

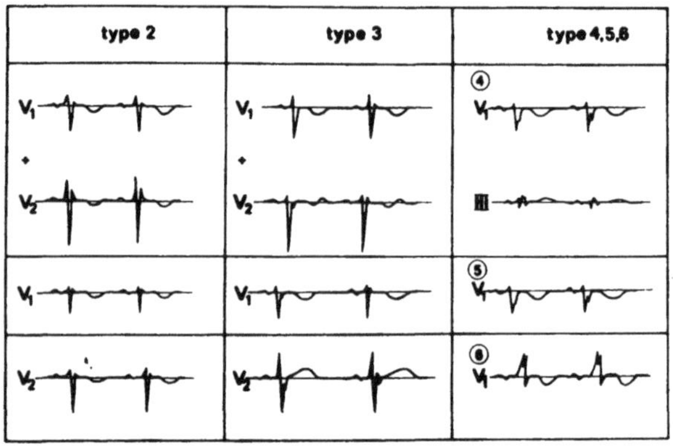

Fig. 1. Morphologically different variants of physiological RVC

1. tracing without characteristics mentioned below, with Rs or rS (RS) configuration in V_1 and/or V_2 (type 1)
2. Q-R interval in V_1 and/or V_2 at a rSr' configuration generally prolonged (type 2)
3. Q-R interval in V_1 and/or V_2 at a partly demonstrable rSr' configuration intermittently prolonged (type 3)
4. S in V_1 and/or V_2 widened and notched and slurred, respectively, QRS complex slurred/singly notched/ multiply notched in EINTHOVEN lead III (type 4)
5. as in type 4 described above, but without a slurred/singly notched/ multiply notched QRS complex in EINTHOVEN lead III (type 5)
6. R in V_1 and/or V_2 notched with prolonged Q-R interval (type 6).

Results (fig. 2.): There was one of the described morphological variants of a physiological RVC of type 2-6 in 39 to 81 per cent in the 23 age groups. The so-called PIRBBB with prolongation of the Q-R interval in V_1 and/or V_2 occurred in 17 to 53 per cent. Considering the age-related percentage prevalence it is evident that during the first year of life there is a continuous increase from a minimum value in the second and third months. Then an obvious decrease is seen. Thereafter, a further discontinuous increase up to percentage prevalences as at the end of the first year of life occurs, with this increase being interrupted by several decreases.

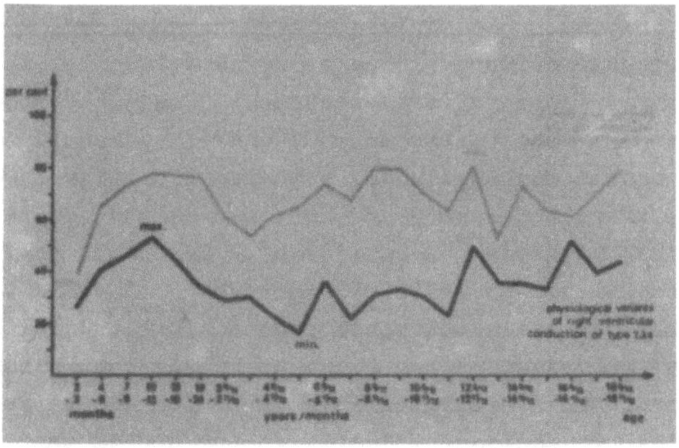

Fig. 2. Prevalence of physiological variants of RVC (type 2-6/2,3,6)

There were no significant sex differences concerning the prevalence of morphologically different physiological variants of RVC of type 2-6 (fig. 3.). In girls it was between 41 and 81 per cent and in boys bet-

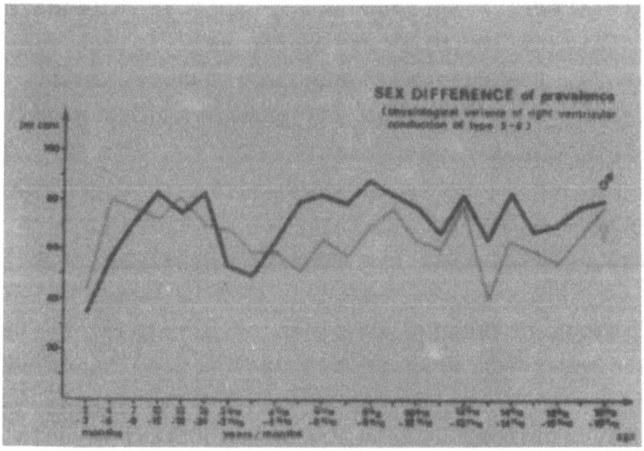

Fig. 3. Sex difference of prevalence of type 2-6

ween 35 and 88 per cent. Both prevalence curves repeatedly cross up to the third year of life. Starting from the fifth year of life the prevalence curve in female probands is always slightly below that of male probands. - We observed rSR' complexes in V_1 and/or V_2 also in healthy probands. According to many authors these complexes are to be considered as pathological incomplete right bundle branch blocks (1,2). In our study we found such patterns predominantly in adolescents actively went in for sports, who were anamnestically and clinically healthy und the ECGs of whom showed no evidence of a right ventricular hypertrophy.

The rSr' configurations in type 2 and 3 seen in WILSON leads V_1 and/or V_2 are analogously also found in the FRANK lead -z. However, simultaneous occurrence both in the conventional and in FRANK leads can't be statistically proved.

<u>Discussion:</u> Prevalence found in our study is evidently higher than given in literature, where it varies between 18 and 26 per cent (2,3). Taking into account that adolescents 17 and 18 years old have almost or already to be considered as adults, prevalence obtained seems to be especially high. Prevalence was 5 per cent in healthy adults (4) and 16 per cent in adult athletes (5) and 19 to 22 per cent, respectively, depending on the kind of sports (6,7). In boys 13-15 years old, who relatively regularly have done endurance sports, longitudinal studies showed an increase in frequency from 26 up to 63 per cent after 3 years (3). The regression of the so-called PIRBBB after finishing training is reported too. Thus, in adolescents going in for sports there can be an a priori existing physiological variant as well as physiological variant of RVC caused by training. Prevalences found in our study can partly be explained by the large number of adolescents actively going in for sports, especially in the older age groups. About 50 per cent went in for sports. An evident increase in the prevalence of physiological variants of RVC of type 2-6 is observed in the first year of life, though paradoxically left ventricular muscle mass increases. The question arises, why there is a following decrease in this prevalence. An answer to both questions could be the highest growth rate in the first year of life. Further cases of a discontinuous increase in the prevalence of the so-called PIRBBB and the different physiological variants of RVC, respectively, show a close relation to the increase in growth rate at the age of 7 and in puberty. Perhaps, effects of centenary acceleration on the cardiovascular system are also underlying causes of the higher prevalence we demonstrated. However, this can't be statistically proved here.

<u>Conclusions:</u> Clinical relevance is shown by a relatively frequent occurrence of physiological variants of RVC in the population of healthy children and adolescents and the necessity of distinguishing a physiological from a pathological RVC. - Prevalence depends both on an exact application of electrodes - increase in prevalence in the third and fourth intercostal space - and the number of probands going in for sports. - In synopsis with anamnestic, clinical and other examination findings and in absence of further signs of hypertrophy in the other ECG leads, a rSR' complex can with great certainty be classified as physiological. - On the other hand, a RVC variant morphologically appearing as a physiological one must not lead to an isolated interpretation, since it can also occur in a cardiopathy.

References:

(1) Gutheil, H.: Kinder-EKG. Georg Thieme Verlag, Stuttgart-New York 1980.

(2) Stoermer, J., and W. Heck: Pädiatrischer EKG-Atlas. Georg Thieme Verlag, Stuttgart 1971.

(3) Kuppardt, H., et al: Ärztl. Jugendkd. 62, 415-423 (1971).

(4) Ritter, O., and V. Fattorusso: Atlas der Elektrokardiographie. VEB Gustav Fischer Verlag, Jena 1981.

(5) Lichtman, J., et al: Arch. internal Med. 132, 763-770 (1973).

(6) Reindell, H., and H. Roskamm: Herzkrankheiten. Pathophysiologie - Diagnostik - Therapie. Springer Verlag, Berlin-Heidelberg-New York 1977.

(7) Rost, R., and W. Hollmann: Elektrokardiographie in der Sportmedizin. Sportherz - Breitensport - Rehabilitation. Georg Thieme Verlag, Stuttgart-New York 1980.

May primary septal hypertrophic cardiomyopathy be responsible for sudden infant death syndrome ? Relevancy of electrovectorcardiographic investigation.

ZIMMERMANN Ch., LEVY J.M., STOLL C., DE GEETER B., HEUMANN G., LUTZ P., ZIMMERMANN Cl.

Hospices Civils de Strasbourg, Institut de Puériculture, France.

SUMMARY.

The mechanism of sudden infant death syndrome remains unexplained in 25 % of the cases. Our procedure reflects a three-step electrovectorcardiographic investigation.

I) The preliminary experimental study included 5 infants suffering from primary septal hypertrophic cardiomyopathy, the diagnosis being made between the intra-uterine stage and the age of 9 months. These patients were treated with a calcium antagonist (Verapamil*) during a period from 2 to 6 1/2 years.

II) The second subject for investigation was provided by 6 newborn infants affected by specifically metabolic septal hypertrophy, secondary to maternal diabetes in 5 cases and to renin hypersecretion in 1 case.

III) In the last investigation 10 "near-miss" infants were concerned.

The study of the vectorcardiographic pattern, focused on septal depolarization, gives the following results :

I) The primary septal hypertrophic cardiomyopathy is conspicuously characterized by the disorganization of the mean septal vector not being influenced by the disappearance of septal hypertrophy due to Verapamil*.

II) Metabolic septal hypertrophy is characterized by the increased magnitude of the septal vector without any distortion of its orientation or rotation.

III) In one surviving "near-miss" infant we noted abnormal orientation and magnitude of the septal vector in the absence of septal hypertrophy.

These findings indicate that the vectorcardiographic investigation of an infant is useful in the detection of septal cardiomyopathy and possibly in the exploration of the unexplained sudden death syndrome.

INTRODUCTION.

The sudden death of an infant is an insupportable event, one which has haunted man for a long time. This type of death remains unexplained in 25 % of the cases. Therefore it seems to us judicious to report the electrovectorcardiographic findings made in a study about primary septal hypertrophic cardiomyopathy.

MATERIAL AND METHODS.

Our electric and ultrasonic results have been determined from 21 infants, using a total of 120 vectorcardiograms. In the course of the explorations, the patients were classified according to three comparative investigations.

I) The experimental study consisted of testing the cardiac reaction of 5 infants to the administration of a calcium antagonist (Verapamil* 7 mg/kg/day). They were all suffering from primary septal hypertrophic cardiomyopathy, 4 of them in the diffuse form (2 obstructive cases and 2 non obstructive cases one of which had right ventricular hypertrophy) and the fifth in a localized non obstructive midventricular form.

II) The second axis of our comparative electric research consisted of exploring 6 new-

born infants affected by specifically metabolic septal hypertrophy.
Five of these infants had diabetic mothers and the sixth was affected by high blood pressure induced by renin hypersecretion.
III) In the final comparative analysis we searched for decisive electric septal signs from 10 infants, survivors of "near-miss" episodes.
Electrovectorcardiographic protocol :
The interpretation of the cardiac electric activity has focused on the QRS vector loop. The analysis of the electrical documents included the study of scalar parameters (duration, amplitude, ratio of the amplitudes of Q and R) from the examination of the electrocardiograms and of the Frank's corrected orthogonal derivations (4th intercostal space). The vectorcardiographic appraisal (vectorcardiogram horizontal even) was based upon voltage criteria, angular indeces (of the 10 ms, initial maximal, 20 ms, 30 ms and maximal vector), chronological references (the times of the initial vector, of the passage from right to left and of the maximal vector's accession), morphological data and unwinding abnormalities. The angles were measured from the left transversal axis. The recording of the QRS loop's integrality was carried out with sensitivities of 2 and 4 cm/mV. A 10 cm/mV scale enabled a better appreciation of the beginning of the septal depolarization and consequently a more precise definition of the initial segment. The time scanning was 2.5 ms for the study of the whole loop and 1 ms for the closer analysis of the initial and final segments. The scalar graphs were recorded with a sensitivity of 1 cm/mV.
RESULTS.
I) Electro-, vector- and echocardiographic effects of a calcium antagonist therapeutic on 5 infants suffering from primary septal hypertrophic cardiomyopathy.
Analogies drawn between certain traces of the horizontal ventricular loop allow us to divide the analysis into two parts.
a) The prevalent position of the QRS vector loop, located anteriorly and to the left, and its counterclockwise rotation characterize the first group. It consists of 3 infants affected by cardiomyopathy, 2 obstructive and 1 non obstructive. Their corresponding septal diseases were diagnosed respectively in utero (familial form) and at the ages of 2 months 21 days and 9 months. As a result of the therapeutic trial, both the disappearance of the pseudonecrotic Q wave and the normalization of the septal vector's magnitude (except in one case) are consistent with the disappearance of the septal hypertrophy. However such a disappearance is opposed by the persistency of the abnormal spatial orientation of the septal vector and by the persistency of the left frontal axial deviation of QRS (0°, + 30°, + 30°).
b) In the second group the discriminative criteria are the median and posterior right position, its clockwise inscription, and the right frontal axial deviation of QRS (+ 180°, + 140°). This pattern is immutable without hemodynamic signs of pulmonary hypertension or right ventricular hyperpressure. To this group belong 2 infants suffering from non obstructive cardiomyopathy, one with the diffuse form combined with right ventricular hypertrophy and the other with localized midventricular lesions. The diagnoses were made respectively at the ages of 16 days and 9 months. The anterior left orientation of the septal vector (azimuthal angle = + 30°) remaining unchanged after the disappearance of the septal and right ventricular hypertrophies, highlights the odd nature of the electric anomalies.

II) Electro-, vector- and echocardiographic data obtained from the 6 newborn infants affected by specifically metabolic septal hypertrophy.

The analysis of the electrical characteristics of the septal hypertrophy, induced by maternal diabetes in 5 cases and by renin hypersecretion in 1 case, indicates a normal evolution. The echocardiographic images of isolated septal hypertrophy due to diabetes vanish by themselves within 2 months. The decline of the vectorcardiographic signs is revealed by the normalization of the septal maximal vector's magnitude (2 mV $\rightarrow$ 1 mV). The septal renin dependent hypertrophy is reduced through treatment with a converting enzyme inhibitor.

III) Electro-, vector- and echocardiographic findings made in the study of 10 "near-miss" infants.

The ultrasonic exploration allows us, in the 10 cases, to eliminate structural, functional, septal and parietal anomalies. The vectorcardiographic study shows in 9 cases a normal evolution of the ventricular loop. The vectorcardiographic abnormalities, discovered during a period of one year, in a syncopal context, in an infant having no septal hypertrophy, require further comments. In effect the median anteposition of the horizontal ventricular loop, the increased magnitude of the septal vector (2 mV, Azimuth : + 105°) and the left frontal axial deviation of QRS (0°), unchanged since birth, combined with a ventricular hyperexcitability (Holter recording) confirm prior clinical fears.

IV) Secondary effects.

Unlike other authors we were not able to observe deleterious electrical or hemodynamic effects during the administration of Verapamil* (1).

COMMENTS.

The difficulties encountered in studying infant sudden deaths on one hand and cardiomyopathy on the other hand can be explained by the multiplicity of factors in the genesis of the former and the differing electrical expressions in the case of the latter. The manipulation of the Ca ion (by Verapamil*) provides an experimental tool for studying the different components of cardiomyopathy (2).

In effect the vectorcardiographic patterns unmasked by the elimination of the septal hypertrophy expose an unusual reality. The steadiness of the QRS loop's position, observed in the 5 cases of septal hypertrophic cardiomyopathy, is astonishing. The exclusively right positioning of the horizontal QRS loop, inscribed clockwise, combined with a right frontal axial deviation in 2 cases reveal a disturbing fact, since in one case there was no right ventricular hypertrophy and in the other case the right ventricular hypertrophy had already disappeared due to treatment with Verapamil*. The left anterior position of the loop, inscribed counterclockwise, combined with a left frontal deviation, monitored in two cases of septal hypertrophy in the absence of either a right bundle branch block or a posterior myocardial necrosis, reinforce the concept of an unusual ventricular depolarization. This unchanging left anterior positioning of the QRS vector loop has been found as well in a "near-miss" infant. This left anterior shifting of QRS, in the absence of defined cardiopathy, could be considered, according to electrophysiological theories, as a mid left septal conductive disorder (3, 4, 5). Moreover the disappearance of the pseudonecrotic pattern, the normalization of the septal vector's magnitude, both concomitant with the normalization of the septal thickness by calcic inhibition, are in contrast with the unchanging unusual spatial orientation of the septal vector : anterior right (azimuthal angle : + 130°) or anterior left (azimuthal angle = + 30°) or almost

perfect superposition with the maximal vector (azimuthal angle = + 80°). Finally, the lack of a neonatal physiological right ventricular predominant vectorcardiographic pattern, observed in two cases of septal hypertrophic cardiomyopathy and in one "near-miss" infant, suggests the potential existence, from birth, of cardiac electric anomalies.
The predominance of the septal aberrations in hypertrophic cardiomyopathy very probably suggests a common denominator, the desorganization of septal depolarization. The reorientation of the depolarization can be attributed to the "whirling architecture" of the septal muscular fibers (6). This hypothesis seems plausible in most cases. However a very recent anglo-saxon anatomopathological study has pointed out the absence of muscular fiber abnormalities in 5 % of the cases of septal hypertrophic cardiomyopathy (7). These findings enable us to infer the possibility of autonomous damage in the septal cardionector system. It is possible to propose the idea of a common embryonal origin of the intraseptal conduction delay and of the metabolic disorders, inducing an added and fluctuating septal hypertrophy. Moreover the suspicion of the implication of a metabolic factor in the building of the septal hypertrophy in primary hypertrophic septal cardiomyopathy is reinforced by the observation of the insensibility to the calcium antagonist in one case of apparently primary cardiomyopathy. Indeed during the evolution of this case, we were able to notice some marks of worn phacomatosis. This observation shows the problem of the differential diagnosis with intraseptal tumors. Moreover the metabolic septal hypertrophy of the infant induced by maternal diabetes or by renin hypersecretion, contrary to the primary septal hypertrophic myocardiopathy, is characterized by the isolated increase of the septal vector's magnitude without orientational abnormalities.

CONCLUSION.

The septal vector's orientational distortions without corresponding hypertrophy represent the fundamental characteristics found during our study of the electrical phenomena in infant's septal cardiomyopathy.
The damage to the intraseptal conduction, shown by the orientational abnormalities of the septal vector, can be considered as an electrical indicator of cardiac vulnerability. The occurence of a ventricular paroxystic hyperexcitability, induced by metabolic disorder, is very likely the cause of some unexplained sudden infant deaths, as revealed by the three critical cases isolated in the present study.

REFERENCES

(1) Epstein S.E., Rosing D.R. : Circulation 64, 437 - 441 (1981).
(2) Zimmermann Ch. et al : XIth International Congress on Electrocardiology, Caen, July 1984.
(3) Kulbertus H.E. et al : Brit. Heart J. 38, 549 - 557 (1976).
(4) Fernando De Padua et al : Adv. Cardiol. 21, 242 - 248 (1978).
(5) Timpone G. et al : 7th International Congress on Electrocardiology, Lisbon, June 1980.
(6) Van Dam R.T. et al : Brit. Heart J. 34, 100 - 112 (1972)
(7) Maron B.J. : Brit. Heart J. 50, 1 - 3 (1983).

Electrocardiography in hypertrophic cardiomyopathy

KIBARSKIS A., RUDYS A.

Department of cardiology, Vilnius State University, USSR

Summary

Hypertrophic cardiomyopathy was diagnosed in 65 patients according to clinical, ECG and echocardiographic data. In 48 cases only hypertrophy of interventricular septum was present, in 8 cases - symmetric hypertrophy of all left ventricle walls, in 8 cases - apical hypertrophy and in I - hypertrophy of the lateral wall. ECG abnormalities were present in all cases, the most often - deep negative T waves in leads V_{2-6}, I and aVL (46 cases). In 3 cases (all with left ventricular outflow tract obstruction) ECG simulated inferior wall infarction. Different changes of T waves were observed during 5 years period.

Introduction

In last decade the diagnosis of hypertrophic cardiomyopathy became routine and this progress is mostly attributible to new methods of investigation (echocardiography on the first place). Despite that, most cases of hypertrophic cardiomyopathy are diagnosed after finding some ECG abnormalities, which are rather common. The purpose of this work was to show different ECG abnormalities in patients with hypertrophic cardiomyopathy and their changes during period of observation.

Material and methods

65 patients, aged from I9 to 75 years (middle 5I), 43 males and 22 female were examined. The diagnosis of hypertrophic cardiomyopathy was based mainly on echocardiographic findings, when there was no other reason of left ventricular hypertrophy (LVH). In 3 cases the diagnosis was verified on autopsy. Echocardiographic examination was performed on Aloka-SSD-II0se in M mode and sector scanning. Examination (clinical, ECG, echocardiography) was repeated after I -5 years (approximately 3 examinations for every patient).

Results

In all 65 patients changes in ECG were noticed. The most often changes were T wave inversion in precordial leads V_{2-6} and I, aVL. In Fig. I ECG of a 50 years old patient with hypertrophic cardiomyopathy is presented. The interval between two tracings is 5 years. Onechocardiographic examination hypertrophy of interventricular septum (IVS) was revealed (about 2 cm), but no hypertrophy of lateral wall or apex was faund. The diagnosis was confirmed by coronaroventriculography. This type of ECG changes shown in Fig. I A was observed in 48 cases. We did not find any relations between degree of IVS hypertrophy and ECG changes in these patients.In 8 cases symmetric hypertrophy of all left ventricle walls and in 4 of them also of the right ventricle was found. The most often ECG changes in these patients were typical LVH with systolic overload

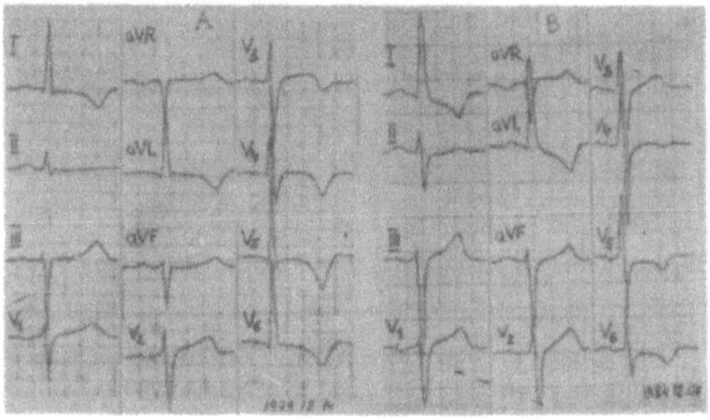

Fig. I. ECG of a patient with IVS hypertrophy.

pattern (5 cases), in the other two patients the ECG changes were low voltage in limb and precordial leads with nonspecific T wave changes (T inversion not exeeding 5 mm). Fig. 2 presents the ECG of a 58 years old patient, admitted to the hospital in terminal stage of cardiac decompensation and with cardiac rhythm disturbance (Fig. 2A). After disappearing of a paroxysm(Fig. 2B) the ECG shows unusualy wide QRS(0,36s) and very high voltage QS form in leads V_{2-4}. The patient died 5hours after admission, on autopsy symmetrical hypertrophy of left and right ventricular walls was found.

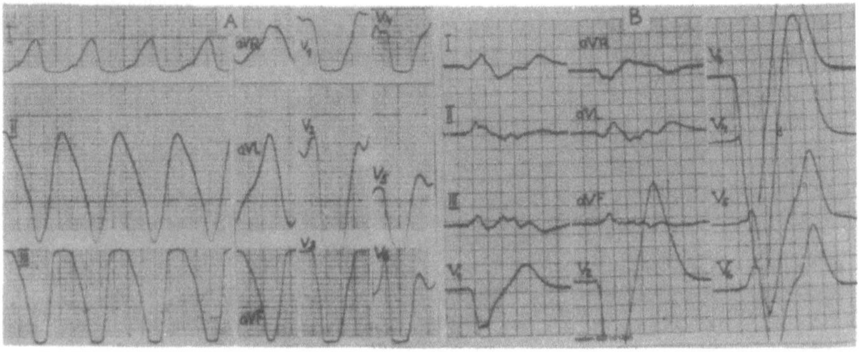

Fig. 2. ECG of a patient with symmetrical LVH during paroxysmal tachycardia (A) and after restored rhythm (B).

In 3 cases ECG changes simulated inferior myocardial infarction. One of these cases is presented in Fig. 3A. The patient was 54 years old male with anginal attacks and systolic ejection murmor on auscultation.

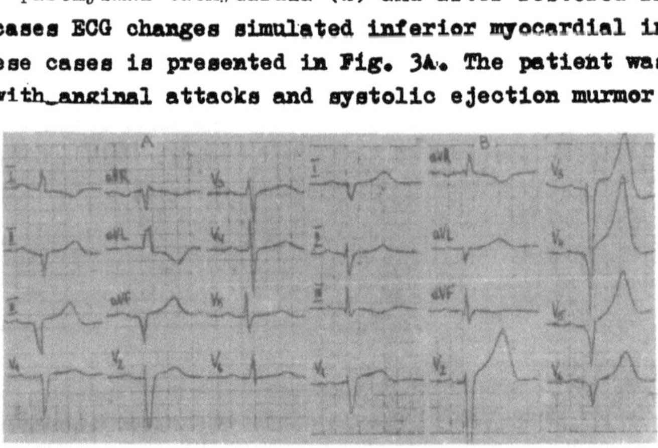

Fig. 3. ECG of two patients showing pseudoinfarctional patterns: A- inferior wall, B- anterolateral wall.

In this case diagnosis was made by echocardiography and verified after coronaroangiographic examjnation. In Fig. 3B another type of ECG changes of patient with hypertrophy of IVS simulating anterolateral MI is shown. This pattern of ECG changes was observed in 2 patients. Examination after I-5 year period showed no changes of Q waves. In 3 cases ECG showed right bundle brunch block pattern. In all these cases on echocardiography was hypertrophy of middle and apical third of IVS with involvement of right ventricular apex in one. In one case after a 5 years period right bundle brunch block disappeared and ECG showed typical LVH pattern. This case is illustrated by Fig. 4. On echocardiography no changes in degree and localisation of IVS hypertrophy were noticed.

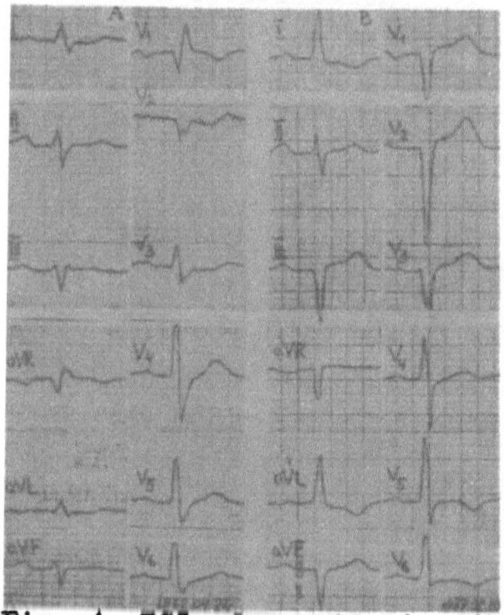

Fig. 4. ECG of a patient with IVS hypertrophy. A- the right bundle brunch block is present, no signs of LVH, B- 5 years later RBBB disappeared and prominent signs of LVH are present.

We did not notice any relation between thickness of IVS and ECG changes. In some cases with minor ECG changes echocardiography revealed markable IVS hypertrophy and vice versa. Such a case is shown in Fig. 5 - minor T wave changes in I9 years old male and IVS thickness about 3 cm.

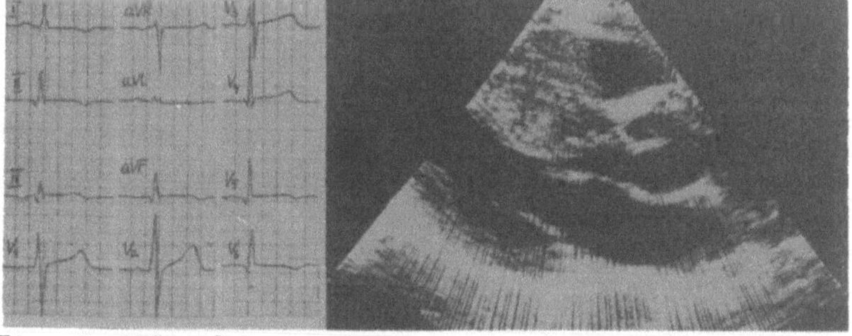

Fig. 5. ECG and long axis parasternal echocardiographic view of a I9 years old male.

Discussion

ECG changes in hypertrophic cardiomyopathy are discussed by many authers (I). Some of investigators found rather high percent of patients with hypertrophic cardiomyopathy without ECG abnormalities(2) . Giant negative T waves are thought to represent apical hypertrophy (3,4). Previously used criteria for the diagnosis of hypertrophic cardiomyopathy are not so reliable now (5). In our group of patients we found no one case without ECG abnormalities. The patients with symmetrical LVH had poor prognosis. No relation was established between localisation of LVH and ECG changes. The same degree of LVH may produce very impressive ECG changes and only minor ECG abnormalities. Dinamicaly observed T wave changes in a 5 years period had no relation to clinical status of patients. Deep negative T waves in precordial leads were noticed more often in IVS hypertrophy than in apical hypertrophy.

References

(I) Goldberger,A.L.: Myocardial infarction. Mosby Comp. (I979)
(2) Kolbel,F. and J.Hradec: Čes.Lek.čes. I24,I473-78 (I985)
(3) Morimoto,S.-I. et al.: J. Cardiography I5,35-5I (I985)
(4) Fujii,J. et al.: J. Cardiography I5,23-33 (I985)
(5) Maron,B.J.: Amer.J.Cardiol. 55,835-838 (I985)

ECG of Postnatally Growing Guinea Pigs with Carbon Monoxide Induced Cardiomegaly

SCHIRMER, E., SCHWARTZE, H.

Institute of Pathological Physiology, Karl Marx University Leipzig, GDR

Summary

Pre- and postnatal chronic exposure of guinea pigs to carbon monoxide (CO) will produce cardiomegaly the type of which should be different at birth or during the following postnatal development. The question was asked wheter ECG parameters are suited to reveal this difference. Daily ECG recordings with off-line computing were made in 9 guinea pigs aged 1-25 days (d) who were exposed pre- and postnatally to 22o ppm CO. The ECG findings consisted in differences between the magnitude curves of the experimental group and a control group showing the signs of a combined hypertrophy of an intergrade type of both the ventricles already at birth. The naturally occuring rightward shift of the early postnatal QRS vector loop is retarded and accentuated in the experimental group versus controls brought about by a retarded decrease of the high neonatal pulmonary vascular resistance. The later postnatal development is characterized by typical ECG signs of a pronounced left heart hypertrophy caused by hypotensive volume loading.

Introduction

Chronic inhalation of carbon monoxide of a sublethal concentration leads to hemodynamic changes described in adult rats (1). Arterial oxygen (O_2) saturation falls by occupying hemoglobin with CO. This produces arteriolar vasodilation which, in turn, causes hypotension in the postnatal circulation. The falling arterial blood pressure provides lower afterload which permits elevated stroke volume and cardiac output. Consequently, an approximate doubling of myocyte numbers in the hyperplastic left ventricle has been found, the greatest increase occuring in newborn rats between birth and 4 d of age.

In contrast, fetal response to CO exposure produces very different hemodynamic mechanisms, responsible for the development of cardiomegaly. Increase of heart mass comes about as fetal pulmonary vascular resistance (PVR) increases strongly following hypoxia and, in turn, partially right ventricular afterload increases. Additionally, even mild tissue hypoxia of the fetus is followed by an increase of the total peripheral resistance (2, 3) so that pressure load affects the whole heart, since both the fetal ventricles eject into the aorta. Accordingly, fresh and dry weights of both the ventricles of rat fetuses exposed to CO in utero were found to be higher than in controls (4). Hence, chronic CO exposure of fetuses which is retained in the born infants will produce cardiomegaly the type of which should be different at birth and during the later postnatal development. The question arose whether electrocardiological parameters are suited to reveal these developmental differences.

Material and methods

Congenital hemodynamic load was induced by chronic exposure of timed pregnant guinea pigs to CO from their midgestation on. Each time 2 female guinea pigs were bred in an exposure box until parturition and subsequantly together with their infants for 25 d. These animals inhaled constantly 2oo ppm CO in room air.
ECG recordings and off-line computing have been made in a longitudinal study technically successful in 9 guinea pigs aged 1-25 d. A modification of the NELSON lead system has been applied (5). For chronic usage, 2o subcutaneously implanted electrodes of steel wire served for daily recordings.The advantage of this particular electrically corrected NELSON system consists in taking care of body dimensions which is essential in growth studies. The respective parameters of body dimensions, such as length as well as diameters and cross sectional area of the thorax influence the calculations of the components of the dipole moment. A total of 144 ECGs has been evaluated.

Results

Our results shall be demonstrated in two parts. Firstly, the beginning and the end of the studied growth period is regarded.

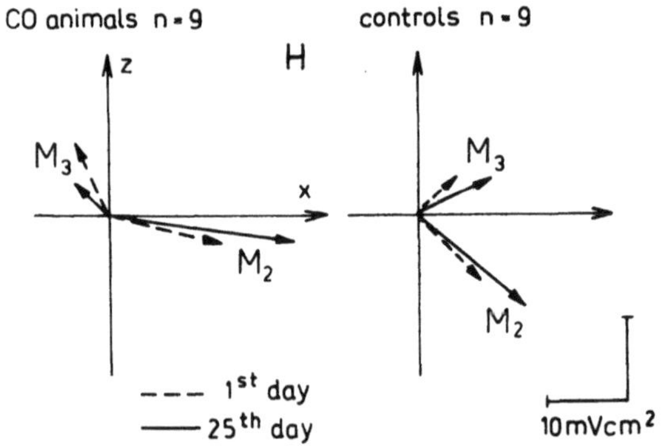

Fig. 1 Horizontal projection of the mean vectors of the peaks M2 and M3, respectively, of the magnitude curves.

Principally, QRS vector loops may have 3 archs corresponding to the 3 waves Q, R, S of the ECG curve and simultaneously to the 3 peak values M1,M2,M3 of the magnitude curve. A magnitude curve is the representation of the amplitudes of all instantaneous vectors over the QRS time.
Figure 1 shows two diagrams of mean vector constructions in the horizontal plane, each of which demonstrates the mean magnitudes M2 and M3, respectively. These two vectors are the diagnostically most relevant ones (6). There is a clear difference between the two groups: while M2 increased in both the differently treated animal groups between d 1 and d 25, the mean magnitudes of the CO group are greater - already at the 1st d - and the vectors are more pronounced directed leftward than in controls. The vectors of M3 are of total different orientations between experimental animals and controls from the very beginning of the postnatal

development on: the early longer M3 and the late short M3 of CO animals, directed to the right, are sharply contrasted to the control groups' results which consist of a short early M3 and a longer late M3, both the vectors being directed to the left.
The 2nd striking finding is the difference between the CO group and the controls during the course of the early postnatal development.

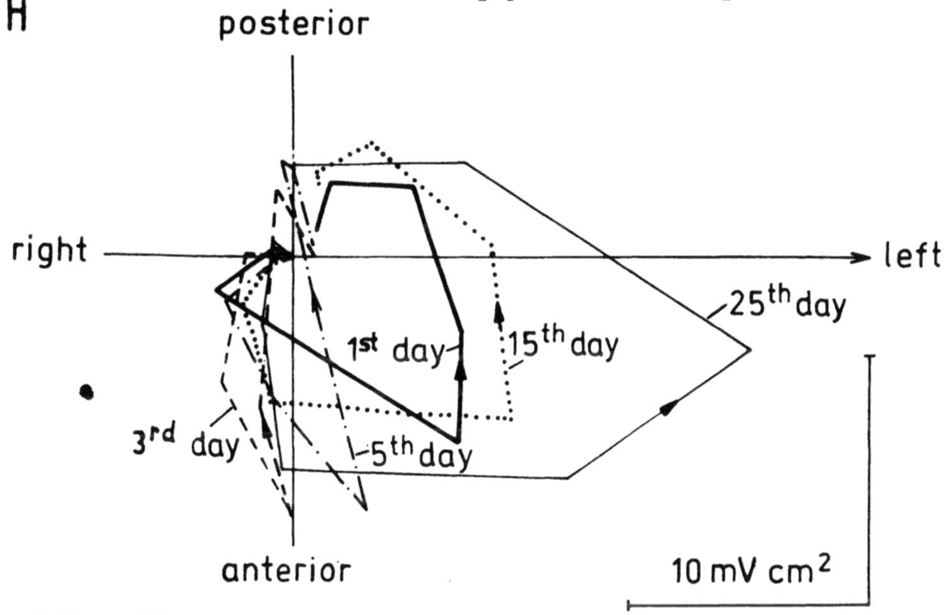

Fig. 2 Mean QRS vector loops of CO animals at several days of the postnatal development.

Figure 2 demonstrates the horizontal projections of time normalised mean QRS vector loops of the experimental CO group at several days of life. Besides the expected increasing enlargement of the leftward directed main parts of the loops with growing age (note the loops of the 1st, 15th, and 25th d), the attention should be focused on the remarkable shift of the loops to the right at d 3 and d 5. At the 3rd postnatal day nearly the complete QRS loop is situated within the right quadrants, but also the loop of d 5 is by far more rightward directed than that of d 1. Also the 2nd days'loop shows yet a very large left part. Whereas the normal neonatal ECG of guinea pigs is rightward accentuated already at the 2nd d of life and reversed up to the 4th d, the more pronounced right type of the ECG of the CO exposed animals developed later during the neonatal period, being residual only until the end of the first week.

<u>Discussion</u>

Although morphological control data are not yet available because of the longitudinal kind of our study we should like to discuss the following interpretation: The ECG type of the newly born CO animals shows characters of a combined hypertrophy of both the ventricles, predominantly of a concentric type. As we may conclude from investigations in spontaneously hypertensive rats with concentric hypertrophied hearts of other authors (6) as well as from results of dynamicly trained infant rats acquiring an eccentric hypertrophy (7), the cardiomegaly of our newborns may not be of a pure type. Instead, some intergrade between these extremes is considered, brought about by hyperplasia following the initially described pressure load of both the ventricles in the fetus, and in part produced by volume loading. This volume load might have two sources: increased stroke volume on the one hand and increased blood volume on the other hand as consequences of the O_2 saturation deficite in the fetus.

The observed accentuation and retardation of the naturally occuring rightward shift of the postnatal QRS loop the normal development of which has been interpreted as an effect of left ventricular enddiastolic volume loading following postnatal decrease of PVR (9) can be discussed briefly: the physiological neonatal ventricular enddiastolic overload could be exaggerated in an abnormally accelerated growing hyperplastic left chamber with reduced compliance. The physiological decrease of pulmonary blood pressure might be retarded by the lesser degree of O_2 saturation in pulmonary blood which would impede a prompt decrease of PVR.

The QRS loops and the magnitude curves of our 25 d old CO animals show the signs of a left heart hypertrophy of an intermediary type originated by physiological left heart growth with lasting hyperplasia (1) in combination with the special situation of hypotensive volume loading.

References

1. Penney, D.G.: Growth of the Heart in Health and Disease, New York, 337-361 (1984)
2. Dawes, G.S.: Foetal and Neonatal Physiology.A Comparative Study of the Changes at Birth, Chicago, 79-100 (1968)
3. Friedman, W.F., S.E.Kirkpatrick: Intrauterine Asphyxia and the Developing Fetal Brain, Chicago, London, 149-165 (1977)
4. Clubb, F.J., D.G.Penney, and M.S.Baylerian: J.Moll.Cell.Cardiol.18, 477-486 (1986)
5. Eifrig, Th., A.Joel, and H.Schwartze: Ergebn.exp.Med. 46, 274-284 (1985)
6. Hodgkin, B.C., C.V.Nelson, and E.T.Angelakos: Am.J.Physiol. 241, H541-H546 (1981)
7. Schwartze, U. and H.Schwartze: this issue
8. Penney, D.G., M.S.Baylerian, and J.E.Thill: Am.J.Physiol. 244, H289-H297 (1983)
9. Dellas, S., Th.Eifrig, A.Joel, and H.Schwartze: Biol.Neonate (1987) in press.

Some quantitative parameters of the QRS complex
obtained from body surface potential maps of normal children

KOZLÍKOVÁ, K., HULÍN, I., [a]SCHUBERT, E., [b]TURZOVÁ, M.

School of Medicine, Comenius University, Bratislava, Czechoslovakia
a/ Institute of Physiology, Humboldt University, Berlin, GDR
b/ Institute of Measurement and Measuring Technique, Slovak Academy of Sciences, Bratislava, Czechoslovakia

SUMMARY

During the puberty there are many physiological changes in the heart concerning both its growth and its electric activity. To obtain more information about these changes the electric heart field in normal children, boys and girls, 9-10 years and 13-14 years old was observed. The potentials were recorded from the whole chest. The body surface isopotential maps of the QRS complex were constructed. Maps of the ventricular breakthrough and the peak maps were chosen for further analysis. The mean values and the areas of the positive and negative potentials were calculated for the whole, and for the anterior and posterior chest parts. The obtained variables were compared for age and sex differences. Also a linear relation between maxima and minima on the maps have been observed.

INTRODUCTION

The activation of the heart ventricles as it can be observed by body surface isopotential mapping was described in many papers. Almost all of them dealt with adults either healthy or with variety of heart diseases. A few of the papers studied the isopotential mapping in children, but almost always from the qualitative point of view (Spach et al., 1966; Flaherty et al., 1967; Spach et al., 1968) or with some quantitative parameters (Liebman et al., 1981; Liebman et al., 1984).

We have studied the electric heart activity in normal children just before the puberty and at its top. The purpose of our study was to find out whether the physiological changes of the heart are manifested in the body surface isopotential maps using chosen quantitative parameters.

METHODS

Eleven children aged 9-10 years (4 boys and 7 girls), and 11 children aged 13-14 years (7 boys and 4 girls) were studied by isopotential body surface mapping. They all were regarded to be healthy and normotensive with normal or slender body habitus.

The electric heart field was investigated using a special measuring and computing system EKKG-80 (Tyšler et al., 1984). The unipolar ECG signals were recorded in

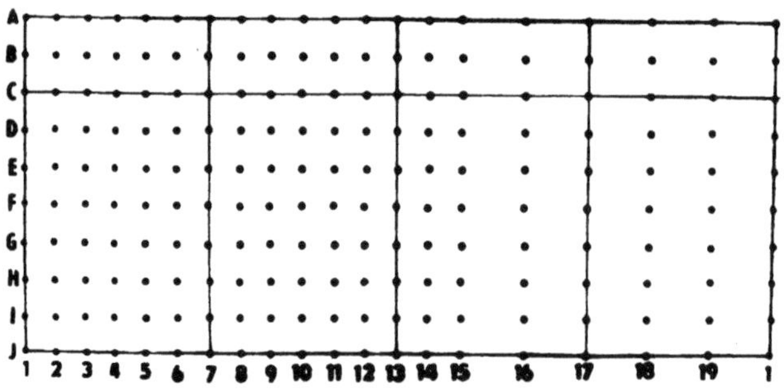

Fig.1 : Points on the chest, from which the unipolar ECGs were recorded. The C row corresponds to the 4-th intercostal space. The columns 1,7,13 and 17 correspond to the right midaxillary and midsternal, left midaxillary and paravertebral lines, resp.

sitting position from the whole thorax in 8 to 10 equidistal planes as it is illustrated in fig. 1. The standard lead II was taken as the reference lead for the time synchronization of the data. The sampling interval was 4 ms for each electrode. The waveforms were filtered and visually checked to eliminate nonlinear baseline drift or other artefacts. Body surface isopotential maps (IPMs) were calculated in every measured time instant during the whole QRS complex and then plotted in form of contour maps using linear interpolation and printed in tabular form. The root mean square (RMS) of the measured potential was calculated in every IPM to represent the magnitude of the obtained potential, which allowed to establish the onset and the offset of the QRS complex. The doubled distance of the electrode columns 15-19 against the columns 1-14 was taken into consideration as well as in all next calculations (fig. 1).

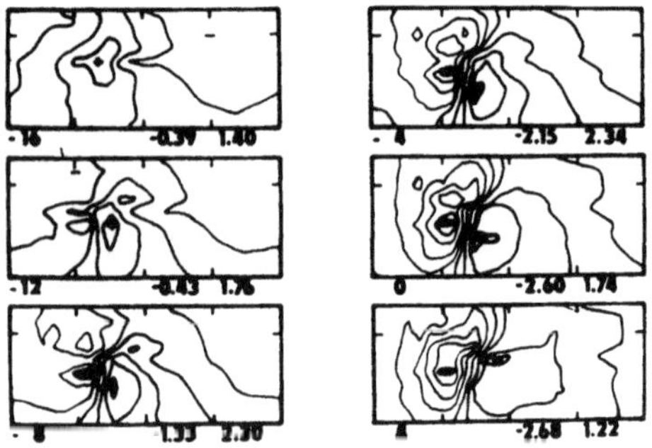

Fig. 2 : A sequence of IPMs of the QRS complex of a 14 years old boy. The numbers under each map mean the time instant, the minimal and the maximal value. The BTM is on the 2-nd, the PM on the 5th place in this sequence. Isopotential lines are drawn with 0.5 mV step.

For further analysis the ventricular breakthrough map (BTM - established as the first appearence of the minumum on the anterior chest - fig. 2) and the peak map (PM - chosen as the map with the maximal RMS value - fig. 2) were taken. In every map the mean positive and the mean negative potential and their corresponding areas as percents of the whole region under investigation were calculated for the anterior chest, for the back and for the whole map.

Each variable in each group was tested for normal distribution and its average value was established. These values were then mutually compared for age and sex differences using Fisher´s distribution for their dispersions and the t-test.

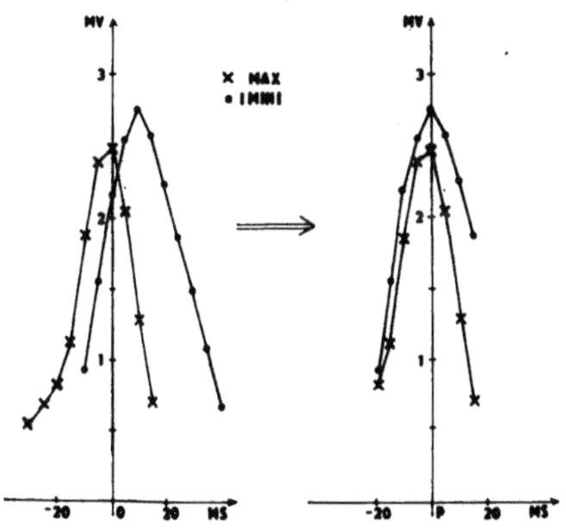

Fig. 3 : The time courses of minima and maxima on the IPM QRS of a 13 years old boy as they were really measured (and smoothed) and after the removal of the delay

In the IPMs QRS we have analyzed the relation between magnitudes of absolute maxima and absolute minima regardless of their position. To eliminate random fluctuations, the time sequences of the extrema were quadratical smoothed always through 5 points. In the measured time course, the minima were delayed after the maxima for 0-20 ms. Therefore, the highest maximum was coordinated to the lowest minimum as it can be seen in fig.3. For the linear relation only those maxima and minima were taken, whose both absolute values were greater than 0.5 mV.

The linear relations were searched in both forms

$$MAX = A_1 \cdot MIN + A_0 \quad \text{and} \quad MIN = B_1 \cdot MAX + B_0$$

using the least squares method separately for the ascending and for the descending branch. The correlation coefficients were computed. The regression coefficients A_1 and B_1 were tested for their difference from zero using t- test and F-test.

RESULTS

From the 12 average values in each of the 4 groups there was no normal distribution in 9 cases. These values were excluded from further statistical tests.

The comparison of the peak maps gave no statistically significant differences. On the breakthrough maps there were significant differences ($p < 0.05$) only between the groups of the younger boys and younger girls. On the anterior chest the boys have higher positive potentials and on a larger area. On the back the boys have lower positive and lower negative potentials. On the whole map the positive area was larger by boys.

The bilateral linear correlation between the maxima and the minima was strong. From 11 boys 5 had better correlation than 99 %, 4 better than 95 % and 2 better than 90% in the ascending branch. In the descending branch the correlation was better than 99 % for all boys.

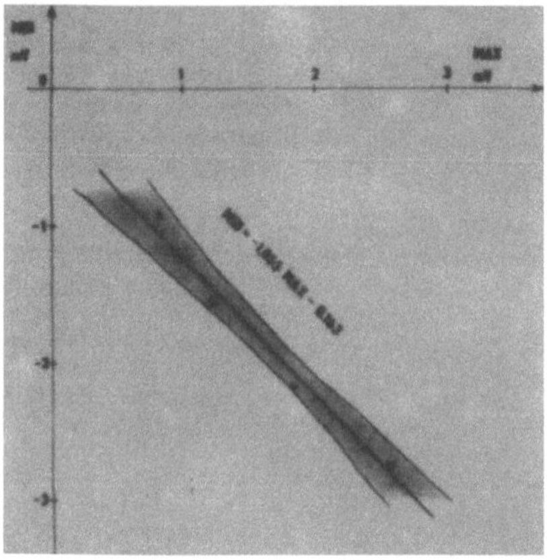

Fig. 4 : The linear correlation between the minima and maxima of the ascending branch depicted in fig.3.

From the 11 girls in the ascending branch the correlation was better than 99 % in 5 cases, and better than 95 % in 4 cases. One case was better than 90 % and 1 better than 80 %. In the descending branch there were 8 cases with correlation better than 99 %, 2 cases better than 95 % and 1 case better than 90 %. The results of the t-test and the F-test were in very good agreement with the correlation coeficients. One linear correlation with the 95 % confidence interval is depicted in fig.4.

DISCUSION AND CONCLUSIONS

In spite of increasing mass and size of the heart we couldn´t find any significant differences on the IPMs of the QRS complex as the dependence of childrens´ age. The study showed that rebuilding procedures concerning anatomical and topographical changes did not influence the way of the heart activation evaluated using described method.

REFERENCES

| 1 | Spach, M.S., Silberberg, W.P., Boineau, J.P., Barr, R.C., Long, E.C., Gallie, T.M., Gabor, J.B., Wallace A.G.: Am. Heart J. 72, 640-652 (1966)

| 2 | Flaherty, J.T., Blumenschein, S.D., Spock, A., Canent, R.V.Jr., Gallie,T.M., Boineau, J.P., Spach, M.S.: Am.J.Cardiol. 20, 29-38 (1967)

| 3 | Spach, M.S., Barr, R.C., Blumenschein, S.D., Boineau, J.P. : Ann.intern. Med. 69, 919-928 (1968)

| 4 | Liebman, J., Thomas, C.W., Rudy, Y., Plomsey, R.: J.Electrocardiol. 14, 249-260 (1981)

| 5 | Liebman, J., Rudy , Y., Diaz, P., Thomas, C.W., Plonsey, R.: J.Electrocardiol. 17, 329-364 (1984)

| 6 | Tyšler, M., Kužmová, J., Kneppo, P., Rosík, V., Kričfaluši, M. : In: Electrocardiology ´83, 160-163 (1984)

Swimming Exercise in Postnatally Growing Rats: Influence on Various ECG Parameters

SCHWARTZE, U., SCHWARTZE, H.

Institute of Pathological Physiology, Karl Marx University, Leipzig, GDR

Summary

The question is open wether prepubescent children can develop an eccentric hypertrophy of the heart by physical training. ECGs were recorded repeatedly in infant rats aged 6-53 days (d), which must swim daily until exhaustion from d 6 to d 3o of life. Main results are: the time normalised mean QRS vector loops of the training group were directed to the left more pronounced and more anteriorly than the loops of a control group. The spatial maximal vector $\vec{R}$ as well as the peak M_2 of the spatial magnitude curve were greater, and the vector of M_2 was directed more leftward in trained animals. Body masses of the 2 groups didn't differ. By comparison of these findings with results in dynamicly trained adult sportsmen of other authors we concluded a symmetrical enlargement of the prepubescent heart by growth adaptation following swimming exercise.

Introduction

The aim of the study consisted in learning means of effective influence on the infantile organism in order to better enable him to tolerate interference factors presumably becoming active on the adult circulatory system. Physical training during childhood might be useful for this purpose. However, mainly due to inadequate training programs (Rowland 1985) the question is open wether already prepubescent children can develop real functionally, morphologically, and biochemically adaptive processes of their hearts to dynamic training. In order to reveal possible enlargement of the heart, electrocardiography as a noninvasive method was used in an exhausting swim training program with infant rats.

Material and methods

The experimental group consisted of 18 rats forced to swim daily until exhaustion at the ages of 6 to 3o d. Each animal swam seperately, the water temperature being gradually lowered from 27 to 2o and finally 15°C because of the improvement of body temperature regulation with growing age. The control group consisted of 1o infant rats growing up uninjured. Electrically corrected ECGs (FRANK lead system) were recorded in trained rats and untrained ones narcotised by ether at 6 different ages: 6, 14, 21, 3o d as well as after the end of the training period at 38 and 53 d of life. Recording and data processing were carried out by subcutaneous needle electrodes and off-line computing of horizontal vector loops and magnitude curves of QRS as well as the spatial magnitudes of $\vec{R}$. Statistical comparison of longitudinal data was done by computation of time normalised mean vector loops; cross sectional data were treated by the U-test ($p \leq 0.05$).

Results

Fig. 1 shows the mean spatial maximal vector $\hat{R}$ of our trained rats and the untrained group in relation to age which is identical with the training period up to d 3o.

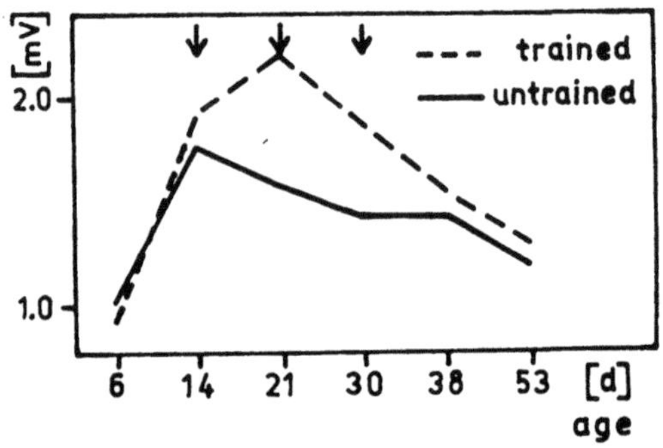

Fig. 1. Arrows indicate significant differences between the magnitudes of $\hat{R}$ in trained rats versus the control group.

The next diagram gives time normalised horizontal mean QRS loops of 7 trained infant rats and 8 control animals. Only in these reduced groups the complete longitudinal data acquisition had been technically successful.

The evaluation of the QRS vector loops included the calculation of those instantaneous vectors which belong to the peaks M_2 and M_3, respectively of the magnitude curves. These vectors are suited as indicators of hypertrophy in spontaneous hypertensive rats (Hodgkin et al. 1981).

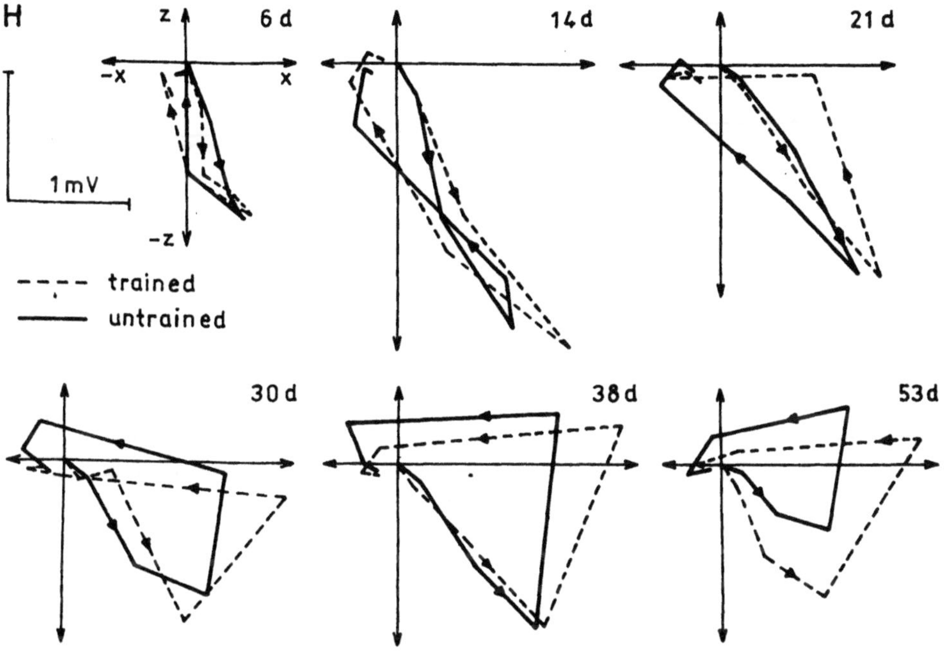

Fig. 2. d 6-14: no remarkable difference between the 2 groups; d 21-53: the QRS loops of trained animals show a clear shift to the left and by 3o d additionally to the front relatively to the controls.

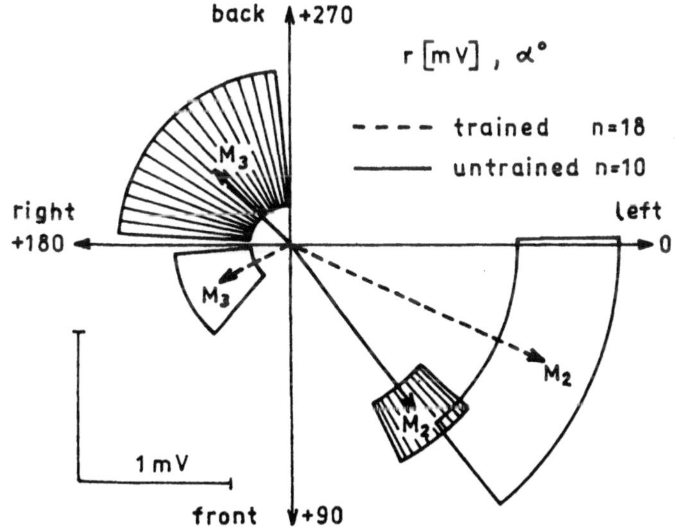

Fig. 3. Length of arrows corresponds to the mean magnitude of $\bar{M}_2$ and $\bar{M}_3$, respectively; arcshaped areas show the standard deviations for projected magnitudes and angles (open areas = 18 trained animals; striped areas = 1o controls).

Fig. 3 shows the horizontal projection of the mean vectors belonging to the peaks M_2 and M_3 of the magnitude curves at d 3o. The mean vectors of M_2 and M_3, respectively show a shift to the left and the mean magnitude of M_2 is significantly increased in training rats versus controls.

Discussion and conclusion

In accordance with different ECG findings in adult sportsmen exercised either by static or by dynamic training - like swimming - (Chignon 198o) we concluded from our results an eccentric hypertrophy of the infant rat heart produced by symmetrical growth processes following the exhausting dynamic training. The respective ECG parameters are: increase of spatial $\vec{R}$, leftward and anterior shift of the QRS loop, and increase of the peak M_2 of the QRS magnitude curve. Since body mass gain has been found to be identical in both, the experimental group and the controls (Schwartze 1987), the ECG alterations must have been evoked by circulatory functional adaptation with following structural enlargement of the prepubescent heart. It is remarkable that the outlined ECG changes produced by the physical strain didn't disappear completely untill 3 weeks after the end of the training period when our animals reached puberty.

References

(1) Rowland, T.W.: Med. Sci. Sports Exerc. 17, 493-497 (1985)

(2) Hodgkin, B.C., C.V. Nelson, and E.T. Angelakos: Am. J. Physiol. 241, H541-H546 (1981)

(3) Chignon, J.C.: in Sportkardiologie; Hrsg.: J.P.Broustet, Stuttgart 198o, pp 24-36

(4) Schwartze, U.: Diss. A, Med. Fak. Karl Marx University 1987

Experimental body surface isopotential mapping in healthy, swimming and sympathectomized young rats

LADISLAV ZLATOŠ, MARIÁN BERNADIČ, ŠTEFAN KARPIŠ

Department of Pathophysiology, Faculty of Medicine, Comenius University, Sasinkova 4, 811 08 Bratislava, Czechoslovakia

Summary

The examinations were carried out on 24 young rats devided in the groups: 1. Controls /C/; 2. Swimming rats /SW/; 3. Sympathectomized rats /G/; 4. Sympathectomized swimming rats /G+SW/. Body surface isopotential maps were recorded on the 42nd day of their life. In groups SW, G and G+SW the voltage of R wave significantly increased. The heart axis was orientated more downward and backwards in groups G and G+SW. The propagation of the ventricles activation was nearly the same in all investigated groups. The potential maximum values in groups G+SW /1.76 mV/ and SW /1.54 mV/ are significantly higher than in the group C /1.10 mV/. We assume that the observed changes of cardioelectric field in experimental groups probably reflect an increase of the number of cardiomyocytes /G+SW/, respectively enlargement of their volume /SW/ and thus the different enlarged area of action membranes in the myocardium.

Introduction

The results of our previous studies showed that increased working load of the heart in the early postnatal period causes more intensive stimulation of the mitotic activity of cardiomyocytes in the newborn animals with sympathectomy in comparison to the nonsympathectomized younglings /Zlatoš et al., 1984, 1985; Slezák and Zlatoš, 1986/. When studying the properties of the cardioelectric field of puppies with experimental cardiomegaly we found the amplitude of the instantaneous vectors of the QRS loop significantly higher in sympathectomized puppies than in puppies without sympathectomy /Bernadič et al., 1986/. These increased amplitude of the QRS vectors we have attributed to the increased number of muscle cells and thus to the enlarged area of activating membranes in the myocardium of the sympathectomized young animals.

The aim of the present work was to verify the assumption we have already introduced, on the model of physiologicaly increased working load of the heart in the early postnatal period. The properties of the cardioelectric field in sympathectomized swimming young rats we investigated by the method of the precordial isopotential mapping.

Material and methods

We investigated 24 young rats devided in these four groups: 1st group - control healthy rats /C/; 2nd group - swimming rats, pups swam from the 15th day of age /SW/; 3rd group - sympathectomized rats, received guanethidine /20 mg.kg^{-1} s.c./ injected daily during the first 21 days of life /G/; 4th group - sympathectomized swimming rats, received guanethidine as pups of the 3rd group and swam from the 15th day of age /G+SW/. The body surface isopotential maps were recorded on the 42nd day of their life in pentobarbital anesthesy. We used 23-leads system which covers the whole precordium and upper portion of the abdomen /Bernadič et al., 1984/. The ECG signals were at first elaborated by an analog-to-digital transfer Codimat /fy Contraves/ and then printed out in form of instantaneous isopotential maps of the chosen sections of the heart depolarization and repolarization. The minimal time interval for construction of the maps was 5 msec.

Results

The average body weight of groups C, SW, G and G+SW was 212.4 g, 182.3 g, 183.7 g, respectively 200.1 g. The average heart weight was 685.4 mg, 761.1 mg, 669.7 mg, respectively 783.8 mg. Heart rate in the groups SW /423.min^{-1}/, G /387.min^{-1}/, and G+SW /429.min^{-1}/, in comparison with the controls /473.min^{-1}/ significantly decreased /p 0.05/. In the groups SW, G and G+SW the voltage of R_{II} wave significantly increased /0.823 mV, 0.930 mV, respectively 0.756 mV/ and the amplitude of S_{III} wave decreased /0.178 mV, 0.025 mV, respectively 0.120 mV/ compared to the controls /R_{II}: 0.654 mV and S_{III}: -0.364 mV/. The duration of the QRS was not changed.

The heart electric axis was orientated more downward and backward in animals of the groups G and G+SW. In all four groups the activation of ventricles starts from the upper left precordium and propagates in a circle downward to the right, continuing upwardly to the left so as to cover the whole precordium /Fig. 1A/. During the repolarization the whole area of precordium is positive. In the group SW inhomogeneity of cardioelectric field with islands of negativity appears and repolarization sequence is late /Fig. 1B/. In the groups G and G+SW is similar course of myocardial activation but without expresive inhomogeneities /Fig. 1C,D/. The vector connecting potential maximum and minimum is orientated downward in the controls but in the groups SW, G and G+SW is orientated upwardly and to the right. The potential maximum values in the groups G+SW /1.76 mV/ and SW /1.54 mV/ are significantly higher /p 0.05/ than in the controls /1.100 mV/.

Discussion and conclusions

Claycomb /1976, 1977/ created the hypothesis about the participation of the maturation of adrenergic innervation of the heart on the mechanism of the decrease and complete cessation of the mitotic activity of cardiomyocytes in the early postnatal period. The observation of Kugler et al. /1980/ supported this hypothesis. They found out that the cytoplasmic DNA polymerase activity was significantly increased in the sym-

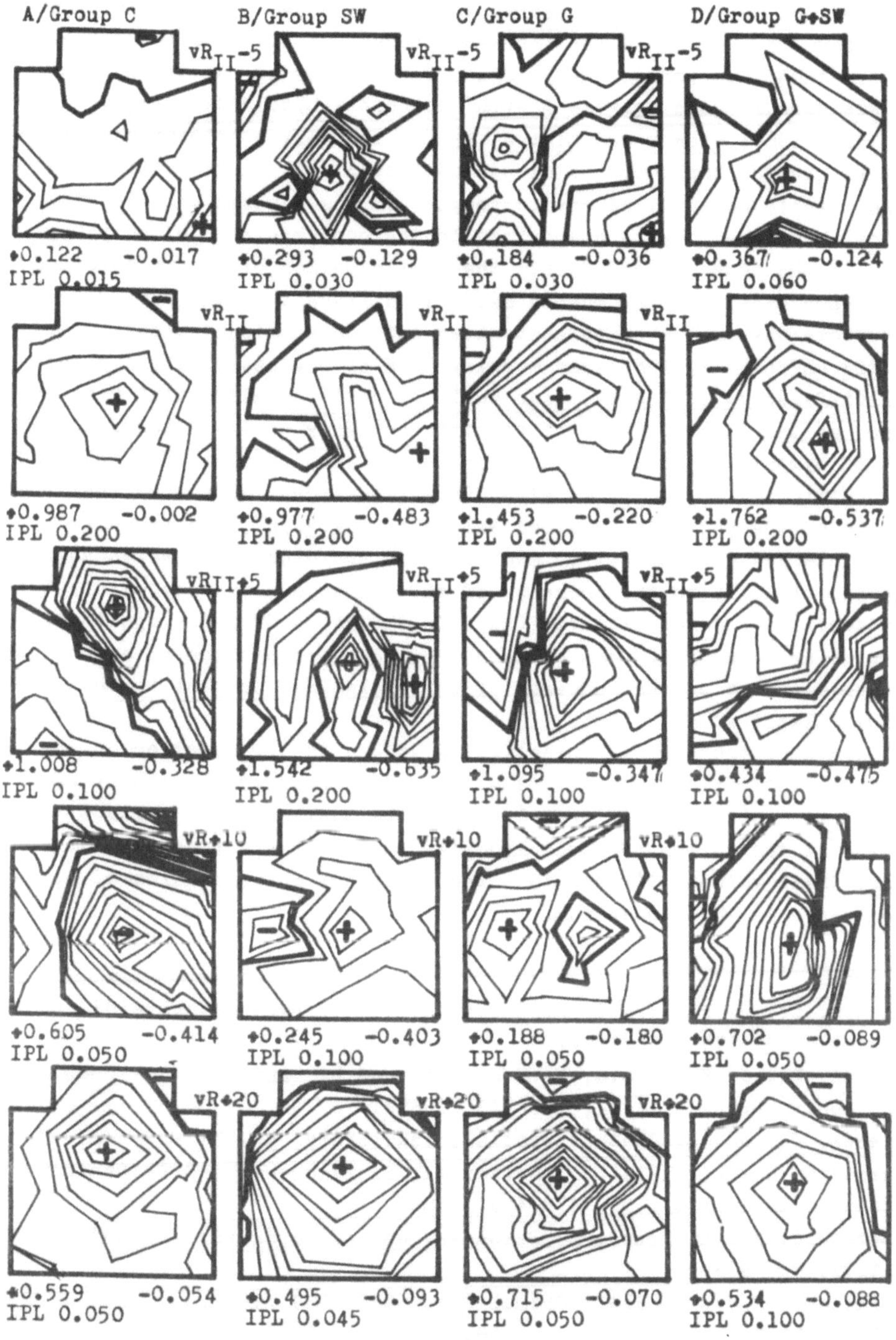

FIGURE 1.
Typical isopotential maps for normal /C/, swimming /SW/, sympathectomized /G/ and sympathectomized swimming young rats /G+SW/. Each map corresponds to a specific instant relativ to max amplitude of R wave of the 2nd standard lead. The zero-potential line is identified by a heavier trace and the plus and minus signs indicate the potentiel maximum and minimum. IPL - isopotential lines differende.

pathectomized newborn rats relative to the controls. The sympathectomized newborn rats also had the increased number of the labelled cardiomyocytes that incorporate ^{3}H-tymidine. The results of our previous studies are also in good agreement with Claycomb's hypothesis /Zlatoš et al., 1984, 1985; Slezák and Zlatoš, 1986/. The work overloading of the heart within the early postnatal period caused more marked stimulation of the mitotic activity of cardiomyocytes in the newborn animals with chemical sympathectomy in comparison to the nonsympathectomized younglings. In the consequence of this the participation of hyperplasia and hypertrophy of myocardial muscle cells is different in the development of cardiomegaly in the sympathectomized and nonsympathectomized pups with the chronically increased working load of the heart. These cytological differences in the cellular basis of cardiac enlargement were expressed at the investigation of electric activity of the hypertrophied heart of sympathectomized and nonsympathectomized puppies with the aortic constriction /Bernadič et al., 1986/. Therefore, we assume that the increase of the potential maximum values in the group G+SW is caused by the enlarged area of action membranes in the myocardium which enlarges proportionally to the increase of the number of cardiomyocytes. The inhomogeneity of cardioelectric field in the group SW /nonsympathectomized swimming young rats/ can be caused by the augmentation of adrenergic structures and so by the increase of catecholamines content in the myocardium /Zlatoš et al., 1986/.

We conclude that in all investigated groups the propagation of the ventricles activation is nearly the same. The observed changes of cardioelectric field in experimental groups the most probably reflect the increase of the number of cardiomyocytes /G+SW/, respectively enlargement of their volume /SW/ and thus the different enlarged area of action membranes in the myocardium.

References

1. Zlatoš, L., J. Holzerová, E. Kvaszová, and Ľ. Danihel: Physiol. bohemoslov., 33, 575-576 /1984/.
2. Zlatoš, L., J. Holzerová, E. Kvaszová, and Ľ. Danihel: Acta Facult. Med. Univ. Brunensis, 92, 137-143 /1985/.
3. Slezák, J., and L. Zlatoš: Bratisl. lek. Listy, 86, 577-592 /1986/.
4. Bernadič, M., L. Zlatoš, J. Holzerová, E. Kvaszová, and Ľ. Danihel: Bratisl. lek. Listy, 85, 478-495 /1986/.
5. Bernadič, M., A. Fízel, M. Bakošová, and E. Sapáková: Bratisl. lek. Listy, 82, 973-982 /1984/.
6. Claycomb, W.C.: J. Biol. Chem., 251, 6082-6089 /1976/.
7. Claycomb, W.C.: Biochem. J., 168, 599-601 /1977/.
8. Kugler, J.D., P.C. Gillette, S.P. Graham, et al: Pediat. Res., 14, 881-884 /1980/.
9. Zlatoš, L., J. Holzerová, E. Kvaszová, and Ľ. Danihel: Bratisl. lek. Listy, 85, 430-443 /1986/.

E X E R C I S E

E L E C T R O C A R D I O L O G Y

Prognostic value of different exercise-ECG-signs, ten years follow-up.
The Erfurt Intervention Study

HOLTZ, H., J. HEINRICH, D. TIETZE, J. KNAPPE, K.-D. DÜCK

Erfurt Medical School, Department of Cardiology,
5020 Erfurt, Gartenstraße 2, GDR

Summary: Out of 1158 middle aged men 687 were apparently healthy. After ten years 19.7 % of them had coronary artery disease (CAD). CAD-rate was lower in subjects with initially normal exercise ECG and higher in those with ECG abnormalities. Combination of exercise induced abnormalities improve the prognostic value which is not greater than that of the classic risk factors.

Introduction: One of the main concerns of preventive cardiology is to find out subjects at risk for coronary artery disease (CAD) to treat them before they are be taken ill. Exercise ECG is an excellent method for clinical use with high specificity (about 90 %) and sensitivity (about 50 %, 1). Because of the lower prevalence of CAD however it is of limited importance in screeening of whole populations (BAYES' Theorem, 2).

It is the aim of our study to find out of whether or not the valuation of exercise induced changes of R-wave and heart rate as well as premature termination of the test additional to the horizontal or downsloping ST-segment depression is able to improve the prognostic value of exercise ECG in middle aged, initially apparently healthy men.

Material and Methods: From 1155 middle aged men (mean age 47.2, range 39 - 59 y) 687 were found apparently healthy. They underwent an exercise test and were followed for on average of ten years. 455 of them accepted our invitation to the final examination , 195 did not, but were alive. Apparently healthy were subjects without angina pectoris, hypertension, heart failure, vitium cordis, infectious diseases, decompensated metabolic disorders, those not taking heart glycosides, antihypertensive drugs and betablockers and subjects without major ECG-findings (Minnesota-Codes 1.1, 1.2, 3.2, 4.1, 4.2, 6.1, 6.2, 6.4, 7.1, 7.2, 8.1, 8.3). Exercise testing was performed on bicycle ergometer in sitting position with 60 r.p.m. Loads were 130 watts for 39 - 49 years old and 140 watts for 50 - 59 years old. This is adequate about 75 % of maximal aerobic capacity (3). Definition of CAD: Fatal or nonfatal myocardial infarction (410, 411, 412, ICD 9th revision) and/or typical exercise induced angina.

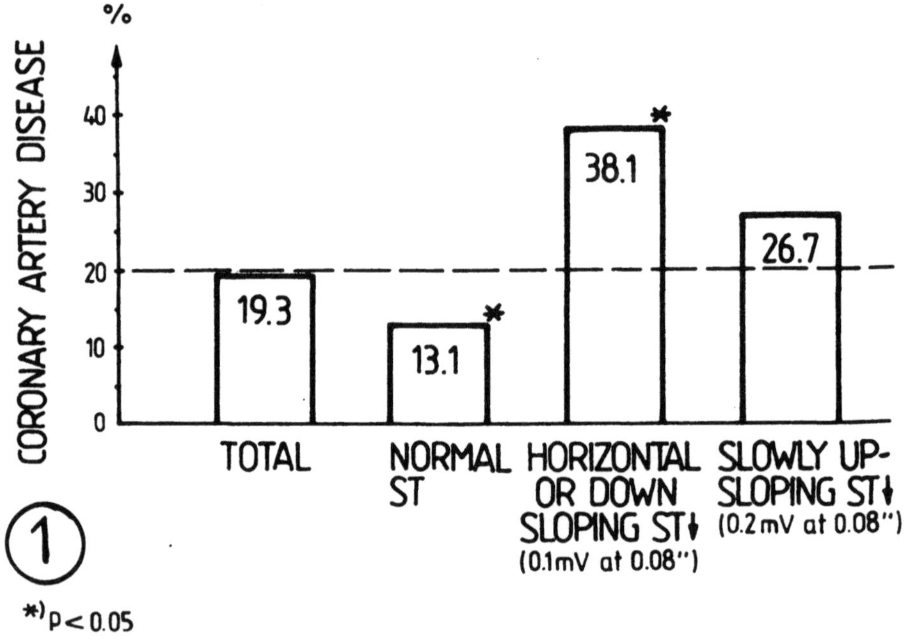

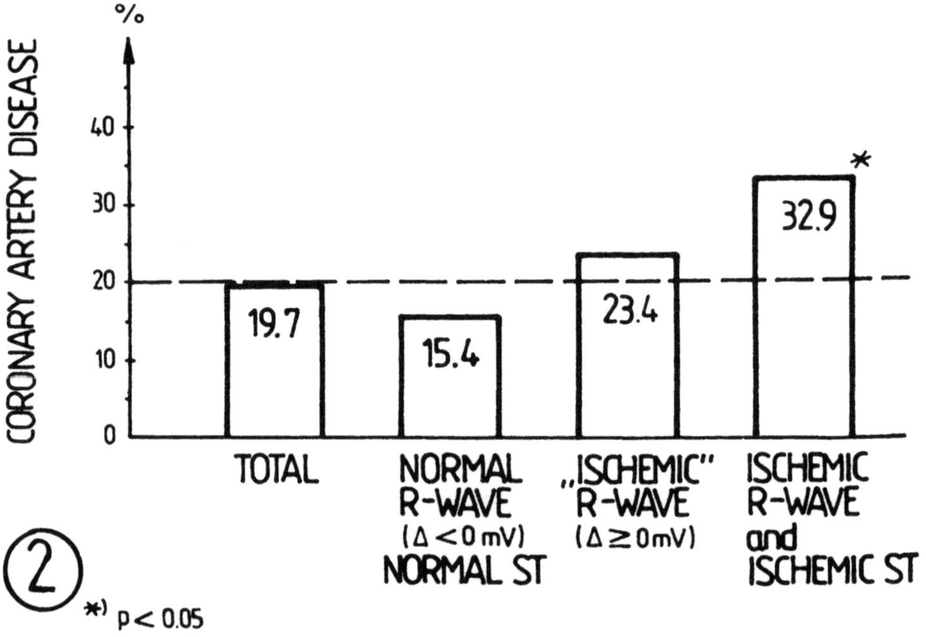

Figures 1 - 3

Frequency of coronary artery disease in subjects with different exercise abnormalities

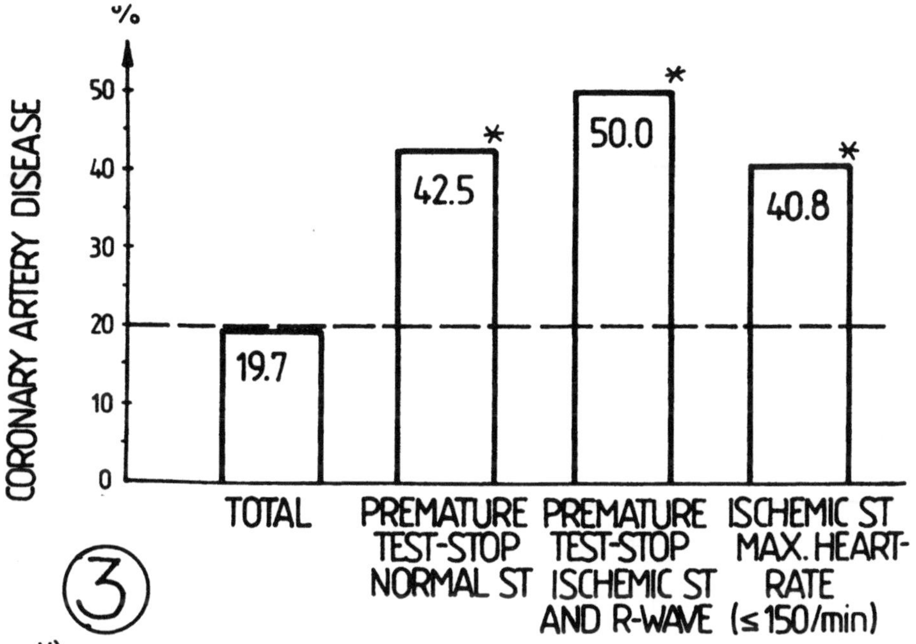

*) $p < 0.05$

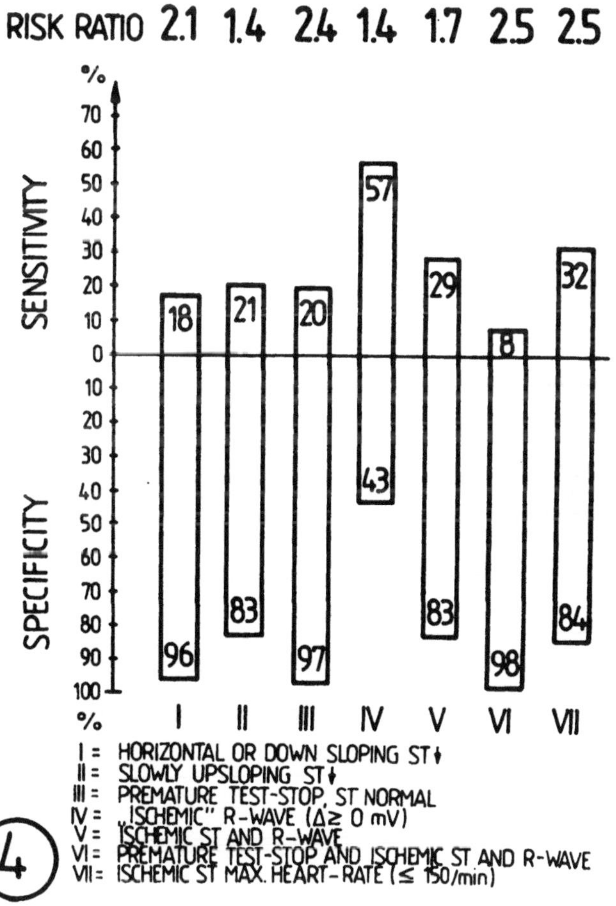

Figure 4

Specificity and sensitivity as well as risk ratios of various exercise incluced abnormalities

Results: Ten years later 19.7 % of initially healthy had suffered CAD. The incidences of CAD in subjects with different exercise abnormalities are presented in figures 1 - 3. Frequency of CAD was lower in subjects with normal ST-segment response and higher in those with exercise ECG abnormalities.

Premature termination of the test with and without additional ECG-signs and the impossibility to reach the predicted exercise heart rate of 150/min in combination with ischemic ST depression were of the greatest prognostic value for later CAD.

Value of horizontal and downsloping ST segment depression alone was smaller but significant whereas slowly upsloping ST segment depression alone was only in tendency but not significant related to later CAD.

Specificity and sensitivity as well as risk ratios of various exercise induced abnormalities are summarized in figure 4.

Risk ratio of hypertension (diastolic > 90 mm Hg), hypercholesterolemia (> 250 mg %) and smoking is about 1.9 to 3. Combination of these risk factors increases risk ratio to 4 - 6 (4).

Conclusions

(1) Combination of exercise induced abnormalities improve prognostic value of exercise-ECG.

(2) Combined exercise ECG abnormalities have low sensitivity, high specificity and moderate predictive value for later CAD in middle aged apparently healthy men.

(3) The prognostic importance is not greater than that of the classic risk factors.

References

(1) Uhl, G.S. and V. Froehlicher. J. Am coll. cardiol. 1 (3), 946-55
(2) Rifkin, B. and W. B. Hood: New Engl. J. Med. 297, 681-7 (1977)
(3) Holtz, H., J. Exner et al.: Dt. Gesundh. Wesen 29, 246-50 (1974)
(4) Commission for Heart Disease Resources: Circulation 42, A-55 (1970)

Improved Diagnosis of Cardiac Dysrhythmias During Stress-Tests Using Bipolar Oesophageal ECG [x]

SCHWELA H., OLTMANNS G., KNORRE M., REISSMANN H.C., BISCHOFF K.H., FRANKE T.

Medical Academy, Erfurt, 5010, GDR

Summary: An improved diagnosis of heart rhythm in stress-testing can be obtained from filtered bipolar oesophageal ECG in addition to the conventional surface ECG. A clear statement on the P wave incidence, determination of irregular P waves, and improved tracing of the atrio-ventricular sequence facilitate differentiation between the supraventricular and ventricular origin of cardiac excitation, especially in the event of stress-induced aberrancies or bundle-branch blocks. The method recommended may be used in routine in stress-tests. Further improvements can be achieved by the method as a basis of an automatic real-time heart rhythm analysis system.

Introduction: The detection of dysrhythmias and their exact classification from the ECG will be impaired in particular when applying physical stress by factors that have an impact on P wave evaluation: reduced signal-to-noise ratio, interference of peripheral muscle potentials, artifacts, base line drift. Aiming at an improvement of the cardiac rhythm analysis, tracing of oesophageal ECG-leads in addition to the conventional surface ECG, was tested in cardial stress tests.

Method: For recording the oesophageal ECG, bipolar 3-5 F pacemaker electrode catheters have proved to be the adequate means. 5 F catheters are appropriate to be safely inserted. For catheters of a smaller diameter it is suggested to use a guiding tube. The catheter may be inserted through the nose and may stay without discomforting the patient. Under monitoring control, the electrode cable must be positioned near the left atrium, from where characteristic P wave patterns can be recorded, the P wave amplitude exceeding that of the ventricular complexes, when using the intraoesophageal bipolar lead. The base line drift and other low frequency interferences may be suppressed by filters of 10 Hz (alternatively also 40 Hz) for the low frequency cut-off. The determination of the P wave incidence and the distinction between different P wave patterns will not be adversely influenced by this. In the examples for demonstration the oesophageal ECG at an amplification of up to 50mm/mV together with a bipolar and three unipolar chest leads is recorded on a Mingograph M81.

Results: The method used permits clearly discernible demonstration of the left-atrial excitation, even under inconvenient conditions induced by stress. Considering that ventricular depolarization is evaluated from the simultaneously recorded surface leads, the activation frequency as well as the activation sequence for the atrium and ventricle can be determined separately and also in their relationship to each other. Even atypical excitation patterns can be identified and evaluated. This becomes clear by ECG recordings which have been made in stress tests.

During tachycardia and in auriculoventricular block very often a fusion of T(U) waves with P waves (Fig.1) can be observed. The clear determination of P incidence permits differentiation between sinus tachycardia (Fig.1 a) and auriculoventricular tachycardia, or in the event of a simultaneous bundle-branch block (Fig.2 b) from ventricular rhythm.

Fig.1a ˣ

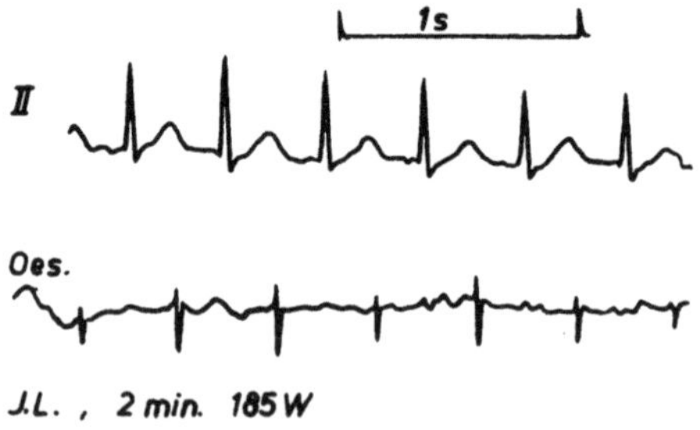

Fig.1b ˣ

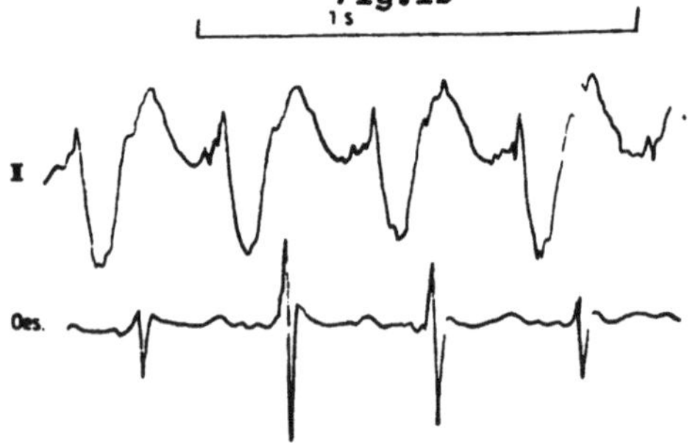

In most cases of coincidence of the atrial and ventricular excitation (Fig.2), the P wave can also be clearly detected both in non-deformed (Fig.2a) and in deformed (Fig.2b) ventricular complexes.

Fig.2aˣ

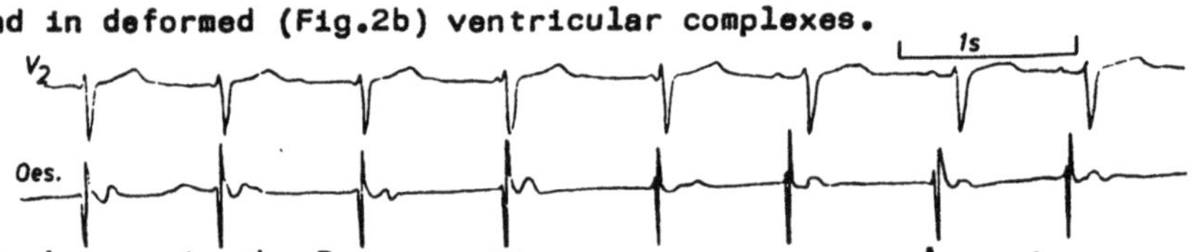

Significant changes in the P wave pattern (Fig.3) are frequently occurring as mirror-image activation patterns. They point to an inversion of the impulse propagation, and mustbe interpreted as supraventricular beats (Fig.3a) or as auricular echoes (Fig.3b). Atrial ectopic excitation may show strongly deformed wave patterns at low amplitudes (Fig.3c), tendencies to repetition and disturbed atrioventricular conduction being often observed.

Fig. 2bˣ

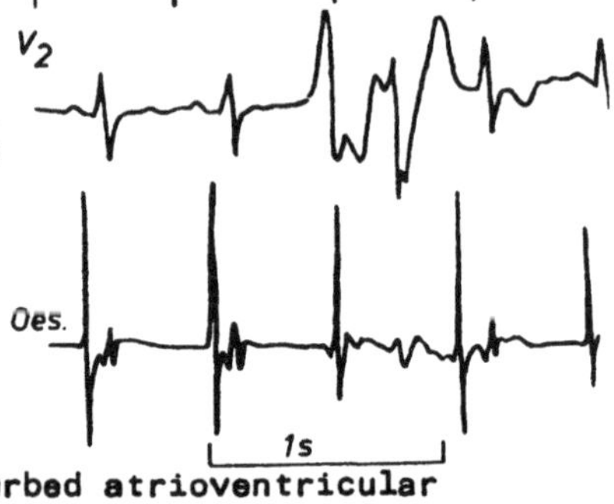

Fig.3aˣ

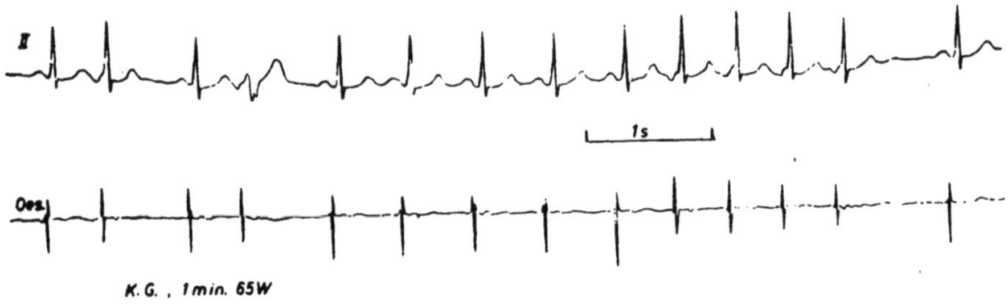

Fig. 3b

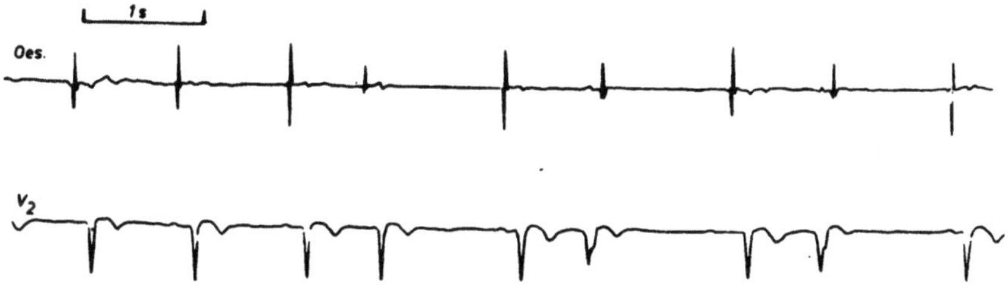

Fig. 3c

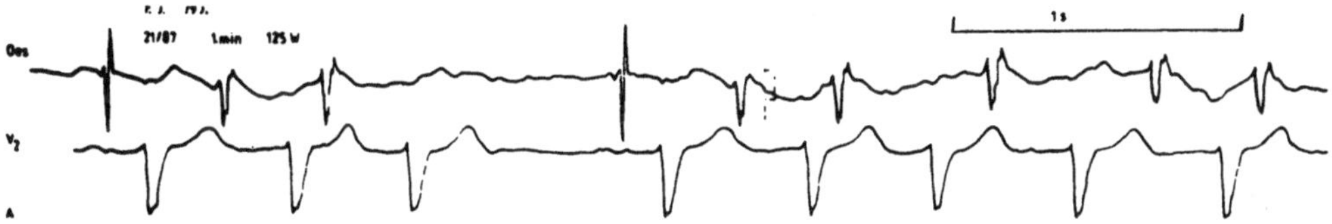

In stress tests not seldom complex dysrhythmias develop which can be analysed more accurately only with the aid of the oesophageal ECG(Figs. 4/5).

Fig. 4a

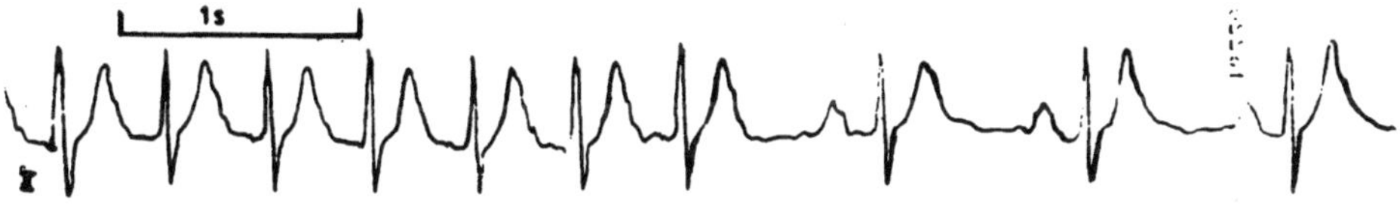

Fig 4b

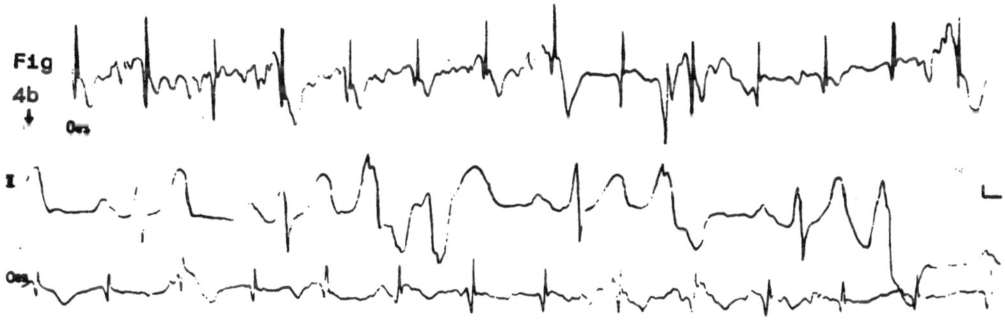

Fig. 4c

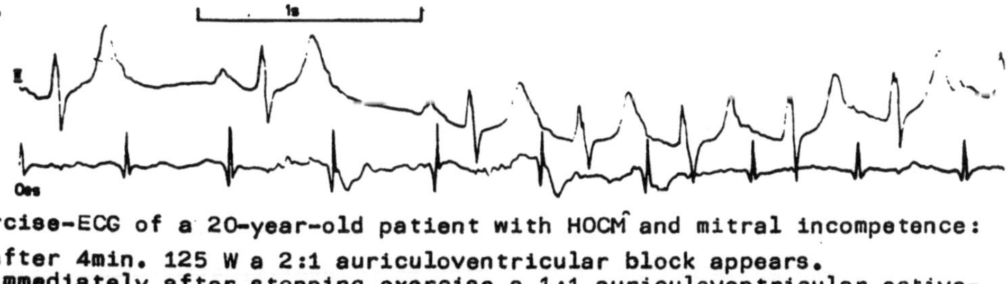

Exercise-ECG of a 20-year-old patient with HOCM and mitral incompetence:

a: after 4min. 125 W a 2:1 auriculoventricular block appears.

b: immediately after stopping exercise a 1:1 auriculoventricular activation sequence at a delayed and aberrant conduction is oberved, then intermittently a sequence of one normal, beat, one aberrant conducted, and one non-conducted atrial activation. When viewing only the surface leads, misinterpretation as paired ventricular extrasystole and intermittend ventricular bigeminal rhythm can be assumed.

c: One minute later regular auriculoventricular conduction reappears.

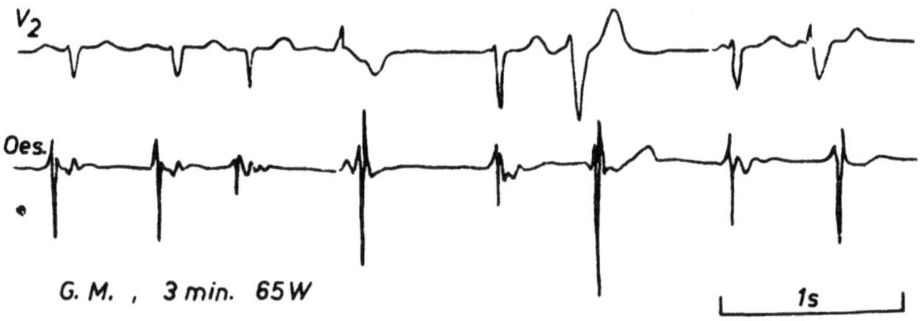

Fig.5

Exercise-ECG of a 56-year-old patient with IHD (3min.65W):After 2 sinus beats a bigeminal coupling as for one supraventricular and one ventricular beat develops intermittently.In the supraventricular excitations the Poes-R distance changes.The ventricular beats are followed by arterial depolarizations at fixed coupling intervals (retrograde conduction).

Discussion: The advancements in differential therapy of cardiac dysrhythmias have led to highly intensifying the diagnostic efforts. Oesophageal electrocardiography offers the advantages of a non-invasive, almost riskless and frequently repeatable approach that even under unfavourable conditions is capable of yielding reliable results (Rübesamen et al.). Its use in cardial stress tests from this point of view seems to be logic. The experience we gathered justifies this step. The diagnostic benefit for the heart rhythm analysis follows from the determination of the P wave incidence and sequence, and from the detection of irregular atrial excitations. The synopsis with the surface ECG permits better tracing of the atrioventricular conduction that frequently is impaired in irregular atrial actions. It moreover permits detection of echobeats and concealed conduction, atrioventricular dissociation, and above, reliable differentiation between ventricular and atrial dysrhythmias with aberrant conduction, or between a bundle-branch block and ventricular ectopic activation. In our view, this makes up for all shortcomings: The characteristic steep-deflecting P wave in the oesophageal ECG only documents excitation in the left atrium. For the determination of the conduction time it must be taken into consideration that dextroatrial excitation starts about 40 ms earlier, in other words, the PQ periods differ by this amount as to compared to the surface ECG. The electrode cable is not fixed within the oesophagus. The position of the electrodes, therefore, may be influenced by the oesophageal peristalsis and by ventilation as well as by heart action. The resulting interfering waves and amplitude variaticions,however,impair the diagnostic power only slightly.We use the method in routine in all stress tests in patients with a known or suspected cardiac dysrhythmia. Further improvements can be achieved by using the computer technique. Application of an identification algorithm for P waves from the oesophageal lead and for the QRS complexes from a surface lead may constitute the basis of an automatic real-time heart rhythm analysis during cardiac stress tests.

Reference:
Rübesamen M.,Reissmann H.C.,Knorre M., Schwela H., Oltmanns G.
In: Electrocardiology'81, eds:Antaloczy Z.,Preda I., Akademia Kiado Budapest, 493-497 (1981).

The importance of ECG to determine the autonomic nervous control of cardiac action during thermal stress

CONRADI, E., BRENKE, R., KAHLBAUM, C.-K.

Clinic of Physiotherapy, Department of Medicine (Charité), Humboldt-University Berlin, Monbijoustraße 2, Berlin 1040, GDR

Introduction

The determination of the cardiac vegetative nerve tone in rest and under load has proved in praxis to solve definite questions. By this means it is possible for example, to determine exactly the course of heart control during adjustment to physical load. Investigations of Schubert and Eckoldt have yielded the basis for a real determination correlating the two parameters of cardiac rhythm: the heart-rate (HR)and variability of HR (Δ HR). The last is defined as the frequency corrected mean value of differences of one after another following period of heart. This can be read of ECG or by electronic data processing. Increase of HR can be caused by enhanced influence of sympathetic nerve tone or decreased of vagustonus. The variation of Δ HR will be caused only by vagus. Above a HR of 120 beats min^{-1} the influence of vagus goes out and Δ HR is near sero about 3 - 5 msec.

In physiotherapy we use besides gymnastic and training bathes and sauna. We suppose a two-part reaction. During the effect of heat a sympathetic influence growes up, followod by vagustone after it. Ott has examined this reaction in sauna which we have confirmed by determination of autonomic heart control. The influence of extreme cold exposition, popular at present, is not yet investigated. Our problem was, to compare the heart control under the conditions of heat and cold to get conclusions for therapy.

Method

We examined ten healthy men, who were 39 years old and participate the study with sauna analog nine persons (5 men and 4 women), who were 17 - 39 years of age, were tested in the icewater of a lake in winter.

The temperature in sauna was in 1,5 m high 83 ∓ 3 %°, the relative air moisture of 7 % ∓ 3. The sublingual temperature increases about 1,5°. The ten persons rested for 10 min, than they stay at sauna for 8 min. After that they go for 1 min into a room with normal-temperature and had cold showers. During this time we continuously registered the ECG to evaluate Δ HR and HR.

The air-temperature in winter was 0 - 3° and the water-temperature 0 - 1°. The ECG was transmitted by telemetry; the blood pressure was measured at several times by Riva Rocci. The subjects, who were habituated to the bathing in winter, first changed sportswear in the open air and had to run for warming up about five minutes. After that they went in the icewater and stayed there for 3 - 5 minutes. After bathing they had a shorthly running. The sublingual temperature decrease about 1°.

The results were tested statistically using the difference t-test or the Wilcoxontest; the degree of probability was $< 0,05$.

Results

The figure 1 showes the course of HR and Δ HR during the two thermal expositions. In both series the reading points before (1), during the first (2,2') and the last minute (3) of exposition and immediatly after that (4) were at the same time. The last value after sauna was 15 minutes later.

Entering sauna HR continuously increased and had reached her maximum in the 8. min. with 112 beats-min^{-1} (s = 12) (3). Already 1 min. later, staying outside, the HR fell down to 88 and after the cold showers to 83 (4). After the rest the HR reached 67/min. Quite the contrary was the course of Δ HR. In rest it was 1,8 min^{-1}; at the end of the trial it decreased to 1,2, this is the smallest value. After the heat exposition HR was nearly normal. After the 20 min. HR reached the level of the beginning.

In the cold air of winter the startinglevel of HR are unusual high (107 min^{-1} (1')). The run to warm up made a further increase to 175/min. In the resting period before intrance in the icewater we find only a decline to 131. Instantly after that HR rises to 148/min. (2), but declines in the first minute (2'). The systolic blood-pressure reached his highest value with 177 Torr. During the cold exposition HR declined to 127 (3) and increased once more after getting out (4). The variability ofΔHR showed the contrary. At the first point it was 3,8. The Δ HR declines during running to 2,6. The lowest figure we see after entering the water was 1,4, but than the Δ HR increase up to 2,03 and at the end to 2,0. After going out Δ HR was 2,03.

Discussion

The results we can arrange in a diagram of Eckoldt which allowes the determination of the vagustonia. The frequency is in its variability

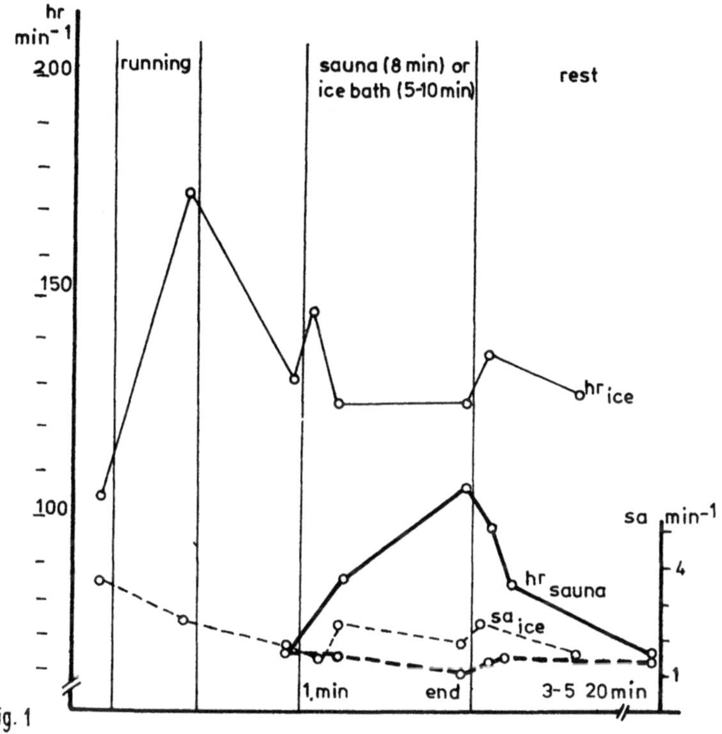

Fig. 1

Heart rate ($\bar{x}$) and sinusarrhytmia ($\bar{x}$) during a sauna and during ice bathing (winter swimming (n = 10 or 9)

heart rate in sauna
sinusarrhytmia in sauna
heart rate in ice bath
sinusarrhytmia in ice bath

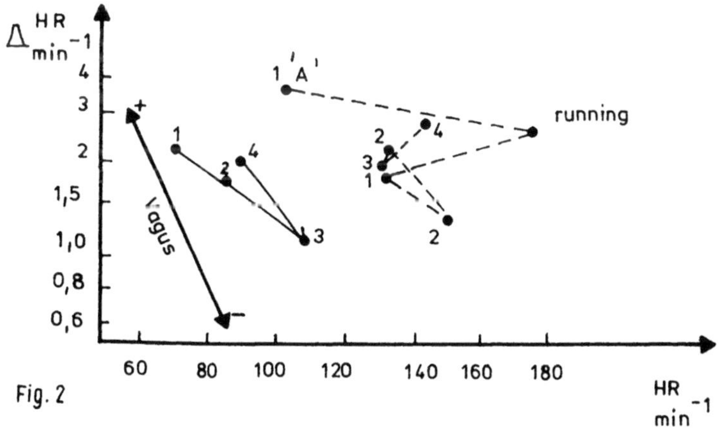

Fig. 2

Courses of the cardiac nervous control in sauna (——) and icewater (— — —)
Explanation in the text.

represented logarithmic. All points shifting parallel to the vagus-curve indicate an in or decrease of vagustonia. All changings parallel to the abszisse are caused by sympathicus. Our inquiry has shown that heat and cold will be answered by the organism in a different way (Fig. 2). In sauna corresponding to the growing up of the body-temperature. HR increases and simultaneous Δ HR falls down. According to Eckoldt HR in the range untill 120/min. will be mainly controled by vagus and less by sympathicus. After the showers the activity of sympathicus declines. A vagussituation like Drexel and Krauß we have not found.
In winterbathing the persons had first a remarcable heat loss by changing their clothes. This makes mainly an increase of HR but no alteration of Δ HR. Therefore we suggest that this is controled by sympathatic nerve. During running the Δ HR falls down and HR rises, so that we conclude a vagus reaction too. Shortly after stepping in the icewater we can suggest once more increasing of sympathicus and decreasing of vagus. In contrary to sauna we observe than an recovering of vagus still remaining in the icewater. The reasons for this repeated variations may be among other things the influence of temperature of the water and the hydrostatic pressure.

Conclusion

1. Heat provoces a decline of vagus and an activation of sympathicus in dependence of heating up the body. This is similar to adaptation to a physical load.

2. In icewater we have in the beginning a short stress-situation but a quickly recovering. We suggest that cold exposition will be a higher stress than heat.

3. For therapy we suggest that cold measures provoce a short sympathicus activation and heat a vagus reduction.

Electrocardiographic Changes in Men Under Hypokinesia and Physical Exercise

YAN G. ZORBAS, GUEORGUI L, NIZAMOV, and HIHASHI N. HITOMI

Hypokinetic Physiology Lab., European Institute of Environmental Cybernetics, GR-162 32 Athens, Greece

It has been suggested that physical exercise (PE) may be used in preventing electrocardiographic changes in men under hypokinesia (diminished muscular activity). Thus, the aim of this investigation was to determine bioelectric activity changes of the heart in 18 physically healthy men aged 19-24 years under 364 days of hypokinesia (HK) with PE and during 76-days of readaptation period (RP). For the simulation of hypokinetic effect the men were kapt under a liberal bed rest regime, that is, the men allowed to stay in bed as they were pleased. They were divided into three groups with 6-men in each. Among the subjects the 1st group of men subjected to HK and intensive PE, the 2nd group submitted to HK and moderate PE and the 3rd group exposed to pure HK, that is, without the use of any preventive measures. Electrocardiographic parameters recorded during the background period (BGP), under HK, and in the RP. Increased heart rate (HR), time of atrioventricular conduction and amplitude of the QRS complex, and decreased amplitude of T wave, primarily in the 1st and 3rd group of men were demonstrated. During the RP an increased HR observed in the 3rd group of men. It was concluded that PE failed to counteract effectively the development of electrocardiographic changes in men under hypokinetic conditions.

INTRODUCTION

Analysis of date in the scientific literature indicates that certain changes developed in the phase structure of cardiac cycle under HK. However, this has not been sufficiently investigated with regard to prolonged exposure to HK, and the available material has not been completely evaluated (1).

Bioelectric activity of the myocardium is required to be tested further under HK, both to assess ongoing health status of men and demonstrate general patterns and mechanisms of changes in bioelectric activity of the myocardium of men under prolonged HK. Thus, the objective of this investigation was to determine the bioelectric activity of the heart of men under HK and PE.

MATERIALS AND METHODS

Experiments performed on 18 physically healthy male volunteers ranging in the age from 19-24 years (weight ranged from 68-74 kg and height from 173-177 cm) under 364-days of HK and a set of PE and during the RP of 76-days. For the simulation of the hypokinetic effect the men were kept under a liberal bed rest regime for 364-days in three 6-bed rooms with an ambient temperature of 22-24 °C and ambient humidity 40-60 %. The range of muscular activity was controlled by the need to move when taken food, by performing the natural wants in the usual way, by recording the different parameters under study and exercising with the designated set of physical exercises. The number of steps taken per day by the men ranged between the 400 to 800. The 1st and the 2nd group of men were subjected to a set of preventive measures (2). Specifically the 1st group of men was submitted to intensive training with a 20-min warm-up period, exercising 60-65 min, twice a day, on a 4-day cycle, that is, 3-days of training, plus 1-day of active rest (3), which performed on an bicycle ergometer in a seated position, as well as combination of athletic exercise that involve the main muscles groups (4). The athletic exercise consisted of 5-8 min warm-up period, 15-20 min pedaling, 15-20 min professional and amateur running on a place, 15-20 min inertial impact load and at the final stages breathing exercises were performed (5). The 2nd group of men was subjected to a moderate set of physical exercise which consisted again of training with a bicycle ergometer and combination of athletic exercise, but it had greater intensity of training alternating with periods of the same volume and greater intensity of exercise and was performed 3-times a week. The calories expended on the set of preventive measures ranged from 400 to 500 kcal/h in different individuals. The 3rd group of men was exposed to pure HK, that is, without the use of any preventive measures and served as control. In an attempt to maintain an adequate level of body hydration under HK all of the men received daily fluid and salt supplements in very small divided doses. Electrocardiographic parameters (corrected orthogonal leads according to Frank) were recorded on a Micrograph-81 apparatus with resisstance-correcting attachement. The electrocardiographic recordings, were made in the morning hours of the study, prior to the intake of breakfast and under conditions of rest. The electrocardiographic recordings were taken several times in the background period of 30-days, on the 15th, 82nd, 140th, 220th, 308th, 344 th day of the hypokinetic period and on the 35th, and 56th day of the RP of 76-days. For the quantitative analysis of electrocardiographic recordings were used the parameters proposed in previous studies (6). In the vector analysis, angles H (azimuth) and E (elevation) were determined with a vectocardiometers (7). The obtained data were submitted to statistical processing by means of two factorial analysis variance of (factor A-duration of HK, factor B-intensity of PE) and S method of multiple comparison using available computers.

RESULTS AND DISCUSSION

The results obtained were indicative of consistent changes in the electrocardiographic parameters of men, which were related primarily to the duration of HK and intensity of diminished muscular activity. Under HK, the mean heart rate feiled to demonstrate statistically significant differences from both the BGP value and between the three groups of men. The least pronounced changes of heart rate observed in the men who were subjected to combined HK and moderate PE. All groups of men exhibited an appreciable increase of heart rate during the RP. The mean value of heart rate exceeded with statistical significance (P 0.05) all previous mean values in the men who were subjected to pore HK, as well as all means characterizing the other two groups of men who were submitted to combined HK and a set of PE of different intensity.

The time of PQ, QRS, QT parameters of the electrocardiograms remained within the normal range in all groups of men. The effect of the factor of duration of HK was statistically significant (P 0.05) apparently for only the PQ interval which increased consistently; however, the difference between minimum BGP value and maximum value between the 308th to 344th days of HK, as well as between parameters of different groups of men, was not statistically significant (P 0.05) under hypokinetic conditions.

The manifestation of alterations under HK in P waves shape, amplitude, duration were consistent, and they did not have any clinical significance. The effect of duration of HK on amplitude parameters of the Q S complex (R_x,+S_y+S_z+ und S_x+R_y+R_z) was statistically significant (P 0.05), and was characterized by a consistent elevation thereof. On the whole, there was a relatively proportional increase in potentials of the ventricles. This, was confirmed by the results obtained by the use of vector analysis, particularly the absence of significant changes in orientation of the QRS vector (angles E and H) according to the time factor. Intergroup differences in size of angles E were only present at certain periods of HK, specifically on the 220th and 344th day.

The mean amplitude of T waves remained within the normal range in all groups of men. A reduction in amplitude of T wave was determined in all leads for the men who were submitted to combined HK and PE of different intensity, and only in the "y" lead for those men who were subjected to pure HK. The statistically significant (P 0.05) difference in amplitude of T wave between the men who were submitted to combined HK and a set of PE of different intensity, which was manifested in the BGP, disappeared under HK as a result of reduction in the amplitude of T_x in the men of the 1st group and elevated in the men of the 2nd group. A maximum reduction in amplitude of T_y in the men who were submitted to pure HK determined by the 220th day of HK, and it was statistically significant (P 0.05) in comparison to analogous parameters for the men who were subjected to combined HK and a set of PE of different intensity. During the RP manifested a considerable increase in amplitude of T_x and T_z waves (it exceeded the BGP values in the 1st and 2nd groups of men). The wave of T_y remained below the BGP level in all groups of men. During the entire experimental period it was not possible to demonstrate any significant changes in amplitude and shape of ST segments that would have made it possible to characterize these changes as being pathological in nature. The amplitude of ST point did not exceed the normal range in any of the examined groups of men. The demonstarted alterations in amplitude of T waves, in the absence of appreciable changes in the shape, as well as in the absence of changes in ST segment and QT intervals, were not such as to would have mede possible to characterize the changes in repolarization process as being pathological. Thus, the demonstrated changes in electrocardiographic parameters were consistent and significant (P 0.05) under the 364-days of HK and a set of PE of different intensity. An increased heart rate observed in all groups of men. An increased time of atrioventricular conductance, increased amplitude of the QRS complex, and decreased amplitude of T wave was also observed in all groups of men. There were not demonstarble any significant distrophic changes in the myocardium of the subjects. Alter the foregoing it can be concluded that hypokinesia induced consistant and significant electrocardiographic disturbances in men, while at the same time it was revealed that PE cannot be used to counteract effectively the development of adverse reactions of bioelectric activity of the heart of men under hypokinetic conditions.

REFERENCES

1. Zorbas, Y. G., and Nizamov, G. L.: in Advances in Electrocardiology, Ed.) P d'Alche, Universite de Caen, Caen(1984), pp 457-459
2. Zorbas, Y. G., and Matveyev, I. O.: in 1st Vienna International Workshop on Functional Electrostimulation, Universite of Vienna, Vienna, (1983), pp 2-6
3. Zarakovskiy, G. M., and Rysakova, S. L.: Kosmicheskaya Biol., 3, 67-71, (1972)
4. Zorbas, Y. G., and Matveyev, I. O.: Int. J. Rehab, Research, 10(1), 63-68, (1987)
5. Stepantsov, V. I., Tikhonov, M. A., and Yeremin, A. V., Kosmicheskaya Biol., 4, 64-68, (1972)
6. Ozol, E. A.: Corrected Orthogonal EKG Leads in Clinical Analysis of Bioelectric Activity of the Heart, USSR Ministry of Health, Kazan, (1972)
7. Kenedi, P.: Orv. Hetil., 113, 997-999, (1972)

FACILITIES OF ECG TELEMETRY IN PHYSICAL MEDICINE

R. BRENKE and E. CONRADI
Clinic of Physiotherapy, Department of Medicine (Charité),
Humboldt-University Berlin (Charité), Monbijoustraße 2, Berlin 1040,GDR

Introduction

Reportedly, an ever increasing number of healthy persons, but also patients with a high cardiac risk wish to do conditioning exercises which have been unusual so far. Sauna, winter swimming (ice bathing) or jogging in the cold count amongst those. Before starting to take on such strain, however, the position regarding the cardiovascular stress as well as any possible risks should be clear. Since measuring the pulse by the patient himself is not sufficient to allow for instance the estimation of a patient with a risk, the ECG telemetry comes to help. Besides watching the situation through the ECG in a particular stress situation it so becomes possible through determination of the parameters heart frequency/sinus arrhythmia to get a judgment concerning the effect by the vegetative influende on the cardionerves. Yet, the clinical possibilities are limited, ECG telemetry cannot be applied to every patient. Additionally, frequent technical interferences (for example under water) complicate a continuous surveillance.

Problem

We tried to find out the degree of cardiovascular stress connected with three rather popular conditioning measures.

1. Jogging in cold air (3 - 5 minutes, air temperature 0 - 3°C)
2. Ice-bathing after jogging (1 - 10 minutes, water temperature 0 - 1°C)
3. Sauna (8 minutes, 83°C)

Method applied

On the example of 9 joggers, 9 winter swimmers and 10 sauna bathers continuous ECG telemetric surveillance was carried out. Visually the actions were permanently watched on the screen, intermittent recordings of the marking line Nehb A took place. The ECG interpretation was done along with determining the heart frequency (min^{-1}) and the sinus arrhythmia ($\Delta\ \overline{Hf}$, min^{-1}).

The cardiovascular stress was evaluated by comparing the measured mean heart frequency data against the standard values as established for the various age groups on the bicycle-ergometer.

Results and discussion

The most essential results are shown in the tables Nos. 1 and 2. Clearly, the highest stress is related to jogging in cold air, in average it is over 200 watt. Ice bathing (winter swimming) bears about 160 watt. The lowest stress relates to the sauna (about 75 watt).
All stresses lead to the decrease of the cardial vagotonus and to the increase of the sympathicotonus. Whilst during jogging and sauna bathing the stress is growing with the time of application continuing, it is particularly high when ice bathing at the moment of entering the water.
Isolated extrasystoles occur especially during jogging, more scarcely they appear with ice bathing or sauna bathing.

Conclusions and summary

The ECG telemetric investigation offers the possibility to estimate the cardiovascular stress along with detecting generally current short-time modifications which from the very outset cannot be anticipated to their full extent. It offers insights into the dynamic of the stress processing.

It is suggested to test some new and unusual conditioning measures in a pilot study by means of telemetry so as to estimate the stress by comparison against the data delivered by the bicycle-ergometer. So, at a later point even without the telemetry it could be possible by means of an orientating ergometry to take the decision whether or not the patient concerned will tolerate the stress anticipated.

Examples presented are stress situations during sauna, winter swimming and jogging in the cold. In average the estimated watt ranges are:

sauna	75 watt
winter swimming	165 watt
jogging in the cold over	200 watt

	heart rate ($\bar{x}$, min^{-1})			sinusarrhythmia ($\bar{x}$, min^{-1})			remarks
	rest	1.min of load	end of load	rest	1.min of load	end of load	
sauna (n=10)	65,7	87,5	108,3 (8.min)	1,86	1,72	1,18 (8.min)	
ice bathing after jogging (n=9)	130,9	147,8	126,9 (1-10 min)	1,88	1,48	2,0 (1-10 min)	In one case ES. Large increase of blood pressure
jogging in the cold (n=9)	106,8		175,4 (3-5 min)	3,81		2,66 (3-5 min)	In two cases ES

tab. 1: Heart rate and sinusarrhythmia in some kinds of fitness training (results from ECG-telemetry)

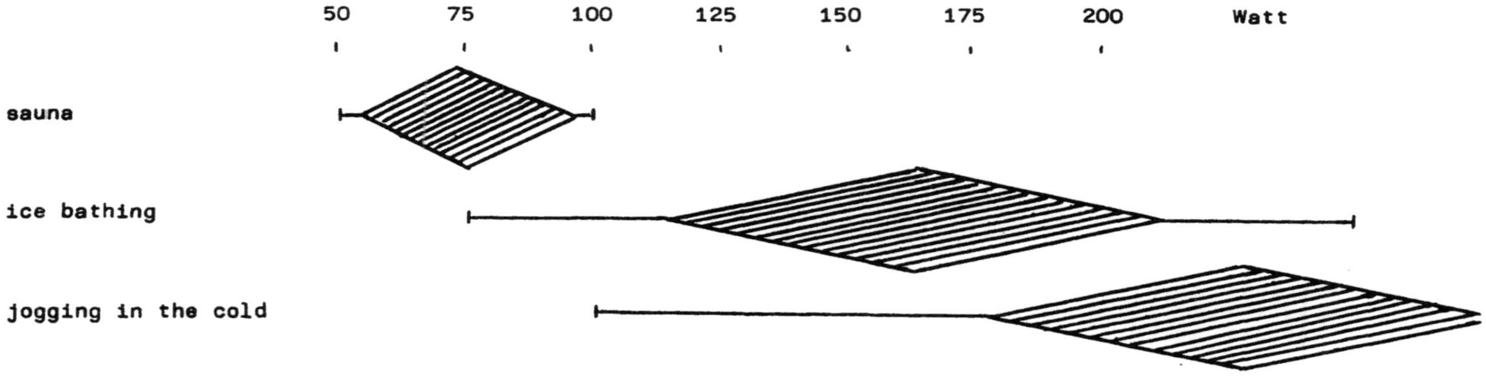

fig. 1: Estimation of the performance in some new kinds of fitness training

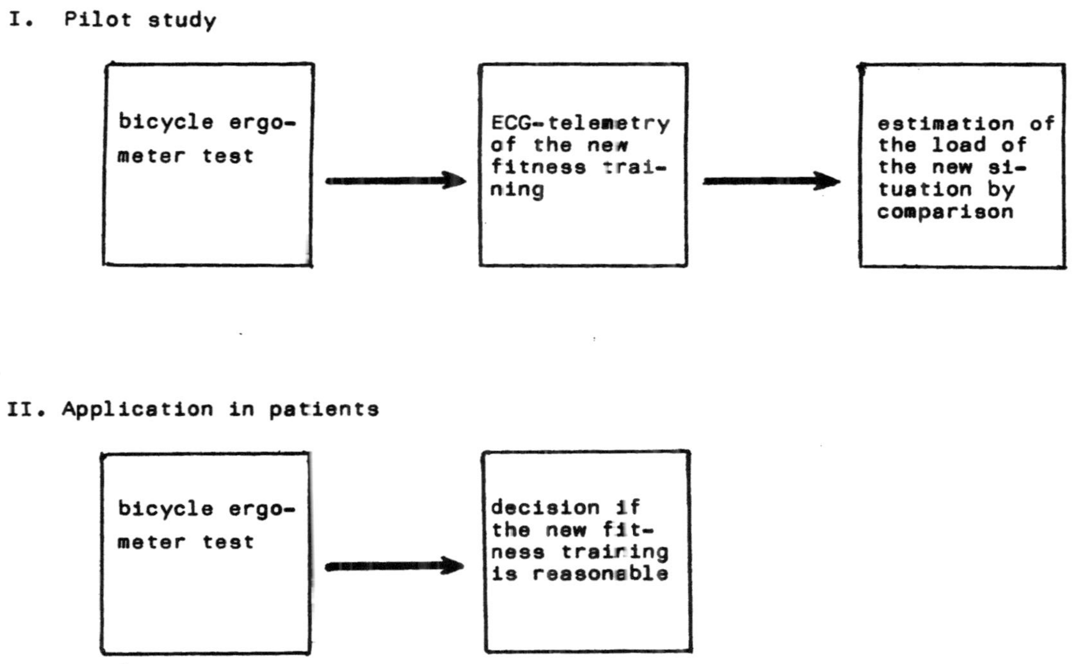

fig. 2: Recommendation: Proceeding in practice in testing a new kind of fitness training

Modified ECG Functional Test for Prognosis of Rehabilitation Effect in Patients after Myocardial Infarction

SIDORENKO G.I., RUSETSKAYA V.G., KOVALCHUK YU.A.
Byelorussian Research Institute of Cardiology, Minsk, USSR

The modified ECG functional test comprises a bicycle double exercise test. Higher tolerance to the second exercise test performed after a 30-minute interval makes it possible to predict positive rehabilitation effect in patients with myocardial infarction.

Individual control over the rehabilitation process necessitates a strictly objective evaluation of coronary circulation, myocardial function and reserve potentialities. The results of traditional exercise tests, e.g. bicycle test, change considerably during both short and long time periods under the influence of 24-hour biorhythm (Oransky I.E. et al., 1978). The tolerance study of healthy individuals and patients with ischemic heart disease to consecutive exercise tests conducted with different time intervals resulted in the modified bicycle double exercise test (BDET).

The aim of the present study is to investigate the BDET informative value for prognosis of rehabilitation effect in patients with myocardial infarction.

BDET methods. The exercise test was repeated 30 minutes after the first one. The preliminary findings showed that no tolerance changes were observed after 5 to 10 minutes interval. Significant changes occurred and maintained during 30 to 180 minutes after the termination of the first exercise test. The optimal time interval preceding second exercise test was found to be equal to 30 minutes which does not prolong essentially time limits of the examination. The exercise test was carried out in continuous stepwise increasing pattern under continuous ECG control (150, 300, 600, 900 Kpm min^{-1}). Each stage was 3 minutes long. Both the first exercise test and the second one were terminated according to the WHO criteria.

The tolerance to physical load was determined by the following parameters total work fulfilled Kpm min^{-1} (A), double product (DP), as well as the cardiac efficiency parameter (CEP), determined as DP upon A ratio. The BDET results were evaluated by comparing the above-mentioned parameters obtained during the first and the second testing with positive, neutral and negative BDET variants singled out. The positive variant was characterised by higher A and better cardiac efficiency in the second test. The negative one was marked by lower values of these parameters, while the neutral variant showed no significant changes in the second exercise.

101 patients with ischemic heart disease after myocardial infarction (average age 47.6 ± 3.4 years) were examined. The patients were divided into functional classes (FC) according to the classification of Canadian Heart Association.

26 healthy men (average age 47.2 ± 2.3 years) made up a control group. BDET was performed at the beginning and 21 day after the health-resort rehabilitation at the end of the cure.

The findings of this study at the initial state are cited in Table 1.

Table 1. Increase in the volume of work fulfilled in the second BDET test as compared to that of the first one (Kpm/min)

Statistical indices	Groups of IHD patients			
	II FC	III FC microfocal myocardial infarction	III FC macrofocal myocardial infarction	IV FC
n	12	25	35	8
M	+ 386.0	+ 338.8	+ 199.3	- 197.9
m	35.4	46.8	24.0	42.7

n - number of examinations

As is seen from Table 1, patients of the II FC and III FC demonstrate better tolerance to the second exercise test, while the tolerance of the IV FC patients to the second exercise test goes down.

Thus, the compensatory cardiac reserves mobilise during the second exercise test in the patients of II FC and III FC. A weaker compensatory response to the second exercise test testifies to the exhaustion of compensatory cardiac reserves.

To study the possibility of the rehabilitation effect prognosis BDET was repeated in 60 patients with myocardial infarction 21 day after their admission to the health-resort and a year after it. The patients were divided into two groups according to their response to the second exercise test (Table 2). The first group comprised 35 patients with the positive BDET variant registered during the first testing at the beginning of rehabilitation.

Table 2. Correlation of health-resort rehabilitation effectiveness with BDET variants

BDET variant	Total number	Rehabilitation effect	
		Positive	Negative
$A_2 > A_1$	35	32	3
$A_2 \leq A_1$	25	4	21

A_1 and A_2 represent total amount of work fulfilled during the first and the second bicycle exercise testing

25 patients with satisfactory state of compensatory reserves made up the second group. These patients showed neutral or negative BDET variant during the first testing at the beginning of rehabilitation. The rehabilitation effectiveness was evaluated by the clinical signs and the tolerance dynamics to physical exercise.

Higher tolerance to the work fulfilled in patients of the first group

with the positive BDET variant was +59 per cent at the end of health - resort cure, while that in the group of patients with the neutral BDET variant at the beginning of rehabilitation was practically negligible by the end of this period (A - 1.5 per cent).
Clinical examinations of patients with positive BDET variant testified to the rehabilitation effect in 32 out of 35 patients.
Favourable rehabilitation effect was observed in 4 out of 25 patients in the group with negative and neutral BDET variant.
To evaluate the rehabilitation follow-up results the return of patients working ability was checked one year after (Table 3). One year after working capacity index and BDET parameters at the beginning of the rehabilitation correlated significantly ($r=+0.96$; $p<0.001$).

Table 3. Return of working capacity to patients with myocardial infarction according to the criteria of exercise termination

Cause of exercise termination	BDET variant	Patients total	Working capacity	
			Restored	Lost
1. Fatigue or ST segment depression below 0.2 mV		20	19	1
2. Either ST segment depression or elevation by 0.2 mV and angina	positive	31	27	4
3. Either ST segment depression or elevation by 0.2 mV and angina	negative, neutral	23	5	18

Adaptation process to the second exercise loads concerns contractile myocardial function too. Better myocardial function, i.e. lower diastolic pressure in pulmonary artery during the bicycle second exercise test, performed after 20 minutes interval, was also observed by A. Westheim (1980). We studied hemodynamic response to the second exercise test, performed after 30 minutes interval (Yu. A. Kovalchuk et al, 1987). Higher values of stroke volume and cardiac output during BDET was found to be expressed in those patients with myocardial infarction, for whom the exercise load was terminated according to the objective signs of transient myocardial ischemia (ST segment depression or elevation). Thus, short-time myocardial ischemia, induced by preceding exercise load, resulted in higher tolerance to the second exercise load and revealed cardiac reserves.
Higher tolerance to the second exercise load was not observed in those cases, when exercise test was terminated prior to the ischemic response onset, for example, either because of fatigue or submaximal heart rate.
It can be concluded, that BDET may be useful not only for rehabilitation effect prognosis and selection of adequate rehabilitation exercise intensity, but it may also shed light on the mechanics of the phenomenon, known as "second wind".

(I) Оранский И.Е.,Селивестрова Г.П.,Крушинина Т.В. и др.:Кардиология, 6,I22–I26 (I978)
(2) Westheim A.,Grendahl H.,Kjershis I.et al.:Europ.Congr.Cardiol., 68 (1980)
(3) Ковальчук Ю.А.,Русецкая В.Г.,Сидоренко Г.И.:Кардиология,4,40–43 (I987)

Comparison of exercise precordial mapping and exercise thallium scintigraphy in the diagnosis of coronary artery disease

István PRÉDA, Ildikó BALOGH, Károly TÓTH, Zoltán ANTALÓCZY, István SZILVÁSI and Ernő BERENTEY

2nd Medical Clinic and Radiological Department of Postgraduate Medical School, H-1389 Budapest, POB.112. Hungary

SUMMARY

71 patients (50 men, 21 women, mean age 42 years) referred for evaluation of chest pain suspected to be coronary in origin were evaluated. None had pain at rest, but 19 had electrocardiographic evidences of previous myocardial infarction. The exercise protocol consisted of 12-lead ECG, 30-unipolar lead ECG-exercise mapping and 201-thallium chloride submaximal exercise scintigraphy as well as selective coronarography and left ventricular angiography.

52 of the 71 patients showed significant (more than 75 per cent) stenosis of one or more major coronary arteries. 7 patients had coronary kinking with a visible slowing of coronary flow and slightly elevated left ventricular end-diastolic pressure (mean 18 mmHg) but the ejection fraction still mentained (mean 0,74). 12 patients had normal coronary artery system, but 7 of them exhibited mitral valve prolapse.

According to the results the sensitivity of both exercise precordial mapping (94 per cent) and 201-thallium scanning (86 per cent) are high and their combination seems to be even more valuable for preselection of patients for coronary angiography. False negative exercise mapping is rare, when it occurs the intramyocardial collateral circulation is well developed. False-positive exercise mapping may happen exclusively in cases with elevated LVEDP and/or mitral valve prolapse. For false-negative scanning the main predisposing factors are the existence of triple-vessel disease and well developed collaterals. False-positive scanning also may occur in cases of elevated LVEDP and mitral valve prolapse.

INTRODUCTION

In the management of patients presenting with chest pain it is important to have a non-invasive test that will accurately identify those with ischemic heart disease. In this aspect, exercise electrocardiograms have now become a standard diagnostic tool, however, a sizable number of false negative tests are still found when the results are correlated with coronary arteriography. The recent introduction of exercise ECG mapping permits measurement of the severity of exercise-induced ST segment changes in the whole precordial area (1-5). Thallium-201 exercise myocardial perfusion scintigraphy is also a safe non-invasive method for identifying stress-induced abnormal myocardial perfusion and, indirectly, significant coronary artery lesions (6-9). In the present study the diagnostic accuracy of combined precordial exercise mapping and thallium scanning was compared with that of 12-lead exercise electrocardiography.

METHODS

71 patients (50 men, 21 women, mean age 42 years) were involved in the study. All patients were referred for evaluation of chest patin suspected to be coronary in origin. None had pain at rest, but 19 had electrocardiographic Q-waves of 0,04 seconds or more in duration confirming a history of prior myocardial infarction. Submaximal graded bicycle ergometer 12-lead ECG exercise tests were obtained one day before the mapping-scanning protocol. Precordial maps were obtained in supine position from 30 unipolar electrodes distributed in a 5x6 matrix covering the anterior thoracic wall from the right mid-clavicular to the left axillary line (10). After recording the resting maps an intravenous catheter was placed into the antecubital vein and each patient underwent the same symptom limited submaximal bicycle ergometer test as was done with 12-lead ECG. One minute before the exercise end-point was reached, 74 MBq of thallium-201 chloride was injected through the established intravenous line and thereafter the exercise map was recorded and processed on-line on a TPA/1 microcomputer. After recovery, scintigraphy was performed with a gamma camera from the anterior, left anterior oblique 45° and left anterior oblique 70° projections and it was repeated 4 hours later to obtain resting (redistribution) scintigrams.
Selective coronarography and left ventricular angiography was performed a few days after the exercise protocol in all of the 71 cases. Significant coronary lesions were those revealing a 75 per cent or greater area of stenosis in at least one major coronary vessel on selective coronary angiography.Detailed results of left ventricular function and the existence of segmental wall motion abnormalities and collateral circulation were also teken into account.

RESULTS AND DISCUSSION

52 of the 71 patients showed significant, more than 75 per cent stenosis of one or more major coronary arteries (Table 1.). 7 patients had a tortuous left anterior descending

Table 1. Overall results of coronary angiography compared with the 12-lead exercise-ECG, exercise precordial mapping and exercise 201-thallium scanning tests.

	No	FALSE-NEGATIVE			FALSE-POSITIVE		
		ECG	M	Sc	ECG	M	Sc
Single-vessel disease							
LAD	6	2	1	1			
LCx	5	3					
RCA	8	3					
Double-vessel disease							
Left main	3						
LAD+LCx	9	3					
LAD+RCA	5	1					
RCA+LCx	7	1					
Triple-vessel disease							
Left main+RCA	2						
LAD+LCx+RCA	7	1		2			
Coronary kinking	7				4	5	
Normal coronary artery	12				5	4	3
	71	14	1	3	9	9	3

or circumflex coronary artery without significant obstruction (coronary kinking), but with a visible slowing of coronary flow. All of them had slightly elevated left ventricular end-diastolic pressure (mean 18 mmHg), but the ejection fraction was still mentained (mean 0,74). 12 patients had normal, or near normal coronary artery system with normal left ventricular systolic and diastolic function, but 7 of them exhibited late-systolic mitral prolapse involving one or both mitral leaflets.

The 12 lead exercise ECG was evaluated by an experienced cardiologist in the usual way. ST-segment changes were considered to be pathological if there was a horizontal or descending ST-segment depression (0,1 mV or more) 80 msec after the J-point. False negativ exercise test occured in 14 of the 52 cases with significant coronary obstruction (sensitivity 73 per cent), whereas 9 tests were false positive.

The precordial exercise mapping test was considered to be positive if the ST-depression after 60 msec of the J-point was more than 0,1 mV in at least 3 neighbouring leads (Table 3.). A false negative test occured in one case (sensitivity 94 per cent) and there were 9 false positive tests, five of these with coronary kinking and impared left ventricular diastolic function and four of these with mitral valve prolapse, but no alteration of left ventricular function. Consequently, all the false positive exercise mapping tests were belonging to a certain pathologic cardiac process showing subendocardial lesion to stress.

Table 2. Characteristic features of left ventricular function and coronary anatomy in the in the cases of false-negative and false-positive exercise precordial mapping tests.

FALSE-NEGATIVE PRECORDIAL MAPPING

N°	PT	LVEDP	EF	DIAGNOSIS
1.	B.L.	7 mmHg	0.80	LAD occlusion

FALSE-POSITIVE PRECORDIAL MAPPING

N°	PT	LVEDP	EF	DIAGNOSIS
1.	L.K.	10 mmHg	0.59	Coronary Kinking
2.	L.E.	23 mmHg	0.71	Coronary Kinking
3.	Z.J.	18 mmHg	0.86	Coronary Kinking
4.	V.K.	14 mmHg	0.86	Coronary Kinking
5.	K.T.	23 mmHg	0.70	Coronary Kinking + Mitral Prolapse
$\bar{x}$		18 mmHg	0.74	
6.	H.S.	8 mmHg	0.81	Mitral Prolapse
7.	B.J.	5 mmHg	0.73	Mitral Prolapse
8.	K.J.	8 mmHg	0.80	Mitral Prolapse
9.	P.M.	15 mmHg	0.79	Mitral Prolapse
$\bar{x}$		9 mmHg	0.78	

In order to analyse the results of 201-thallium scintigraphy stress and resting pictures were compared qualitatively (analogue scinti-photos) and quantitatively (circumferential analysis with Goris-Watson background subtraction). False negative tests occured in 3 patients (sensitivity 86 per cent), two of them with triple-vessel disease and one with a case of vasospastic angina. In all of the three false-negative cases a collateral circulation between the right and left coronary artery system were also evident in the coronary angiograms.

Combination of precordial exercise mapping and 201-thallium scanning tests resulted in the elimination of false negative cases (sensitivity 100 per cent considering the 71 patients investigated), but the number of false positive tests is relatively high (4 from 19) giving a 79 per cent specificity. The relatively low specificity may be misleading because all the patients investigated exhibited characteristic anginal chest pain and consequently small vessel disease or metabolic cardiac disorder cannot be excluded.

Table 3. Sensitivity and specificity figures in ischemic heart disease obtained with different exercise tests.

	SENSITIVITY	SPECIFICITY
12-lead ECG	73 per cent	63 per cent
MAPPING	94 per cent	63 per cent
SCANNING	86 per cent	86 per cent
MAPPING+SCANNING	100 per cent	79 per cent

REFERENCES

1./ Maroko,P.R. et al: Precordial S-T segment elevation mapping: an atraumatic method for assessing alterations in the extent of myocardial ischemic injury. The effects of pharmacologic and haemodynamic interventions. Am.J.Cardiol. 29:223, 1972.

2./ Fox,K.M. et al: Precordial electrocardiographic mapping after exercise in the diagnosis of coronary artery disease. Am.J.Cardiol, 43:541, 1979.

3./ Hinsen,H. et al: Computer analysis of multiple lead stress tests for predicting coronary artery disease. Electrocardiology'81, eds:Z.Antalóczy and I.Préda,Akadémia, Budapest, pp:263-267, 1982.

4./ Kubota,I.: Body surface distributions of ST-segment changes after exercise in effort angina pectoris without myocardial infarction.Am.Heart J. 110:949-955, 1985.

5./ Macfarlane,P.W. et al: 16-lead exercise electrocardiography: in:Advances in Electrocardiology, ed:P.d'Alché, Publications de l'Université de Caen, pp:179-181,1985.

6./ Botvinick,E.H. et al: Thallium-201 myocardial perfusion scintigraphy for clinical clarification, abnormal and equivocal electrocardiographic stress tests.Am.J.Cardiol 41:43, 1978.

7./ Verani,M.Z. et al: Sensitivity and specificity of thallium-201 perfusion scintigrams under exercise in the diagnosis of coronary artery disease.J.Nucl.Med. 19:773, 1978.

8./ Wada,M. et al: Exercise stress body surface isopotential map in patients with coronary angiographic and stress myocardial perfusion scintigraphic findings.Jap.Circ.J. 45:1203, 1981.

9./ Mizuno,Y. et al: Exercise stress body surface ST-potential distribution in ischemic heart disease. Comparison with myocardial stress perfusion scintigram and coronary angiogram.Advances in Body Surface Potential Mapping, eds:K.Yamada,K.Harumi and T. Muscha,Nagoya Press pp:235-242, 1983.

10./ Préda,I. et al: System for 32-channel on-line exercise mapping. in:Electrocardiology 83, eds:I.Ruttkay-Nedecky and P.Macfarlane, Excerpta Medica,Amsterdam,pp:164-166, 1984.

Frequency analysis of ECG during bycicle exercise in patients with ischaemic heart disease

KOLÁŘOVÁ, N. JANOTA, M.

Institute of clinical and experimental medicine, Vídeňská 800, Prague 4, 146 22

Summary

The object of this report is the explanation of the relationship between the decrease of T wave and occurence of higher frequencies in ECG records spectra in patients with ischaemic heart disease. For the analysis of this phenomenon the Fast Fourier Transform has been applied, by means of which the ergometric ECG records have been transformed from the time area into the frequency area. For the analysis of the obtained "estimates" of spectra the approach has been chosen which principally belongs to the group of methods of cluster analysis. Even the visual analysis of the graphic representation of spectra by means of the compressed spectra array method shows obviosly that, in contrast to healthy individuals, in these patients there does not occur the synchronization of local maxima of spectra during the ergometric load. The explanation of this phenomenon in the time area of the signal will be discussed on the basis of comparison of the frequency pictures of ECG records of healthy individuals with application of antiarythmic agents, of heparin NOVO and of sportsmen.

1. Introduction

Acute ischaemic disease results in significant changes in metabolism of free fatty acids that exert an immediate effect on the structure of the cardiac cell membrane and its function. A number of investigators in this field |1| assume a causal relationship between the changes in free fatty acids, products of their metabolism, and the electrophysiological peculiarities due to the onset of ischaemia. Discussion on whether it is possible--in order to study the electrophysiological manifestations of ischaemic disease--to use the heart hypothesis on their products has persisted to date. While the hypothesis cannot be refuted altogether, there is still lack of clinical evidence confirming it. All these facts can be summed up into a single question, that is, whether there are any mutually distinguishable principles governing the changes of electrical heart activities produced by changes in the level of free fatty acids in the body.

The aim of this study was develope and test a method of assessment of ECG recordings that would make it possible to answer this question on the basis of their objective processing.

2. Materials and methods

Before initiating the trial, it was necessary to design and carry out experiments involving the administration of drugs that significantly change the levels of non-esterified fatty acids (NEFA) in the body.

To carry out initial experiments, the subjects were given heparin and a polarization solution glucose-insulin-potassium (GIP). Heparin was chosen because its administration led to a significant increase in the level of free fatty acids. An opposite phenomenon was observed during administration on the GIP polarization solution.

Whereas, in the GIP experiment, glycaemia rises significantly and, on the contrary, during exercise it decreases rapidly down to hypoglycaemic values. This is associated with a decrease in the level of free fatty acids (NEFA).

In the experiment involving heparin administration, while glycaemia does not change virtually, the levels of NEFA, however, are significantly increased troughout the experiment.

The design of the study, performed in seven total of healthy men aged 18 years, was as follows:

1) 500ml of 20% and 12 u. of insulin + 10mmol K^+ (i.e., 10ml of 7.46 KCl solution) were administred during 60 minutes.

2) This was followed by 60-minute infusion of 500ml of isotonic solution of KCl with 10000 u. of NOVO heparin.

3) On the basis of results yielded by these studies tests, another group of five volunteers was again administred infusion of saline with heparin, with 10ml of 1% mesocain infusion on the same day.

The infusion were given using an INFUSOMAT pump fy Braun. Their sequence was different in each subject. Once infusion was over, the volunteers were requested to sit immediately on an ELEMA ergometer and subjected to 8.5 minute workload of 1.5W/kg b.w. after 4 minutes. ALL experiments were carried out in the morning with fasting volunteers under precisely defined laboratory conditions.

Another group of subjects were top performance sportsmen, 4 cyclists and 5 weight lifters. These sportsmen were subjected to three-step ergometry with regular periods of rests to let them return to almost initial resting heart rate values. 20 minute ECG recordings were obtained from each cyclists. Suprisingly, the athletes were unable to cope with this type of workload and had to discontinue the test even though they did non reach physical load.

In collaboration with the Laboratory of cardiology of the Department of Medicin II of the Institute for Clinical and Experimental Medicine in Praque, the ECG recordings of patients with documented ischaemic heart disease and those with suspected ischaemic heart disease were obtained. A total of 20 patients were examined.

To analyse the above phenomena, a mathematical procedure was chosen based on the transcription of the ECG recording from a time area to a frequency area using in algorithm of the Fast Fourier Transform (FFT). The design and actual application on the method can be divided into three stages:

a) ECG signal pre-processing
b) ectraction of informative signs from the ECG signal
c) use of cluster analysis to classify experimental situations in agreement with á priori information about the inclusion of individual recordings to their respective classes.

a) ECG recording pre - processing

A ECG recording was fed into the input of the analog part of a hybrid EAI - 690 computer system from a tape recorder cassette. The ECG recording was discreted into a sequence of instantaneous values, i.e., into a data organization for futher computer- assisted processing. Sampled signal was evenly segmented into 5.12s parts. The FFT was applied to each segment. In this manner, we obtained the frequency estimates of spectra corresponding to individuals segments. To obtain graphic representation of the estimates of ECG spectra, the method of compressed spectra array was used.

b) Extraction of informative signs from the ECG signal

To outline significant frequency components of the signal, the so called loupe was used, that is, cutting of all spectra at the bottom by a respective fraction of the amplitude of the peak of spectrum and respective shiftint of the zero level. In the time spectrum sequence, the time segment was found in which the spectra were stabilized, that is, alligned. The ECG signal in that area is periodical with a constant heart rate value. That interval, that is, steady state, yielded 20 consecutive spectra for subsequent processimg to obtain an average spectrum assessed by computer. The frequency range of this spectrum was divided into three intervals whose length were determined using the optimalization procedure. To express the nature of the average, we chose quantitative description using the number of local peaks in these intervals obtained by optimization.

c) Use of the method of cluster analysis

Each interval correspnds to a computer-assessed number of peaks giving the lenth of of coordinate to the vector in the image space of signs representing the ECG recording of each subject examined. This vector is shown in the vector space by coordinates x,y,z.

3. Results of application of the method in real ECG signal

An assessment of representatives of each group is given.Fig. 1. shows a typical feature of a resting ECG recording, that is, disarray of the spectra. The moment of onset of workload is associated with their synchronization, that is, alingment. Administration of GIP leads to a predominance of low frequency components in the spectra (primarily around 2Hz). Increased use of free fatty acids enhances the spectral components with substantially higher frequencies (about 6Hz).

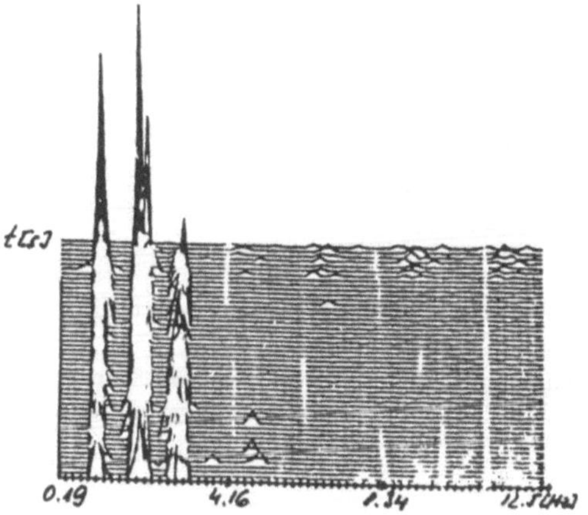

Fig. 1 Administration of polarization solutin GIP

Fig. 2 shows the frequency pattern of an exercise ECG recording with heparin administration and subsequent administration of mesocain. Apparently, the more potent the drug, the poorer the ECG spectrum in higher frequency components of the signal and, vice versa, richer in low frequency.

In patients with confirmed ischaemic

heart disease, the frequency pattern of ECG signal is visually very similar to that in persons with heparin administration, that is, in those with a significant increase in the levels of free fatty acids in the body, this, however, only from the point of view of distribution of frequency spectra components. While, just in healthy persons, stabilization of the shape of wave components of the ECG curve does not occur. This is actually what makes them differ from subjects free of ischaemic heart disease (Fig. 3).

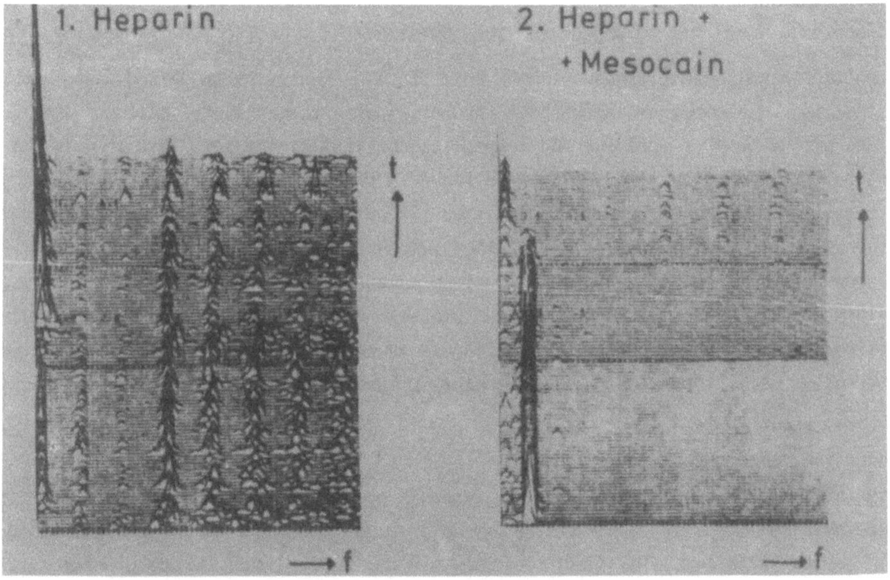

Fig.2

Frequency pattern of an exercise ECG regording with heparin administration and subsequent administration of mesocain.

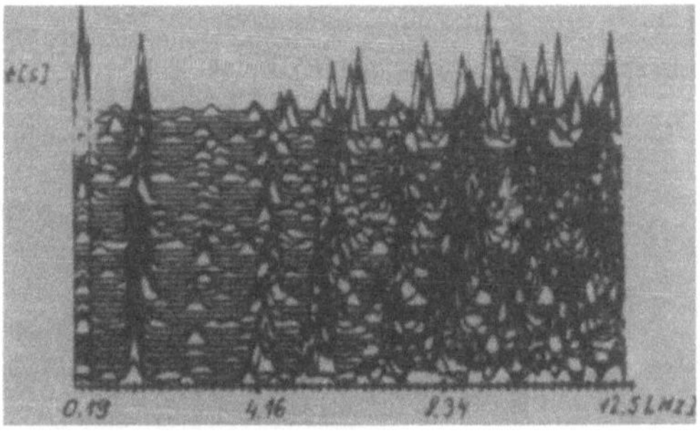

Fig. 3

Frequency pattern of an ECG recording of patients with ischaemic heart disease.

|1| Fozzard, H.A., Haber, E., et al.: The Heart and Cardiovascular System, Scientific Foundation, Raven Press, New york, 1986

Significance of the ascending type of ST-segment depression during diagnostic exercise ECG in patients with ischaemic heart disease.

MÜLLER, S., GEISSLER, W., FÖRSTER, A., FRANZ, N.

Humboldt-University, Medical School (Charite), Clinic of Internal Medicine, Berlin, German Democratic Republic

Summary

Resting ECG and ECG during bicycle exercise testing were investigated in comparison with the coronary angiographic findings in 280 patients (pts.). In 50 pts. (18 %) the ascending type of ST-segment depression (asc. ST↓) was observed exclusive in exercise ECG. These pts. exercise ECG were analyzed by selected parameters. It was found that a ischaemic response exist when the following three characteristics have been fulfiled: 1. ST↓ 0,08 sec after the J point ≥ 0,15 mV, 2. S-type (slowly asc. ST↓ reaching the isoelectric line at the beginning of the T-wave), 3. when previously is seen a asc. ST↓ in resting ECG this asc. ST↓ increases in the exercise test at least 0,1 mV. In 25 pts. with a asc. ST↓ of so called ischaemic type in the exercise test 20 pts. (80 %) showed haemodynamic critical stenoses respectively fastening in the coronary angiographic findings. The results have proved that the ascending type of ST-segment depression also can demonstrate a ischaemic reaction in the exercise test.

Introduction

The opinion on the diagnostic significance of the different types of ST-segment changes for the diagnosis and evaluation of coronary heart disease is not uniform. Commonly, the exercise test was considered positive for ischaemia when ST-segment depression (ST↓) was descending or horizontal (4). This study was undertaken to assess if the ascending ST-segment depression (ST↓) also can indicate ischaemic reaction. Therefore several electrocardiographic criteria of asc. ST↓ were analyzed in comparison with the coronary angiographic findings.

Material and method

The subjects of this retrospective study were 200 patients (pts.), mean age 47 years, 242 men and 38 women. The coronary obstructions observed by coronary angiographic evaluation were classified into three groups: 1. Normal coronary arteries, 2. Haemodynamic not significant stenoses (≤ 50 %), 3. Haemodynamic significant stenoses and total obstructions (> 50 %). The findings of the exercise test were divided into five groups: 1. ST-segment elevation (ST↑) ≥ 0,1 mV, 2. Horizontal or descending ST ↓ ≥0,1 mV, 3. 1. and 2., 4. Only asc. ST↓, 5. No ST-segment changes. The ST↑ or ST↓ was measured 0,08 sec after the J point and only in leads without signs of myocardial infarction. Asc. ST↓ were analyzed using six specific criteria:

1. ST-segment depression 0,08 sec after the J point
   pathological: $\geq$ 0,15 mV (5)

2. a) b)

   Pattern of R- (a) and S-type (b) (5)
   a) slowly asc. ST↓ which crosses the baseline before the beginning of the T-wave
   b) slowly asc. ST↓ not reaching the baseline before the beginning of the T-wave

3. Pattern of asc. ST↓ the ST-ascent considered (8)
   pathological: J point depression at least 0,1 mV the ascent of the ST-segment not more than 1,0 mV/s

4. Pattern of asc. ST↓ in the sec half between beginning of S-wave and peak of T-wave
   1. beginning of S-wave
   2. half between S-wave and peak of T-wave
   3. peak of T-wave
   pathological: ST↓ $\geq$ 0,2 mV (7)

5. QT - ratio (QT_r)

$$QT_r = \frac{QT_a}{QT_c} \qquad QT_c = k \cdot \sqrt{R - R} \qquad k = 0,4$$

   pathological QT_r: $\geq$ 1,07 (3)
   QT_a = actual QT-time
   QT_c = frequence related QT-time

6. QX/QT - ratio
   pathological: $\geq$ 0,5 (3)
   X = crossing point of ST-segment and baseline

Statistical methods

Significant differences were analyzed by Chi-squar test.

Results

In 50 subjects of the investigated 280 pts. the exercise test demonstrated asc. ST↓ . Table 1 presents the results of the analyzed asc. ST↓ using six electrocardiographic criteria. The data have shown significant differences between pts. with ST↓ of S-type and $\geq$0,15 mV 0,08 sec after the J point and those with ST↓ of R-type and $<$0,15 mV 0,08 sec after the J point. Of the 50 pts. six pts. showed an asc. ST↓ in resting ECG. This asc. ST↓ increases in the exercise test at least 0,1 mV when there was observed a pathological coronary angiographic finding. Therefore an asc. ST↓ was considered as a ischaemic reaction (ischaemic-type): (1) ST↓ 0,08 sec after the J point $\geq$ 0,15 mV; (2) slowly asc. ST↓ which does not reach the baseline before beginning of the T-wave (S-type); (3) in the presence of asc. ST↓ at rest, an additonal 0,1 mV of ST↓0,08 sec after the J point. These three criteria having not been fulfilled asc. ST↓ characterized as a normal-type. In comparison with angiographic findings we could find only in one patient a false positive exercise test result. In this patient a small vessel disease diagnosed by myocardial biopsy. False negative electrocardiographic responses occured

Table 1. Correlation of different electrocardiographical criteria of asc. ST↓ with coronary angiographic findings

Electrocardiographical criteria of asc. ST	Normal coronary arteries	Coronarangiogram Haemodynamic not significant stenoses	Haemodynamic significant stenoses/total obstructions	Total	Statistical significance
1. ST↓ 0,08 sec after the J point					
$<$ 0,15 mV	11	3	7	21	significant
$\geq$ 0,15 mV (pathological)	5	4	20	29	$p = 0,05$
2. R-type	9	0	1	10	significant
S-type (pathological)	7	7	26	40	$p = 0,01$
3. ST-ascent in 1 sec					
$>$ 1 mV	14	5	21	40	not
$\leq$ 1 mV (pathological)	2	2	6	10	significant
4. ST↓ in the sec half between beginning of S-wave and peak of T-wave					
$<$ 0,2 mV	15	7	22	44	not
$\geq$ 0,2 mV (pathological)	1	0	5	6	significant
5. QT - ratio					
$<$ 1,07	3	2	6	11	not
$\geq$ 1,07 (pathological)	13	5	21	39	significant
6. QX/QT - ratio					
$<$ 0,5	2	2	1	5	not
$\geq$ 0,5 (pathological)	14	5	26	45	significant

in ten pts.. Seven pts. survieved myocardial infarction. In ten pts. the exercise test must be stopped because of subjective symptoms.

Discussion and conclusions

The diagnostic value of different types of ST↓ is controversial (7). In the own study was shown that asc. ST↓ also ca indicate a ischaemic reaction in the exercise test using the following three electrocardiographic criteria: 1. ST↓ 0,08 sec after the J point ≥ 0,15 mV, 2. S-type: slowly asc. ST↓ reaching the baseline at the beginning of the T-wave, 3. If asc. ST↓ is present in the resting ECG, this asc. ST↓ increases in the exercise test at least 0,1 mV. In 280 pts., application of the exercise test conventional ST criteria gave a sensitivity of 52 % and a specifity of 63 %, using the ischaemic-type of asc. ST↓ as the criterion to evaluation the exercise test sensitivity was 61 % and specifity 60 %. False positive results were found in women but without special frequency in women with only asc. ST↓ in the exercise test (1). There were false negative results in pts. with myocardial infarction or when the test had to be stopped because of subjective symptoms (2, 6).

References

1. Eriksen, J., I. Enge, K. Forfang, O. Storskin: Circulation 54, 371 - 376 (1976)
2. Kattus, A. A.: Amer. J. Cardiol. 33, 721 - 731 (1974)
3. Master, A. M.: Amer. Heart J. 75, 809 - 837 (1968)
4. Pellinen, T.J., K. S. Virtanen, M. Valle, M. H. Frick: Clin. Cardiol. 9, 315 - 322 (1986)
5. Punsar, S., K. Pyörälä, P. Siltanen: Ann. med. int. Fenn. 57, 53 - 63 (1968)
6. Salem, B. I., M. Terasawa, V. S. Mathur, E. Garcia, C. M. De castra, R. J. Hall: Progr. cardiovasc. Dis. 5, 384 - 390 (1978)
7. Schmidt, F. E.: Med. Clinic 69, 1942 - 1950 (1974)
8. Timmis, G. C., D. C. Westveer, S. Gordon R. G. Ramos, V. Gangadharan: J. Electrocardiol. 12, 241 - 248 (1979)

D I A G N O S T I C   O F

M Y O C A R D I A L   I N F A R C T I O N

Effect of infarct location on the incidence of silent myocardial ischemia in patients with transmural myocardial infarction.

MANUELA FIUZA; FRANCISCO CORREIA-JUNIOR; JOSÉ CORREIA and FERNANDO DE PÁDUA.

Cardiology Center - University of Lisbon (LA3), CECP (INSA) and INCP, Lisbon, Portugal

Summary

Eighty nine patients (pts) survivors of first myocardial infarction (MI) were studied by Ambulatory Dynamic ECG, after hospital discharge, in order to study the incidence of silent myocardial ischemia (SMI) according to infarct location. SMI was detected in 13 pts (15%) and was more frequent in single ventricular wall infarction, although it could be found in any location.

Women had more episodes of SMI than men.

SMI presented a circadian variation, being more frequent during sleep hours and first morning hours, that is to say, between 6 and 9 hours a.m.

Purpose of the study

To study the incidence of SMI according to infarct location, in ambulatory patients survivors of acute transmural M.I., after hospital discharge.

Material and methods

Eighty nine ambulatory pts, survivors of a non complicated transmural (Q wave) MI, were studied using 24 hour Ambulatory Dynamic ECG recordings.

Seventy one were male (mean age: 57 ± 10 years) and 18 female (mean age: 63 ± 9 years) Total mean age: 58 ± 10 years.

The infarct location was classified as: inferior (33 pts); anterior (27 pts); combined (29 pts).

All patients presented with regular sinus rhythm and no patient was taking digitalis. Intraventricular conduction disturbances were excluded.

An Avionics 447 recording system with two channels (two pairs of bipolar leads) was employed.

For the 1st channel was used a V5-like position and for the 2nd channel an aVF-like position.

Ischemic episodes were defined as: ST depression ≥ 1 mm at J point and at 80 msec thereafter, for at least 60 seconds.

Results

None of the 89 pts refered symptoms during the 24 hour recording period. Nevertheless in 13 pts, ischemic episodes were detected (15%).

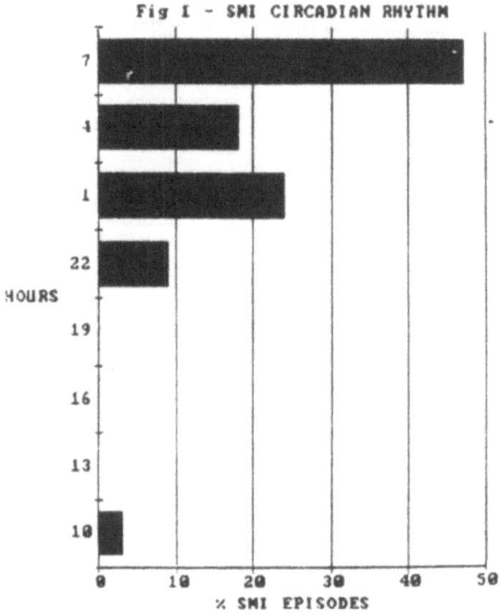
Fig 1 - SMI CIRCADIAN RHYTHM
7
4
1
22
HOURS
19
16
13
10
0
10
20
30
40
50
% SMI EPISODES

Fig 1

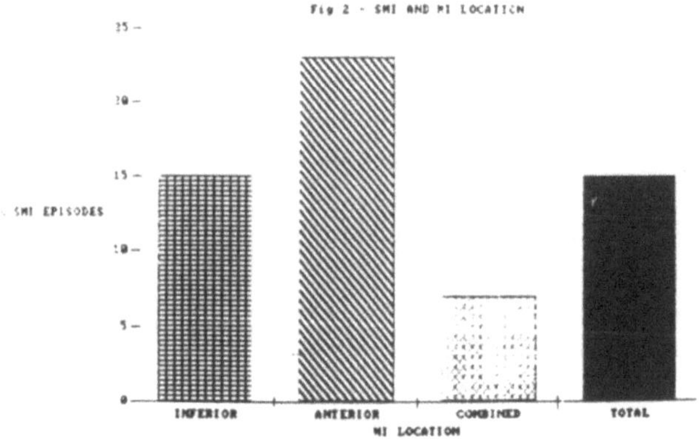
Fig 2 - SMI AND MI LOCATION
15
5
0
SMI EPISODES
INFERIOR
ANTERIOR
COMBINED
TOTAL
MI LOCATION

Fig 2

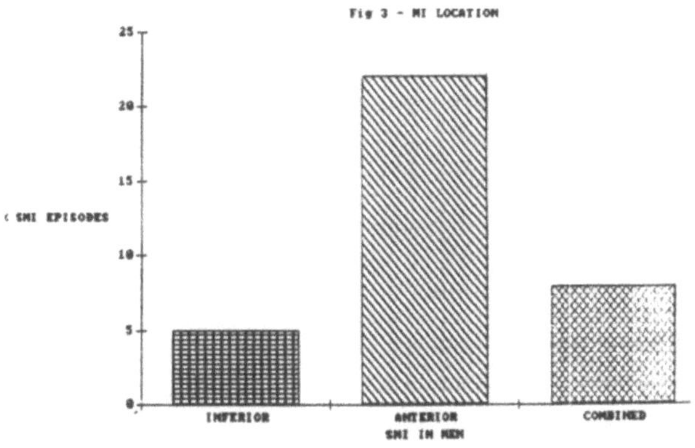

Fig 3

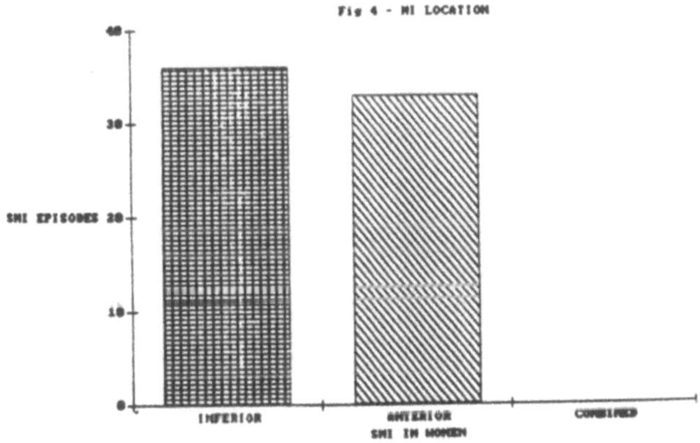

Fig 4

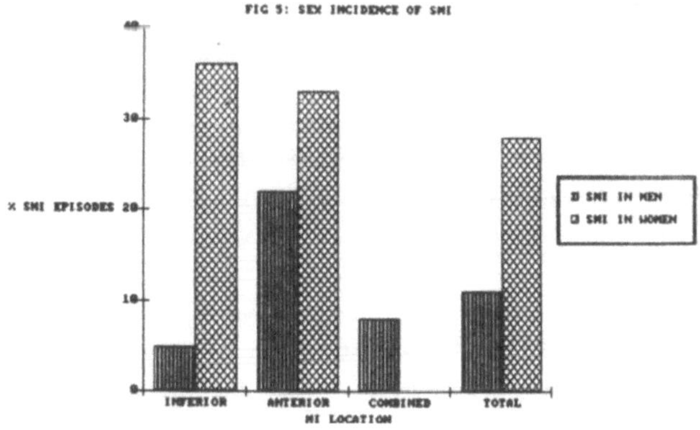

Fig 5

SMI was present almost exclusively during rest time and in particular during sleep, with a peak incidence between 6 and 9 hours a.m, **(fig. 1)**.

No difference was observed between sexes. As far as infarct location is concerned, SMI was detected in every location. However it was more frequent in single ventricular wall than in combined infarctions **(fig. 2)**.

Among men, SMI episodes were more frequent in anterior wall infarction (22%) **(fig. 3)**, while among women they were detected in inferior wall (36%) and anterior wall (33%) and not in combined MI **(fig. 4)**.

When the different incidence of SMI between sexes was studied, women were found to have more episodes than men (28% vs 11%). The difference was significant in inferior MI (36% vs 5%) **(fig. 5)**.

Discussion

There are few studies concerning the incidence of SMI in assymptomatic pts survivors of non complicated MI. Cohn et al (1, 2, 3) estimated the prevalence of SMI in those pts as being around 20-30% (however exercise testing was also included). In our study, using exclusively ambulatory ECG recordings for a period of 24 hours, the prevalance of SMI was 15%.

Interesting enough, the episodes of SMI seem to follow a circadian variation, already mentioned in previous studies (4, 5, 6, 7). In our patients a peak incidence was noticed between 6 and 9 hours a.m., resembling that observed for myocardial infarction and sudden cardiac death. No difference was observed between sexes, possibly because the hormonal influence is overshadowed in these older women post MI. This marked increase in ischemic activity during the first morning hours is of importance and may imply newer schedules for medical treatment.

Women appear to have more episodes of SMI than men, the prevalence in our study being 28% vs 11%. This same difference was also observed in the Framingham study, where unrecognized MI were more frequent in women than in men (35% vs 28%), at all ages (8).

In regard to infarct location, SMI was detected in any location. However it was more frequent in cases of single ventricular wall infarction.

The possibility of spatial cancellation of the electrical potentials in combined infarction can not be excluded.

Conclusions:

In 89 post transmural MI ambulatory patients, SMI was found in 15%.

SMI was more frequent during rest time, with a peak incidence between 6 and 9 hours a.m.. Women were more affected than men, specially in inferior wall infarctions.

SMI must be kept in mind in every post myocardial infarction patient. It may identify a subset of patients at higher risk of another major coronary artery event and/or sudden death. Most probably SMI indicates the need of closer and more aggressive management.

References:

1- Cohn, F. P.: Mod. Conc. Card. Disease 56, 1-5 (1987)

2- Cohn, F. P.: Am. J. Cardiol 59, 3C-6C (1987)

3- Cohn, F. P.: Circulation 75, II-2 (1987)

4- Rocco, D. M.; Nabel, G. E.; Selwyn, A. P.: Am. J. Cardiol. 59, 13C-17C (1987)

5- Rocco, B. M.; Barry, J.; Campbell, S.: Circulation 75, 395-400 (1987)

6- Muller, J. E.; Stone, P. H.; Turi, Z. G. et al: N. E. J. Med. 313, 1315-1322 (1985)

7- Correia-Junior, F.; Fiuza, M.; Correia, J. and Pádua, F. "Ambulatory ST segment changes and related incidence of silent ischemia". J. Electrocardiology 20(1), 1987,75.

8- Kannel, W. B.: Cardiol. Clinics, 4, 583-591 (1986)

Discriminant body surface potential map patterns in anterior and inferior myocardial infarction.

FRED KORNREICH, TERRENCE J. MONTAGUE, MIKHAIL KAVADIAS, JORIS SEGERS, PENTTI M. RAUTAHARJU AND MILAN B. HORACEK.

Unit for Cardiovascular Research and Engineering, Free University Brussels (VUB), Brussels, Belgium.

SUMMARY

Sequential body surface potential maps from 236 normal subjects, 114 patients with anterior myocardial infarction and 144 patients with inferior myocardial infarction (MI) were expressed as linear combinations of 12 orthonormal map distributions (basis maps), producing expansion coefficients associating each map with the respective basis maps at each instant. Corresponding time-varying coefficients were averaged over the normal, anterior MI and inferior MI groups, respectively. By subtracting normal coefficient waveforms in turn from corresponding anterior and inferior MI waveforms and standardizing the resulting differences, discriminant instants and features were identified. The anterior MI group was characterized by loss of potentials in the anterior torso during the first part of QRS and the late portion of T; in the inferior MI group, loss of potentials was observed in the inferior right anterior chest and lower left flank at mid- and late QRS and in late T.

INTRODUCTION

Statistical analysis of body surface potential maps (BSPM) requires considerable reduction of the amount of data generated by the recording of over 100 surface ECG signals. Several strategies for achieving data-reduction have been developed and have resulted in:

- the reduction of the number of leads for optimal signal representation (1, 2)
- the reduction of the number of leads for optimal diagnostic information (3)
- the compression of BSPM data along temporal and/or spatial basis patterns (4, 5, 6).

The present study aims at assessing quantitatively and in a compact form, characteristic map distributions in anterior MI (AMI) and inferior MI (IMI).

MATERIAL AND METHODS

BSPM were recorded from 120 electrode sites in 236 normal subjects (N) and 258 patients with initial evidence of AMI (114 patients) or IMI (144 patients). QRS and ST-T waveforms were time-normalized separately and represented by 70 and 180 points, respectively. In each patients, maps at each instant were represented as a linear combination of 12 orthonormal map distributions (basis maps) previously computed from maps of the entire study population .

Corresponding expansion coefficients from each instant in each individual were averaged over the N, AMI and IMI groups respectively, yielding 12 group-mean time-functions (coefficient waveforms); each function represents for the population, the time-varying amount of a particular basis distribution.

By subtracting from AMI and IMI corresponding N coefficient waveforms and dividing the resulting differences by the standard deviations of the population considered for each bigroup comparison, statistically significant differences were demonstrated. Discriminant analysis was also performed in order to separate AMI and IMI patients from N, using expansion coefficients as variables.

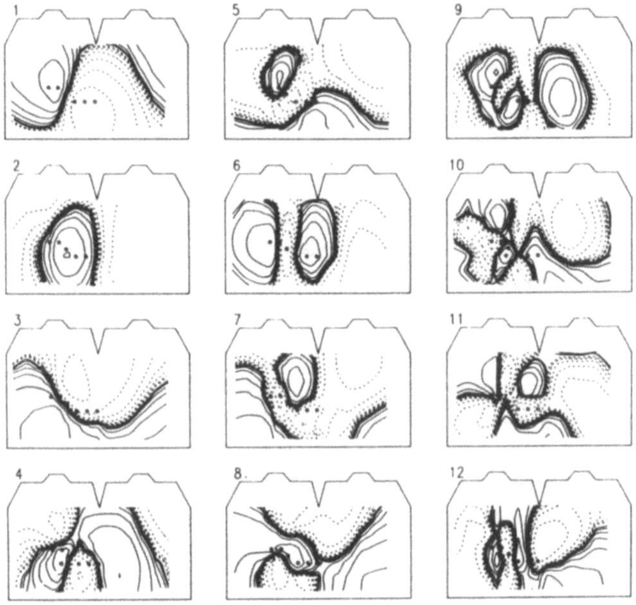

Figure 1. *The first 12 basis maps (numbered from 1 to 12 in decreasing order of eigenvalue amplitude) are represented.*

RESULTS

Figure 1 depicts the first 12 basis maps, accounting for 99% of the total available signal information: each map in each individual is represented as a linear combination of these 12 common basis distributions. Only the expansion coefficients vary from instant to instant and from subject to subject; as such they can be used in discriminant analysis as measurements univocally characterizing each individual.

Figure 2 shows the 2 best discriminant features in maps from the AMI population. In the upper row, the map pattern representing mainly left hemithorax positivity is present in increasing amounts throughout the first half of QRS in N while it is affected with a negative coefficient in AMI during the entire QRS duration. At the time of peak difference between coefficient waveforms of N and AMI, the actual maps show a positive potential distribution over the left hemithorax and the inferior anterior border of the chest in N and a negative voltage distribution covering practically the entire anterior torso in AMI. The lower row represents another discriminant pattern peaking in early QRS and corresponding to the loss of potentials in the upper left precordium in AMI.

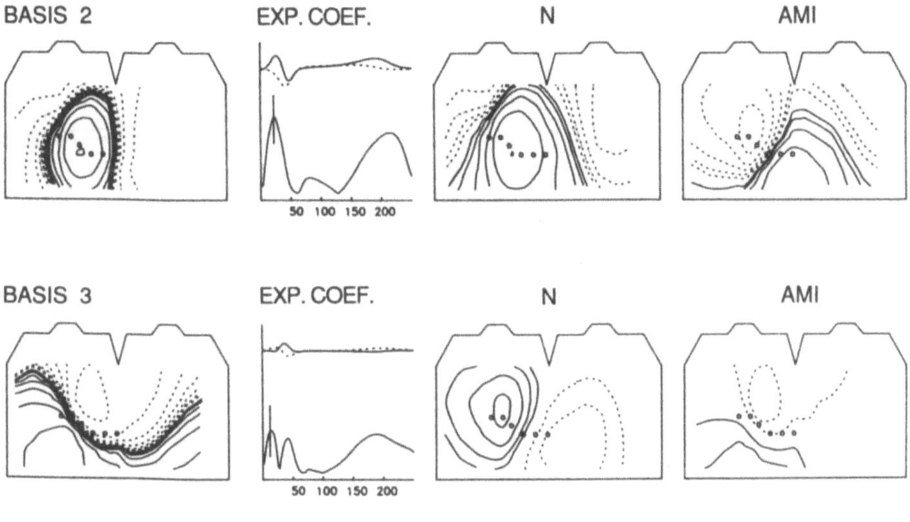

Figure 2. *Upper row: left: basis map 2; middle: group-mean coefficient waveforms superimposed for N and AMI with the time-varying discriminant capability at the bottom (standardized difference); right: group-mean N and AMI maps at instant corresponding to peak discrimination.*
Lower row: left: basis map 3; middle: group-mean coefficient waveforms and discriminant curve; right: N and AMI maps at instant of peak discrimination.
Contour lines are drawn at the following μV values: ±20, 40, 80, 160, 320, 640, 1280. Solid lines: positive voltages; dotted lines: negative voltages.

Figure 3 illustrates the 2 best discriminant features in maps from the IMI population. The upper row shows the varying amounts of the bipolar distribution present in the first basis map. In N, large negative quantities of that pattern (negative coefficient) result in prominent positive voltages for T in the left hemithorax and negative T voltages in the upper right anterior torso and most of the back; in IMI, the anterior T potentials are of lower magnitude and only very small negative T voltages are noticed elsewhere. The lower row depicts another discriminant pattern in IMI: while the entire inferior border around the thorax remains positive in N during the middle part of QRS, it becomes negative in the right hemithorax and in the back in IMI; reciprocal positivities are also observed in the upper left precordial region.

Stepwise discriminant analysis was performed in order to separate AMI and IMI patients from N. Using 6 expansion coefficients for each bigroup comparison (AMI vs N and IMI vs N) and keeping the specificity at 95%, 96% of AMI and 93% of IMI were correctly classified.

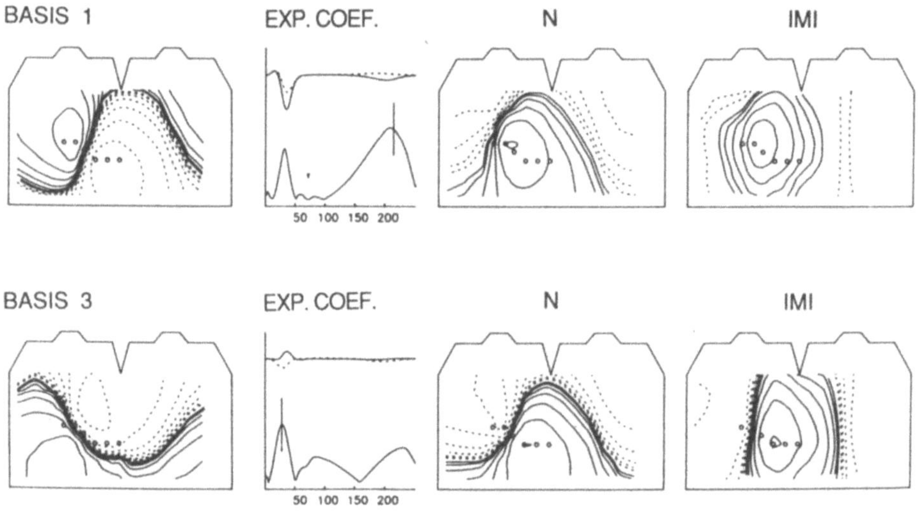

Figure 3. *Upper row: left: basis map 1; middle: group-mean coefficient waveforms for N and IMI and discriminant curve; right: N and IMI maps at instant of peak discrimination. Lower row: left: basis map 3; middle: coefficient and discriminant waveforms for N and IMI; right: actual N and IMI maps at selected instant.*

CONCLUSION

The expansion of complex BSPM distributions into various amounts of common building blocks permits data-reduction and quantification of individual map patterns; this approach is therefore well suited for statistical analysis. It can also help interpret maps in terms of underlying electrophysiological events by pinpointing those features that are significantly different from normal in particular diagnostic entities. The use of expansion coefficients together with their associated map distributions allows identification of sites and instants of loss of potentials in AMI and IMI. Used as parameters for discriminant purposes, they achieve very high rates of correct classification.

REFERENCES

(1) Barr RC, Spach MS, Herman-Giddens GS. : IEEE Trans Biomed Eng, 18, 125-138 (1971)
(2) Lux RL et al. : Circulation 2 , 356 - 363 (1979)
(3) Kornreich F et al.: Am. J. Cardiol. 58 , 863 - 871 (1986)
(4) Uijen GJH, Heringa A, Van Oosterom A. : IEEE Trans Biomed Eng, 31, 706 -714 (1984)
(5) Lux RL et al. : Circ. Res. 49 , 186 - 196 (1981)
(6) Evans AK et al.: Circ. Res. 49 , 197 - 203 (1981)

Correlation of myocardial infarction development character and disturbances of coronary blood flow

YA.S.VASILTSEV, I.V.MAXIMOV, V.I.VARVARENKO, V.A.MARKOV, A.L.KRYLOV

Tyumen Branch of All-Union Cardiology Research Center, USSR

Summary

The dynamics of myocardial necrosis focus development was studied in 40 patients suffering from transmural anterior MI with the help of precardial mapping (PM) of ECG (35 leads), serial determination of CPK activity and myoglobin (MG) concentration in blood serum. Fourteen patients underwent selective coronarography. The determined two types of MI final size formation depended upon the manifestation and dynamics of coronary blood flow disturbance.

Introduction

As the focus of ischemic affection of myocardium arises, its characteristic feature is the natural dynamics of development, demonstrating the evolution of ischemic pain into necrosis with the following transition to reparative processes of the affected myocardium. A number of factors both of coronarogeneous and noncoronarogeneous nature may influence the dynamics of myocardial infarction (MI) focus development. The purpose of the investigation was to study coronarogeneous factors (occlusion of coronary artery (CA) or its subtotal stenosis) influencing the MI focus development.

Material and methods

The dynamics of myocardial necrosis focus development was studied in 40 patients suffering from transmural anterior MI. They were examined with the help of PM of ECG, serial determination of CPK activity and MG concentration in blood serum. In the period of acute MI 14 of the 40 patients underwent coronarographic examination. To determine the dynamics of myocardial necrosis focus formation we analyzed the time of peak value achievement of the indices PM (nQS-index, the total area of the waves R, Q and QS complexes (ΣSR, ΣSQQS), CPK activity, MG concentration and the rate of their change.

Results

The evaluation of dynamics of MI focus formation showed that it is different in the cases with the examined patients. A rapid type of MI focus formation was observed in 25 patients. The shortest development time was characteristic of this type according to the data of PM for nQS 9,0 ± 0,5 h, ΣSR 10,7 ± 1,0 h, ΣSQQS 10,7 ± 0,6 h; according to the data of serial CPK activity analysis 14,6 ± 1,2 h, MG concentra - tion 6,8 ± 0,5 h. In 15 cases a delayed type of MI focus formation that unlike the rapid type had the development time according to the same data, was determined: for nQS 22,3 ± 1,7 h, ΣSR 21,1 ± 2,0 h, ΣSQQS 22,0 ± 1,9 h; MG 10,8 ± 0,7 h ($P < 0{,}001$) and CPK 22,8 ± 2,0 h (Fig.1). Provided these groups of patients had no differences in the value of cartographic and biochemical markers of necrosis between the types of rapid and delayed MI focus formation there were differences in the rate of indices change: nQS 1,67 ± 0,2 vs 0,8 ± 0,1 cartographic units/hour (CU/h) ($P < 0{,}001$), ΣSR 18,0 ± 3,6 vs 7,0 ± 1,7 mm^2/h ($P < 0{,}01$) (Fig.2); MG concentration 113,8 - 12,5 vs 60,8 ± 2,0 ng/l/h ($P < 0{,}01$) respectively (Fig.3).

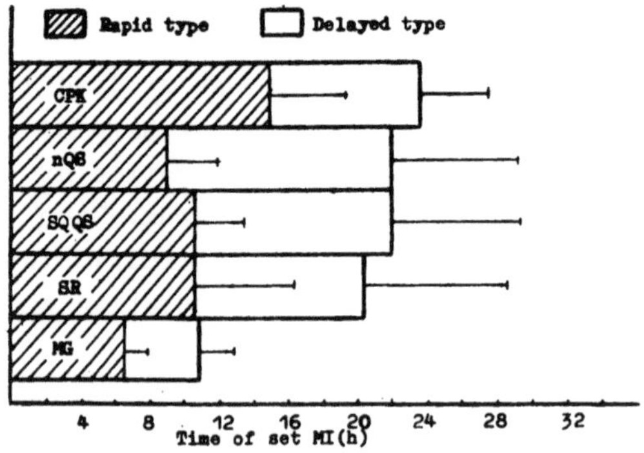

Fig.1. Time of peak value achievement of the indices CPK, MG, nQS, ΣSQQS, ΣSR at different types of MI formation.

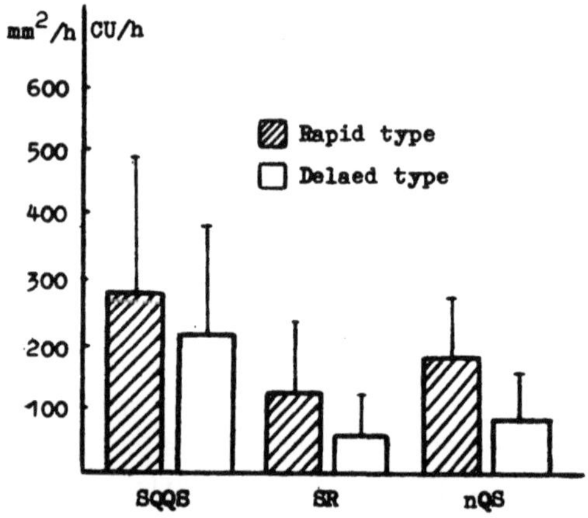

Fig.2. The rate of PM indices change at different types of MI formation.

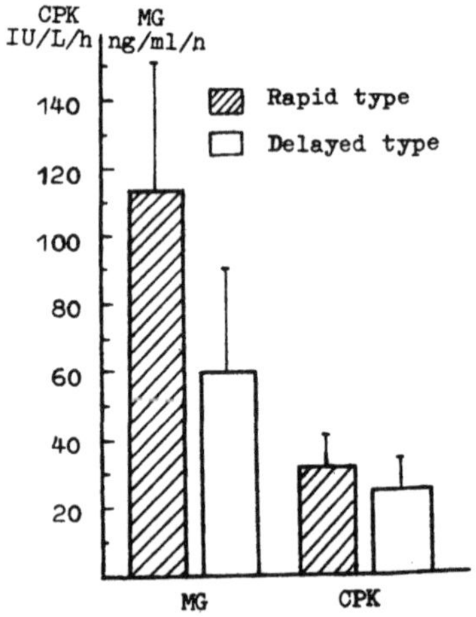

Fig.3. The rate of CPK and MG concentration change at different types of MI formation.

In 27,3% of cases episodes of MI recidivities were revealed. The re - curring course was observed 3 times as frequent (47% vs 16%) in the group of patients with a delayed type of MI necrosis focus formation. The comparison of coronarographic examination data with those of MI focus development demonstrated that 5 (71,4%) of 7 patients suffering from subtotal CA stenosis had a delayed type of necrosis focus formation and the same number of patients manifested episodes of MI recurring. Five of 7 patients having CA occlusion showed a delayed type of necrosis focus formation. To evaluate the degree of relation of manifestation of coronarographic features (occlusion, subtotal CA stenosis) and those characterizing the necrosis focus forming type (rapid or delayed) we determined the correlation coefficient between them by using the Baies hypothesis formula. The analysis revealed a considerable correlational dependence between the above mentioned features (r=0,452), that creates the necessary prerequisites for solving the problems of prognosis by using the evaluation of coronary blood state according to the data of indirect control methods over the MI focus development. Thus, the type of myocardial necrosis focus formation (rapid or delayed) and the character of its following dynamics depended on those of coronary blood flow disturbances: the presence of occlusion or subtotal stenosis, recanalization or reocclusion of CA.

Discussion and conclusions

According to the angiographic data the marked residual stenosis of CA observed in the majority of patients with MI was combined with a delayed formation of the final MI size after the thrombolysis by means of intracoronary streptokinase infusion (1,2,3,4). Such a stenosis may become "critical" as a result of vascular tonus alternation (5) and cause the necrosis of some extra myocardial areas even when the patient is at rest. This fact is also related to a considerable sensitivity increase of vascular smooth musculation and to various influences in the points of their atherosclerotic injury (stenosis). Besides that, a dynamic variability of artery lumen in the point of its atherosclerotic injury caused now by the initial thrombosis formation, now by its spontaneous thrombolysis may also be important (6). The data obtained give us the grounds to find the optimum treatment of patients having MI with different types of its formation.

The type (rapid or delayed) of the final MI size formation primarily depends upon the manifestation degree of coronary blood flow decrease in a certain area (occlusions, reocclusions, subtotal stenoses of coronary artery). Recurrence episodes of MI are observed in the majority of patients with a delayed type of necrosis formation.

References

(1) Merx W. et al. Amer. Heart J. 102, 1181-1187 (1981)
(2) Ganz W. et al. Amer. J. Cardiol. 53, 1209-1216 (1984)
(3) Schmutzler H. et al. Herz, N 1, 1-8 (1986)
(4) Vasiltsev Ya. et al. Ter. Arkh., N 11, 108-112 (1986)
(5) Raffenbeul W., Lichtlen P.Z. Kardiol., 71, 439-444 (1982)
(6) Feiter P. et al. Circulation, 67, 1039-1043 (1983)

Contribution of the on-line computer ECG mapping to the rapid diagnostics of myocardial infarction size and localization.

SLAVOMÍRA FILIPOVÁ, STANISLAV CAGÁŇ

Department of Internal Medicine, School of Medicine, Komensky University, Bratislava, Czechoslovakia

Introduction.

The surface electrocardiographic mapping has given the possibility to study of cardioelectric field changes caused the focal abnormalities in various regions of atrial and ventricular myocardium. In presence of ischemic heart disease this method has the importance for clinical purposes only if it has given the rapid information about the locality and the size of ischemic process and about the time factor of its origin.

The aim of presented study has been the elaboration of the rapid clinical procedure for the evaluation of myocardial infarction size and localization with the microcomputer system.

Material and methods.

The computer system for the surface ECG mapping KARDIO-SMEP 01.0 (figure 1) has been developed in the collaboration with the Research Institute of Computer Technique and Slovac Faculty of Technology. It has enabled the simultaneous recording from 34 leads and on-line data processing in several elected regimes, that the doctor has gained the colour map information on the display and printer immediately after examination of pacient.

We have examined 82 pacients: a- with the acute myocardial infarction (M.I.) of various placements; b- with the old M.I.; c- the M.I. accompanied with intraventricular pathway disturbances (bundle branch blocks, preexcitation).

We have used the own normal data of cardioelectric field distribution during the ventricular depolarization and repolarization (Filipová, Cagáň, 1986) and the informative division of the body surface into areas according to Toyama and co-workers (1982).

Results.

In the figure 2 are placed the maps of pacient with the acute M.I. The infarction lesion has been located at the inferior apical wall, inferior wall of the left and right ventricle (19.5 ms of QRS). For the purpose to analyze the acute phase of myocardial infarction we have studied the repolarization maps, too. At the peak T wave map the abnormal negative area covered almost the same region as in the early QRS period.

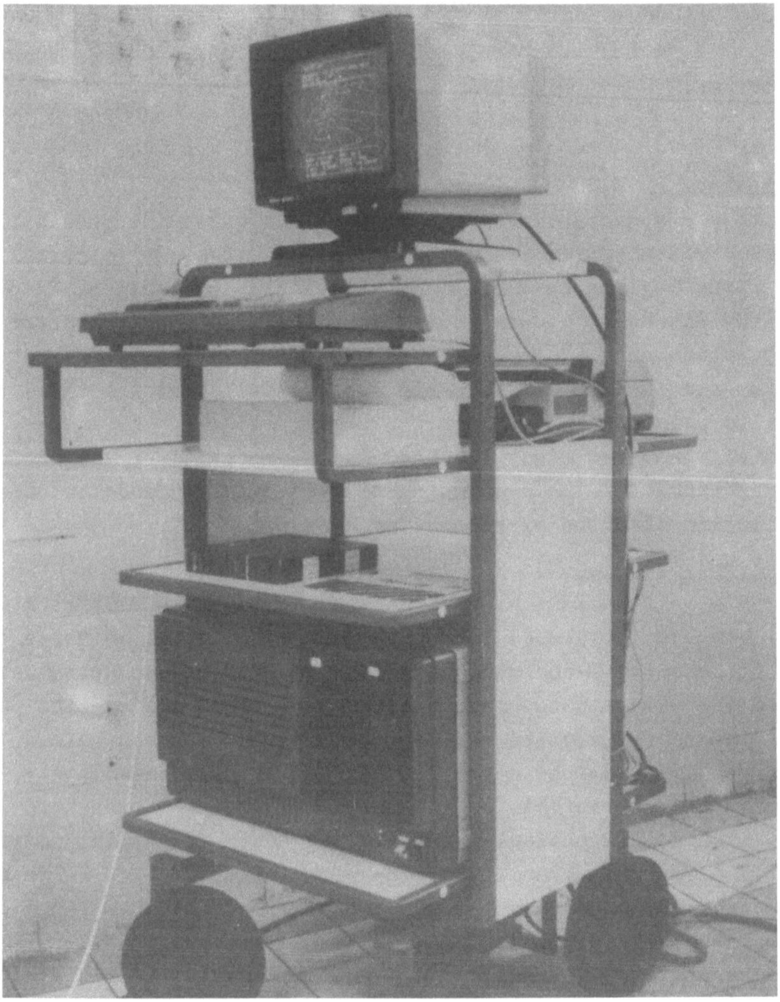

Fig. 1

Photograph of the colour display system of the body surface ECG-mapping KARDIO-SMEP 01.0 with the line printer.

In the figure 3 it is demonstrated the map at 10.5 ms QRS of patient with the history of 3 myocardial infarctions (inferior, anterolateral and inferior reinfarction) and with the development of CLBBB during the third coronary acute lesion. On the basis of 12-lead ECG it was not possible to evaluate the anterosepta M.I. With

M6-
ac.M.I.

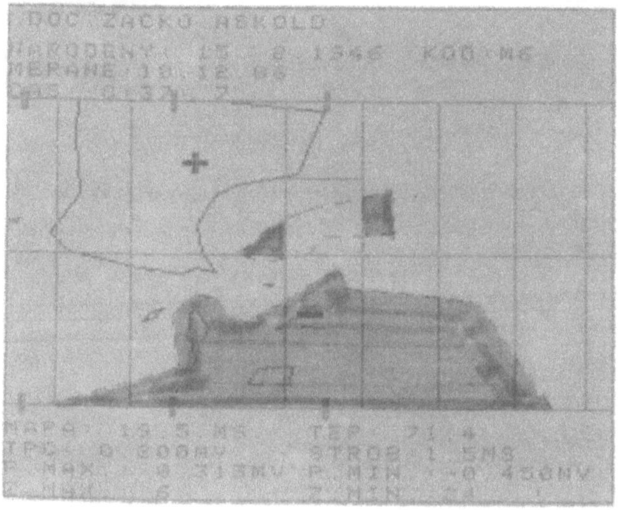

19.5 ms QRS

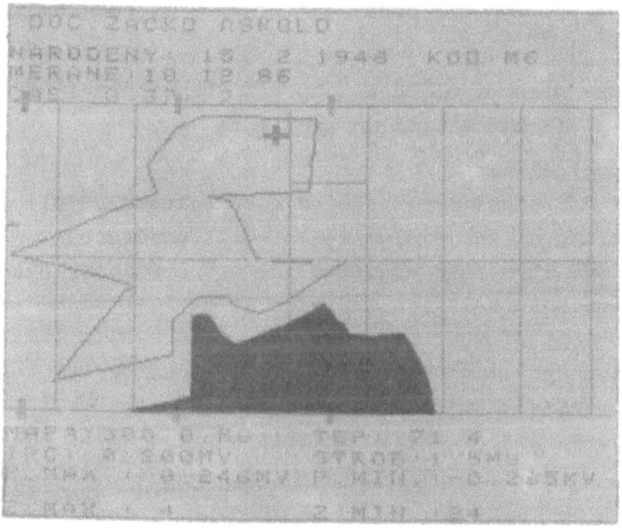

300.0 ms T

Fig. 2

Pacient M6 (40 yrs old) with the acute M.I. Maps of 19.5 ms QRS complex and of the peak of T wave. The abnormal negative potential regions are indicated.

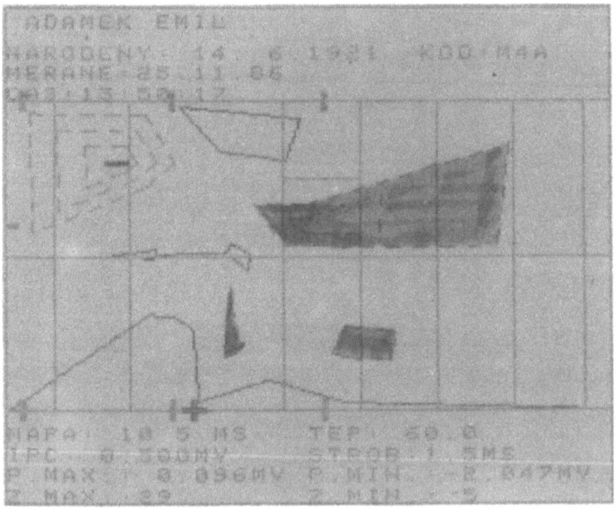

M4A
CLBBB
+
3 OLD M.I.s

10.5 ms QRS

Fig. 3

Patient M4A (65 yrs old) with the CLBBB and after 3 myocardial infarctions during the last 7 years of life.

the ECG mapping by the side of CLBBB we can see the abnormal negative regions belonged to 3 old myocardial infarctions.

Discussion and conclusions.

We have found out the significant concordance between results of 12-lead ECG and ECG mapping at the evaluation of M.I. presence and localization. The surface ECG maps have acquired the extraordinary significance, when the other ECG abnormalities are present at 12-lead ECG, which complainted of assessment of M.I. lesions. This method with the utilization of computerized system of recording and evaluation has indicated clinically noninvasive advantageous procedure for the rapid assessment of character and extent of cardioelectric surface field abnormalities.

References.

(1) Filipová,S., Cagáň, S.: Vnitř.Lék. 32, 1162-1172 (1986)
(2) Toyama, S. et al.: J.Electrocardiol. 15, 241-248 (1982)

VCG semi-quantitative evaluation of infarcted area in the acute phase of MI and after 6 months of follow-up: clinical and prognostic correlations.

PALMIERI M., GOTTI G., ZILIO G., CATTARINI G., MORATTI P.

Servizio di Cardiologia e CCU - Ospedale Provinciale Monfalcone (Italy)

Summary

In order to check the evolution of infarcted area, 28 pts who entered the CCU within 4 hours after onset of symptoms of MI underwent repeated Frank-VCG recordings: every 6 hours for 48 hours; then every 12 hours up to discharge from CCU, after 6 months of follow-up. The electric forces of QRS (time of onset, voltage and spatial position) were evaluated with the method of integrated score of trapetium area, and compared with the Peel Index (P.I.) and the CPK release curve. After 6 months of follow-up two groups of pts were recognized: group A: 14 pts(50%) aged 49-81(mean 62.2), P.I. 3-14(mean 7.5), 7 of them(50%) treated with i.v. Streptokinase (SK:1.500.000 I.U.), presented VCG modifications suggestive of partial reduction of the previously evaluated infarcted area. Group B: 14 pts(50%), aged 45-80(mean 58.6), P.I. 3-14(mean 10.5), 8 (57.1%) treated with SK, in whom a progressive loss of electric forces in the infarcted area was observed. The acute clinical course was better in Group A pts as reflected by the P.I.; and after one year of follow-up clinical events as post-MI angina, congestive heart failure (CHF) and re-infarction occurred in 5 out of 14 (33.3%) pts of Group A and in 10 out 14(66.6%)pts of Group B. Conclusions: the Frank-VCG seems to be a useful diagnostic and prognostic tool in the evaluation of the infarcted area, in the acute phase and during the clinical course of MI.

Introduction

VCG examination has been utilized as a simple, reliable, non-invasive procedure in the early diagnosis of MI, especially when ECG findings are questionable in presence of non-transmural myocardial infarction, intraventricular conduction disturbances(IVCDs) as CLBBB, RBBB associated with left anterior-or posterior fascicular block, or when the necrotic area is localized in the terminal part of QRS (1,2,3). Another important field of application of the VCG is the monitoring of the infarcted pt in order to perform a semiquantitative assessment of the infarcted area (4,5). VCG has demonstrated a good correlation with the events of ventricular activation and the spread of electric potentials on the body surface. The electric field of the heart generates a complex distribution of potentials on the surface areas and these electromotive forces are reduced to tree equipotential ortoghonal leads in the spatial VCG. The magnitude and the temporo - spatial orientation of these forces depend upon the site of the activated area in that instant. When myocardial ischemia causes a loss of viable myocardium, this results in an important shift of vectorial forces from the inert zone to a direction opposite to that of the MI. The monitoring of the S-T and QRS changes in the acute phase of MI allows the progressive evaluation of the reversible injury and the extent of myocardial cell death characterized by irreversible damage(6,7). The aim of this study has been to check the acute phase of MI for an indirect semi-quantitative evaluation of the myocardial cell loss resulting in an im portant shift of QRS vectors recorded in the Frank VCG.At the same time,the total CPK release curve has been performed in subsequent times,and correlations have been researched between these two parameters of myocar - dial cell damage and the Peel Index (P.I.) values,considered of prognostic importance in the acute stage of MI.The follow-up at 6 months permitted some clinical and technical considerations upon the evolution of MI as reflected by the VCG and the clinical status of pts.

Material and methods

28 pts admitted in the CCU within 4 hours after onset of symptoms of MI undewent repeated recordings of VCG and blood samples for the total CPK release curve (see Table 1).

Table 1 N. PTS 28 MEN:24(85,7%) WOMEN:4(14,3%)

Age range: 42-81 (mean 59,7)

These patients were classified as follows:
- INFERIOR MI: 13 pts;
- ANTERIOR MI: 13 pts;
- INFERO-ANTERIOR MI: 1 pt;
- NON-TRANSMURAL MI: 1 pt.

The selection excluded other pts not meeting the following criteria: 1)coronary time lower than 4 hours after onset of symptoms(mean 2.24 ± 1.10);2)No previous history or past ECG signs of MI,along with the absence of previous or subsequent IVCDs and intra-infarction blocks causing a prolongation of QRS superior to 0,80 ms;3)ECG recordings lacking Q necrotic waves.Entering the CCU the ECGs and VCGs were recorded and blood samples drawn for total CPK determinations. The monitoring of these parameters comprised one check every 6 hrs for the first 48 hours;and then,every 12 hours up to the discharge of pts from CCU to a sub-intensive area (50-100 hours).After 6 months from the acute episode,all pts were evaluated for clinical and VCG investigation in our out-patient clinic.The complete history of pts and the follow-up data were taken by direct inquiry and by talks with the family phisicians.

Analysis of data. In all VCGs the voltage of QRS vectors has been measured every 2,5 ms in each planar loop, in order to obtain the projection of the electromotive forces in the orthogonal leads X, Y, Z, in that very instant. The electrical forces of QRS (time of onset,voltage,spatial position)were plotted as a function of time and evaluated by the method of integrated score of trapetium area,according to the formula:

$$\int_a^b f(x)\,dx = dx/2\ (y0 + 2y1 + 2y2 \ldots\ldots + 2y_{n-1} + y_n)$$

In the VCG procedure,when dx is considered the time unit 0,10 ms,the formula is simplified in the sum of the vectorial voltages in single instants,that is: $A=(V_1+V_2+\ldots\ldots V_n)$ ms · mV

The square root of the 3 areas obtained for X, Y, Z, results in the spatial deviation of vectors according to the following: $\sqrt{dx^2 + dy^2 + dz^2}$

The modifications in the area variations have been changed in percent indices of variation,according to :

$$(Ai - Af/Ai) \cdot 100$$

The absolute and percent values of these data have been matched with the total CPK Max and the Peel Index respectively,as this index is considered the more reliable and comparable among others.The confrontation differences were obtained by registration in the hyperacute phase of MI,those performed at discharge from CCU and after 6 months of follow-up:the first being chosen as reference and the others vectorially subtracted from this to obtain the "QRS vector difference".

Results

The confrontation of the spatial position of QRS in the second stage of MI with respect to the spatial orientation in the hyperacute phase not only demonstrates a 100% shift in a direction opposite to that of the infarcted area,but furthermore,shows important shiftings of the VCG forces even though not evident in the standard ECG.For example:

1) 2 pts out of 13 with inferior MI had an important forward shift of QRS even if an overt necrosis of the posterior wall was not evident in the standard ECG.Other 3 pts of them presented an important deviation to the right without the evidence of RBBB.
2) In pts with anterior wall MI was especially noteworty the upward shift of QRS in 8 out of 13,frequently realizing a trans-septal picture of MI.

In both groups of pts a leftward shift of QRS was noted in 8 cases of evident left ventricle enlargement with congestive heart failure (CHF).In the acute phase of MI a regression curve has been built regarding the confrontation of QRS vectorial variation and the P.I., as demonstration of the close correlation between the percent variation of spatial vectors and the P.I. values (coefficient of correlation : r=0.5).Another significant correlation has been found comparing total CPK Max curve and the absolute values of the area shifting in the VCG recorded in the subacute phase of MI (r=0.7).

Follow-up: the comparison of the VCG findings after 6 months of follow-up allowed the recognition of two groups of pts: Group A: 14 pts (50%),aged 49-81(mean 62.2),P.I. 3-14 (mean 7.5),7 of them (50%) treated with i.v. Streptokinase (SK) 1.500.000 I.U., presented VCG modifications suggestive for a partial reduction of the previously evaluated infarcted area.The site of the MI in these pts was: Inferior in 8 pts,Antero-septal in 4,Antero-lateral in 1,Non-transmural in 1. Group B: 14 pts(50%),aged 45-80(mean 58,6),P.I. 3-14 (mean 10,5),superior 38.6% with respect to P.I. of the group A, 8 of whom (57,1%) treated with i.v. SK, in whom a progressive loss of electric forces was observed.After one year of follow-up important clinical events as post-MI angina, congestive heart failure (CHF), and re-infarction occurred in 5 out of 14 (33.3%) pts of Group A;and in 10 out 14 (66.6%) pts of Group B.

Discussion and conclusions

After the evaluation of our data in the acute phase and after the follow-up period of the MI,these comments can be made. The timed recording of VCG spatial variation of QRS in the acute stage of MI allows a useful and reliable monitoring of the progressive modifications of the infarcted zone and the ischemic area with their possible variations under several therapeutic interventions.In most cases,the initial spatial shift of the QRS forces obviously recorded in the VCG is not apparent in the standard ECG.These results are particularly important as close correlations have been found between "QRS vector difference" subtractions and the prognostic Index of Peel,as well as, with the total CPK Max. The P.I. being considered a reliable prognostic tool and the evidence of high CPK values a very important parameter playing for the extension of the infarcted area (5,7,8,9).

From the prognostic point of view,the same considerations can be made after the follow-up period of the two groups of pts taken into consideration. In fact,even though the number of pts is not so high to permit a complete poliparametric statistical study,there is clear evidence that at distance,pts with high P.I. values in the acute stage more frequently present a further trend of vectors shifts suggestive for the expan sion of the infarcted area;and along with a worse acute clinical course they present more frequently an in cidence of major complications,as CHF,post-MI angina,re-infarction. On the contrary,the other group presents better VCG findings and P.I. values during the acute MI,and subsequently a minor incidence of clinical complications and a trend of a VCG reduction of the previously evaluated infarcted area. Even if the mechanism of this finding remains as yet speculative,its clinical interest cannot be overlooked,especially when the prognostic formulation of the pt is considered.From this point of view,the informations given by the VCG may be considered of rilevant importance as other non-invasive procedures (scintigraphy,ECO-2D)for the diagnostic and prognostic assessment of pts in the acute stage of MI(4,5,6,10).

In conclusion,even if our data must be supported by a larger number of pts undergoing the same study protocol and a coronary angiography, we can summarize the followings:

1) The evolution of VCG data in the acute phase of MI permits the monitoring of the infarcted area and of the ischemic lesion at risk for necrosis, with its implications for the prognosis and the observation of the therapeutic interventions to reduce the necrotic area.
2) When the site and evolution of MI are concerned, the VCG data are sufficiently comparable with those of myocardial scintigraphy and ECO-2D (4,5,6,10),because the shift of the QRS forces in the subsequently recorded VCGs represent a semi-quantitative evaluation of the anatomic lesion and correspond to the clinical manifestations of the pts.
3) Even if not always a coronary angiography has been performed in our pts,a strong correlation was demonstrated between QRS vectors amplitude variation,the absolute total CPK samples and the P.I. values for an indirect semi-quantitative evaluation of the infarcted area.

References

(1) Palmieri,M.,G.Gotti,L.Borgioni,P.Moratti,R.Chiozza,MT.DellaMea,G.Zilio,R.Magris,E.Barducci: Proceedings XIth Int.Congr.Electrocardiol., 285-287 (1984)

(2) Palmieri,M.,G.Gotti,L.Borgioni,P.Moratti,R.Chiozza,MT.DellaMea,G.Zilio,R.Magris,E.Barducci: Proceedings XIth Int.Congr.Electrocardiol., 347-349 (1984)

(3) Polu,J.M.,J.M.Gilgenkrantz,G.Faivre: Arch.Mal.Coeur, 9, 1041-1044 (1972)

(4) Wickline S.A.,J.J.McNamara: Circulation, 57, 910-920 (1978)

(5) Sederholm,M.,P.Grøttum,L.Erhardt,J.Kjekshus: Circulation, 68, 1006-1011 (1983)

(6) Wikswo,J.P.Jr.,S.C.Gundersen,W.Murphy,A.K.Dawson,R.F.Smith: Circul.Research, 49, 1055-1062 (1981)

(7) Bleifeld,W.,D.Mathey,P.Hanrath,H.Buss,S.Effert: Circulation, 55, 303-311 (1977)

(8) Grøttum,P.,J.K.Kjekshus: J. Electrocardiol., 19, 337-346 (1986)

(9) Kronenberg,M.W.,M.Hodges,T.Akiyama,D.L.Roberts,D.Ehrich,L.Biddle,P.Nyu: Circulation, 54, 756-761 (1976)

(10) Piccolo,E.,P.Delise,G.Zuin,A.Bonso,S.Romano,V.Ricciardiello,D.Fischer,F.Tani,C.Forleo,V.Portulano,L.Tini Brunozzi,L.Meniconi: G. Ital. Cardiol., 17, 57-62 (1987)

ECG Patterns in Subjects with Self-Reported Old Myocardial Infarctions
Results from a Cross-Sectional Population Study

PERZ, S., GEHRING, J.*, PÖPPL, S.J., STIEBER, J.

GSF - MEDIS Institute, D-8042 Neuherberg, FRG
*Klinik Höhenried for Cardiovascular Diseases,
D-8139 Bernried, FRG

Agreement of self-reported old myocardial infarctions (MI) with ECG signs of MI was analysed comparing the questionnaire information derived from 4003 participants of the Monica Augsburg Survey (cross-sectional population study of a random sample of 5312 citizens aged 25-64) with the results of computer-processed twelve lead resting ECG reviewed by a cardiologist. The rate of self-reported positive MI beeing simultaneously reported as confirmed by a physician was 2.9 % (59/2014) in men and 0.9 % (14/1489) in women respectively. 68 % (50/73) of those with self-reported MI declared, that their MI was treated in a hospital; 30 % (22/73) declared, that they suffered from more than one MI. The average time interval between the latest MI event and the date of the Monica data collection was 7 years (s=5.7). Depending on the ECG criteria used, percentages of MI signs ranged from 1.6 % (32/ 2014) - 7.4 % (150/2014) in men and 0.2 % (3/1989) - 4.6 % (92/1989) in women.
Only 46 % (27/59) of all males and 29 % (4/14) of all females with self-reported MI showed any ECG signs of MI. On the other hand 58 % (18/31) of the men and all women (n=3) with ECG signs characteristic of MI were unaware of any MI. Sex and hospitalization were found to be factors affecting significantly the ECG evidence of self-reported MI.
Conclusion: The majority of subjects with self-reported MI did not show any MI signs in the ECG; on the other hand the majority of those with ECG signs characteristic of MI were unaware of MI.

Introduction

It is well-known that myocardial infarctions (MI) may occur in the absence of symptoms /1/. This phenomenon labelled as silent MI is receiving considerable attention as a factor with prognostic significance due to increased mortality risk /2/. According to the absence of symptoms silent myocardial infarction may be detected by a routinely taken electrocardiogram (ECG). On the other hand MI may occur without any typical ECG changes because of the limited sensitivity of the ECG. Agreement of self-reported old MI with ECG signs of MI was analysed using the data of the First MONICA Augsburg Survey, a cross-sectional population study, which is part of the multinational WHO-MONICA Project /3/.

Material and methods

The study area of Augsburg is situated in the southern part of the Federal Republic of Germany. It contains a population of about 530000 people. 5312 men and woman aged 25-64 were randomly selected for the first Survey 1984/85. The components of the screening procedure /4/ included also the twelve lead resting ECG, which was derived from 4003 survey participants from October 1984 until May 1985.

ECG analysis

Computerized ECG analysis was performed using the MEDIS ECG Analysis Program which was implemented on stand-alone ECG data acquisition and analysis system of type SICARD 803 /5/. The ECGs were additionally reviewed by a cardiologist. This combined method was expected to improve the ECG interpretation taking advantage of both the consistency of computerized ECG interpretation and the experience of an independent ECG expert. The cardiologist's ECG criteria for old 'definite MI' are described in table 1. Criteria for 'possible MI' and 'MI cannot be excluded' were smaller Q waves (Q duration) in limb leads and precordial leads and reduced R wave progression in the precordial leads including T wave inversion for the lateral site.

Table 1. ECG criteria for old 'definite' myocardial infarctions used by the cardiologist (twelve lead resting ECG)

Localisation	Criteria
Anterior site	Q duration $\geq$ 0.03 sec in at least two of the precordial leads
Inferior site	Q duration $\geq$ 0.04 sec in at least two of the leads II, III, aVF or Q duration at least 0.04 sec in lead aVF plus Q/R amplitude ratio > 1/4
Lateral site	Q duration $\geq$ 0.03 sec in leads I and aVL plus negative T waves in lead aVL

MI Self-reporting

The interview of the Survey included questions concerning the history of MI confirmed by a physician, time of onset and hospital admission.

Results

The rate of self-reported MI was 2.9 % (59/2014) in men and only 0.9 % (14/1989) in women. As shown in table 2, percentage of self-reported MI was markedly increasing by age; 81 % (48/59) of self-reported MI were found in men aged 55-64 and 70 % (14/1989) of all in women.

Depending on the ECG criteria used percentages of ECG signs of MI ranged from 1.5 % (31/2014) to 7.4 % (150/2014) in men and 0.2 % (3/1989) to 4.5 % (90/1989) in women. All age-groups taken together, percentage of self-reported MI was found to be similar to that derived from summarizing ECG signs of 'definite MI' and 'possible MI'. However, the age trends of self-reported MI were most similar to that of ECG signs of 'definite MI' which were also rapidly increasing in the age-group 55-64.

Comparison of self-reported MI with ECG signs of MI is shown in table 3. The majority of subjects with ECG signs of MI was unaware of any MI, even if only 'definite' ECG signs of MI were considered: 58 % (18/31) of the men and all women (n=3).

Table 2. Prevalence of self-reported old myocardial infarctions and ECG signs of myocardial infarctions by age and sex

Age	N	Self-reported MI (%)	ECG signs of MI (%)			
			Any	Definite	Possible	Cannot be excluded
MEN	2014	2.9	7.5	1.6	1.5	4.4
25-34	461	0.2	1.1	-	0.2	0.9
35-44	485	0.8	4.5	0.8	0.6	3.1
45-54	539	1.1	8.0	0.9	1.7	5.4
55-64	529	9.0	15.1	4.4	3.2	7.6
WOMEN	1989	0.7	4.6	0.2	0.9	3.6
25-34	460	-	0.4	-	-	0.4
35-44	522	-	1.5	-	-	1.5
45-54	513	0.8	4.9	0.2	0.6	4.1
55-64	494	2.0	11.5	0.4	2.8	8.3

Table 3. Self-reported old myocardial infarctions vs. ECG signs of myocardial infarction in men and women

Self-reported MI	MI by ECG				
	Definite	Possible	Cannot be excluded	Negative	Total
MEN					
Positive	13	7	7	32	59
Don't know	1	1	3	16	21
Negative	18	22	78	1815	1933
Total	32	30	88	1863	2013*
WOMEN					
Positive	0	1	3	10	14
Don't know	0	2	0	5	7
Negative	3	14	69	1881	1967
Total	3	17	72	1896	1988*

* One man and one woman have been excluded due to missing data.

Discussion

When discussing discrepancies between self-reported MI and ECG signs of MI, it has to be taken into account that both sources of information, interview as well as ECG, have limited validity, also that the analysed data have been derived from a population with low MI prevalence.

To improve the validity of the questionnaire information, self-reported MI should have been confirmed by a physician. In the case of symptoms which usually precede a physician's MI diagnosis, the number of subjects

who, at the time of the interview, ignore previous MI events should be small. Reliability of self-reported MI is rather confined, first, by the physician's diagnosis and, secondly, by its understanding and replication by the patient; this may have resulted in an overrating of only suspected MI. Colditz et al. /6/ described an overreporting of self-reported MI validating questionnaire information by independent means. However, silent MI was ignored within that study, and the data were gathered from nurses only. In our study, electrocardiographic manifestation of self-reported MI was found more frequently in men than in women ($p < 0.05$). On the other hand, the validity of self-reported diagnoses is affected by the use of the diagnostic tools that are available in the health care system of the study area and have been, over the years, subject to rapid change. This fact has to be taken into account as the average time interval between our data collection and the latest MI event was 7 years ($s=5.7$). ECG signs of MI were more common in subjects with hospitalized MI as compared to non-hospitalized ones ($p < 0.01$). Though not significant, there was some evidence for other factors which may have affected the validity of self-reported MI. Having divided the cases with self-reported MI into two almost equally sized groups, we found ECG signs of MI less common in cases with self-reported MI having occurred before 1980 as compared with those having occurred from then onwards. In addition to that, positive ECG were more likely to be found in subjects with recurrent infarctions. Agreement of self-reported MI with ECG signs of MI is, of course, also limited by the specificity and the sensitivity of the ECG; the latter resulting from events such as MI occurring without any electrocardiographic manifestation or with subsequent regression of specific ECG abnormalities /7/. From the clinical point of view, 'definite' ECG signs of MI are considered quite reliable, i.e. highly specific. However, low prevalence of MI in the average population requires a specificity of almost 100 % of the ECG criteria used to detect a reasonable rate of true positives as shown by Rantaharju /8/.
To what extent asymptomatic cases with 'definite' ECG signs of MI could be called 'silent MI' should be clarified in our follow-up study by including the results of additional diagnostic procedures. Furthermore the availability of an MI register in the study area will provide additional important long-term information.

References

/1/ Kannel, W.B. and Abbot, R.D.: N.Engl.J.Med., 18, 1144-1147 (1984)
/2/ Medalie,J.H. and Goldbourt,V.: Ann.Intern.Med., 84, 526-531 (1976)
/3/ Tunstall-Pedoe, H.: WHO Chronicle, 39, 3 - 5 (1985)
/4/ GSF Report 20/85: Monica Augsburg Survey - Manual of Operations
/5/ Pöppl, J.S. et al.: Electromedica, 52, 111 - 121 (1984)
/6/ Colditz, G.A. et al.: Am J. Epidemiol., 123, 894 - 900 (1986)
/7/ Burns-Cox, C.J.: Am Heart J., 4, 572 - 574 (1968)
/8/ Rantaharju, P.M.,in: Willems,J.L., van Bemmel,J.H. and Zywietz,C. : Computer ECG analysis (North Holland, Amsterdam), 315 - 322 (1973)

Repolarization wave abnormalities and symptomatic coronary artery disease

F.U.HUWEZ and P.W.MACFARLANE.

University Department Medical Cardiology, Royal Infirmary, Glasgow, Scotland.

Repolarization wave abnormalities are recognized features of coronary disease (CAD) particularly when they are associated with pathological Q waves or ST segment deviations. However, T wave abnormalities without pathological Q waves and ST segment deviations are not uncommon and their interpretation in relation to CAD needs to be clarified especially in the inferior leads, and particularly aVF. A wide angle between the QRS and T wave axis has been claimed to separate normal and abnormal T wave changes in the frontal plane. In particular, Schamroth (1) suggested that a QRS-T angle > 60° is an indication of myocardial disease including ischemia. This is supported by Chung (3), but Rowlands (11) suggests that an angle > ± 45° between the QRS and the T wave axis is abnormal. Therefore, it was decided to study the role of QRS-T angle in a group of patients with documented symptomatic CAD with particular emphasis on T wave abnormalities in the inferior leads and to compare the findings with those derived from a group of apparently healthy individuals.

METHODS.

Patients who had symptomatic CAD for which they were to undergo coronary arteriography were considered for inclusion in the study provided that they had (i) isolated T wave inversion without pathological Q waves and/or ST segment deviations in lead aVF with or without T wave inversion in lead I, (ii) no history of old myocardial infarction, (iii) no acquired or congenital heart disease that might cause T wave inversion. Only preoperative ECGs were included. The electrocardiograms were recorded either by a Siemens Mingorec 4 or by a locally developed computer compatible electrocardiograph (9). All leads were recorded simultanously and the degree of T wave inversion in the inferior leads as well as the QRS-T angle were measured by computer using a locally developed program described elsewhere (2).

As a part of an ongoing study (12) of 1500 apparently healthy normals, 12 lead ECGs were previously recorded from 397 individuals 40 years old and over (244 men and 153 women). All subjects were screened by a physician and were regarded as being free from any disease likely to affect the cardiovascular system.

RESULTS.

12 patients (9 male, 3 female, age range 49-66 with a mean age of 58.7 years) with symptomatic coronary artery disease and T wave abnormalties in the limb leads but no pathological Q waves and/or ST segment deviations, were found over a period of six months. All had significant CAD on coronary angiography (narrowing ≥ 70%)

TABLE 1	CRITERION	QRS-T > 60°	QRS-T > 45°
	SENSITIVITY:	5/12 (42%)	7/12 (58%)
	SPECIFICITY:	377/397(95%)	356/397(90%)
	PREDICTIVE VALUE:	5/25 (20%)	7/48 (15%)

which revealed that 10 had triple vessel disease. The remaining two had double vessel disease; one of them had disease of the left anterior descending and circumflex arteries while the other had right coronary and circumflex arteries affected.

The QRS-T angle measurements were as follows:

1. The mean QRS axis from all patients was +14.5 with a range of -13 to +146° while their mean T wave axis was -15.6° with a range of -89 to +174°.
2. A narrow QRS-T angle below 60° was found in 7 of 12 (58%) patients. They included 6 men and 1 woman with a mean age of 61.2 years and a range of 55-66 years. Their mean QRS axis was +5.4° with a range of -6 to +18°. The mean T wave axis in these patients was -25.7° with a range of -9 to -59°.
3. A QRS-T angle exceeding 60° was found in 5 of 12 (42%) patients (Table 1) who included 3 men and 2 women with an age range of 49-60 years and a mean of 55.2 years. The QRS axis of 4 of them ranged from -13 to +46° with a mean of +23° and their T wave axis ranged from -15 to -89 with a mean of -45.5°. One patient had a QRS and T wave axis of +44 and +174° respectively, on account of T wave abnormalities in lead I.
4. A QRS-T angle less than 45° was found in 5 of 12 (42%) patients. Their QRS axis ranged from -6 to +18 with a mean of +5.8° while the T wave axis ranged from -9 to -20 with a mean of -16.4°.
5. A QRS-T angle greater than 45° was found in 7 patients. The QRS axis in 6 of them ranged from -13 to +46 with a mean of +16.8° while their T wave axis ranged from -15 to -89 with a mean of -46.6°.

TABLE 2 QRS-T ANGLE (NORMAL MALES)

AGE	n	MEAN QRS-T	RANGE
18-29	265	16.6 ± 23.9	-39 - 71
30-39	220	7.2 ± 27.3	-61 - 59
40-49	117	-4.8 ± 26.3	-67 - 37
> 50	125	-13.0 ± 27.1	-82 - 40

6. The normal range of QRS-T (Table 2) and the criterion of QRS-T > 60° was also assessed in a population of 397 apparently normal individuals aged 40 years and over and was found to be 95% specific for myocardial disease as 20 of these apparently normal people had a QRS-T angle exceeding 60° (Table 1).
7. The criterion of QRS-T angle > 45° was also assessed in both groups, as shown in Table 1. As expected, this increased sensitivity but decreased specificity of

TABLE 3	CRITERION:	QRS-T >60° AND T < 0°	QRS-T >45° AND T < 0°
	SENSITIVITY:	4/12 (33%)	6/12 (50%)
	SPECIFICITY:	397/397(100%)	397/397(100%)
	PREDICTIVE VALUE:	4/4 (100%)	6/6 (100%)

reporting myocardial ischaemia.

8. All the patients had T wave inversion in lead aVF with a range of -50 to -148 microvolts and a mean of -84.4 microvolts. 11 had a T axis <0° and hence the combination of QRS-T > 60° and T < 0° was assessed as was the pairing of QRS-T > 45° and T <0°. Results are shown in Table 3.

DISCUSSION.

T wave inversion simulating myocardial ischemia may occur in healthy individuals as a normal variant. Examples include the persistence of the juvenile pattern which is more commonly seen in black women (4) and the benign T wave inversion of healthy young adults, especially in young black and trained athletes (5-8). However, in all the above reported types of T wave inversion found in young people, the T wave inversion was mainly in the precordial leads and occasionally associated with such changes in the inferior leads. It is also well known that premenopausal women may exhibit non-specific T wave changes particularly in the inferior leads.

Myocardial ischaemia may be defined electrocardiographically as a condition in which (i) the depolarization process takes place normally, (ii) repolarization is delayed in a particular area, and (iii) the polarization is normal in the same area during diastole (10). The repolarization sequence of the ventricles is directed from the epicardium to the endocardium while the repolarization vector points in the opposite direction to that of the repolarization seauence (in contrary to depolarization). The QRS and T vectors are therefore both directed from the endocardium to the epicardium, i.e. in the same direction in a normal heart. Therefore, the direction of the QRS and T axes are normally similar so that the QRS-T angle < 60° (1).

In the presence of myocardial disease - commonly ischemia - the T wave axis tends to deviate from the ischemic region whereas the QRS axis remains normally directed or even may deviate in the opposite direction. Therefore, a QRS-T angle greater than 60° is thought to be a sensitive index of significant T wave abnormality and myocardial disease and is more reliable than the empirical observation of T wave changes in isolated leads (1).

In this study all patients had symptomatic ischaemic heart disease proved by coronary angiography. They all were selected on the basis of having T wave inversion in Lead aVF and one had T wave inversion in Lead I in addition. It is clear from the results that a wide QRS-T angle on its own is insensitive as a criterion and on the other hand, is an unnecessary requisite for the diagnosis of ischaemic heart disease in the presence of inverted T wave in the inferior leads. Nevertheless, from a study of the apparently healthy individuals, the use of a criterion such as the QRS-T angle exceeding either 45 or 60° would be somewhat non-specific. It therefore seemed sensible to improve criteria by adding the requirement that the T axis in the frontal plane should be superior to 0°. When this was done as shown in Table 2, it was found that the sensitivity decreased slightly but the specificity improved markedly to 99%. Thus a new criterion of a T axis < 0° and QRS-T > 45° is proposed as consistent with myocardial ischaemia. It was possible to assess this on a test group of 940 younger apparently healthy individuals aged from 18-39 years of age, consisting of 493 males and 447 females. In this group only 6 individuals had a QRS-T angle in excess of 45° together with a T axis superior to 0°. This provides a test specificity of over 99% in a group where non-specific T wave abnormalities are not uncommon.

In conclusion, the use of a wide QRS-T angle on its own as an index of ischaemic heart disease is somewhat insensitive and is certainly not a prerequisite for the diagnosis particularly as QRS axis moves superiorly with increasing age. On the other hand, the combination of a wide QRS-T axis exceeding 45° together with a T axis superior to 0° provides an added degree of specificity and a modest improvement in sensitivity. Its application to subjects with or without symptoms of ischaemic heart disease can be recommended. Indeed, further assessment shows that the simple criterion of T < 0° is highly specific being in excess of 99% for those over 40 and the 940 normals under 40. In addition, it was in fact more sensitive than the combination of a superiorly directed T wave axis and a wide QRS-T angle, being 58% sensitive.

The overall conclusion would seem to be that the use of a wide QRS-T angle is of little relevance in the diagnosis of ischaemic heart disease when a more simple criterion involving T axis alone appears to be sensitive and specific.

REFERENCES

(1) Schamroth, L: 5th (ed). Blackwell Scientific Publications, 5th ed, 104-105 (1976).
(2) Macfarlane, P.W. et al: In: Computer ECG analysis; Towards Standardization. North Holland, 2-5 (1986).
(3) Chung, E.K: Harper and Row. 2nd ed, 3-29 (1980).
(4) Thomas, J., Harris, E., Lassiter, G: Am J Cardiol. 5, 468 (1960).
(5) Gottlieb, R.S., Duca, P.R., Kasparian, H. et al: Am Heart J. 90, 451 (1975).
(6) Hane-Paparo, N., Wendkos, M.H., Brunner, T: Am Heart J. 81, 743 (1971).
(7) Lichtman, T., et al: Arch Int Med. 132, 763 (1973).
(8) Dafilzadeh M., et al: Dis Chest. 52, 101 (1967).
(9) Watt, M.P., Shoat, D.B: Journal of I.E.R.E. (In press).
(10) Lipman, B.S,. Massie, E: Year Book Med. Pub. USA. 5th ed. 216-66 (1965).
(11) Rowlands, D.J: In: Understanding the Electrocardiogram. ICI Ltd. 56-57, 1980.
(12) Macfarlane P.W., et al: In: Advances in Electrocardiology. University of Caen, France, 160-63 (1985).

Transtelephonic 12-lead ECG service centers in the Netherlands.

H.A. HOLTKAMP and N.H. VAN BOXEL.

H.A. Holtkamp, cardiologist, Sophia Ziekenhuis, NL8025 AB Zwolle
N.H. van Boxel, GP, Oude Delft 128a, NL2611 CG Delft.

SUMMARY A new and practical ECG modem has been developed for transtelephonic transmission of standard 12-lead ECGs. The ECGs were made at the primary health care level (GP's office or patient's home). The interpretation was done by a cardiologist in a general hospital. The study measured positive and negative effects on diagnostics and referral. It was shown that:

- it is a reliable, simple and widely applicable method,
- diagnostic efficiency is greatly improved,
- negative side effects are hardly present,
- the ECG should be accompanied by patient's case history and personal data,
- co-operation between GP and cardiologist benefits through the method and
- incidence of myocardial infarction may be substantially higher than indicated by official statistics.

In the Netherlands ECG service centers are quickly expanding. The method is now also in use to obtain earlier - i.e. at the patient's home - intervention with thrombolytic therapy like tPA or streptokinase.

INTRODUCTION

In the Netherlands patients with complaints suggesting ischaemic heart disease usually contact their GP. The GP filters out those patients without cardiac disease (the majority) and takes adequate measures for the others (1). Cardiologists only see the outcome of the filtering and most think there is room for improvement of the GP filter function. Some even allow patients to bypass the GP and go directly to the hospital (free call). From a logistical point of view it seems unwise, both in terms of net health care results and cost-effectiveness, not to make use of the highly qualified GPs. Although at first transtelephonic ECG centers gave hopeful results (2), nevertheless none was still operational in the Netherlands by 1975. Together with the National Institute of General Practice (N.H.I.) the "Zwolle Cardiophony Project" was initiated.

The aim of this study was: 1) to find the optimal organization for a transtelephonic ECG center, 2) to put such a center into use and 3) to describe and evaluate the results.

MATERIAL AND METHODS

The hardware and the organization for a transtelephonic ECG center were optimized by an adaptive trial and error method between 1975 to 1980. From 1980 16 GPs participated in the trial with a total patient population of 47000. For each transmitted ECG a registration form was used (3). To give the cardiologist extra information and to prevent biasing of the answers of the GPs by the outcome of the ECG, most answers were recorded on the answering device of the receiving station immediately after ECG transmission. The ECGs were read by a cardiologist and described according to the thesaurus of table I.

Table I. Grouping of ECG diagnoses by mutual arrangement with GPs and cardiologists.

Category 100: combines diagnoses and normal ECGs which have no consequences as regards treatment.
(101) normal ECG, (102) no distinct abnormalities, (103) minimal tachycardia, (104) minimal bradycardia, (105) supra-ventricular premature beats, (106) few ventricular premature beats
Category 200: contains the ECG diagnoses appropriate to mild disorders which can usually be treated by the GP.
(201) atrial fibrillation, (202) atrial flutter, (203) nodal rhythm, (204) many ventricular premature beats, (205) complete left bundle branch block, (206) complete right bundle branch block,(207) first-degree atrioventricular heart block, (208) left anterior block, (209) left atrial overload, (210) right atrial overload, (211) hypertrophy of left ventricle, (212) hypertrophy of right ventricle, (213) repolarization distur bance possibly indicating: myocardial ischaemia, (214) ditto: digitalis, (215) ditto: hypokalemia, (216) ditto: pericarditis, (217) aspecific repolarization disturbance, (218) suggestive of cor pulmonale, (219) old infarction
Category 300: contains the ECG diagnoses appropriate to severe disorders which generally require specialist treatment.
(301) sino-atrial block, (302) sinus arrest, (303) supraventricular tachycardia, (304) Wolff-Parkinson-White syndrome, (305) distinct left ventricular hypertrophy with repolarization disturbances, (306) second-degree atrioventricular block, (307) abnormal ST/T segment, with suspected infarction, (308) unexpected old infarction
Category 400: contains the ECG diagnoses appropriate to a disorder requiring urgent specialist treatment and/or hospitalization.
(401) ventricular tachycardia, (402) ECG suggesting new infarction, (403) total AV heart block, (404) frequent multifocal premature beats Category 500: (501) miscellaneous

The data on the answering device were taken into consideration and the cardiologist gave a "filter-advice" in one of the categories : (21) no abnormalities, (22) treatment by GP, (23) referral indicated and (24) immediate hospitalization necessary. Also an objective verification method was created to measure correctness of advice and referral. In the follow up all referred patients underwent a complete cardiological examination and were filtered to preset criteria. If the cardiologist had given advice (23) or (24) but the patients were not referred, they were recovered from the GP's files. A random sample of 10% of the negatives (no referral and advice (21) or (22) given) was taken to calculate false negatives, sensitivity and specificity. Statistical methods used: Chi square test, sign test, Cohens Kappa, point estimation with 95% confidence intervals.

RESULTS

Hardware

Eleven successive versions of hardware were developed and tested. The final version was a lightweight, battery operated, portable ECG modem for acoustic coupling to the telephone network. Pushing one button automatically transmits a standard 12-lead ECG in 48 seconds together with an identification code of the modem. The fully automatic receiving station used an answering device and a 50 mm thermosensitve ECG writer operated by codes from the transmitter.

Organization

Initially the GPs were not satisfied with a mere description of the ECG according to the thesaurus but asked for a real advice from the cardiologist. The cardiologists, not having seen the patient, were reluctant to comply, but finally four categories of advice were given with full responsability remaining for the GPs. The cardiologists only took responsability for the description of the ECG. An immediate consultation by telephone was allowed to GP and cardiologist. Otherwise the ECG, its description and the advice were mailed to the GP the same day.

Trial year (1980)

In the trial year 801 ECGs were transmitted (17 per 1000 patients). Seventeen were not accompanied by an appropiate registration form and 29 were repeat ECGs. In 100 cases (12%) an additional telephonic consultation took place. These consultations certainly led to better understan ding and cooperation. The most frequent indications for the GPs were chest pain (33%), atypical pain (45%),arrythmia (27%), hypertension (28%), reassurance GP (28%) and reassurance patient (47%). The advice expected by the GP was significantly less serious than the advice given by the cardiologist (Cohens Kappa rating 0.346, $p<0.001$, "fair correlation"). A justified conclusion seems that the GP tends to underestimate the cardiac complaints of the patient.

Referral policy.

The referral policy of the GP showed an impressive change as a result of the advice of the cardiologist:

Table II.

		GP's actual referral	
		yes	no
GP's referral intention	yes	89	147
	no	61	422
	?	6	30

Follow up

All referred patients had a standard follow up examination. Only 2 patients of the random sample refused the standard follow up examination. None of the other 58 had positive criteria. None of the fourteen patients with advice "not to refer" but nevertheless referred had positive criteria. From this results a point estimation of zero false negatives with 95% confidence intervals of 0 to 22 (0-4%). Since the other data were exactly known the following table was established:

TABLE III. Improvement of diagnostic quality and GP filter function.

	Diagnostic quality		Filter function	
	advice expected	advice given	intended referral	actual referral
sensitivity x 100	35-48	87-99	47-63	63-72
specificity x 100	76-79	91	68-77	91
% false positives	60-71	28	56-71	33
% false negatives	16-20	0- 4	12-18	7-10

The double figures represent the 95% confidence intervals. A single figure means that this interval is smaller than 1.

DISCUSSION

The transtelephonic ECG center described differed on two points from previous centers: its new hardware and an organization that demanded more commitment by cardiologist and GP. The high quality of the advice given by the cardiologist on such limited data as ECG, indications and short patient history came as a surprise.

The diagnostic power of the GP increased in accordance with the quality of the advice. The GP filter function attained the specifity of the cardiologist's advice but, surprisingly, sensitivity was not significantly increased. In part this was caused by the uncertainty for 36 patients regarding referral intention, but analysis showed too that a GP takes many more factors into consideration in his decision to refer a patient than only cardiological disease. Most factors are quite logical, like very old age, other concomitant diseases such as terminal carcinoma, or the refusal of the patient to go to the hospital. Therefore it can be concluded that the method improves the filter function of the GP in all four aspects. An often expressed fear for an increase in false negatives by availability of expert ECG-reading to the GP (4) was not confirmed in this trial. In fact false negatives decreased significantly.

Extension.

In 1981 the number of participating GPs was increased to 57. From 1982 other hospitals followed. Now ten centers of this type are operational in the Netherlands. About 5.5 % of all Dutch GPs now have an ECG modem. In two centers in the Netherlands the method is used for another application. The ECG modem is carried in all ambulances in the area. Two trials are currently set up to measure the influence of avoiding transportation delay on thrombolytic therapy. The patient is injected tPA or streptokinase at his home before transportation. ECG reading then is necessary to obtain at least two criteria of MI.

Myocardial infarction

The part of the protocol concerning MI stipulated that the GP would transfer the patient and NOT the ECG to the hospital. Nevertheless 39 MIs were unexpectedly found in the first year. In 8 cases the GP intended hospitalization without having a correct diagnosis. With the other 31 there were apparently so few clinical symptoms that the GP did not raise the alarm. If extrapolation of this fact is allowed, the official MI incidence statistics should probably be increased in the order of 30 percent.

References.

(1) Does, E. van der, and J. Lubsen; Acute coronary events in general practice: the Imminent Myocardial Infarction Rotterdam study. Doctorate thesis Rotterdam (1978)

(2) Schilperoort, J., The applicability of electrocardiographic diagnosis in general practice. Doctorate thesis Utrecht (1977).

(3) Holtkamp, H.A., Cardiophony. A new method of 12-lead ECG transmission as a part of the communication between GP and cardiologist for early diagnosis of cardiac complaints. Doctorate thesis Groningen(1986).

(4). Short, D., An electrocardiogram reporting service: Its role and its risks. Br Heart J:31,531-535 (1969).

ECG criteria and thrombolysis in acute myocardial infarction

PARSI, E., R.A. PARSI, and K. KOTHE
Medical Clinic, Charité Hospital, Humboldt University, Berlin, GDR

Summary

In 28 patients (16,5 % of total number of patients with acute myocardial infarction (AMI)) admitted to CCU up to four hours after onset of chest pain thrombolytic therapy was performed.

The ECG changes at admission, two hours and 8 - 20 hrs. after thrombolysis were analysed. The sum of ST elevation and contralateral ST depression were measured in corresponding leads as well as the changing of Q waves.

The ST elevation in anterior and inferior infarctions was significantly reduced 2 hrs. after thrombolysis ($p < 0.01$). Its was nearly normalized at 8 - 20 hrs. (anterior AMI: $p < 0.05$; inferior AMI: $p < 0.01$). The ST depression was normalized at 8 - 20 hrs. too (anterior AMI: $p < 0.01$; inferior AMI: $p < 0.05$).

The beginning of thrombolysis under 2 hrs. leads more frequent to non-transmural and after two hrs. to transmural infarctions ($p < 0.02$).

It can be concluded: 1. the ECG is the most important criterion to indicate thrombolysis in AMI, 2. the beginning of this therapy determines the development of infarction, 3. the ST elevation is rapidly reduced after thrombolysis, 4. thrombolysis does not prevent myocardial infarction but limits its size, 5. to clear up the significance of reciprocal ST depressions in further studies is necessary.

Introduction

The thrombolytic therapy in AMI is already an accepted intervention. In the reported studies intervall from onset of chest pain to intervention as well as ECG changes are different (1, 2, 3, 4).

The aim of our study was to investigate in a well-defined group of patients with AMI the ECG changes at admission, 2 hrs. and 8 - 20 hrs. after thrombolysis.

Patients and methods

170 patients with AMI who had entered the CCU of Charité Hospital between January 1986 and May 1987, were investigated. From these were admitted 28 patients (25 males, 3 females, average age 54.0±5.9 yrs.) (16,5%) within 4 hrs. after onset of chest pain and showed following inclusion criteria (tab. 1). The location of AMI was inferior in 8 and anterior in 20 patients.

Patients with thrombolysis later than 4 hrs. after onset of chest pain, and ECG patterns of bundle branch block, W P W syndrome, A V block third degree, and escape rhythm were excluded.

The criteria of abnormal Q wave were used after Bar et al. (4).

Tab. 1: Inclusion criteria for thrombolysis in AMI

• Chest pain > 20 min	• No Q wave in leads with ST elevation
• Onset of symptoms < 4 hrs	• serum enzymes normal
• ST elevation ⩾ 1 mm in 1 extremity lead or > 2 mm in ⩾ 1 precordial lead	• no contraindications for thrombolysis

The extremity leads I - III, aVR - aVF and the chest leads V_1 - V_6, V_7 - V_9, $V_{r3,4}$ were registred before, 2 hrs. and 8 - 20 hrs. after thrombolysis. The ST elevation and depression were measured in mm (1 mV = 10 mm). The mode of thrombolysis was in 19 patients an ultra short time lysis with 750 000 U streptokinase/ 30 min i.v. and in 9 patients an intracoronary thrombolysis.
The statistical analysis was done by paired t test.

Results

The sum of ST elevation in anterior infarction was significantly reduced 2 hrs. ($p < 0.01$) and 8 - 20 hrs. ($p < 0.05$) after thrombolysis. The sum of contralateral ST depression was only 8 - 20 hrs. later significantly reduced ($p < 0.01$).
The sum of ST elevation in inferior infarction was significantly reduced 2 hrs ($p < 0.01$) and 8 - 20 hrs. ($p < 0.01$) after lysis. The ST depression was significantly reduced 8 - 20 hrs. after therapy (fig. 1).
Significant differences could be found between starting of thrombolysis after onset of chest pain and related infarction type (tab. 2).

Tab. 2: Development of AMI after onset of thrombolysis

non - transmural	1.6 ± 0.4 hrs	$p < 0.02$
transmural	2.3 ± 0.7 hrs	

In total the outcome of 28 patients with thrombolysis were the evolving of non-transmural infarction in 9, transmural in 19 patients. 4 of them died: 1 caused by reperfusion arrhythmia and 3 by pump failure.

Discussion and conclusions

While the Q waves have been used as a sign of myocardial necrosis and in farct size, the ST elevation gives information on severity of ischemic injury (5, 6).
Therefore we have excluded in line with other authors (1, 2, 3) patients who have had at admission pathological Q waves. Although the salvage of myocardial tissue by thrombolysis could be achieved in these patients too (4).
The development of abnormal Q waves after thrombolysis was defined as transmural and its absence as non-transmural infarction. Although we are

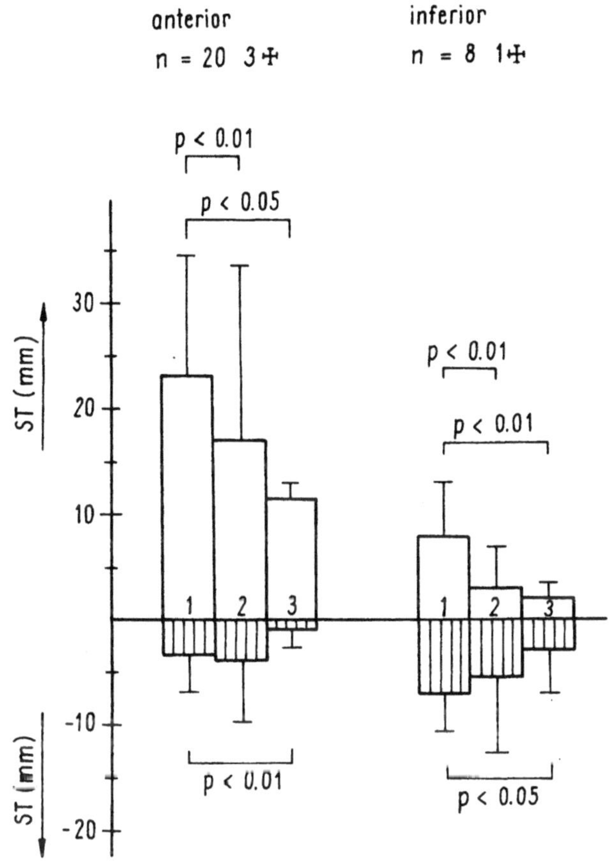

aware of the discussion on the non-specifity of the ECG for distinguishing anatomically transmural from non-transmural infarctions (7,8).
The subgroup with chest pain less than 2 hrs. at admission has had after thrombolysis significantly less abnormal Q waves than patients who entered after 2 hrs. the CCU. This finding is in accordance with the results of others (4) who found a prominent infarct size limitation in most patients arriving the hospital within 2 hrs. after onset of chest pain.
The ST elevation was reduced significantly within 2 hrs. after thrombolysis. Three patients with persisting ST elevation have died due to pump failure.
The returning of ST elevation after thrombolysis is a sign of limitation of infarct size. The reciprocal ST depression disappeared with the regression of ST elevation. Therefore in accordance with Little et al.(9) the ST depression can be regarded as a mirror image of ST elevation. The origin of this ST depression is not cleared ultimately and needs further investigations.

It can be concluded: 1. The ECG is the most important criterion to indicate thrombolysis in AMI, 2. the startof therapy under 2 hours leads significantly more frequent to non-transmural and after 2 hours to transmural infarctions, 3. the ST elevation is rapidly reduced after thrombolysis, its persistens suggests a not successful treatment, 4. thrombolysis does not prevent myocardial damage but limits the infarct size.

References

(1) Kennedy,J.W., J.L. Ritchie, K.B. Davis, J.K. Fritz: New Engl. J. Med. 312, 1073 - 1078 (1985)

(2) Mathey,D.G., K.H. Kuck, V. Tilsner, H.J. Krebber, W. Bleifeld: Circulation 63, 489 - 497 (1981)

(3) Rentrop,K.P., F. Feit, H. Blanke, P Stecy, R. Schneider, M. Rey, S. Horowitz, M. Goldman, K. Karsch, H. Meilma, M. Cohen, S. Siegel, J. Sanger, J. Slater, R. Gorlin, A. Fox, R. Fagerstrom, W.F. Calhoun: New Engl. J. Med. 311, 1457 - 1463 (1984)

(4) Bar,F.W., F. Vermeer, C. de Zwaan, M. Ramentol, W.T. Hermens, A. van de Laarse, F.W.A. Verheugt, H.Krauss, H.J.J. Wellens: Amer. J. Cardiol. 59, 6 - 13 (1987)

(5) Wagner,G.S., C.J. Freye, S.T. Palmeri, S.F. Roark, N.C. Stack, R.E. Ideker, F.E. Hareel, R.H. Selvester: Circulation 65, 342 - 347(1982)

(6) Muller,J.E., P.R. Marokko, E. Braunwald: Circulation 52, 16-- 27 (1975)

(7) Phibbs,B.: J. Am. Coll. Cardiol. 1, 561 - 564 (1983)

(8) Spodick,D.H.: Amer. J. Cardiol. 56, 913 - 915 (1983)

(9) Little,W.C., E.W. Rogers, M.T. Sodums: Ann. intern. Med. 100, 226 - 229 (1984)

The Quantitation of Regional Ischemia
Criteria from a Fine Grid Computer Simulation of QRS-T

RONALD H. S. SELVESTER, JOSEPH C. SOLOMON, and GIL D. TOLAN

University of Southern California, Rancho Los Amigos Campus, Downey 90242, CA, USA
and USAF School of Aerospace Medicine, Brooks Air Force Base, TX 78235-5301, USA

SUMMARY: Criteria in the ST-T of the electrocardiogram (ECG) for quantitating the severity of regional ischemia were developed from a comprehensive fine grid (1 cu mm) simulation of excitation and recovery (QRS-T). Realistic cardiac and torso anatomy, and electrophysiologic properties were incorporated into the model that produced an ECG total body surface map (BSM). This led to the specific hypothesis that additional leads on the upper and lower torso, and back, are required to optimize the quantitation and localization of ischemia and infarction. The combination of the leads in which the QRST changes occur and the severity of the change provide a testable set of hypotheses for predicting the size, extent, severity and location of areas of infarction, resting and exercise ischemia, resting and exercise perfusion defects, and coronary obstructions.

INTRODUCTION: The digital computer simulation of the human ECG BSM was constructed from measured torso anatomy, resistivities, and electrophysiology [1,2]. The simulation of the excitation wave was developed at a 1 cu mm grid resolution based on Huygens principle of wave construction using a distributed dipole model of the electromotive surface [3], and measured heart and infarct geometry. The electromotive surface activity was then projected to the centroid of 20 regional generators imbedded in a realistic inhomogeneous male torso that included intracardiac blood mass, and lungs. Transfer impedances generated by the Gelernter-Swihart solution [3] projected the 20 sources to the torso as a 1300 point BSM. The 12 lead ECG and any vectorcardiographic (VCG) lead system is a subset of the map. This simulation contains all the first order variables known to influence the QRS of the human ECG. Numerical experiments with the model led to a set of VCG criteria and an ECG QRS score (1 point = 3% of the left ventricle) for quantitating infarct size in all heart locations [4,5]. Working with the Duke University group the QRS infarct size score was validated in a series of classic pathoanatomic studies [6-8].

We have recently automated the incorporation of individual myocardial action potential (MAP) wave forms into each 1 cu mm "cell" of this simulation [9]. Programs for displaying the excitation-recovery sequence on a set of cross sections of the heart in a high resolution colorgraphics 3D perspective, as well as ECG/VCGs, have been developed for a normal heart, or any combination of regional ischemia or infarction. We also reported [10] on a minimum set of chest leads which optimized the sensitivity of the model to regional ischemia. These findings have been confirmed by Kornreich et al [11]. It is the purpose of this paper to present typical examples of recent color graphic and 12 lead ECG outputs and to propose criteria from the simulations for localizing and quantitating ischemia (and infarction) in each coronary distribution.

METHODS AND RESULTS: Each MAP generator was derived from an equation containing 3 arbitrary parameters and 4 constants. Thus each discrete point within the myocardium was represented by a unique waveform. These parameters and constants were found by table-look-up that incorporated the endo-epicardial and apex to base gradient in MAP durations and refractory periods. This allowed the specification of local areas of injury/ischemia/infarction by their known effects on local MAPs. Individual MAPs from each 1 cu mm "cell" were then projected to the 20 regional equivalent cardiac generators and via the Gelernter-Swihart heart-to-chest transfer impedances to 1300 torso points. The MAP parameters were adjusted within physiologically realistic bounds such that numerically computed body surface QRST distributions were made to agree with those measured on normal subjects. Myocardial infarcts were then simulated using the quantitative planometric pathology of such lesions from the Duke validation studies provided by Dr. R. Ideker. Figure 1 is the 12 lead ECG from the simulation of a large anterior infarct. In

LARGE ANTERIOR MI

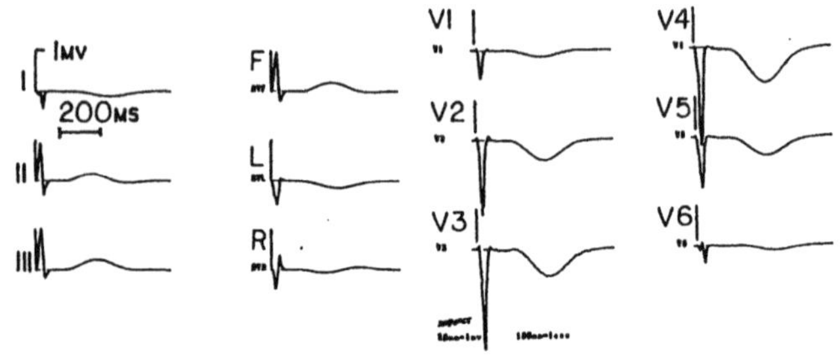

FIGURE 1.

this case no alterations to simulate ischemia in the border zone or other areas were introduced. The changes are typical of those seen clinically in the chronic phase of such large anterior infarcts.

DISCUSSION: One of the major strengths of a simulation constructed from anatomic and electrophysiologic information is that it can be used to generate testable hypotheses regarding the process simulated. We are now at that stage in the model development. If electrode sites are chosen that are relatively specific for each local region the amplitude of STT in that lead can be normalized to 1) the surface R wave voltage of a local unit dipole from the simlulations [10], 2) the mean local R voltage of normals such as Kornreich's normal BSM data [11], or 3) the mean voltage in the usual exercise testing reference lead V5 (ie, 1.3mv) as done by Hollenberg [12]. When this is done, the same amplitude of local ST-T change in each surface lead shown in Figure 2 now represents, hypothetically, the same degree of regional ischemia.

Table 1 presents our proposed criteria for regional subendocardial ischemia in each of the main coronary artery distributions. Simple measurements of ST segments at J, and ST 60ms or 80ms after J produced by maximal stress testing, are proposed initially with the ST normalized to an R amplitude of 1.3 mv in leads with R/S=>0.5.

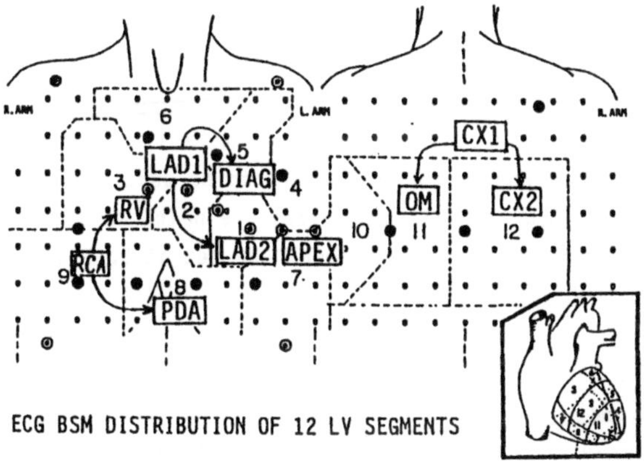

ECG BSM DISTRIBUTION OF 12 LV SEGMENTS

FIGURE 2: RECOMMENDED LEAD LOCATIONS: 20 simultaneous leads recorded as follows:

A. 6 limb leads: Computed from 2 simultaneous limb leads;

B. 18 simultaneous precordial and back leads located as follows:

1. 6 standard precordial leads V1-V6: Records left anterior descending (LAD) area, anteroseptal wall and apex (other regions poorly shown).
2. 3rd ICS chest leads V3ICS3 and V5ICS3: Records DIAG/LAD area, ant-superior wall.
3. Right and lower chest leads; V1ICS2, V4R and 7th ICS leads V4RICS7, VFXRICS7 (ParaXiphoid Rt ICS7), VPXICS7, and V4ICS7. Records right coronary and posterior descending (RCA/PDA) arterial area (RV and inferior wall of both).
4. Back leads V8, VMB (Mid Back), V8R, and VSR (Scapula, Right acromion in MCL). Records left circumflex (LCX) arterial area (posterolateral wall).

TABLE 1: CRITERIA FOR QUANTITATION OF REGIONAL ISCHEMIA:

A. General -- severity of subendocardial ischemia in any location or lead set (normalized voltages); criteria for J, ST60, and ST80 as follows:

	J and ST60 depressed and ST flat or downsloping and		or ST upsloping and	
Borderline:	depressed	=>100uv	depressed	=>150uv
Probable:	"	=>125uv	"	=>175uv
Mild but def.:	"	=>150uv	"	=>200uv
Moderate:	"	=>200uv	"	=>250uv
Severe:	"	=>300uv	"	=>350uv

B. Specific -- Predicted local segment: The probable risk area and coronary artery is based on the local leads in which change occurs as follows:

1 Vessel disease, abnormal ST change in following leads:

- LAD distal to the DIAGonal: Leads V3-V5 and V4ICS7.
- DIAG: Leads I, AVL, V3ICS3, V5ICS3, and V6.
- LAD proximal to the DIAG: Distal LAD Leads + DIAG Leads ± V2.
- LCX: Leads V8, VMB, V8R, and VSR (Scapula,Rt Acromion, MCL)*.
- PDA/RCA: Leads II, III, AVF, V4RICS7, VPXRICS7, and VPXICS7*.

*Note: Ischemia in LCX or PDA/RCA leads plus APICAL leads I, V5, V6, and V5ICS7 but not ANT leads V1-V4 is indicative of more extensive LCX or PDA/RCA ischemia.

VALIDATION STUDIES: Subjects who have stress test abnormalities or other indications for coronary angiography and who have normal coronary arteries at angiography provide the normal controls for specificity studies. Those with definite exercise perfusion defects in one coronary distribution who have 70% or more narrowing of that artery are the study population with which to validate the proposed quantitative criteria for regiona ischemia. The specific criteria from Table 1 will need to be adjusted for optimal specificity and sensitivity for the population in which they are being used. In the low incidence apparently healthy groups the specificity should be set at 96-99%, using this lead set, for exercise testing to be an effecive screening tool in this population.

POSSIBLE LIMITATIONS: Some 20-30% of patients with totally occluded coronary arteries do not have regional wall motion abnormalities at rest. About half of such patients, in most series, do not have perfusion defects or wall motion abnormalities with exercise. It follows that this subset of subjects in the proposed validation studies will have significant coronary obstruction but normal ST segments on multilead exercise ECGs and normal perfusion studies with exercise. One can postulate however, that 1) such patients would not have pain or ST change with balloon occlusion at angioplasty, 2) the functional impairment would be minimal or insignificant, and 3) the long term morbidity and mortality would be significantly better in this subset.

BIBLIOGRAPHY:

1. Selvester RH, Kalaba R, Collier CR, Bellman R, Kagiwada H: Am Heart J 74:792, 1967.
2. Selvester RH, Solomon JC, Gillespie TL: Circ 38:684, 1968.
3. Solomon JC, Selvester RH: Am Heart J 85(4):518, 1973.
4. Selvester RH, Sanmarco ME: Proc 4th Int Congress ECG, 1978
5. Selvester RH, Sanmarco ME, Solomon JC, Wagner GS: in Myocardial Infarction: Measurement and Intervention. Wagner GS, ed, Martinus Nijhoff, The Hague, 1982
6. Palmeri ST, Harrison DG, Cobb FR, Morris KG, Harrell FE, Ideker RE, Selvester RH, Wagner GS: N Engl J Med 306(1):4, 1982.
7. Wagner GS, Freye CH, Palmeri ST, Roark SF, Stack BA, Ideker RE, Harrell FE, Selvester RH: Circ 65(2):342, 1982.
8. Ward RM, White RD, Ideker RE, Hindman NB, Alonso DR, Bishop SP, Bloor CM, Fallon JT, Gottlieb GJ, Hackel DB, Hutchins GM, Phillips HR, Reimer KA, Roark SF, Rochlani SP, Rogers WJ, Ruth WK, Savage RM, Weiss JL, Selvester RH, Wagner GS: Am J Cardiol 53:706, 1984.
9. Solomon JC, Selvester RH, Tolan GD: Eng Found Conf, Computerized Interpretation of the ECG XI, Bailey JJ ed, Eng Found, NY, 146, 1986
10. Selvester RH, Solomon JC, 3rd Int Symp Body Surface Mapping, van Dam RT, van Oosterom A, eds, Martinus Nijhoff, Dordrecht, Boston, 1985
11. Kornreich F, Montague JM, Rautaharju PM, Block P, Warren J, Horacek BM: Am J Cardiol 58:863, 1986
12. Hollenberg M, Zoltil JM, Go M, Yaney SF, Daniels W, Davis RC, Bedymer J: N Engl J Med 313(10): 600, 1985

Comparison of vectorcardiographic, electrocardiographic, ventriculographic, echocardiographic and coronarographic findings in patients with stenocardia

I. RIEČANSKÝ, J. KASPER, I. RUTTKAY-NEDECKÝ, L. PLACHÁ, J. MIŠEKOVÁ, K. HAVLÍNOVÁ, J. ZELENAY

Institute of Cardiovascular Diseases, Bratislava, Partizánska 2, CSSR;
Institute of Normal and Pathological Physiology, Centre of Physiol. Sci. Slovak Academy of Sciences, Sienkiewiczova 1, Bratislava, CSSR

Summary

50 patients with complaints of stenocardia, aged 22 to 59 years (9 women, 41 men), underwent vectorcardiographic (McFee lead system), echocardiographic, electrocardiographic (12 standard leads), coronarographic and ventriculographic investigations. If isolated positivity of either of these methods was considered as false positivity and the presence or absence of positivity in the combination of at least two methods (ECG excluded) as true positivity, or true negativity, then vectorcardiography ranked first in sensitivity (96%), negative predictive value (80%) and overall predicitivity (83%), while echocardiography ranked last with 53%, 36%, and 64% respectively. On the contrary, in specificity and positive predictive value echocardiography ranked first with 100% and vectorcardiography last with 62% and 83%, respectively. The combination of vectorcardiography with echocardiography, versus positivity of coronarography and/or ventriculography, had a sensitivity of 89%, specificity of 80%, positive predictive value of 89%, negative predictive value of 80% and overall predicitivity of 89%, considering more than 50% stenosis as the criterion. If obstruction was required, the figures were 93%, 75%, 83% and 86% respectively. Vectorcardiography and echocardiography are complementary non- invasive methods with a fair predictive value when looking for presence of focal myocardial injury.

Introduction

Focal myocardial lesions are detected by recording various functional and morphological changes in the coronary circulation and in the ventricular myocardium. None of the currently used methods gives per se a complete picture. The aim of this study was therefore to investigate their relations and their mutual predictive values.

Material and methods

The study group comprised 50 patients (41 men, 9 women, aged 22 to 59 y.) with chest pain, referred for diagnostic investigation.

Selective coronary arteriograms (CA) were evaluated using a I to V scale according to Vlodaver et al.(1). Biplane left ventriculography and echocardiography (VG, ECHO) were employed to detect ventricular motion disorders (dyssynergy). Standard 12 lead electrocardiograms (ECG) were evaluated by the Minnesota code. Vectorcardiograms were recorded (VC) with the Hewlett-Packard vectorcardiograph system 1520A, using the McFee axial lead system in seated subjects and photographed from the oscillo-

scope screen. After optical enlargement the QRS loops were evaluated with respect to signs of focal lesions of the myocardium.
Positive results of the above diagnostic methods were regarded as subsets of the set of all investigations.

Results

Consensus of all methods was found in 40% of patients if considering more than 50% stenosis as criterion of coronary artery disease. If the presence of total obstruction of at least one coronary vessel was required, consensus was found only in 36% of patients.
Table 1 shows positive results of diagnostic methods with respect to the outcome of coronary arteriography.

Table 1

Percentage of agreement between VG,ECHO,VC and 2 criteria of CA

positivity	50% stenosis	obstruction
VC	10	10
ECHO	0	0
CA	6	4
VG	2	4
VC+ECHO	4	6
VC+CA	4	4
VC+VG	4	8
ECHO+CA	0	0
ECHO+VG	0	2
CA+VG	4	2
VC+ECHO+CA	6	4
ECHO+CA+VG	0	0
VG+VC+ECHO	4	8
VG+VC+CA	16	12
ECHO+VC+CA+VG	24	18

Using the 50% stenosis as CA criterion, 16% of patients had all results negative. Using the obstruction as criterion, this figure was 18%.
Results of coronary arteriography, vectorcardiography and echocardiography (ventriculography omitted) are shown as Venn diagrams on Fig.1.
From Table 1 it is evident, that vectorcardiography alone was positive in 10% of cases, demonstrating a rather high incidence of abnormal ventricular conduction in patients with stenocardiac complaints, but with only less than 50% coronary artery stenosis and without impairement of ventricular kinetics. Isolated positivity of coronary arteriography was found in 6% of cases, of ventriculography in 2%, and of echocardiography in none. Vectorcardiography was negative in no case with positive CA,VG and ECHO. On the contrary, negative echocardiographic results were in 8 patients (16%) with positive CA, VC and VG.
If isolated positivity of one method was considered as false positivity and the presence or absence of positivity in the combination of at least two methods as true positivity or true negativity, then vectorcardiography ranked first in sensitivity, negative predictive value and overall predictivity (96%, 80%, 83%), while echocardiography ranked last with 55%, 36% and 83%, respectively.

On the contrary, echocardiography ranked first in specificity (100%) and positive predictive value (100%) and vectorcardiography last (62% and 83%).

The combination of vectorcardiography and echocardiography versus positivity of coronary arteriography and/or ventriculography had a sensitivity of 90%, specificity of 80%, positive predictive value of 90%, negative predictive value of 80% and overall predictivity of 86% if more than 50% stenosis was considered as criterion. If obstruction was required, the figures were 94%, 75%, 83%, 90% and 86% respectively.

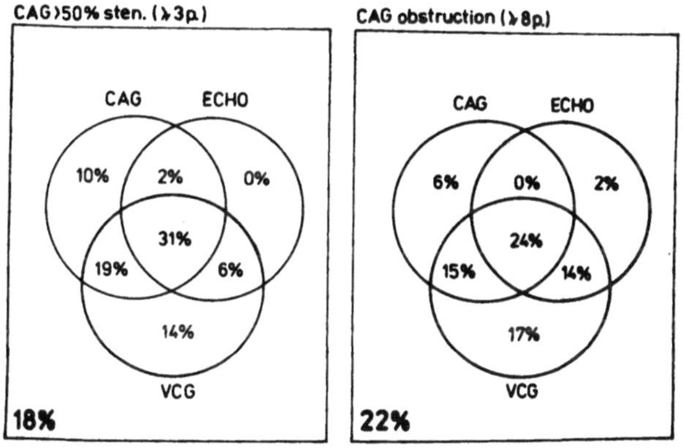

Fig.1.Venn digrams of positive results obtained by coronary arteriography (CAG), echocardiography (ECHO) and vectorcardiography (VCG). The whole set of results is represented by squares. Left:criterion for CAG positivity at more than 50% stenosis.Right:presence of obstruction as criterion.Numbers indicate percent of subjects.

Positivity of the 12 lead ECG was assessed by finding Minnesota codes 1-1, 1-2 or 1-3. Table 2 shows the comparison of ECG and VCG with respect to presence of more than 50% stenosis or obstruction as documented by CA.

Table 2.

ECG and VC versus more than 50% stenosis on CA

	Sensitivity	Specificity	Positive predict.	Negative predict.
ECG	50	41	63	29
VC	79	44	72	53

Overall predictive value of electrocardiography was in this relation 47% of vectorcardiography 67%.

Sensitivity of the ECG with respect to more than 50% stenosis of one, two or three vessels was 57%, 20% and 59%, of the vectorcardiogram 71%, 83% and 88%. Sensitivity of ventriculographically ascertained hypokinesis or akinesis of the left ventricular wall was in the same respect

86% in one vessel disease, 67% in two vessel disease and 81% in three vessel disease.

Discussion and conclusions

The limitations of this study lie in the nature of our patient population and in the inherent limitations of electrocardiologic, echocardiographic, coronarographic and ventriculographic techniques.

None of them is specific for the detection of a circumscribed myocardial lesion.

No attempt was made to correlate the localization and the extent of focal lesion as seen by the diagnostic methods used.

Evaluation of the 12 lead electrocardiogram and of the vectorcariogram was based on the QRS complex only.

The decision rules for diagnostic assessment of the vectorcardiogram were built on the spatial localization of instantaneous vector endpoints (2). The best-discriminative QRS vectors and vectorcardiographic plane projections were: the horizontal plane projection of the 10ms vector for anteroseptal and anterolateral infarctions, the sagittal plane projection of the 20ms vector for posteroseptal infarctions, the horizontal plane projection of the 20ms vector for lateral wall infarctions, the sagittal plane projection of the 30ms vector for diaphragmatic infarctions and the 30-50 ms sagittal and horizontal plane vector projections for posterolateral wall infarctions.

Evaluating the two non-invasive diagnostic methods: vectorcardiography and echocardiography, it may be concluded that they are complementary in predicting the outcome of the invasive methods of coronary arteriography and ventriculography.

They have a practically acceptable predictive value when looking for the mere presence of ventricular myocardial injury.

References

(1) Vlodaver,Z.,K.Amplatz,H.B.Burchell and J.E.Edwards: Coronary Heart Disease.Springer,New York,Heidelberg ,Berlin,1976, p.584

(2) Ruttkay-Nedecký,I.,V.Szathmáry,and S.Cagáň:Adv.Cardiol.19,185-186, (1977).

Diagnostic possibilities of electrocardiotopography and mathematical model in myocardial infarction

VORONTSOVA L. A., TRUBNICOV G. V., CHUMACOVA G. A., CHERNICOV S. Ju.

Altai Medical Institute, Barnaul, Lenin-street 40, USSR

Summary

The most traditional and fundamental method of myocard's estimation in myocardial infarction is the electrocardiography and the most informatical is the electrocardiotopographical.

But the clinical practice shows us, that the development of heart failure as the main cause of mortality in MI is connected not only with the necrosis mass, but with the features of haemodynamic acute MI. Pathogenesis of heart failure in acute M. I. as known is heterogeneous and includes three components.

1. The first component is connected with preceiding heart changes and more static.
2. The sec. component depends on the mass of necrosis.
3. The most labial component depends on the character and expression of primary adaptation and stress reactions of organism.

It can be redeveloped and differs from the first and the second. So, the main role in heart failure development in MI in 24 hours plays the third component - the degree of compensatory hyperfunction of intact cells. But to the moment of necrosis mass stabilisation (wo three days) the mass of necrosis focus.

Introduction

The task of the following investigational fragment is the establishment of the connections between the degree of affection with MI according to ECG and haemodynamical changes.

Material and methods

Here we show the materials of haemodynamical and electrocardiotopographical parallels about 25 MI patients in age from 45 to 72. There were 23 men and 2 women. All of them had acute large-facal anterior MI. 5 patients had acute heart failure as a result of MI (cardiac dropsy), 3 got acute anewrism of the left ventricle. 22 became well, 3-died, We investigated the patients, admitted to the hospital within 6 hours of the attack.

The degree of the development of the necrosis mass was found by means of electrocardiotopography in 35 leads. The necrosis mass was calculated according to formula. According to the cartograms we apreciated the following points:

- The leads quantity with QS and pathological Q waves.
- The summary square of QS and pathological Q waves.
- The lead's quantity with ST-segment elevation from 1mm and higer.
- The summary square elevation of ST-segment.
- The summary amplitude and R waves square.
- The necrosis mass.
- The investigations of the central haemodynamics were used in a complex, including measuring of cardiac output by tetrapolar reography, the measuring of arterial and mean arterial blood presure with tachocyclography, central venous pressure - by direct method. We developed the invasive and non-invasive variants of monitoring, according to the cateterisation of magnistral vesselswhether to use it or not. We used the method of mathematical model cardiovascular system. By means of computering system "Iskra-227" we calculated the follo ing points: haemodynamic loading of left ventricular - its capacity ($C_{1\ v}$ Y), elasticity of arterial (E_a) and venous vessels (E_v) of the large circle of circulation, peripheral resistance of vessels and cor pumping coefficient.

Results

Retrospective analysis of the results showed, that after 6 hour's development of chest pain attac or the moment of patients investigation in the block of intensive treatment, appeared 3 groups of patients: according to level haemodynamical load.
The level of mean arterial pressure of patients of these groups didn't differ. The quantity of the cardiac index in groups with hyper and aukinetic circulation differed much.
The simultanious investigation of MI size by means of precordial cartography showed that in the groups of patients didn't differ withing 6 hours of MI, and up to 24 hours the groups of patients differed in variants of circulation.
So, patients with hyperkinetic type of circulation had the necrosis square up to 24 hours became $541{,}2 \pm 52{,}3$ mm^2, but the patients with hypocinetic circulation had it 1,5 less, with normocinetic circulation - 2,1 times less.
The size of ishemic damage of miocard, inderectly measured by the point of ST withing the group of patients with hyper - and hypodynamic variants didn't differ at all (was the same) and has more than 2 times within the group of patients with normocinetical variant.
After 2-3 days of MI, patients with hyperdynamic variant of circulation hed the second peak of ST segment elevation. It is shown that within 36-42 hours haemodynamical load of heart vaised ($C_{1\ v}$).
We supposed that these peaks are connected with necrosis mass extention. But the mass was practically the same ($46{,}3 \pm 3{,}8$ gramms and

48,2 ± 4,2 g). Extention of necrosis and damage squares was accompanied by the increase of leads number of cartogramme with following changes. So the correlations - summary square of Q and QS waves devided by number of Q waves. And summare elevation of ST segment devided by number of ST elevation don't changes.
So, we can suppose, that repeated peaks are not symptoms of prolonging MI, as others consider, but point to dilatation of left ventricle to 2-3 days of hyperdynamic syndrome.
But we admit that future investigation is needed. The same conclusion is true in the case with 3 patients with developed acute aneurism of left ventricle. These patients had the constantly high level of haemodynamic leading capacity ($C_{1\,v}$) from first days of ilness (0,84w/m^2) combined with expressed dynamism of precordial cartogramm indexes, expressing necrosis square, but constant MI mass in comparison to first measures.
The analysis of haemodynamical determinants of hypercinetical circulation on the mathematical model, showed that it may be different on different MI stages.
So in first hours of MI development, patients with hypercinetical circulation are characterised by developing C_{1v} by means of cor pumping work (2 thirds of patients).
Up to the end of 24 hours, the number of patients is reduced to 1 thirds (1/3).

Conclusion

In conclusion parallel use of precordial cartogramme and mathematical model of central haemodynamic showed the possibility of haemodynamic leading index use as the early characteristic, which shows the extention of necrosis zone. Extention of C_{1v} can be explained by different of computory monitoring became the basis of treatment.
Treatment can lead to heart load reduction and after all to prophylaxis of necrosis zone extention.

Electrocardiotopography value in myocardial infarction and stenocardia.

ANDREICHEV N.A.

The Kazan State Medical Institute, Propedeutics of Internal Diseases Department, Butlerov st., 49, Kazan, USSR.

Summary. The peculiarities of potentials distribution in microfocal myocardial infarction (IM) and stenocardia were studied in 116 patients using integral topography (IT) technique. Three projections of zero zones location in microfocal IM were revealed. In patients with angina pectoris IT method revealed 14,5% of focal lesions without changes in 12 classic leads. The electric field characteristics in patients with angina pectoris with determined focal lesions approach the parameters of microfocal IM. Seven types of focal myocardial lesion projections were revealed. Additional leads were recommended, increasing the exactness of focal myocardial lesions (MNL) diagnosis in patients with angina pectoris by 8,7-11,6%.

The presentday electrocardiology is characterized by wide application of multiple leads in clinical picture (R.Z.Amirov [1,2,3], M.M.Mirrachimov [7], Khodzhaeva, Andreichev [4,5,6], Toyama [8]). The possibilities of IT methods for increasing the exactness of IHD diagnosis were studied.

Material and methods. Heart electric activity was studied in 116 patients with acute and chronic IHD (27 persons with microfocal IM, 89 persons with IHD with angina pectoris attacks, FC_{II-IV}). 49 practically healthy persons formed a control group. Electrocardiography according to R.Z.Amirov's method was used. To draw the IT the system of monopolar leads according to Wilson was used drawing the ECG from 84-110 points of body surface. Together with the visual analysis of ECG the peaks value was calculated, the results were displayed on the maps of electropositivity (EP) (R and R' peaks) and electronegativity (EN) (Q and S peaks). After the mapping of IT heart electric field characteristics were studied (the maximus, overlapping zones, zero zones).

Results and Discussion. Microfocal IM is characterized by the following regularities: 1) zero zones registration in EP beyond the limits of 12 classic leads; 2) zero zone registration in EP in upper right anterior and posterior chest without hypertrophy of left ventricle; 3) QR zone registration in atypical place of localization if compared with normal, without hypertrophy of right ventricle (q-type of hypertrophy in IT); 4) low anterior Q wave beyond the limits of 12 classic leads; we must mention here that the deepening of Q wave on posterior part of chest by its upper levels of registration is more typical for hypertrophy of left ventricle; 5) the dynamics of T-peak /its inversion, the deviation of T-peak in an atypical place of localization/ has a great meaning. Patients with microfocal IM were divided into 2 groups: 1) patients with ECG signs of microfocal IM in 12 classic leads - 10 persons; 2) patients without ECG signs of myocardial lesion in 12 classic leads - 17 persons. We must note, that all these patients had microfocal IM, but IT registrated it only on the 3rd-4th weeks of the infarction or in more remote postinfarction period. For the first froup of patients the IT registrated the diffusion of microfocal IM; beyond the limits of 12 classic leads the infarction had a transmural character of lesion. In the second group of patients the IM was either small in diffusion, or IT registrated it in more remote postinfarction period, so 12 classic leads had no sighs of myocardial lesion. The IT beyond the limits of commonly accepted ECG registrated the myocardial lesions foci, the projections are displayed on Fig.I.

Fig.I. Microfocal myocardial lesions foci projections.

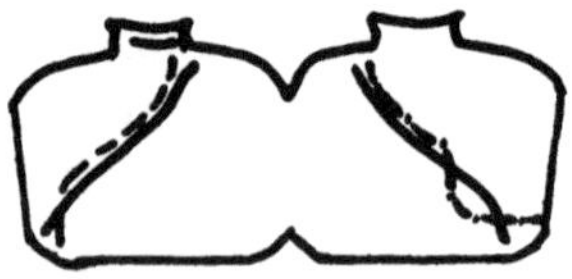

1) upper right anterior chest and right posterior chest - 4 persons ———

2) upper right anterior chest-2 persons - - - -

3) upper right posterior chest-7 persons —·—·—·—

So in 13 persons of 17 (76,47%) with previous microfocal IM the IT method reveals the signs of IM, absent in 12 classic leads.

The group of patients with IHD was of special interest because the majority of patients had in anamnesis often, sometimes prolonged (15-20-30 min) angina pectoris attacks, FC_{II-IV}, critical picture of disease, had repeatedly received stationary treatment, had been hospitalized with suspected coronary pathology, but in the majority of cases the usual ECG investigation in dynamics revealed no focal myocardial lesions. The comparative analysis of 12 classic leads information was done as well as 3 orthogonal Frank's leads with the exchange of "Z and IT. (Table I).

Table I. Frequency of focal myocardial lesions revealing in patients with IHD with angina pectoris attacks by usual methods.

	12 + IT :	12 + 3 IT :	3 + IT :	IT	:
12 classic leads	3,37%	12,35%	-	-	15,72%
3 orthogonal Frank's leads	-	12,35%	8,99%	-	21,34%
IT	3,37%	12,35%	8,99%	14,58%	39,29%

Table I shows that patients with IHD with angina pectoris attacks having normal ECG in 12 classic leads need special attention. Revealing 14,58% of focal myocardial lesions without ECG signs of myocardial lesions in 12 classic leads in patients with IHD with angina pectoris attacks testifies for the lack of correspondence between clinical and ECG signs of IHD.

So it is adbisable to use IT technique for diagnosis of the most complicated cases as it is more informative. The electric activity of myocard in patients with IHD with angina pectoris attacks was studied the signs of MNL were revealed. The patients were divided into 4 groups (Table 2).

Table 2. Heart electric field characteristics in patients with IHD with angina pectoris attacks in focal myocardial lesions and microfocal IM.

	Overlapping zones area		Zero zones area		Maxima values		Area variations overlapping zones		Area variations zero zones		Maxima values variations	
	EP	EN	EP	EN	EP	EN	EP	EN	EP	EN	EP	EN
12+3+IT	4,00	4,27	0,54	6,90	17,81	10,95	0-9	0-18	0-40	0-30	11-26,5	6-17
12+IT	0,66	1,00	12,0	5,00	14,33	15,33	0-2	0-3	4-21	4-6	7,5-23	7-15
3+IT	2,00	2,25	15,25	5,75	17,11	14,37	0-12	0-10	2-43	0-14	9,5-28	11-20
IT	0,92	2,69	13,46	4,46	18,46	14,61	0-4	0-14	8-23	0-14	10,5-32	8,5-30
Microfocal IM	3,40	3,36	9,12	3,63	15,56	14,22	0-29	0-18	0-24	0-16	9-28	6,5-38
Igr.MIM	2,11	3,77	12,44	4,65	15,05	10,50	0-6	0-10	0-24	0-16	18-28	6,5-20
IIgrMIM	3,05	3,33	8,66	3,24	15,91	16,61	0-29	0-18	0-24	0-12	11-28	9-38

The parameters obtained are very close to the heart electric field characteristics of microfocal IM which testifies for the focal myocardial lesion in patients with IHD with angine pectoris attacks. For all groups of patients the analysis of the zero zones on chest surface was carried out. As IT method revealed the focal lesions in all groups of patients with IHD with angina pectoris attacks and zero zones projections on chest surface were located in the same or very close leads, we considered it advisable to unite all these topograms in one scheme. The projections of zero zones location on chest surface according to the focal myocardial lesions revealed by IT are as follows (Fig.2): 1) in EP right anterior and posterior zero zones are registered - 12 persons; 2) in EP upper right posterior chest is registered - 13 persons; 3) in EP upper anterior and posterior registration levels are registered - 2 persons; 4) in EP upper anterior registration level zero zones are registered - 2 persons; 5) in EP right anterior zero zone is registered - 2 persons; 6) in EN right anterior and posterior low registration level R type zone is registered, in EP - isolated zero points with corresponding posterior upper registration levels QS by EN are registered-2 persons; 7) QR zone is registered with pathologic anterior Q peak in upper registration levels - 2 persons.

Fig.2. Lesion foci projections in patients with IHD with angina pectoris attacks.

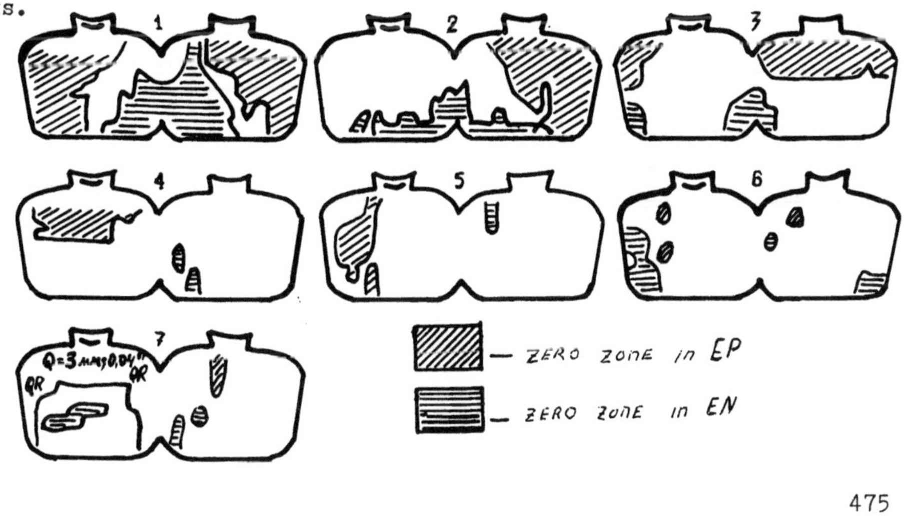

In a single patient zero zone by EP and EN is located within determined areas on chest and testifies for the presence of lesion focus. During the analysis of topograms of patients with IM and angina pectoris the most informative points were determined, where the change of depolarization phase most frequently occurs, i.e. QS complex in IM is registered beyond the limits of 12 classic leads. 2 additional lead modifications were recommended (6 and 12) to increase the exactness of diagnosis of focal myocardial lesions and to reveal the diffusion of IM and the rate of lesion (intramural and transmural). Normal time and amplitude parameters of these leads and their changes in IM were obtained. The use of new additional leads helps to improve the diagnosis of focal myocardial lesions in patients with angina pectoris in the first modification by 8,7%, in the second modification by 11,6% without ECG signs of myocardial lesion in 12 classic leads.

Conclusion. 1. IT reveals 14,58% of focal myocardial changes in patients with IHD with angina pectoris attacks (FC_{I-IV}).

2. In focal myocardial lesions registration heart electric field in patients with angina pectoris attacks does not differ in parameters from potentials distribution in MIM. 7 types of zero zones projections focal myocardial lesions were revealed.

3. The use of new additional leads increases the exactness of focal myocardial lesion diagnosis by 8,7-11,6% in patients with IHD with angina pectoris attacks.

R e f e r e n c e s

1. Amirov R.Z. Integral topograms of heart potential. M."Science",1973.
2. Amirov R.Z. In: International congress on electrocardiology. 12. Abstract book. Minsk, 1985, 8-9.
3. Amirov R.Z. Electrocardiotopography actual questions. M. Cardiology, v.XXVI, 6, 1986, 14-17.
4. Andreichev N.A. In: International congress on electrocardiology. 12. Abstract book. Minsk, 1985, 118-119.
5. Khodzhaeva D.K. and Andreichev N.A. Adv.Cardiology, vol.28, 64-66, Karger.Basel, 1981.
6. Khodzhaeva D.K., Andreichev N.A., Galyavich A.S. In: International congress on electrocardiology.12. Abstract book. Minsk, 1985, 237-238.
7. Mirrachimov M.M., Vimbor U.B., Kenenbaev K.K. M. Cardiology, vol.XXI, 9, 1981, 52-57.
8. Toyama S., Susudi K., Koyana M. Jap.Curculat.J., 45, 10, 1981, 1218-1220.

ECG changes and load tolerance in patients after myocardial infarction

MIKEŠ,Z., J.KOLESÁR, J.LIETAVA, A.DUKÁT, J.KRIŠTÚFEK

Department of Physical Medicine, Comenius Univ.School of Medicine and Research Institute for Human Bioclimatology, Mickiewiczova 13, 813 69 Bratislava, Czechoslovakia

Summary.

The aim of the study was to analyse the type of ECG changes in patients after acute myocardial infarction and to compare them with the changes in physical fitness. The autors examined 218 patients with acute myocardial infarction after discharge from hospital. Resting ECG and graded exercise ECG test on the bicycle ergometer was carried out. Examination technique was in accordance with the WHO recommendations. Statistical evaluation was performed by the Wilcoxon-Mann-Whitney U-test. The load intensity in patients who showed ECG changes of a transmural myocardial infarction was not different in comparison with persons with non-transmural lesion (70,0 W versus 71,7 W). When evaluating the relation between the site of the ECG changes and the load intensity the autors found that, the lowest tolerated load was in those cases where ECG changes suggested an extensive damage of the myocardium (53,5 W, $P < 0,05$). The authors conclude that, the extent of established ECG changes after myocardial infarction is more important in view of physical fitness damage than its classifying to the type Q or non-Q.

Introduction.

Myocardial infarction represents an intervention into the integrity of the cardiovascular system and is connected with a disturbance of the heart function. Nowadays there is no agreement in evaluating the importance of different types of myocardial infarction. Until lately non-Q infarctions were considered as a milder form of the disease. The studies of Maisels et al. (1), Hutter et al. (2) and Conolly et al. (3), however, are pointing out that a long-term prognosis of a non-Q infarction may be even worse than in cases with a developed Q wave. On the other hand Karnegis et al. (4) have found a lower grade dysfunction of the left ventricle in persons without pathological changes of the Q-QS wave in comparison with persons who showed such changes.
The aim of our study was to find out if there were any differences in physical performance between patients with an ECG of the Q-type or those with a non-Q infarction.

Table 1 : Type and localization of the myocardial infarction (MI)

Type of MI	Localization	Steady state reached yes	no	Total	Load (W)	
		n	n	n		
Q	anteroseptal	28	7	35		
	posteroinferior	50	7	57		
	anteroextensive	7	0	7		
	other	40	10	50		
	all Q together	125	24	149	62,33	N.S.
Non - Q		54	15	69	61,23	
All MI		179	39	218		

Table 2 : Maximal load level in various groups (patients, who reached steady state at least at 25 W)

Type of MI	Localization	Maximal load (W)	SE	n
Q	anteroseptal (AS)	78,57	6,52	28
	posteroinferior (PI)	69,50	3,29	50
	anteroextensive (AE)	53,37	8,50	7
	other (O)	57,5	4,83	40
	combined localization (2S) (included in O)	48,08	5,53	26
	all Q together	70,0	2,57	125
Non - Q		71,76	3,49	54

P		
	Q - non Q	N.S.
	AS - non Q	N.S.
	AE - non Q	< 0,05
	AE - AS	≈ 0,05
	AE - PI	≤ 0,06
	AE - all Q	< 0,05
	2S - non Q	< 0,0005
	2S - Q all	< 0,0005
	2S - AS	< 0,0005
	2S - PI	< 0,0005
	2S - AE	N.S.

Material and methods.

We had examined 218 patients discharged from hospital after acute myocardial infarction. The average age of the patients was 51,1 years, the examination protocol was in accordance with the WHO recommendation. The initial load 25 W had been increased every 6 minutes by 25 W till 85% of the maximum heart rate or other criteria for the load interruption. The criteria of load interruption and contraindication of the examination had been published in the past and they did not differ from the currently recommended criteria (5). When localizing infarction according to ECG we followed the commonly used criteria. The statistical evaluation of the results was performed by the Wilcoxon-Mann-Whitney U-test.

Results.

The patients were divided depending on the infarction type as is seen on the tab.1. To the non-Q type belonged 69 persons, 149 patients had ECG criteria corresponding for attribution to the Q type.
From the group Q 35 persons had an anteroseptal localization, 57 a posteroinferior one and 7 an anteroextensive one. The remaining group of 50 persons had other localizations (e.g. septal, apical two sites combination etc.).
In evaluating the load level (tab.2) we did not find any difference in the tolerance between the group of Q and non-Q infarctions. While the maximum load level was evaluated in persons tolerating at least the minimum load level during steady state conditions, lower tolerated loads were seen in persons with ECG signs of anteroextensive infarction in comparison with other localizations, The load level is lower also in cases where there are ECG signs of two sites impairment in comparison with the impairment of one segment.

Discussion and conclusions.

There were several methods suggested to determine the function of the left heart ventricle in patients after myocardial infarction by means of ECG (6,7,8,9), nevertheless with rather limited success (4,10). The terms transmural an subendocardial have been used for many years in the ECG classification of myocardial infarction. Though the newer term Q and non-Q wave describes much more precisely the electrocardiographical characteristics of the attack, there is only a week correlation between the ECG and the pathological finding (2). Neither exists a uniform opinion about the difference in clinical importance of both types. Maisel et al.,e.g.(1) report even a higher mortality rate during hospitalization in cases of infarction extension, as well as during one year lasting follow-up in non-Q types. On the contrary, Karnegis et al.(4) have found in Q-wave infarction explicitly higher occurence of ventriculographically determined dysfunctions of the left ventricle.

The left ventricle function is substantial with regard to physical performance. Therefore it was of interest if there would be found a difference in the physical performance level between the booth infarction types. Our results did not confirm the expected difference in load tolerance between the Q and non-Q infarction. However, an interesting finding was the low level of load tolerance in the grouph with an affliction of two heart segments and in the group with anteroextensive infarction, i.e. in cases with extensive impairment, given by ECG. This finding is in accordance with the finding of Karnegis et al.(4) who found in the Q-wave type a correlation between the infarction extent and the number of segmental wall motion abnormalities during ventriculography.

On the basis of our results we conclude that, the extent of established ECG changes after myocardial infarction is more important in view of physical fitness damage than its classifying to the type Q or non-Q.

References.

(1) Maisel, A.S., S.Ahnve, E. Gilpin, H. Henning, A.L. Goldberger, D. Collins, M. LeWinter, and J. Rose: Circulation 71, 211-217 (1985)

(2) Hutter, A.M., R.W. DeSanctis, T. Flynn, and L.A. Yetman: Am.J.Cardiol 48, 595 - 602 (1981)

(3) Connolly, D.C., V. Fustes, M. Danielson, and R.L. Frye: Circulation 54, (suppl. II), 77 - 78 (1976) abst.

(4) Karnegis, J.N., J. Matts, N. Tuna, K.Amplatz, and the POSCH Group: Am.J.Cardiol. 58, 309 - 405 (1986)

(5) Kolesár, J., and Z. Mikeš: Ergometria v klinickej praxi. 1, 1 - 224 (1981) Publisher Osveta Martin

(6) Askenazi, J., A.F. Parisi, P.F. Cohn, W.B. Freedman, and E. Braunwald: Am.J.Cardiol. 41, 494 - 499 (1978)

(7) Gottwik, M.G., A.F. Parisi, J. Askenazi, and D. McCaugham: Am.J.Cardiol. 41, 9 - 13 (1978)

(8) Rautaharju, P.M., S.W. Warren, U. Jain, H.K. Wolf, and C.L. Nielsen: Circulation 64, 249 - 256 (1981)

(9) Wagner, C.S., C.J. Freye, S.T. Palmeri, S.F. Roark, N.C. Stack, R.E. Ideker, F.E. Harrell Jr., and R.H. Selvester: Circulation 65, 342 - 347 (1982)

(10) Babbitt, D., F. Marcus, G.S. Wagner, and R. Serokman: Am. Heart J. 108, 1426 - 1430 (1984)

RHYTHM AND RHYTHM DISTURBANCES

Circadian variation of the sinus arrhythmia

K. ECKOLDT, H. LOESER, J. BERLIN

Inst. Med. Physics and Biophysics, Humboldt University, Berlin, GDR

Summary:
The circadian variations of heart rate (HR) and its beat-to-beat variability (sinus arrhythmia: SA) were analysed in a group of 17 normal men at their usual lifestyle conditions. Most dayly cycles represent a significant cosinuslike variation in HR as well as in SA ascertained by cosinor analysis. The same holds for the group mean in HR but not in SA. In HR the mean amplitude was found to be 5.5 % of the dayly mean value and the acrophase appears at 14.36 h. In SA no significant mean amplitude and acrophase could be evaluated due to the fact that the individual circadian rhythmicity is not synchroneous neither intraindividually nor interindividually.

Introduction:
Heart rate (HR) and its spontaneous beat-to-beat fluctuations, called sinus arrhythmia (SA), are measures to judge indirectly the cardiac vegetative tonization (1, 2, 3, 4). The cardiac innervation strength is altered in some pathophysiologic circumstances as cardiac related diseases or diabetic neuropathies and the amount of disturbance can be evaluated by HR and SA. On the other hand, most of the vegetative parameters show a distinct circadian variation, as it is well known from body temperature, arterial blood pressure or HR. Up to now, no information has been available concerning the circadian variability of the SA. It was to be expected, that there must be a clear circadian course which should be responsible for a part of the known considerable inter- and intraindividual variability of the SA. If there is a predictable circadian rhythmicity the measured result gained at different times could be corrected to eliminate the circadian rhythmicity. Furthermore, a close relation of the SA to the HR was to be expected because of the mostly reciprocal sympathetic and parasympathetic tonization of the heart.
The aim of our study was to quantify the kind and extent of the circadian variation of the SA under normal lifestyle conditions because diagnostic analyses were also usually done at non-standardized circumstances.

Material and methods:
From 17 healthy male subjects at the age between 17 and 34 years the ECGs were recorded by an Holter storage device over 24 hours, in 2 subjects the recordings were repeated 4 times. After application of the device the subjects went about their usual work. At a certain time every

hour they were forced to sit down quietly and to switch on the apparatus for 15 min. During the night the recordings were done continuously. Each hour 5 minutes of these traces were analysed. HR and SA were evaluated by a special purpose microcomputer after removing possible artefacts. The SA was quantified as the mean of successive differences of instantaneous heart rates:

$$\Delta HR = \frac{1}{n} \sum_{i=1}^{n} | HR_i - HR_{i-1} | .$$

The individual dayly mean values of HR and Δ HR were calculated and the percentual deviations built from it at each hour. These values were treated statistically (mean, standard error, WILCOXON-pair test, Cosinor-analysis).

Results:

Mean values as well as variability coefficients $v = s/\bar{x}$ of HR and Δ HR of all measuring times in 24 hours and during the day hours between 8.30 and 17.30 h of the group (n = 17) and from the two repetition experiments (sbj. 1 and sbj. 2) are displayed in table 1. The variability of Δ HR is about twice that of HR. The intraindividual variability is not smaller than the interindividual one. The variability of the measurements at day hours is not essentially smaller than that over 24 h.

Table 1: Mean values $\bar{x}$ as well as mean coefficients of variability $\bar{v}$ of HR and Δ HR

	24 h		8.30 - 17.30 h	
	HR	Δ HR	HR	Δ HR
Group $\bar{x}$ (min^{-1})	69.3	2.56	72	2.65
(n=17) $\bar{v}$ (%)	10.1	22.5	7.0	16.7
Sbj. 1 $\bar{x}$ (min^{-1})	62.1	1.90	67.1	1.99
(n=5) $\bar{v}$ (%)	10.8	18.2	11.6	18.8
Sbj. 2 $\bar{x}$ (min^{-1})	59.9	2.48	62.7	2.54
(n=5) $\bar{v}$ (%)	8.0	13.8	8.8	11.4

The time course of the group mean values and its standard error from HR and Δ HR is depicted in fig. 1. Thick points and bars mean significant differences from the dayly mean (= 100 %). HR show low values at night and high values in the afternoon with a significant cosinor approximation (amplitude: 5,5 %, acrophase 14.36 h). Δ HR is high in the morning between 6 and 9 p.m. and low in the evening between 6 and 9 a.m., the cosinor approximation is not significant. The reasons for the different behaviour of both parameters can be seen from fig. 2 where the individual cosinor results are displayed. In most cases a significant individual cosinor approximation was possible (14/17 in HR, 12/17 in Δ HR) but whereas in HR the acrophases show essentially similar directions (14/17 between - 180 and - 270° ~ 12-18 h), in Δ HR the acrophases show no distinct preference direction. A relation between the acrophases in HR and Δ HR resp. could not be found. Similar results are obtained from the repetition analysis of the two subjects: constancy of the individual acrophases in HR, different directions in Δ HR.

Discussion and conclusions:

At normal lifestyle conditions the heart rate showed similar circadian rhythmicity as in standardized chronobiological laboratory experiments (e.g. (5)) with maxima in the afternoon and minima in the second half of the night and a cosinor amplitude of 5.5 %. All but 3 of the examined subjects had similar time courses. The total average variability was found to be 10.8 %, that means half of this could be attributed to the predictable circadian rhythmicity. In contrast to this, the circadian rhythm of the sinus arrhythmia showed much more individual differences, so that no significant mean course could be confirmed. In this parameter the total average variability amounts to 22 % interindividually and is intraindividually in the same order of magnitude. It was found to be impossible to reduce this value in order to improve the reliability of SA estimations.

If we attribute the SA to the strength of parasympathetic innervation and the HR to that of sympathetic and parasympathetic one (1) we must assume that the sympathetic innervation exhibit a clear and stable circadian rhythmicity but the vagal one does not or it is much more sensible to actual influences, presumably changes in the respiratory pattern, which provoke masking effects.

Surprisingly, no correlation was found between the individual acrophases in HR and Δ HR. The phase lag between both parameters varies in the 17 subjects between - 170 and 190° ($\sim \pm\pi$) with a mean of 1.1° ± 128°. That means that the cardiac vegetative innervation is not clearly reciprocal in the course of the day but to a certain degree independent.

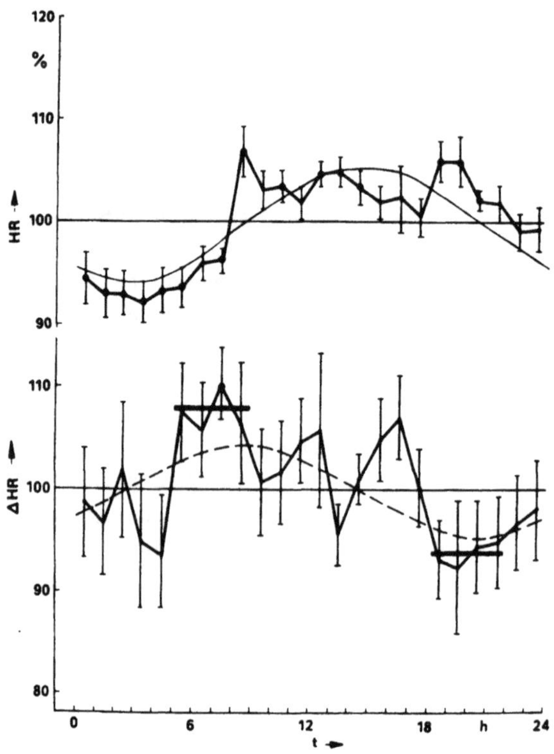

Fig. 1: Time course of HR (above) and Δ HR with cosinor approximation (see text)

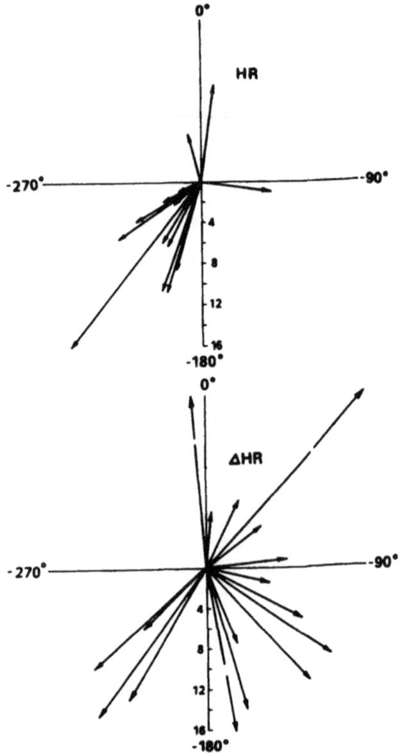

Fig. 2: Individual cosinor amplitudes and acrophases for HR (above) and Δ HR

References:

(1) Eokoldt, K.: Dt. Gesundh.-Wesen 39, 856 - 863 (1984)
(2) Eckoldt, K.: Ergebn. exp. Med. 46, 106 - 116 (1985)
(3) Eckoldt, K.; W. Braun, and V. Lange: Chronobiol. a. Chronomed. Basic research a applicat., Edit.: Hildebrandt, G., R. Moog, F. Raschke Frankfurt/Main; Lang 1987; 181 - 186
(4) Katona, P.G., and F. Jih: J. appl. Physiol. 39, 801 - 805 (1975)
(5) Goldmann, B.: Dissert. Med., Marburg 1980

On the characteristic frequency of sinus arrhythmia

LANGE, V.

Institute of Medical Physics and Biophysics, Humboldt-University, Berlin, GDR

Summary

In addition to the heart rate (HR) and the total amount of sinus arrhythmia (SA), a mean frequency (f) of the HR-fluctuations is an elementary feature of the sinus rhythm of the heart. f may be evaluated as the weighted mean frequency of the power density spectrum. It influences implicitely the values of some measures of SA. We analysed HR, SA and f in 21 healthy male students under conditions of rest and of psychic load. There was no correlation between f and HR and SA resp. at rest condition. With load we found a significant increase of f correlated to a decrease of SA. This response can already be seen during minor demands and does not grow with drastically increased levels of loads. The reliability of the individual measurements of f is low like that of the SA, calculated as root mean square differences of the instantaneous heart rate.

Introduction

Basic measures for the description of time series are the mean level, the effective value and the features of the spectral distribution, in the simplest case a characteristic frequency. Regarding the sinusarrhythmia, such an integral frequency is suitable, because spectral distributions of spontaneous heart rate fluctuations show a strong intersubject variability and their spectral components only partly reflect specific physiologic functions. In the literature one may frequently find the measure "Number of sign changes" as used and calculated as the third main component in factor analyses /1, 2, 3/. Our analyses of sinusarrhythmia measure relationships resulted in the finding of three basic measures. One of them is a characteristic frequency defined by the Fourier spectrum. Properties of this measure regarding activity indication under psychic loads shall be demonstrated and compared with those of the effective value of heart rate variation (sinusarrhythmia) s_{HR}.

Material and methods

A simple relation exists between the measure of variability of a time series s_x and that of the time series of successive differences $s_{\nabla x}$, if the main power density lies below half the Nyquist-frequency.

$$\frac{s_{\nabla x}}{s_x} = \frac{2\pi f_c}{\bar{F}}$$

f_c = characteristic frequency (1)
$\bar{F}$ = mean sampling frequency

$$\text{mit } f_c = \sqrt{\frac{\sum f_i^2 \cdot a_i^2}{\sum a_i^2}}$$

f_i = frequency of the i-th Fourier spectral term (2)

a_i = rms-value of the i-th Fourier spectral term

Values of f_c were estimated by using equation (1). Before measuring the standard deviation s_{HR}, the time series of instantaneous heart rates was digitally high-pass-filtered for suppression of heart rate trends.

$$F(i\omega) = \frac{i\omega T}{1 + i\omega T} \quad , \qquad T = 5 \text{ s}$$

All values belong to 3 min-periods. Under conditions of rest and psychic load the mean heart rate $\overline{HF}$, the standard deviation of the instantaneous heart rate s_{HF} and the characteristic sinusarrhythmia frequency f_c were measured. Using five-minute load periods, the experiments involved a gradual increase in demand and a demand of medium range repeated ten times. Subjects had to distinguish and indicate two kinds of variously marked circles under time pressure. The demand intensity was increased by means of a four-stage reduction of the interstimulus intervals from initial 1.7 s to 1.0 s. In the sixth period, the circles were presented at randomly distributed time intervals. The gradually increased demand experiments involved 21 and the ten times repeated medium range demand experiments 15 healthy male subjects who were medical students aged 20 to 30 years. The medium range demand was realized by an interstimulus interval of 1.3 s.

Results

No changes were found of the group mean of the characteristic sinusarrhythmia frequency f_c and sinusarrhythmia s_{HF} within the sequence of rest periods, within the sequence of the gradually increased demands and within the sequence of identically repeated demands. But there was a significantly increased characteristic sinusarrhythmia frequency from 0.15 Hz at rest to 0.19 Hz under load conditions and a decreased sinusarrhythmia s_{HR} from 4.1 min^{-1} under rest to 2.8 min^{-1} under load conditions. To demonstrate the individual positions in fig. 1 with a diminished intraindividual variability, values from six rest periods as well as from six load periods were averaged.

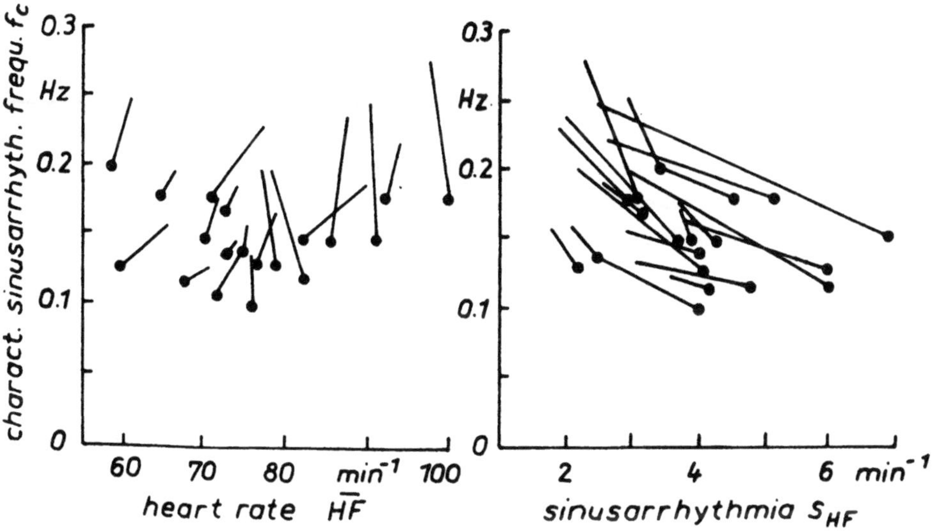

Fig. 1: Distribution of individual values of the heart rate $\overline{HF}$, the sinusarrhythmia s_{HF} and the characteristic sinusarrhythmia frequency f_c under conditions of rest and of psychic load. Each value represents the mean from six 3-minute time series periods.

Neither under conditions of rest nor of psychic load does a correlation exist between f_c and $\overline{HR}$ or f_c and s_{HR}. But the decrease in the sinusarrhythmia $\Delta s_{HF_{rl}}$ under psychic load correlates with the increase of the characteristic sinus arrhythmia frequency $\Delta f_{c_{rl}}$ ($r_s = 0.7$).

Table 1: The table shows the intra- and intersubject variability and the reliability of the heart rate level $\overline{HR}$, the sinusarrhythmia Δs_{HR} and the characteristic sinusarrhythmia frequency Δf_c obtained under conditions of rest (r), of psychic load (l) and as the difference between them (rl).

measure	mean intrasubject variability $\bar{s}_i$	intersubject variability s_z	reliability $G = s_z^2/s_z^2 + \bar{s}_i^2$
$\overline{HR}_r$	2.6 min^{-1}	12.0 min^{-1}	0.96
$\overline{HR}_l$	2.8 min^{-1}	12.0 min^{-1}	0.95
$\Delta\overline{HR}_{rl}$	1.5 min^{-1}	3.1 min^{-1}	0.81
s_{HR_r}	0.7 min^{-1}	1.3 min^{-1}	0.78
s_{HR_l}	0.7 min^{-1}	0.7 min^{-1}	0.50
$\Delta s_{HR_{rl}}$	15 %	12 %	0.39
f_{c_r}	0.020 Hz	0.028 Hz	0.66
f_{c_l}	0.020 Hz	0.028 Hz	0.82
$\Delta f_{c_{rl}}$	0.030 Hz	0.027 Hz	0.45

The reliability of the measures s_{HR} and f_c is small, particularly that of the activiation measures $\Delta s_{HR_{rl}}$ and $\Delta f_{c_{rl}}$.
In contrast, the mean heart rate shows a higher reliability. Significant changes occurred when the psychic load was gradually increased or identically repeated for the group mean as well as for single values. No significant correlation exists between rest-load differences of the respiratory rate ΔRR_{rl} and the characteristic sinusarrhythmia frequency $\Delta f_{c_{rl}}$.

Discussion

In reference to inequality between $2s_y^2$ and $s_{\nabla y}^2$ a trend is seen by some authors /4, 5, 6/ in the time series level, particularly of the heart rate. The equality is valid for unrelated elements of the time series and this is equivalent to noise properties up to the Nyquist-frequency of 0.5 Hz. As Hyndman /7/ found, about 80 % of the spectral power lies below 0.2 Hz. Whereas the above-mentioned relation will not be valid under this condition and that even without any trend, equation (1) is a better approximation of the given reality. It denominates the characteristic sinusarrhythmia frequency f_c. Because no correlation exist between rest-load differences of the characteristic sinusarrhythmia frequency $\Delta f_{c_{rl}}$ and respiratory rate differences ΔRR_{rl} we suppose the increase of f_c as produced by a load conditioned decrease in the high power density of sinusarrhythmia, specifically in the lower frequency range. In this case, compared with the sinusarrhythmia s_{HR}, f_c hardly signals a separate response activity.

References

/1/ Opmeer, C.H.J.M.: Ergonomics 16 105-112 (1973)
/2/ Eriksson, C.G.: Göteborg Psychol. Rep. (Univ.) 5 (1975)
/3/ Müller, K.W.: Univ. München Diss. 1980
/4/ Heslegrave, R.J., J.C. Ogiloie, J.J. Furedy: Psychophysiology 16 151-157 (1979)
/5/ Wastell, D.G.: Psychophysiology 18 88-90 (1981)
/6/ Sharit, J., G. Salvendry, M.P. Deisenroth: Ergonomics 25 107-120 (1982)
/7/ Hyndman, B.W., R.K. Mohn: Automedica 1 239-252 (1975)

HYPERTROPHIC CARDIOMYOPATHY AND MYOCARDIAL INFARCTION: A CHRONOBIOLOGICAL STUDY OF HEART RATE AND PREMATURE BEATS

R. Vergassola, P. Cinelli, M. De Scalzi, R. Idini, V. De Leonardis, A. Becucci, C. Gremigni, A. Triarico, F. Bandini, F. Calzolari

Department of Cardiology - Hospital of S. M. Annunziata, Florence, Italy

SUMMARY

We studied circadian rhythms (CR) of heart rate (HR) and premature beats (PB) in 12 patients (ps) with hypertrophic cardiomyopathy (CM), 12 healthy subjects (HS) and 11 with previous myocardial infarction (MI). Continuous 24-48 hour ECG recording was done using a Holter system with a two-channel recorder that uses CM5 and Lewis modified leads. We found CR of HR and of PB in all the subjects; CR of HR also showed a group rhythm, while CR of PB are dispersed throughout the 24 hours.

Amplitude of the CR of HR in HS was significantly higher than that of patients with MI and lower than that of patients with CM, even if this last difference was not statistically significant.

We can suppose that MI results in reduced sinus-node function and CM may result in abnormal sympathetic stimulation.

INTRODUCTION

Chronobiologic information about CR (24$\pm$4) of electrical cardiac functions may be interesting from a physiopathologic, and also from a therapeutic, point of view. We studied chronobiologic patterns of HR, PAB and PVB in healthy subjects and also in patients with coronary artery disease and hypertrophic cardiomyopathy.

MATERIAL AND METHODS

Thirty-five hospitalized, but not bed ridden, subjects (mean age: 63.1 + 11.6) with premature atrial beats and/or premature ventricular beats were studied. Twelve of these were considered to be normal on the basis of their medical history, ECG recorded at rest and during exercise, and ecocardiogram; eleven had suffered previous myocardial infarction, and twelve had a hypertrophic cardiomyopathy.

All the subjects were given a standard 1,900 Cal. diet (divided into 3 meals taken at 08.00 a.m., 12 noon and 17.00 p.m.); they slept between 23.30 p.m. and 06.00 a.m., and had not taken any drug since five days before the ECG study.

Continuous 96-hour recording of the ECG was done with a Holter system with a 2-channel recorder, using CM5 and Lewis modified leads. The tape reading was stopped every 15 minutes and the number of ventricular beats, PVB and PAB displayed by the scanner were stored. The measurements obtained were chronobiologically evaluated by the least square method to fit 2 cosine functions to the data, in order to prevent a set of rhythm parameters descriptive of the CR rhythmicity. The first one was a 24-h cosine function, and the second one, a cosine function with a period variable within the most significant spectral region computed by the Fast Fourier Transformance. Two kinds of cosinor were performed: "single cosinor", applied to individual time series; and "population mean cosinor", applied to parameter estimates derived from the individual time series, in order to assess the rhythm characteristics of a population.

Statistical evaluation of amplitudes and acrophases of group rhythms was performed by analysis of variance (Manova) and linear discriminant test. The two groups were compared by Student's T test for unpaired data.

RESULTS

1) CH : single cosinor

HR : all the subjects showed a highly significant CR in HR with acrophases occurring between 12.34 p.m and 16.52 p.m.

PVB : only 7 HS, 6 MI and 8 CM patients showed a significant CR of PVB with acrophases occurring between 07.05 a.m. and 19.50 p.m.

PAB : only 5 HS, 3 MI and 7 CM patients had a significant CR of PAB with acrophases occurring between 07.04 a.m. and 18.01 p.m.

2) CR : population mean cosinor

HR : all three groups showed a significant CR of HR, with acrophases occurring between 14.11 p.m. and 14.52 p.m. No significant difference between the mesor of the groups was demonstrated by Student's T test; while analysis of variance (Manova) showed a significant difference, and linear discriminant analysis demonstrated that the difference between the HS and MI groups was due to rhythm amplitude.

Amplitude of HS was higher than that of MI patients; amplitude of HS was lower than that of CM patients, even if this last difference was not statistically significant. (Fig. 1)

PVB and PAB : the analysis by "population mean cosinor" failed to demonstrate a significant rhythm due to the dispersion of the acrophases.

DISCUSSION AND CONCLUSION

The most important finding is the highly significant difference in the amplitude of the CR in HR between HS and MI patients. The reduction in amplitude in patients with MI can be due partly to the normal "aging" process of the S.A. node: as we have demonstrated (1-7), the amplitude of the CR of HR is reduced with age, as are reduced the frequency of the S.A. node and its excursions with exertion and stress. In part, however, we think that the reduction in amplitude of the CR of HR in MI patients is due also to ischemic processes of the S.A. node, due to arteriosclerosis even of small vessels.

The increase in amplitude in patients with CM, although not significant on a statistical level (p 0.2), shows however a "tendency" which could be due to an abnormal sympathetic stimulation; on the other hand, it has been hypothesized that this disease is the consequence of a congenital anomaly of the sympathic (8).

This study failed to demonstrate a group rhythm for PAB and PVB, so a chronopharmacological approach must always be individual.

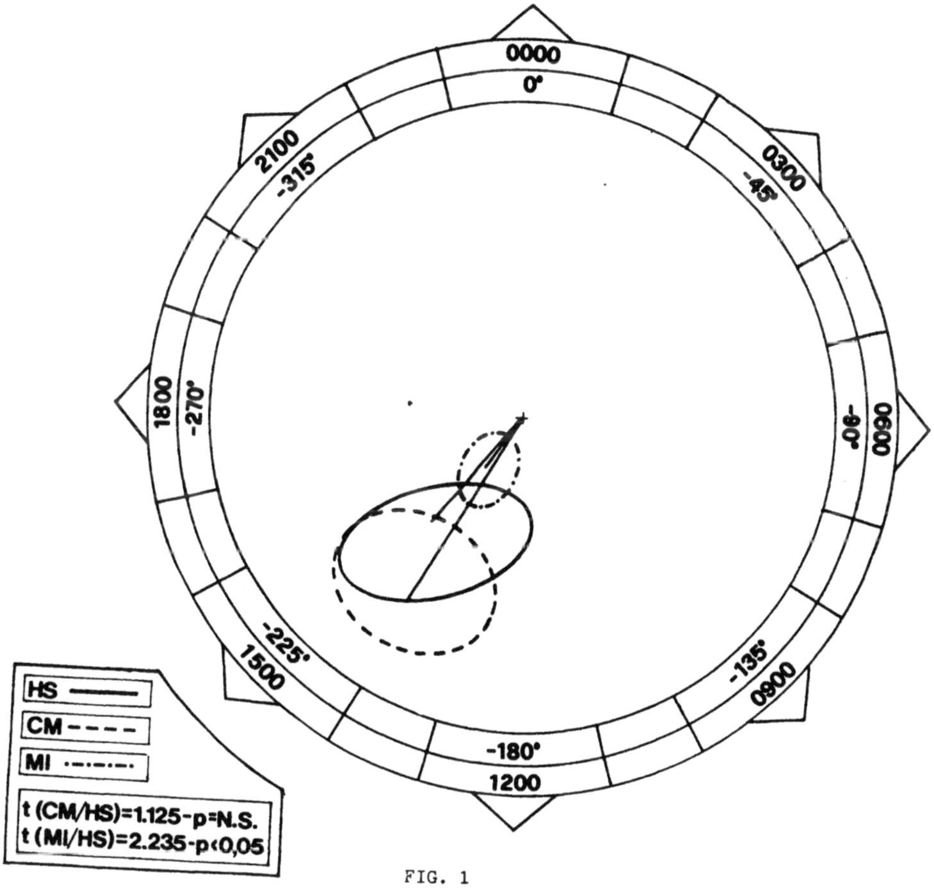

FIG. 1

REFERENCES

1) Cinelli, P., F. Calzolari, V. De Leonardis, L. Chiodi, M. De Scalzi, M. Barchielli, R. Vergassola: Fattori di rischio coronarico e cronobiologia: l'età. Congresso Nazionale di Cardiologia -ANMCO- Bologna, 1983 - P52.
2) Cinelli, P., M. De Scalzi, F. Fabiano, M. Buffoni, V. De Leonardis: Risk factors in chronoelectrocardiology: age. IRCS Med. Sci, 11: 361 (1983).
3) De Leonardis, V., P. Cinelli, F. Capacci, M. De Scalzi, S. Citi: Circadian rhythms in dynamic electrocardiography. J. Electrocardiol., 16: 351 (1983).
4) Vergassola, R., V. De Leonardis, M. De Scalzi, F. Calzolari, M. Barchielli, L. Chiodi, F. Fabiano, P. Cinelli: Cronobiologia dei battiti prematuri atriali. Congresso Nazionale di Cardiologia -ANMCO- Firenze, 1984 - C72.
5) De Scalzi, M., V. De Leonardis, F. Calzolari, M. Barchielli, L. Chiodi, F. Fabiano, P. Cinelli, R. Vergassola: Heart rate and premature beats: a chronobiologic study. Gior. Ital. Cardiol., 14: 465 (1984).
6) Cinelli, P., M. De Scalzi, V. De Leonardis, S.M. Manca, E. Chegai-Spitali, A. Becucci: "Can heart rate be taken as a marker of biological age?" In: B. Tarquini, R. Vergassola: "Social Disease and Chronobiology", Centro Stampa Palagi, Firenze (1986).
7) Vergassola, R., V. De Leonardis, M. De Scalzi, F. Fabiano, F. Calzolari, M. Barchielli, L. Chiodi, P. Cinelli: Circadian and ultradian rhythms of supraventricular premature beats. d'Alché P., editor - Electrocardiology; Caen, 1985, page 207.
8) Perloff, J.K.: "Pathogenesis of hypertrophic cardiomyopathy: hypotheses and speculations". Am. Heart J., 101: 219 (1981).

Measurement of periodic heart rate variability for investigation of the vegetative level during the induction of anaesthesia

MIKOLEIT, J., H. GEIKLER and K. ECKOLDT *

Bezirkskrankenhaus Magdeburg, Max-Otten-Str.11-15, 3040 Magdeburg,GDR
*Institut fuer medizinische Physik und Biophysik der Humboldt-Universitaet zu Berlin, Invalidenstr. 42, 1040 Berlin, GDR

Summary
During the induction of anaesthesia the heart rate variability was studied off-line with fast fourier transformation in 60 patients. The calculated power density spectra show three rhythms. Their increasing or diminution allow valuation of vegetative level. In case of anaesthesia with hexobarbital the vegetative level is more changed than after use of dehydrobenzperidol and fentanyl (NLA). The parasympathetic tone was found increased after administration of succinylcholine.

Introduction
The study of the periodic variability of heart rate allows conclusions on the tone of vegetative cardiac nerves. Animal experiments are known from literature that indicate a close relationship between the parasympathetic tone and spontaneous fluctuations of heart rate. The study of heart rate variability of man appears to be a good indirect method for determining the vegetative cardiac tone. SAYERS [1] succeeded in showing that 70 to 90 % of heart rate fluctuations are periodic. Numerous authors have shown that three dominating rhythms can be detected in the heart rate power spectrum. These rhythms have period durations of 2.5 to 6 seconds, 6 to 20 seconds and 0.5 to 4 minutes, respectively. They are called respiratory, circulatory and minute rhythmic modulations of heart rate. Particularly AKSELROD et al.[2] have shown that the degree of circulatory and respiratory rhythms is proportional to the parasympathetic tone, while minute rhythmic fluctuations depend largely on the level of sympathetic tone. Information on cardiac tone of the parasympathetic and sympathetic systems is of great importance for anaesthesists and surgeons as life-threatening situation can arise through cardio-circulatory reflexes in case of the dominance of parasympathetic system during anaesthesia induction and operation.

Material and methods
In our studies, heart beat periods of about 60 patients who had to undergo surgical treatment were continuously recorded during the initial phase of anaesthesia and then evaluated by means of a computer. A trigger pulse that modulates a 1000 Hz frequency in amplitude in the rhythm of heart beats is formed synchronously with the patient's QRS complex. This signal is stored on magnetic tape. After that the computer calculates interbeat intervals and, using the fast fourier transformation, the power spectrum. According to various authors, power spectra were divided into three fixed regions for this study and the respective integral sums were calculated. This offers the possibility to compare quantitatively individual amounts of subrhythms.

Results
Figure 1 shows the integral values of the three rhythms of a patient group who were examined during the induction of neurolept-analgesia (NLA). Prior to the induction of analgesia, the modulation of heart rate by respiration and circulation is still distinctly marked. As soon as anaesthesia has reached the nessesary depth, these rhythms greatly diminish and only the minute rhythm is still distinctly present. Compared with results by AKSELROD et al.[2], this phenomenon can be explained by a decrease of parasympathetic activity.

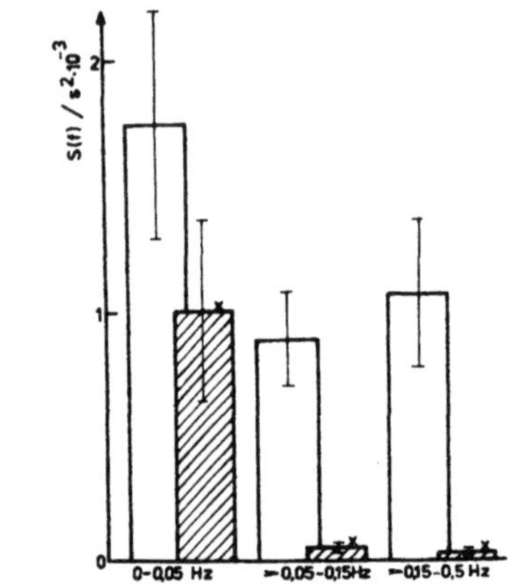

Fig.1
Integral power densities of three rhythms of heart rate variability during induction of neurolept-analgesia.
Free area: prior NLA-induction
Dashed area: after NLA-induction (same distinctive marks in all figures)

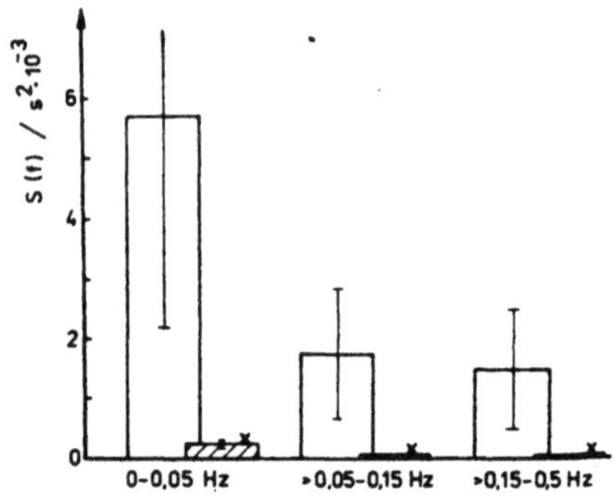

Fig.2
Integral power densities of three rhythms of heart rate variability during induction of anesthesia using hexobarbital.

If one compares that to spectra of a group of patients whose anaesthesia was induced using hexobarbital (Fig.2), one recognizes that, after the necessary depth of anaesthesia is reached, all three rhythms have greatly diminished. Here, too, one can assume a decrease of parasympathetic activity. As the patients' heart rates rose, however, up to 135 beats per minute with this kind of anaesthesia, one can suppose an increase of sympathetic tone. These results were obtained in groups in which breaks lasting 5 to 10 minutes between individual injections were kept.

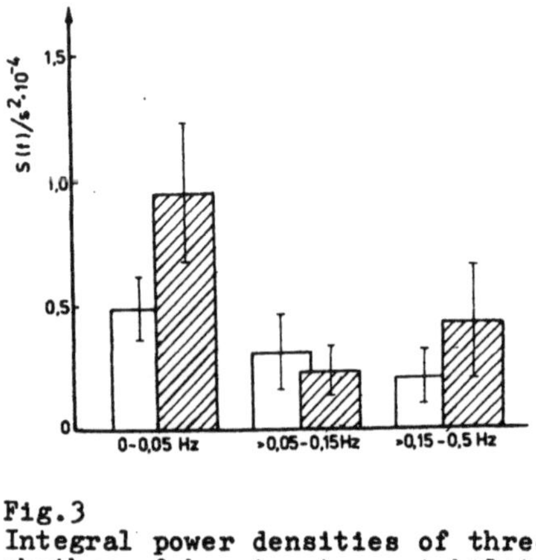

Fig.3
Integral power densities of three rhythms of heart rate variability during NLA-induction and a longer break after succinylcholine injection.

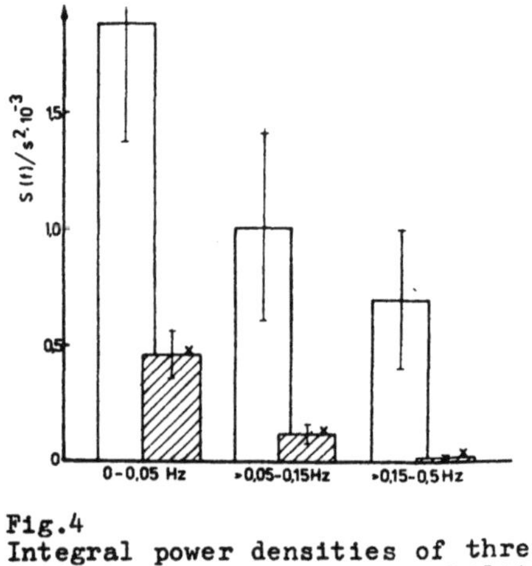

Fig.4
Integral power densities of three rhythms of heart rate variability during induction of anesthesia using hexobarbital and a longer break after succinylcholine injection.

Figure 3 shows the integral power densities of the tree rhythms of a group of patients who got neurolept-analgesia with a longer break after the administration of the shortacting relaxant succinylcholine. It is clearly recognizable that, in this study, the contributions of respiratory and circulatory rhythms to total variability do not decrease. After succinylcholine injection, the modulation of heart rate is even more pronounced than before. Similar results are obtained with patients whose anaesthesia was induced using hexobarbital if a break is inserted after the succinylcholine injection, too. The integral power densities of this patient group are shown in figure 4. Circulatory and respiratory heart rate modulations are not so greatly reduced as in the case of the same induction of anaesthesia within a temporal routine scheme. From literature it is known, that the administration of succinylcholine results in a rise of parasympathetic tone. The present results clearly confirm this fact.

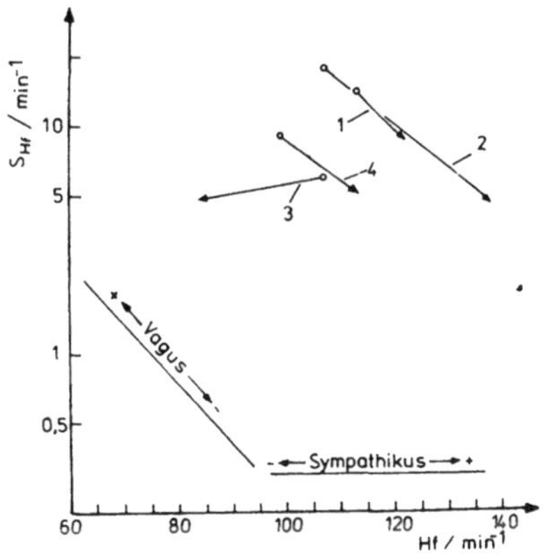

Fig.5
Variability-rate diagram according to ECKOLDT [3] for determining changes of autonomous cardiac nerve tone.

Discussion and conclusions
The results can be consistently included into the variability-rate diagram as used by ECKOLDT [3] for determining changes of autonomous cardiac nerve tone (Fig. 5). In this way, the relative heart rate standard deviation is plotted versus the average heart rate of the patient group. The arrows drawn connect the respective rate and variability values before and after the experiments done. In connection with entered, experimentally obtained action lines of the parasympathetic and sympathetic nerves and considering the slopes and directions of arrows, one can take conclusions concerning the proportional changes of cardiac nerve tone. Every arrow must be regarded as a resultant vector whose components parallel to action lines are proportional to changes in tone of the sympathetic and parasympathetic nervous systems. The numbering of arrows corresponds to the order of the experiments presented here. The induction of neuroleptic analgesia in a temporal routine scheme (arrow 1) causes exclusively a reduction of parasympathetic tone. The induction of anaesthesia using hexobarbital (arrow 2) produces, as was supposed above, a great reduction of parasympathetic tone accompanied by an increase of sympathetic tone. Effects resulting from an extended active period of succinylcholine are represented by arrows 3 and 4. The drug effects at the parasympathetic nerve are distinctly discernible, the reduction of the variability is less pronounced.
Studying the vegetative tone using the heart rate power spectrum represents a good method for clinical practice. Particularly for patients who run the risk of suffering shock (e.g. in case of gastro-intestinal haemorrhages or intense pain) this method enables accurate premedication and thus optimal tone adjustment of the autonomous

system. This is impossible in case of the customary drug dosage based on body weight. We have reported earlier on the influence of premedication on the vegetative cardiac tone in various publications [4,5].

References

[1] Sayers, B.: Ergonomics 16,17-32 (1973)
[2] Akselrod, S., D.Gordon, F.A.Ubel, D.C.Shannon, A.C.Barger, and R.J.Cohen: Science, 213, 220-222, (1981)
[3] Eckoldt, K.: Dt.Gesundh.-Wesen, 39, 865-863 (1984)
[4] Mikoleit, J., K.Eckoldt, and H.Geikler: Z.ges.inn.Med.,40, 122-126 (1985)
[5] Mikoleit,J.,K.Eckoldt, and H.Geikler: Anaesthesiol.u.Reanimat.,10,51-59 (1985)

The influence of beta-adrenergic blockers propranolol and talinolol on ECG in young men

WITTEK, G.; MÜCKE, D.
Children's clinic of the Military Medical Academy, Bad Saarow, GDR

Summary: A total of 68 young men with a sound heart having a normal ECG corresponding to age was subjected to a beta-adrenergic blocker test. 36 probands took 50 mg of propranolol and 32 probands 150 mg of talinolol. A body surface ECG was recorded before and one hour after drug administration and comprehensively evaluated. As a result of the statistical analysis of parameters measured and documented, it was ascertained that propranolol in the chosen dose caused larger modifications of the ECG than talinolol.

Introduction: Effects of vegetative nervous system influencing the electrocardiogram play a large role in infancy, childhood, adolescence and adulthood. The differentiation of vegetative from organically caused changes in electrocardiograms presents problems also to experienced doctors now and then. Cardiac arrhythmias as extrasystoles, sinus arrhythmias, sinus tachycardia and sinus bradycardia as well as morphological ECG changes especially in the repolarisation phase are counted as such changes. S-T depression, flattening and inversion of T waves and high T waves are belong to them. The effects of the vegetative nervous system can be so unusual that they can simulate a pathological ECG and lead to wrong therapeutical decisions, if it is incorrectly interpreted. The propranolol test has been used in adult and child's electrocardiography for a longer period of time to differentiate vegetative from organically caused repolarization disorders (Delius 1967; Pfeifer 1974; Hille 1980). The question whether diagnostic possibilities could be improved by using relatively cardioselective beta-adrenergic blocking agents is still not clear.

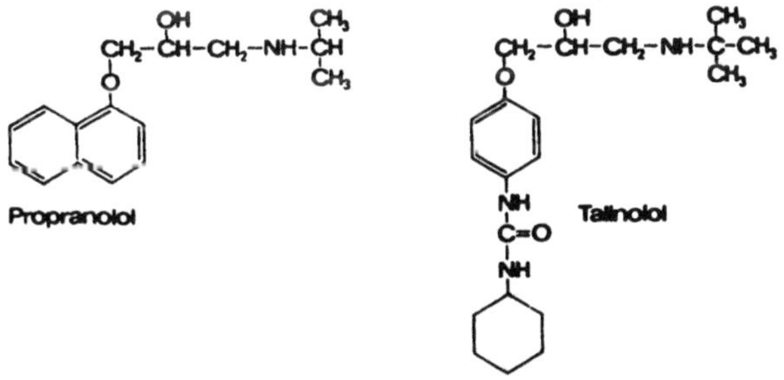

Figure 1. Structure of propranolol and talinolol

Propranolol has a blocking effect on $beta_1$- and $beta_2$-adrenergic receptors. Talinolol is a specific $beta_1$-adrenergic blocker. There have been no results concerning the usability of a talinolol test so far. We saw the necessity of carrying out investigations to answer to question what changes in normal electrocardiograms at rest are caused by the inhibition of the sympathetic tone. We were especially interested in the influence on heart rate and the morphology of the repolarization phase. In addition to this, changes in the electrocardiogram caused by the beta-adrenolytic substances propranolol and talinolol are to be commented on. Comparing the effect of a $beta_1/beta_2$-adrenergic receptor blocker with that of a relatively cardioselective beta-adrenergic receptor blocker, we expected further information about the genesis of ECG changes caused by false regulations of the autonomic nervous system and about the possibilities of influencing them.

Material and methods: 36 probands were subjected to a propranolol test and 32 probands to a talinolol test. Young men 18 to 25 years old with normal weight were concerned. All probands were clinically healthy and had normal electrocardiograms. There was no competitive athlete among the probands. Tests were carried out in the morning between 9 and 12 o'clock. Probands didn't have either alcohol, nicotine and coffee or sports and heavy physical activities before and during the examinations. Oral dose of the test substance was 50 mg of propranolol and 150 mg of talinolol, respectively. A body surface ECG was recorded before and one hour after drug application. Leads I, II, III, aVR, aVL, aVF and precordial leads V_1 - V_6 were recorded. Paper speed was 50 mm/sec. Fifteen cardiac cycles were included in the investigations. Tracings were visually evaluated according to usual principles.

Heart rate analysis: The mean R-R interval was obtained from 15 successive R-R intervals.

$$\overline{RR} = \frac{1}{n} \sum_{i=1}^{n} RR_i$$

Analysis of cardiac rhythm variability: by Echoldt (1984): The difference in R-R intervals was determined from cardiac cycle to cardiac cycle. The mean value of the absolute values of differences is the mean difference of R-R intervals.

$$\overline{|\Delta RR|} = \frac{1}{n} \sum_{i=1}^{n} |RR_i - RR_{i+1}|$$

Amplitude values of all waves were measured in limb and precordial leads. Time parameters belonging to minimal and maximal R-R intervals were measured in lead II. The arithmetical mean of measured values was considered as the mean time value.

Results: Cardiac rhythm: An evident influence on heart rate could be observed both under propranolol and talinolol. The application of propranolol leads to a statistically significant average increase in the mean R-R interval of 0,134 s (+ 14.2 %). Talinolol causes an increase of 71 ms (+ 9.3 %). The increase in the mean R-R interval corresponds to an average heart rate decrease of 8 (propranolol) and 6 (talinolol) beats/minute, respectively. An increase in sinus arrhythmia existing can be observed under both drugs too. The mean difference in R-R intervals increases by 32 ms (+ 58.5 %) under propranolol and by 12 ms (+ 19.7 %) under talinolol. In figure 2 the more pronounced effect of propranolol on the mean R-R interval and sinus arrhythmia is seen.

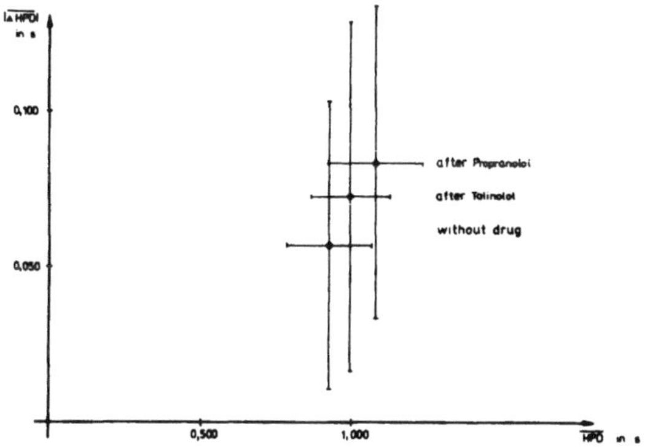

Figure 2. The influence of propranolol and talinolol on mean R-R interval and sinus arrhythmia

Amplitude parameters: Both beta-adrenergic receptor blockers cause an evident increase in T wave amplitudes. Propranolol has a more obvious influence on the electrocardiogram than talinolol. In precordial leads T wave amplitude is increased on an average by 17.9 % under propranolol and 10.5 % under talinolol. All the other amplitude values remained unchanged.

Time parameters: Propranolol caused a statistically significant prolongation of the absolute P-Q duration of 11 ms on an average (+ 7.7 %). A statistically non-significant prolongation of this parameter of 2 ms on an average only was observed after talinolol application. The relative P-Q duration is scarcely influenced by both drugs. Even though the absolute Q-T duration was not affected by both substances, an evident shortening of the relative Q-T duration could be recorded. This effect is more pronounced under propranolol, and is due to the constancy of Q-T interval with decreasing heart rate. Our investigations show that in normal vegetative tone beta-adrenergic receptor blocker application has an evident effect on both cardiac rhythm and morphology of the repolarization phase of the electrocardiogram. Propranolol causes a stronger ECG modification than talinolol. Despite of a relative cardioselectivity talinolol has to be considered as less suitable for its use as test substance. Now as before, one has to give preference to propranolol on account of its obviously more complex beta-adrenergic receptor blocking effect.

References:

(1) Delius, W.: Med. Klinik 62, 1128 - 1136 (1967).

(2) Pfeifer, E.; H. Schneider and P. Thiele: Dtsch. Gesundh.wes. 29, 1756 - 1759 (1974).

(3) Hille, R.: Dtsch. Gesundh.wes. 35, 1141 - 1145 (1980).

(4) Echoldt, K.: Dtsch. Gesundh.wes. 39, 856 - 863 (1984).

"Warming-up" Phenomenon
Differential Diagnosis and Quantitative Study

JAROSLAV JEDLIČKA

Cardiac Laboratory, IInd Department of Medicine, Charles University
U nemocnice 2, 128 08 Prague 2, Czechoslovakia

SUMMARY: Differential diagnosis of this phenomenon is presented. In two representative cases a quantitative study was performed diagrammatically. In the case of A-V junctional rhythm, a cumulative effect of its suppression by the dominant sinus rhythm was ascertained. On the other hand, the opposite was observed in sinus rhythm intermitently discharged by paroxysmal supraventricular tachycardia; this is interpreted as sign of its depression by the first ectopic beat only and its protection during the paroxysm establishing S-A dissociation.

"Warming-up" phenomenon can be defined as acceleration of the previously depressed cardiac pacemaker until its intrinsic rate is attained. Thus, both depression of the pacemaker and its "warming-up" represent two facets of one condition, two phases causally linked together. Synonymic denominations of the latter are: rhythm of development (for idioventricular rhythm - Gaskell), acceleration of the subsidiary pacemaker, from German Treppe-Phänomen: treppo phenomenon or staircase phenomenon, "warm-up" phenomenon. The differential diagnosis of this pattern has to consider similar cycle length changes in (1) shifting of the pacemaker - in the case of sinus rhythm, esp., (2) vagally induced heart frequency fluctuations, (3) shortening of A-V junction refractoriness during atrial fibrillation, and (4) gradual alleviation of a high-grade exit block of the dominant or parasystolic tachycardic pacemaker (1).

The main purpose of this study was to ascertain the anticipated impact of repeated discharges of the dominant rhythm (which represent an analogy of artificial "overdriving"), i.e., the influence of the degree (duration) of discharging on the degree of depression and on the "warming-up" pattern. Two representative cases giving opportunity to correlate both phenomena are presented in detail.

C a s e 1 . Female 41 years old, with atrial septal defect, not digitalized. Fig. 1 shows respiratory sinus arrhythmia with S-A block and S-A dissociation (2) with ensuing 16 instances of sinus pauses and one to ten A-V junctional escapes, most of them with retrograde atrial activation. The intervals between consecutive last conducted P waves before block measure 4 s or multiples of 4 s which evidences the role of respiration 15 per minute giving rise to blocking. The longer was the

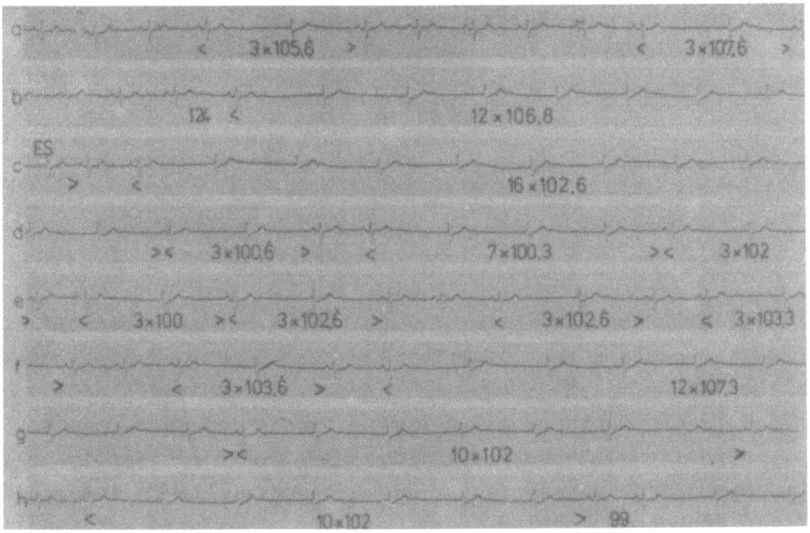

Fig. 1. Case 1. Continuous record of Lead I. Time in s/100. Respiratory sinus arrhythmia: longest P-P in b (124), shortest P-P in h (99). S-A block with junctional escapes, sinus pauses expressed as multiples of 100 - 107,6 s/100.

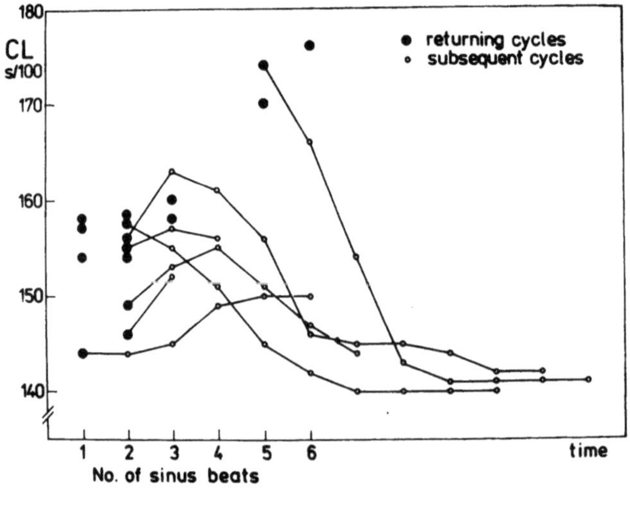

Fig. 2. Case 1. Correlation of the duration of sinus rhythm (1 - 6 on x axis) and the duration of returning cycles of junctional escapes (CL = cycle length on y axis) followed by time histograms (open circles). Discussed in text.

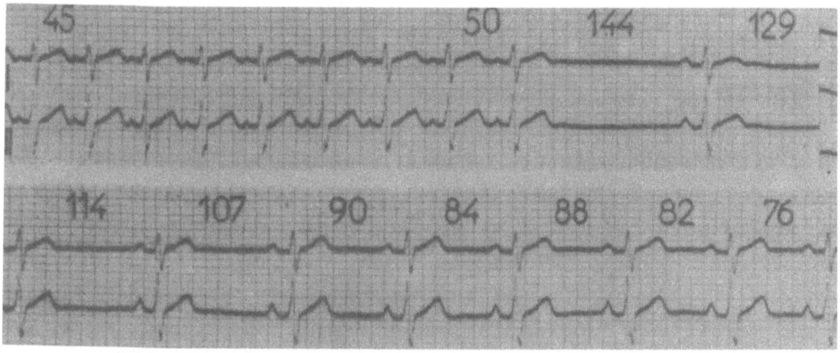

Fig. 3. Case 2. Continuous record. Time in s/100. The end of paroxysmal supraventricular tachycardia followed by sinus rhythm exhibiting "warming-up" phenomenon.

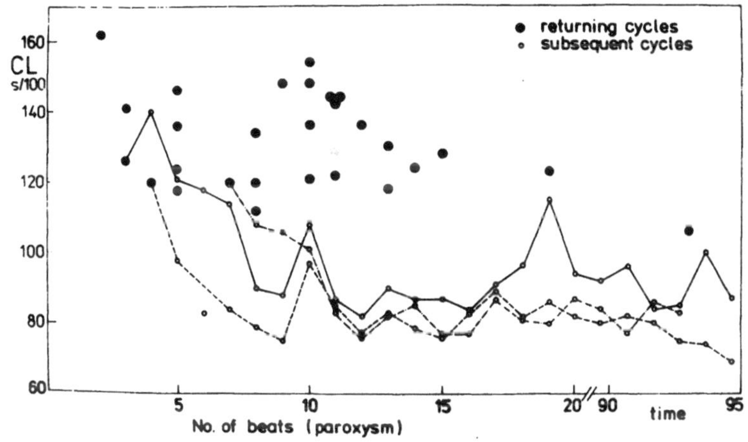

Fig. 4. Case 2. Correlation of the duration of the paroxysms (x) and returning cycles of sinus rhythm (CL = cycle length on y axis). Discussed in text.

period of sinus rhythm discharging the A-V junctional focus, the longer was the returning cycle of the first junctional escape; this follows from Fig. 2 correlating the number of sinus beats with subsequent returning cycles. Respective time histograms of each period of junctional escapes demonstrate the prevalence of the "warming-up" phenomenon as well as the fact that the longer the returning cycle was, the steeper was the "warm-up" curve.

C a s e 2 . Male 16 years of age, with intractable paroxysmal supraventricular tachycardia and a pathological EEG finding. During paroxysms the cycle length prolonged, whereas short interspaced periods of sinus rhythm exhibited the "warming-up" phenomenon. Often only one or two sinus beats were present between consecutive paroxysms; this and the "cooling-down" of the paroxystic cycle length and the fact that some paroxysms were iniciated by a sinus beat favour the interpretation that sino-atrial reciprocation was their mechanism. Fig. 3 shows the termination of tachycardia and the "warming-up" phenomenon of the restored and relatively longlasting sinus rhythm. Similarly as in Case 1 for junctional rhythm, the correlation of the duration of tachycardia and the returning cycles of the sinus rhythm was performed (Fig. 4). Ten records with 28 episodes of paroxysm were analyzed. Surprisingly, the opposite was found as compared with Case 1, Fig. 2: the shorter was the duration of paroxysm, the longer was the sinus returning cycle. "Warming-up" phenomenon was seen in all instances; for clarity, only three respective time histograms are drawn in Fig. 4.

Thus, two different aspects in two different situations are to be discussed. As anticipated, in the case of the ectopic (junctional) rhythm the duration of the returning cycle was proportional to the duration of antecedent discharging (the same was seen in idioventricular rhythm). The opposite behaviour in Case 2 may be explained this way: S-A node activity was depressed by the first ectopic beat as well but thereafter both rhythms were dissociated (2) and S-A node cycle length immediately started to return to normal values without any cumulative effect of further depression. In other words, as documented by Fig. 4, the shortest paroxysm was followed by the longest sinus cycle length and in the wake of longest paroxysms the shorter returning cycles were found.

There is a significant difference in the shape of "warming-up" curves; for the ectopic rhythm (Fig. 2), the returning cycle was the longest cycle in each period in 28% while this pattern in sinus rhythm amounted to 80% of respective time histograms (Fig. 4). Again, this demonstrates the cumulative effect of repeated discharges. When its maximum is attained (174 s/100 in Fig. 2), "warming-up" starts immediately with the resumption of the slower rhythm.

These observations represent a contribution to the notion of "secondary pauses" (3). Furthermore, the depression of the dominant rhythm by a single ectopic beat may mimic a fully compensatory pause. Finally, from the clinival point of view, they suggest a quantitative evaluation of artificial "overdriving" of tachycardias.

REFERENCES: (1) Jedlička, J.: in "Advances in Electrocardiology" (Ed.: P. d'Alché), Univ. de Caen, 1985, p. 380 - 382. - (2) Jedlička, J.: S-A block ... (in this Volume). - (3) Schmidt, G., S. Mashima, T. K. Shen, K. Takayanagi, and S. Murao: J. Electrocardiol. 17, 79 - 84 (1984).

The comparative study of 24-hour ECG monitoring in patients with different forms of angina pectoris and myocardial infarction

DOBROTVORSKAYA T., ABDULLAEVA T., MUSTAFAEV F.

123836 Barrikadnaya street, 2. The I caphedra of therapy, Central Institute for advanced medical studies, Moscow,USSR

Summary 24-hour Holter ECG monitoring was carried out during the first day of hospitalisation in three groups of male patients of similar average age; 86 with unstable rest angina (I gr), 30 with stable angina of effort (II gr) and other 30 with acute myocardial infarction (III gr).The study documented the higher prevalence of different arrhithmias, especially complex VPB, and transitory ST-segment changes in patients with unstable rest angina pectoris.

During the past several years there has been widespread interest in ventricular arrhythmias and sudden death(7).Technical advances, especially 24-hour Holter ECG monitoring, have improved our ability to record continuous ECG. Although the significance of "complex" premature ventricular beats is still discussed, the majority of authors (1-6) agree about their prognostic role in sudden death,especially in patients with ischemic heart disease (IHD). The diagnosis and prediction of clinical states, which can lead to myocardial infarction and sudden death, remains one of the important problem in cardiology (3).
The main purpose of our study was:1)to analyse the frequency and types of ventricular and supraventricular premature beats (VPB and SVPB) among patients with different forms of IHD; 2) to compare the frequency of transitory ECG changes during the repolarisation phase of cardiac cycle in patients with different forms of angina pectoris.
Material and method: 146 male patients about 38-59 y.old (the average age was 52,9±2,4 y.old), hospitalised in cardiology department with IHD, were studied; Unstable rest angina was diagnosed in 86 patients (I gr); stable angina pectoris of effort in 30 patients (II gr),acute myocardial infarction - in 30 patients (III gr). The age-differences among groups were not significant. 24-hour Holter ECG monitoring was carried out on the first day being in clinic, and after on the 7,14-th and 21 days. During the monitoring all of the patients received only long-acting nitrates, nitroglycerine sublingual, the patients of I and III gr. - 20-40 mg of nitroglycerine a day intravenously. Among the I gr. 31 patient had the recent onset of angina pectoris, 55 suffered with stable angina of effort about 2-10 years; the unstability appeared during last 7-10 days and that was the reason of their hospitalisa-

tion. The number of heart affacks was about 8-23 a day, nitroglycerine intake about 14-40 tabl. Patients of II gr suffered with IHD during several years and had 2-4 heart affacks a day. All of the patients in III gr. before acute myocardial infarction suffered with IHD during 2-12 years.

Results. First of all we should line to sign the advantages of 24-hour ECG monitoring in detection of arrhythmias, especially VPB, in patients with IHD: during routine ECG-recording VPB were detected in 3,6; 10,4 a. 34,3%% of patients in I, II and III gr. respectively, while the 24-hour ECG monitoring detected the VPB in 96,5; 76,6 a. 93,3%% of patients (table 1). It was found out that either VPB or SVPB were registered in the majority of patients and these data did not depend upon the clinical form of IHD. But as for the frequency of "high grade" VPB and average number of different types of VPB, these data correlated with the severity of angina: among I and II gr. infrequent uniform VPB occured in 11,6 a. 43,3%% of patients respectively frequent in 84,9 and 33,3%%, multiform - in 32,6 and 13,3%%, pairs - in 29,1 and 10,0%%, R-on-T in 23,3 and 6,7%% of patients.

Table 1. The frequency of cardiac arrhythmias in patients with different forms of IHD (during 24-hour ECG monitoring)

Type of arrhythmias	Unstable rest angina I gr. n=86	Stable angina of effort II gr. n=30	Myocardial infarction III gr. n=30	P_{I-II}	P_{I-III}
Ventricular premature beats:	96,5%	76,6%	93,3%	0,05	0,05
unfrequent	11,6"	43,3"	10,0"	0,01	
frequent	84,9"	33,3"	83,3"	0,01	
multiform	32,6"	13,3"	26,7"	0,05	
douplets	29,1"	10,0"	40,0"	0,05	0,05
R-on-T	23,3"	6,7"	26,7"	0,05	
Combinations	39,5"	16,7"	56,6"	0,05	0,05
Supraventricular premature beats	94,2"	86,7"	96,7"		
Ventricular flutter (short periods)	1,2"	-	3,3"		
Atrial flutter (short periods)	2,3"	-	10,0"		

The frequency of detected arrhythmias in patients with unstable angina was sometimes even more then in patients with myocardial infarction. Among III gr infrequent VPB were detected in 10,0%, periods of frequent VPB - in 83,3%, multiform - in 26,7%, pairs - in 40,0%, R-on-T - in 26,7% of patients (table 1). In patients of I and III gr. the combinations of 2 or 3 types of high grade PVB were usually found.

The average number of any VPB in I gr. was significantly higher than in II gr. and was close to the number of VPB in patient of III gr. So in patients of I, II and III gr. during 24-hour monitoring, the average number of VPB was about 1545±234; 207±48 and 1225±138; of multiform: 24±4; 4±1 and 20±5; of pairs: 55±9; 7±3 and 93±14; of R-on-T: 28±4; 7±2; 38±13 (p I-II 0,01; p. I-III 0,05).

The average number of SVPB daily was also significantly higher in patients of I gr. (417±66), than in II gr.(127±44) and even in III gr. (367±102) (p I, II 0,05).
Besides the mentioned arrhythmias, the significant differences in ST-segment and T wave transitory changes in two groups were found: among patients with unstable angina the periods of transitory ST-segment elevation were recorded in 46,5%; ST-segment depression - in 39,5%; these changes were at the same time combined with complex VPB in 19,8% of patients. As for the group with stable angina pectoris, the ST-segement elevations were detected in 13,3%, ST-segment depression - in 20% of patients. The periods of coronary negative T-wave about 3-15 mm were found in 13% of patients I gr. These periods continued from a few up to 40 minutes long and were always accompained with ST-segment changes.
We suppose, that the combination of ST-segment elevation periods with negative T-wave during 24-hours recording is of a great importance, because all the patients of I gr. with such abnormalities (5,9%) developed acute myocardial infarction during the first week of hospitalisation. Among II group the periods of negative T wave about 2-3 mm were found only in 3,3% of patients.
The dynamic ECG-monitoring revealed, that the improvement in clinical state of patients with unstable angina, that is the dissappearence of severe heart attacks due to intensive treatment with nitrates only in cardiology department, correlates with great diminishing of cardiac arrhythmias and ST-T changes.
So, the major value of our study was the documentation of higher prevalence of different arrhythmias, especially VPB, and transitory ST-segment changes in patients with unstable rest angina. The data obtained emphasize the necessity of simultaneous severe antianginal and antiarrhythmic therapy during the period of unstability in such patients.

REFERENCES

(1) Biagini A., M.Mazeri et al.: Am.Heart J., 103, 13-17 (1982).
(2) Johnson S., D.Mauritson et al.: Amer.Heart J. 4, 103-108(1982).
(3) Mazur N.: The sudden death, p.186, Medicina, Moscow (1985).
(4) Mooss A., V.Aronow et al.: Clin.Cardiol.,6, 435-439 (1983).
(5) Oliva Ph.: Ann.Intern.Med.,100, 424-440 (1984).
(6) Russel R., Ch.Racker and N.Konchoukos: Circulation, 65, 73-76(1982).
(7) Winkle R. Progr.Cardiovasc.Dis., XXII, 99-126(1980).

Behavior of the QT_c-interval at multiple praecordial ECG-leads in healthy persons and patients with different heart diseases

KASSEL,P.,I.ASSMANN

Dept. of Cardiology
Clinic of Internal Medicine, Medical School Erfurt, GDR

Summary

According to LOWN, the electric instability of the myocard is the key element in the genesis of the sudden cardiac death and in 70 - 90 percent is the cause the ventricular fibrillation. The mechanism of such a rhythm disturbance may - among others be an inhomogenous repolarization. Starting from this fact, the clinical interpretation of the QT-time and the frequencycorrected value, but also of its lengthening became very actual again. QT_c-lengthenings were also described in patients with coronary artery disease, ventricular tachyarrhythmias, arterial hypertension, acute myocardial infarction, WPW-syndrome. There was the question: If there are only global or also regional different QT_c-intervals and if the use of muliple praecordial ECG-leads gives better results. There were, however distinct variations in regard of the height of the medium values and also of the single vaules between the different examined clinical pictures. The lowest mean values of QT were revealed by the 10 examined patients with supraventricular extrasystoly, the highest values were observed in the patients with ventricular extrasystoly of severity degree II.

Introduction

World-wide, the high prevalence and incidence of heart diseases have resulted in the development of control strategies. in this connection, the sudden cardiac death also represents one of the most urgent health-political problems.

According to LOWN, the electric instability of the myocard is the key element in the genesis of the sudden cardiac death and in 70 90 percent is the cause the ventricular fibrillation. The mechanism of such a rhythm disturbance may-among others-be an inhomogenous repolarization. Starting from this fact the clinical interpretation of the QT-time and the frequency-corrected value, but also of its lengthening became very actual again. Lengthenings of QT_c may be congenital, or it occurs, in case of special syndromes and processes where some patients have tendencies to ventricular tachyarrhythmias- (ANDERSON et al, ASSMANN et al, FASER et al, HAYNES et al).

Material and methods

There was the question: If there are only global or also regional different QT_c-intervals and if the use of multiple ECG leads in the body surface ECG are better than conventional leads. By means of a six canal-electrocardiograph, the limb leads were registered according to Einthoven, the praecardial leads according to NEHB and WILSON. The center of examinations was the enlarged praecordial surface ECG with altogether 36 points.

In this paper, there are evaluated the global and regional QT resp. QT_c (Bazett's formula) behaviors of the conventional ECG leads in healthy persons (HP) (n = 106) as well as in patients (pts) with different cardiac diseases: 96 pts with coronary artery diseases (CAD-NYHA II), 11 pts with myocardial infarction (MI), 35 pts with arterial hypertension, 85 pts with ventricular extrasystoles (VES) (LOWN I and II), 5 pts with WPW-syndrome, and 10 pts with supraventricular extrasystoles (SVES).

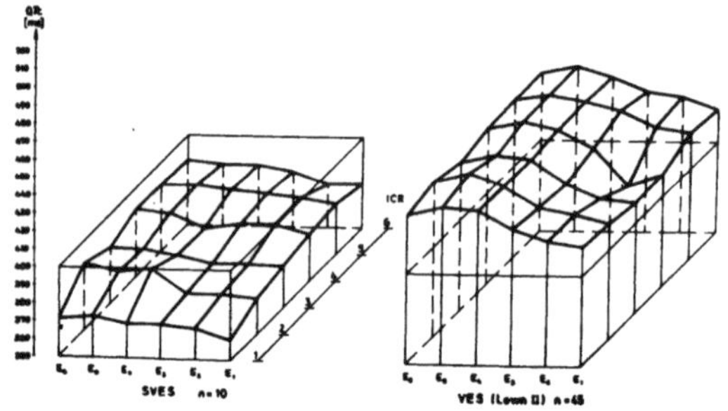

Fig. 1 QT_c-intervals (multiple praecordial ECG-leads) in pts with SVES and pts with VES LOWN II
(ICR = intercostal space, E = lead point)

Results

In all examined patients we have observed the longest QT_c-values in the lead according to NEHB A and in the left praecordial lead points. There were however distinct variations in regard of the height of the mean values and also of the single values between the different examnined clinical pictures. The lowest mean values of QT_c were reveald by the 10 pts with SVES. (Fig 1) In HP, the QT_c-intervals were nearly of the same duration (440 ms) in the praecordial and the standard leads. There were only slight differences between the 1st and 2nd ICS right parasternal and the 4th and 5th ICS left parasternal. On the latter, we found the longest QT_c-intervals. (Fig 2)

Pts with CAD and arterial hypertension showed nearly the same distribution of the QT_c-intervals, but the values were slightly longer. (Fig. 3). When comparing these QT_c-values of the 96 CAD-pts with that ones of the 45 patients with ventricular extrasystoly LOWN II we got an impressive picture in regard of the duration of QT_c-values and the repolarization picture. We found in a great number of examined pts pathological increased QT_c-intervals and thus differences between 20 and 56 msec were strinking. (Fig 4) In pts with MI, there were significant longer QT_c-intervals too and the values often showed great differences between two adjoining praecordial points. The longest QT_c-intervales were seen in pts with WPW-syndrome.

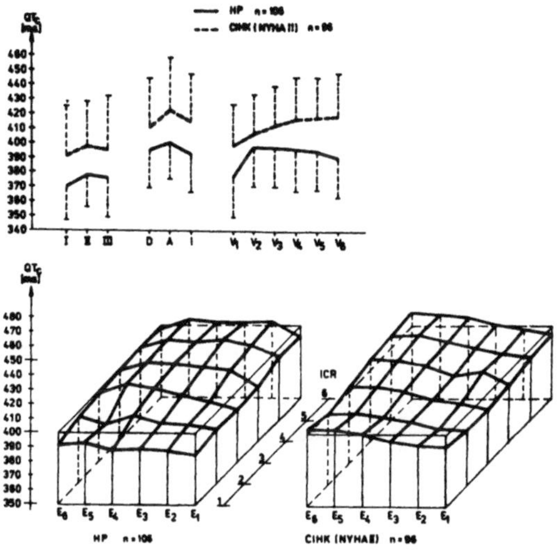

Fig 2 QT_c-intervals (conventional ECG and multiple praecordial ECG) in healthy persons and pts with CAD-NYHA II

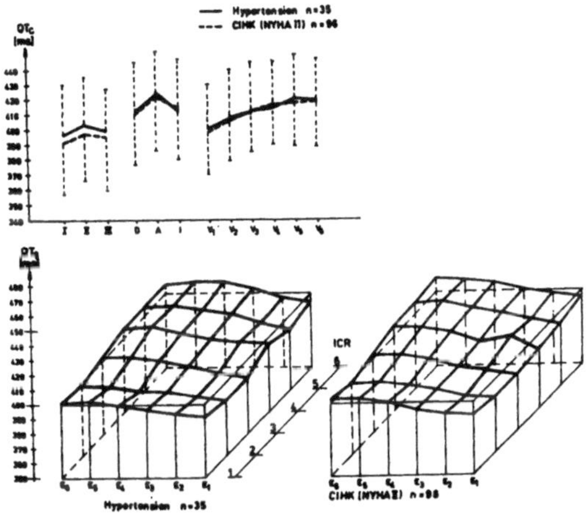

Fig 3 QT_c-intervals (conventional ECG and multiple praecordial ECG leads) in pts with hypertension and CAD-NYHA II

Discussion and conclusions

The results show that in pts with certain cardiac diseases, the repolarization may be prolonged not only globally but also regionally, and this can also be the expression of an in homogenous repolarization. In risk - pts e.g. after MI or pts with ventricular dysrhythmias the QT-interval measurement at multiple points should also be performed to avoid errors.

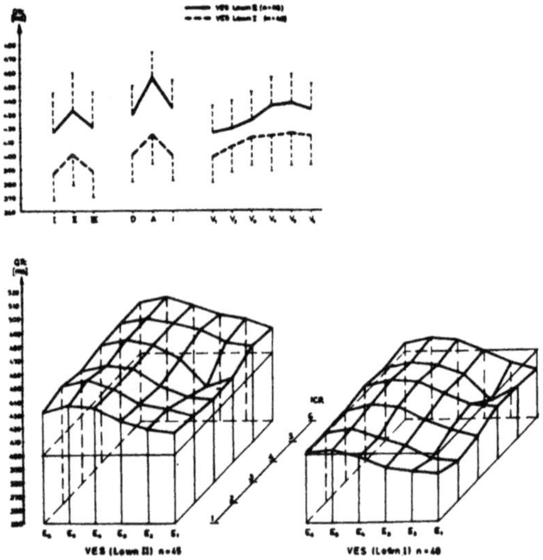

Fig 4 QT_c-intervals (conventional ECG and multiple praecordial ECG leads) in pts with VES

References

(1) Lown, B. Am.J. Cardiol. 43, 313-328 (1979)
(2) Lown, B. Circulation 60 , 1593-1599 (1979)
(3) Anderson, P., L. Lundkwist Acta med. scand. 206, 73-76 (1979)
(4) Aßmann,I., H. Fiehring, K.H. Stock Dt. Gesundh.-wesen 38 ,336-340 (1980)
(5) Faser, P., P. Frogatt, T.N. James Quart.J.Med. 33 , 361-385 (1964)
(6) Haynes, R.E., A.P. Hallström, C.A. Cobb Res. 25 , 1430-1431 (1977)

Bundle branch reentrant tachycardia treated by transvenous catheter ablation of the right bundle branch

KÜHNERT, H.; VOLKMANN, H.; DANNBERG, G.; HEINKE, M.
Division of Cardiology, Department of Internal Medicine,
Friedrich Schiller University, Karl Marx Allee 101, Jena-Lobeda,
DDR-6902

Summery

Recurrent episodes of ventricular tachycardia not responding to medical treatment occurred in a 56 year old man. Electrophysiologic investigation showed ventricular tachycardia due to bundle branch reentry. Using a method similar to catheter ablation of the atrioventricular junction, an ablation of the right bundle branch was performed by an electric shock of 250 J. While before the ablation ventricular tachycardia occurred several times a day and its induction by programmed ventricular stimulation was facilitated by the administration of antiarrhythmic drugs, no initiation of ventricular tachycardia was possible after ablation of the right bundle branch. Over a follow up of 22 months the patient has not suffered from tachycardia and the artificial right bundle branch block persists.

Introduction

Ventricular tachycardia (VT) always are emergencies and one of the major risks of sudden cardiac death. Electrophysiologic testing has been widely accepted as a standard technique for prospectively evaluating drug regimens for treatment of patients with recurrent ventricular tachyarrhythmias. VT refractory to antiarrhythmic drugs requires surgery or the implantation of antiarrhythmic devices. A new and interesting method is the use of intracardiac catheter electrodes for delivery of destructive electric energy to the tachycardia site. Although the final role of this experimental form of therapy remains undetermined, there are sufficient data to justify continuing investigations.
This is the report about the first successful management of a recurrent VT due to bundle branch reentry by ablation of the right bundle branch.

Case report

The 56 year old man suffered from frequent syncopes and attacks of palpitations combined with dizziness, perspiration and nausea, but no angina. The ECG showed a left anterior fascicular block and a first degree AV block with a PR interval of 500 ms; intermittently a second degree AV block appeared. It was necessary to install an external transvenous pacemaker. Because of paroxysmal VT with a rate of 230/min some DC shocks were applied, for Lidocaine 200 mg as bolus was ineffective. Lidocaine therapy as infusion 3 mg/min was not successful either, since the tachycardia recurred.

During sinus rhythm the ECG showed a first degree AV block with a PR interval ranging from 470 to 560 ms, intermittently a second degree AV block Mobitz type I. The QRS complex duration was 100 ms and the axis was directed to -45 degrees. During the VT the QRS pattern was similar to the left bundle branch block, the duration was 160 ms, the axis deviated to -40 degrees and the rate was 230/min.

Electrophysiologic findings

Electrophysiologic investigation was performed in the usual way. Lidocaine therapy was discontinued 24 hours before the testing. The stimulation protocol consisted of single and double extrastimuli at spontaneous rhythm as well as four basic drive cycle lengths (600, 500, 400, 330 ms) and two right ventricular sites.

The VT was initiated regularly at a basic cycle length of 320 ms and a single extrastimulus S_1S_2 260 ms and was terminated by rapid ventricular stimulation S_1S_1 220 ms.

For the induction it was important to obtain a critical prolongation of the retrograde conduction of the Purkinje's fibres, i.e. the V_2H_2 interval.

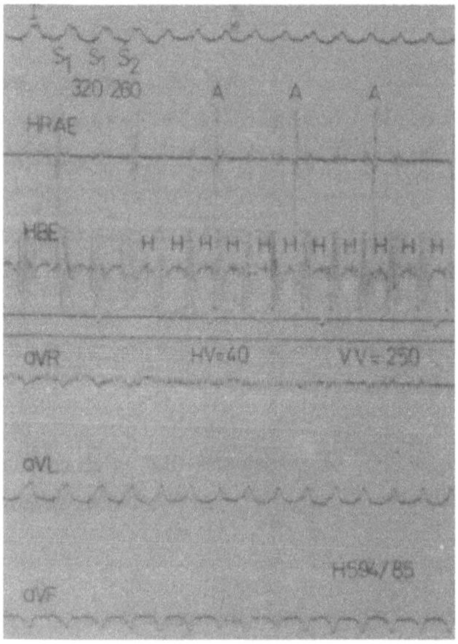

Fig. 1

Initiation of the ventricular tachycardia by ventricular stimulation at a basic cycle length of 320 ms and a single extrastimulus S_1S_2 260 ms. The QRS pattern is similar to that of right ventricular pacing. Each ventricular complex is preceded by a His potential.

The pattern of the induced tachycardia was similar to that of right ventricular pacing and identical to the spontaneous VT. The HV interval was identical, too. These findings suggested a bundle branch reentry. Further pathologic results were the prolongation of sinus node recovery time (3750 ms) and the AV conduction (AH 460 ms and more).

Pharmacologic testing of Procainamide, Disopyramide, Mexiletine, Diphenylhydantoine and Amiodarone by programmed ventricular stimulation showed a better inducibility of VT, only the heart rate decreased. Ajmaline and Propranolol did not have to be tested at all, because of frequent recurrence of VT during intravenous therapy.

Technique of ablation

As the frequency of VT under antiarrhythmic drug therapy increased, on the one hand, and a potential curative therapy was available, on the other hand, the ablation or fulguration of the right bundle branch was attempted. After information of the patient and his written consent the ablation was performed using a method similar to catheter ablation of the atrioventricular junction. A tripolar electrode catheter (USCI) was positioned near the His bundle where recording of the spike of right bundle branch was possible. The distal electrode was connected to the cathodal output of a defibrillator and an oesophageal cylindric electrode (diameter 10 mm, length 50 mm) positioned in the projection of the intracardiac catheter was connected to the anodal sink. After the patient was anesthetized, one shock of 250 J was delivered in synchronized fashion. Because of an asystole a ventricular pacing was necessary, but half a minute later the first degree AV block occurred again, showing no changes in AH interval. The HV interval was prolongated from 40 to 110 ms and a right bundle branch block was existing. 60 min after ablation a programmed ventricular stimulation was performed on the same way, but tachycardia was not inducible and this proved to be so 5 days later.

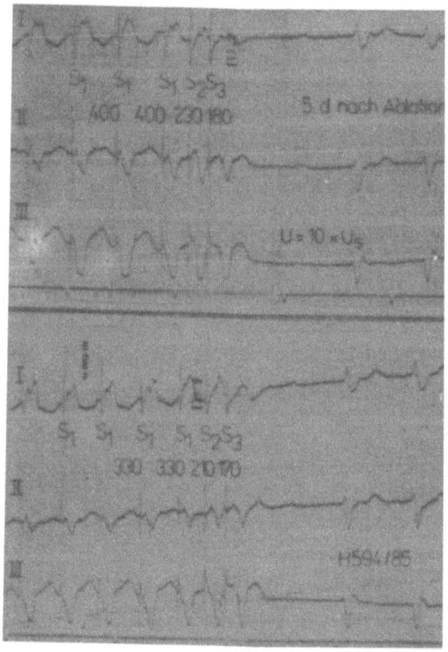

Fig. 2

Programmed ventricular stimulation 5 days after ablation. Ventricular tachycardia is not inducible by double extrastimuli at basic drive cycle length of 400 ms (upper panel) and 330 ms (lower panel). The artificial right bundle branch block is shown on the right.

Because of the sinus node dysfunction and the conduction disturbances a DDD pacemaker was implanted.
Since that time the patient has not had any complaints and has been free of tachycardia without antiarrhythmic drug therapy for 22 months.

Conclusion
While investigations concerning electric ablation of atrial and atrioventricular tachycardias refractory to antiarrhythmic drugs have been made by many authors recently and the catheter technique has been shown to be as effective as surgical ablation of the His bundle, reports about ablation of ventricular tachycardias are still rare. In most cases it was attempted to destroy the focus of arrhythmia, but the results often proved to be negative. If the tachycardia circuit can be determined exactly and if there is only one unimorphic tachycardia, the possibility of successful ablation is given. Although the final role of this experimental form of therapy remains undetermined and a number of complications will not be avoidable yet, a nearly curative therapy in some special cases has become possible.

References

(1) Gallagher, I., R. Svenson, I. Kasell, L. German, G. Bardy, A. Broughton and G. Critelli: N. Engl. J. Med. 306, 194 - 200(1982)
(2) Scheinman, M.: PACE 9, 551 - 564 (1986)
(3) Volkmann, H., H. Kühnert, M. Heinke and F. Meier: Z. Klin. Med. 40, 541 - 544 (1985)
(4) Volkmann, H., H. Kühnert, M. Heinke, G. Dannberg and F. Meier: Z. Kardiol. 75, 628 - 633 (1986)

Clinical Studies on Post-Tachycardia Syndrome

KAZUO OHNISHI, KIYOHARU SAITO
and KIICHIRO TANEMOTO

Kobe Rosai Hospital, Department of Internal Medicine
4-1-23, Kagoike-Dori, Chuo-ku, Kobe, 651, Japan.

(Summary)

In order to clarify clinical features and ECG changes in post-tachycardia syndrome (PTS), 72 patients with paroxysmal supraventricular tachycardia (PSVT), were examined with serial ECG changes and laboratory findings. Of 72 cases with PSVT, 6 males without heart disease showed PTS which was characterized by prominent transient inverted T waves without any changes of QRS complexies after termination of the attack. The maximum change of altered T wave was observed immediately or 3-5 days after termination of the attack, and these changes recovered gradually and normalized in 24±8 days. During paroxysms, heart rate was 210±20/min., and all were showed bundle branch block pattern. The duration of the attack was 66±64 hours.

After termination of the attack, the increased value of WBC, GOT, GPT, LDH and BUN were observed and these values returned to normal in 3 weeks. These phenomena were also experimentally produced in normal dogs with rapid cardiac pacing. A possible explanation was thought that ECG changes of PTS was repolarization anomaly following to unusual ventricular depolarization.

(Introduction)

An electrocardiographic syndrome consisting of transient inversion of T wave after the cessation of paroxysmal tachycardia in normal hearts has been reported as PTS. However, this syndrome has not been generally recognized.

In this paper, in order to clarify clinical features and the mechanism of ECG changes in PTS, 72 patients with PSVT were examined with serial ECG changes and laboratory findings. And experimentally induced transient T wave inversion as the same as PTS in normal mongrel dogs was also studied to certify the clinical features and laboratory findings.

(Subjects and Methods)

Among 72 cases of PSVT examined, 6 cases fulfilled the following criteria were selected : no evidence of cardiac disease ; follow-up of serial ECG after cessation of the tachycardia ; and well-demonstrated transient T wave inversion wih the absence of other ECG changes suggesting cardiac disease. And serial ECG changes, serum enzyme lebel and the response for exercise tolerance test were observed after the cessation of tachycardia in these cases.

And experimentally, serial ECG changes and enzymatic changes were also studied in the PTS induced 6 dogs afte termination of rapid atrial pacing of 300/min. for 72 to 120 hours.

(Results)

The Table 1 summarizes the findings in our 6 cases. The age of the patients varied from 28 to 51 years old with mean of 34, and all were males. ECG findings in the non-paroxysms were, WPW pattern in one, slight ST depression in V5,6 in one and remains 4 were normal. In the attack of PSVT, cardiac rate ranged from 180 to 260 per minutes with mean 210. The duration of the tachycardia varied from 7 to 202 hours with mean 67 hours.

Table 1. ECG Findings in 6 cases with post Tachycardia Syndrome

Case	Age	Sex	ECG atrest	Attack of PSVT			T wave inversion after the attack		
				Heart Rate	ECG pattern	Duration (h)	ECG leads	Maximum ECG change	Recovery (days)
(1) S. A.	25	M	Normal	260	RBBB	202	I, II, aVF, $V_{4,5,6}$	immediate	24
(2) M. T.	25	M	WPW (B)	200	RBBB	57	II, aVF, V_1	immediate	13
(3) K. W.	28	M	Normal	190	RBBB	35	I, II, aVF, $V_{4,5,6}$	3 days after	29
(4) Y. K.	36	M	Normal	180	RBBB	7	I, II, aVF, $V_{5,6}$	5 days after	38
(5) S. K.	51	M	ST dep. $V_{5,6}$ Flat T $V_{5,6}$	230	LBBB	50	I, II, aVF, $V_{4,5,6}$	next day	20
(6) K. N.	48	M	Normal	210	RBBB	48	I, II, aVF, V_{1-6}	immediate	24

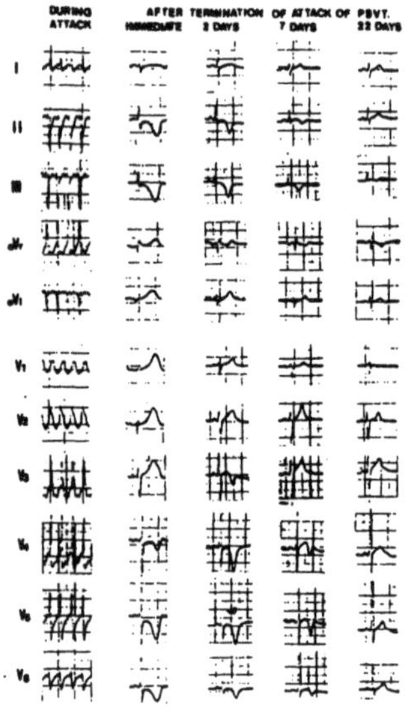

Fig. 1. Serial ECG changes after termination of the attack in case 1.

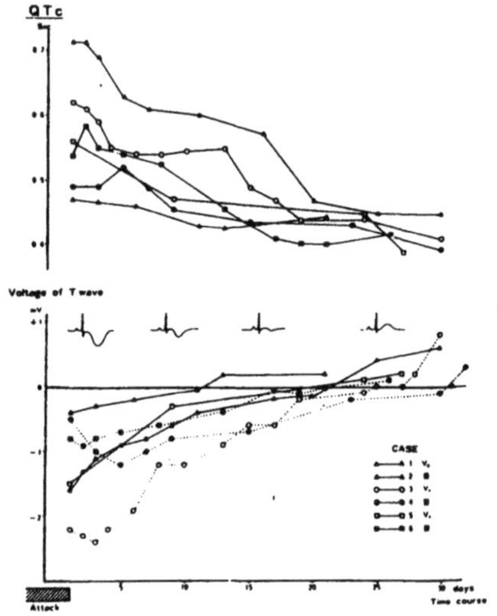

Fig. 2. Normalization of inverted T wave after termination of the attack

The ventricular complexies had the configuration of complete right bundle branch block with left axis deviation in 5 cases and left bundle block with left axis deviation in one.

The ECG changes after reversion to sinus rhythm were conspicious T wave inversion in leads 2,3, aVF, V4 to V6 and associated ST segment depression without abnormal Q waves. The maximal T wave inversion were observed immediately after termination of the attack in 3 cases, 1 to 5 days after in 3 cases. Gradual regression of the T wave inversion occured in all cases. The ECG became normal or the same before the attack in 13 to 38 days with mean 26. In the analysis of QT interval, prolonged QTc was observed in all cases immediately after the cessation of the attack with no relation of the method for termination. These prolonged QTc returned to normal in 20 days. (Fig.1,2).

During the recovery perid, exercise tolerance test revealed accelerated regression of T wave inversion as shown in Fig.3.

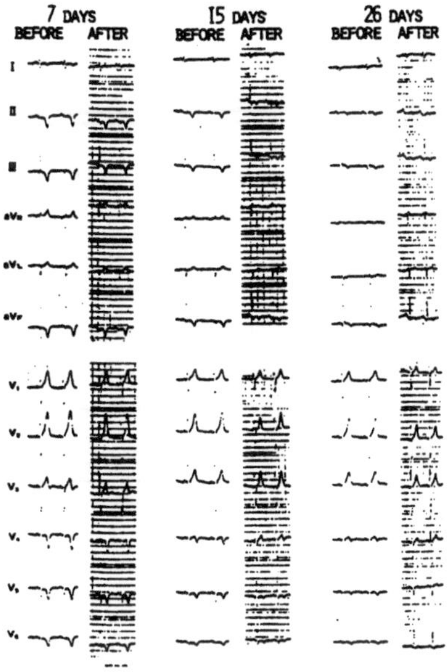

Fig. 3. Accelerated regression of T wave inversion by exercise tolerance test

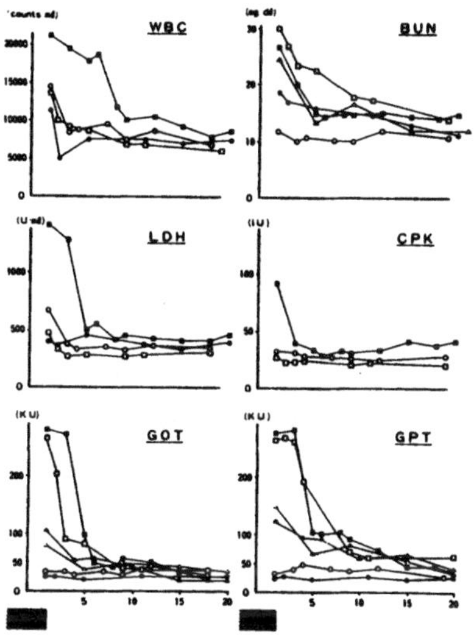

Fig. 4. Serial changes of laboratory findings after termination of the attack

The increase value of WBC, GOT, GPT, LDH and BUN were observed after termination of the attack. WBC counts rised over 10000 with neutrophilia in 3 out of 4 cases immediately after the attack and returned in 3 days. BUN levels increased to 20 mg/dl in 4 out of 5 cases, and returned to normal in 5 days. CPK was normal in 2 out of 3 cases, and slightly increased value was measured in one. LDH were increased in 3 out of 6 cases and returned in 5 days. Serum GOT and GPT level were increased in 4 out of 6 cases immediately after termination of the attack and returned gradually to normal level in parallel with the improvement of ECG changes except late recovery of GPT (Fig.4). No other examination data was normal.

The occurance of transient abnormalities of the T waves in ECG and biochemical changes of blood were induced by rapid atrial pacing experimentally. T wave inversion was observed in 6 dogs in leads 2, 3, aVF and V5,6 and these inversion returned to normal in 4 days. Increased value of WBC, GOT, GPT, LDH, BUN and CPK were observed as seen in clinical cases and returned to normal level in 2 to 4 days.

(Discussion)

It is not known how frequently PTS follows PSVT. In our study, among 72 cases of supraventricular tachycardia, only 6 cases appeared PTS.

In this paper, all PSVT were wide QRS figures as reported by Sargin et al. and Kernohan. Although, the differencial diagnosis between paroxysmal ventricular tachycardia and PSVT with wide ORS complexies is sometimes extremely difficult, PSVT were diagnosed by esophageal lead during the attack, vagal stimulation or electrical provocating test with His bundle ECG in our cases.

The anomalies of the T wave after disappearance of a particular electrocardiographic aspect can occur in some circumstances whose common point as an abnormal initial ventricular depolarization such as ventricular pacing, left bundle branch block and ventricular pre-excitation. Since, in the PSVT with wide QRS, initial ventricular depolarization thought to be abnormal, abnormal T vave inversion, which was abnormal ventricular repolarization, would be determined. PTS after cessation of PSVT with narrow QRS complexies, which was thought no depolarization abnormality in the ventricle, were also reported by Myerson et al. and Geiger. These fact may indicate that the mechanism of PTS is affected by multiple factors such as subendocardial ischemia or local tissue damage. Furthermore, it might be considered that accelerated regression of inverted T waves by exercise tolerance test during the recovery period indicated the possibility of participation of autonomic cardiac nerves in repolarization abnormality.

In our 6 cases, prolonged QTc with inverted T wave and its gradual recovery was observed. T wave abnormalities could be related to antiarrhythmic drugs. Indeed, quinidine or procaine amide prolongs QT and/or T wave duration, but does not, however, reverse its polarity. In our series, the same anomalies of T wave occured after termination by eye ball compression as well as after drug injection. The prolongation of QT interval was considered a part of ECG changes of PTS, but not inevitably required. These anomalies of T wave were suggested repolarization abnormality as observed in patients with subarachnoid hemorrhage.

The elevated values of WBC, GOT, GPT, LDH, CPK and BUN were noted in our clinical observation and these changes were also produced in animal experiments. In the previous reports, these biochemical changes were not reported. The mechanism of these changes were considered to attribute to congestion of liver or dysfunction of multi organs because there was a relationship between the degree of elevated value and the duration of the paroxysms in case 6 which had three attacks with PTS.

The mechanism of post-tachycardial T wave inversion is still unknown. Cassio and others attributed the changes to enlargement of the heart or ventricular strain. Currie postulated that the changes were caused by a completely reversible process indicating some degree of exhaustion or strain of the heart musle. Dubbs and Parmet attributed the transient T wave inversion to fatigue and exhaustion of the myocardium resulting from prolonged tachycardia. Geiger offered the hypothesis of myocardial ischemia associated with a marked diminished output. Recently, Rosenbaum suggested that electrotonically modulated T wave changes show accumulation and memory, and may persist for days or weeks after the provoking stimulus (the change in the activation sequence) is discontinued.

The problem remains unsolved. In this investigation, it seems likely that unusual ventricular depolarization exerts an important role in repolarization process in a manner similar to ventricular pacing or ventricular tachycardia.

(References)

(1) Sargin, C.O. and Demirkol, L.C.C. : Diseases of the Chest 48, 321-323 (1965)
(2) Geiger, A.J. : Amer. Heart J. 26, 555-560 (1943)
(3) Kernohan, R.J. : Brit. Heart J. 31, 803-806 (1969)
(4) Myerson, R.M. and Clagett Jr. A.H. : J.A.M.A. 148, 193-196 (1952)
(5) Rosenbaum, M.B., Blanco, H.B. Elizari, M.V., Lazzari, J.O. Davidenko, J.M. : Amer. J. Cardiol. 50, 213-222 (1982)
(6) Cossio, P., Gonzalez, S.L., Berconsky, I. : Rev. argent de cardiol. 8, 168-170 (1941)
(7) Currie, G.M. : Brit. Heart J. 4, 149-153 (1942)
(8) Nicolai, P., Medvedowsky, J.L., Delaage, M., Barnay, C., Blache E., Pisapia, A : J. Electrocardiology 14, 295-300 (1981)
(9) Surawicz, B. : Amer. J.Cardiol. 50, 363-364 (1982)
(10) Bella, P.D., Grazi, S., Cipolla, C.M., Fabbiocchi, F., Rimondini, A., Sganzerla, P. Guazzi, M.D. : Brit. Heart J. 57, 118-124 (1987)
(11) Dubbs, A.W. and Parmet, D.H. : Amer. Heart J. 24, 272-275 (1942)

Pacemaker Inverse Problem
Computer Supported Diagnosis of Electrocardiograms of Paced Patients

MAREK MALIK, A. JOHN CAMM

Department of Cardiological Sciences
St. George's Hospital Medical School
Cranmer Terrace, Tooting, London SW17 ORE, England

SUMMARY

Similarly to the Electrocardiographic Inverse Problem, the objective of which is the algorithmical analysis and diagnosis of the electrocardiographic record (ECG), the Pacemaker Inverse Problem means the computerized analysis of the ECG in order to establish exact details of the heart - pacemaker interaction (HPI) and to diagnose the pacemaker failures. The solution of this problem is of great importance, since it is often extremely difficult to evaluate the paced ECG records clinically. The ECG patterns of natural extrasystolic heart depolarisations and paced events are often hardly distinguishable and very many combinations of pacemaker state changes have to be taken into consideration.

A computer system providing the automatic analysis of the HPI has been developed. The system is based on the ECG data elaboration and uses a complex algorithm which enables the evaluation for all possible combinations of the heart and pacemaker events. For each of these combinations, the system establishes its correspondence to the specified pacemaker algorithm and parameters.

The first version of the system has been tested with algorithms of the dual chamber cardiac pulse generator AUTIMA II (Telectronics). The interactive input of the system consists of pacemaker algorithm specification and of the analysed ECG in the form of timing of 'definite' and 'possible' sensing events and pacemaker pulses. The performed analysis establishes whether the device operates correctly within its permitted error. Should one or more explanations of the elaborated case be found, the system prints simplified pattern of the eleborated ECG accompanied by simulated marker channel.

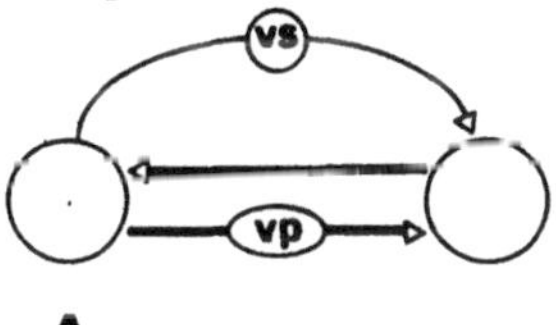

A

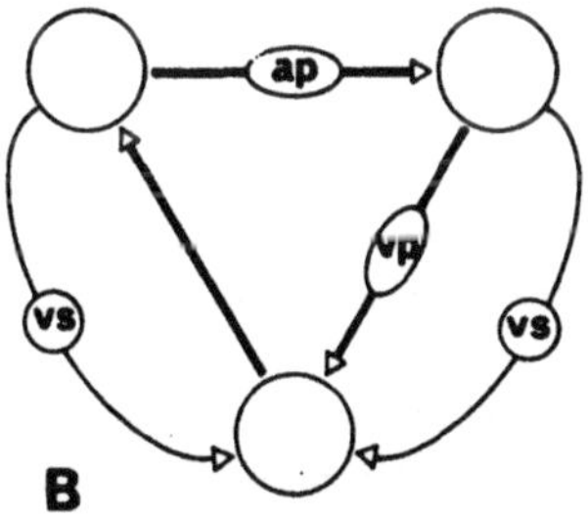

B

Fig. 1. The state diagrams of VVI (A) and DVI (B) pacemakers. The bold arrows indicate implicit changes, the fine arrows describe explicit changes. Some implicit changes are associated with atrial (ap) or ventricular (vp) pacing; the explicit changes are caused by ventricular sensing (vs).

INTRODUCTION

The current implantable cardiac pulse generators employ (1) very complex internal algoritms. These sophisticated modes allow pacemakers to respond properly in most anticipated cases of cardiac rhythm disorders. However, the complexity of pacemaker function limits our ability to evaluate HPI for the diagnosis of device's faults and possible technical failures. The more sophisticated algorithm is used in the pacemaker, the more complex considerations are necessary to predict its behaviour under peculiar situations.

At the same time, understanding of HPI is important in clinical situations. Each unusual episode of the HPI has to be explained in detail since proper reprogramming of pacemaker's internal parameters might prevent more serious disorders which may potentially develope in future.

Manufacturers improve the process of understanding the HPI by introducing the so called marker channel (2). The same electronic device which is used to program the pacemaker (i.e. to modify its mode and internal parameters) is able to produce an ECG record accompanied by special marks tracing and explaining the pacemaker actions and the way in which the device responses to natural cardiac activity. If a marker channel is produced, understanding the HPI is rather easy and causes no difficulties. However, many unusual ECG episodes are recorded in paced patients when this technical support is not available or not in use. Then the mechanisms of the HPI may be difficult to understand. The pacing artefacts indicating pacemaker's activity can fuse with other ECG patterns, records of natural heart depolarisations can imitate the paced beats, etc. In such cases, the evaluation of HPI requires very many possibilities and their combinations to be taken into account. The number of such combinations can be enormous and restricts our ability to evaluate the HPI mentally by logical considerations.

Device type specified : Autima II D.D.D.

Lower ventricular rate	bpm :	60	accuracy (0.001) :	80
Atrio-ventricular delay	ms :	200	accuracy (0.001) :	90
Upper ventricular rate	bpm :	100	accuracy (0.001) :	50
Post vntr. atrial refractory period	ms :	475	accuracy (0.001) :	80
Ventricular refractory period	ms :	250	accuracy (0.001) :	100

Fig. 2. System output summarizing the specified pacemaker mode and its accuracy.

At the same time, the rules of HPI evaluation can be nearly exactly specified. For instance, each pacing impulse which does not fuse with a natural depolarisation or fall in the refractory period of the tissue, should be followed by excitation of the corresponding cardiac chamber, etc. Such general principles enable the HPI evaluation algorithms to be created. Hence, the mental evaluation is complicated by the extent of the problem and not by a principal absence of the necessary information. Therefore, it has been possible to develope a special mathematical theory of the HPI and to create a computer system which performs an automatic analysis ot the paced ECG data.

COMPUTER SUPPORT SYSTEM

Special mathematical means enable each pacemaker algorithm to be specified in a uniform way (3). From the functional point of view, each pulse generator occurs in several different states (atrioventricular delay, refractory period, blanking period, etc.) and the changes between these states are performed instantaneously. The changes of states can be divided into two groups: 'explicit' (external) changes performed in response to a sensed natural depolarisation, and 'implicit' (internal) changes associated with zeroing an internal time counter of the device. At some of these changes, atrial or ventricular pacing pulses are generated, while other changes are restricted only to the internal pacemaker's electronics. The terms of pacemaker states and state changes enable each pacing mode to be described by an operational diagram (Fig. 1.).

SPECIFIED ECG DATA

Definite atrial sensing	...	from	100	till	160
Definite atrial sensing	...	from	720	till	785
Definite atrial sensing	...	from	1000	till	1060
Definite atrial sensing	...	from	4650	till	4710
Definite atrial sensing	...	from	5300	till	5360
Possible atrial sensing	...	from	2700	till	2810
Possible atrial sensing	...	from	3600	till	3710
Definite ventricular sensing	...	from	220	till	320
Definite ventricular sensing	...	from	1250	till	1350
Definite ventricular sensing	...	from	2950	till	3060
Definite ventricular sensing	...	from	3850	till	3960
Definite ventricular sensing	...	from	4850	till	4960
Definite ventricular sensing	...	from	5490	till	5590
Possible ventricular sensing	...	from	2000	till	2140
Definite atrial pacing	...	from	80	till	120
Definite atrial pacing	...	from	4630	till	4670
Possible atrial pacing	...	from	980	till	1020
Possible atrial pacing	...	from	5280	till	5320
Definite ventricular pacing	...	from	1235	till	1265
Definite ventricular pacing	...	from	2935	till	2965
Definite ventricular pacing	...	from	3825	till	3855
Definite ventricular pacing	...	from	4825	till	4855
Definite ventricular pacing	...	from	5535	till	5565
Possible ventricular pacing	...	from	280	till	320
Possible ventricular pacing	...	from	1780	till	2020

Fig. 3. System output summarizing the specified ECG data.

Since the developed system under description is designed to serve a later off-line analysis of ECG traces recorded in paced events, its ECG input is based on manual distinguishing the separate ECG events. The diagnosis of the

Fig. 4. A hypothetical ECG record in a patient with a DDD pacemaker. Four paced ventricular complexes and two paced P waves are clearly visible. The other patterns (a-f) permit different explanations.

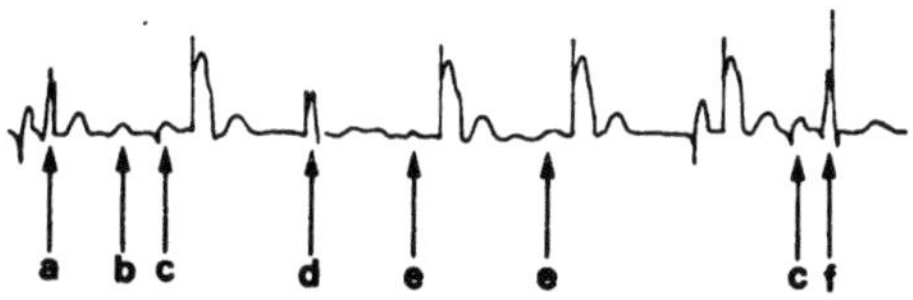

HPI requires only four types of events to be considered and recognised within the analysed ECG: atrial and ventricular pacing pulses, and atrial and ventricular cardiac depolarisations which can be sensed by the pacemaker and influence its performance. We have already mentioned that exact distinguishing between separate ECG patterns can be difficult. Therefore, the system enables to postulate that some HPI events definitely occured, while others are only possible. Similarly, the timing of events cannot be exact and must be specified as a time interval during which the event occurred. Moreover, the timing intervals of several events may occur simultaneously or may partly fuse.

The main evaluation phase of the system establishes whether there exists an appropriate correspondence between the specified algorithm of the pacemaker and the events recognised in the analysed ECG. This requires to find an exact representation of the uncertain ECG data, which means: I. for each of those events which are specified as possible, an establishment whether it did really happen; II. for all events which occurred, a localisation of the occurrence within the specified time interval.

COMPUTER EXPERIMENTS

The first version of the system has been implemented on an IBM PC AT computer. The program is written in Turbo Pascal and its source text has more than 11000 lines. This first version is designed to cope with a real clinical pulse generator AUTIMA-II (Telectronics) (4). However, this restriction refers to the pacemaker specification part only, other segments of the system have already been developed in a universal way and are prepared to accept any pacing mode.

The system output summarizes the specified pacemaker mode (Fig. 2.) and prints a simple table listing out the specified ECG events (Fig. 3.). This makes it possible to check the input data.

Then the system reproduces the specified ECG in a simplified graphical form. If one or more different interpretations of the HPI are found, the reproduced ECG is accompanied by a artificial marker channel indicating the timing of sensing and pacing events. To make more detailed considerations of the pacemaker behaviour possible, another technical marker

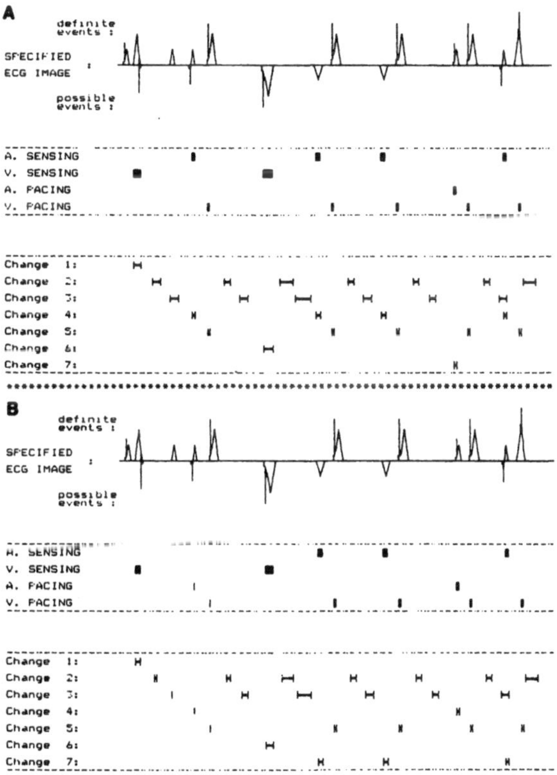

Fig. 5. Computer elaboration shown in Fig. 4. Cases A and B show two of several different explanations. These two cases differ in interpreting the first pattern 'c' as natural (A) and paced (B). The internal changes 1-7 (ordered differently in both cases) refer to the specified pacemaker algorithm.

channel is also produced. It supports the clinical marker channel by tracing the explicit and implicit changes of the pacemaker algorithm. The system has been tested with many complicated artificial ECG records (Fig. 4. and 5.) which proved its clinical relevance. Clinically (5), the system can be used to evaluate various episodes in paced ECG traces (Fig. 6. and 7.).

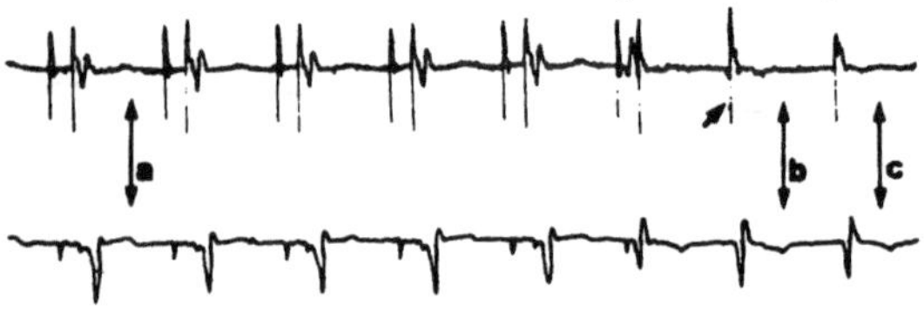

Fig. 6. Example of a rhythm episode recorded in a patient with a non-comitted DVI pacemaker.

DISCUSSION

The currently implemented version of the system has several important technical limitations and clinical disadvantages. The next version of the system must be redesigned to accept more different pacing modes. From the clinical point of view, the most important restriction of the system lies in its diagnostics possibilities. When a discrepancy between the pacemaker mode and the ECG trace is foud, the system declares this situation but does not discuss or classify the possible mechanism which may cause the pacemaker to behave improperly.

Despite of these restrictions, the developed system performs a clinically relevant evaluation of complicated episodes observed in paced ECGs. It demonstrates the possibility of computerizing the diagnosis of the heart pacemaker interface.

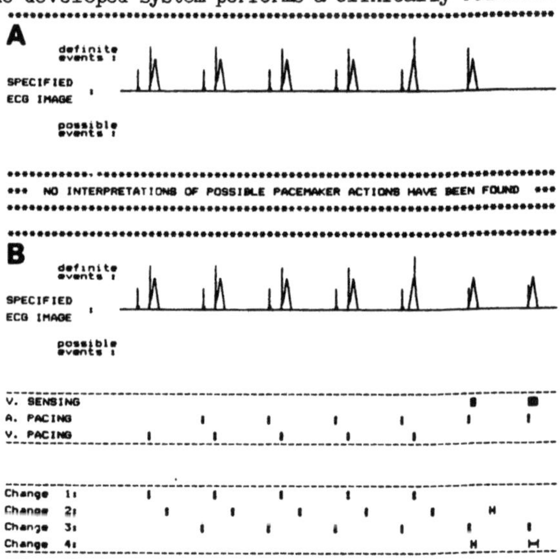

Fig. 7. Computer evaluation of the episode shown in Fig. 6. The result A corresponds to the a-b interval, the result B to the a-c interval. In the case A, the pacing spike indicated by arrow is treated as ventricular pacing, in the case B as atrial pacing. The system diagnoses that atrial pacing causes ventricular depolarisation.

REFERENCES

(1) Barold SS, Falkoff MD, Ong LS, et al: In: Satini M, Pistolese M, Alliegro A (eds.): Progress in Clinical Pacing, Rome 1986, pp. 276

(2) Kruse I, Markowitz T, Ryden L: PACE 6, 801 (1983)

(3) Malik M., Camm AJ.: Comput. Biomed. Res. submitted (1987)

(4) AUTIMA-II, technical manual, Telectronics Ltd., London

(5) Malik M., Camm AJ.: Cardiovasc. Res. submitted (1987).

Optimal setting of programmable cardiac pacemakers by means of radionuclide ventriculography

GUNKEL,H., PUNDRICH, R., OTTO,H.-J., GÜNTHER, K.-F., SCHMIDT, H., HÖFS, R., SAAD, B.

Clinic of radiology, Department of Nuclearmedicine and Clinic of Internal Medicine, Department of Cardiology
Medical Academy Magdeburg, GDR

Summary

In many cases the possibilities of programmable pacemakers are not used in the full extent because there are scarely noninvasive investigations to prove the optimal setting of program (1). We determined the best frequency respectively by DDD-systems also the atrioventricular delay by means of radionuclide ventriculography (RNV).
In 32 of the 41 pts. the pacemakers were reprogrammed. Follow-up studies after 1 years was especially valuable in 5 cases with congenital or early aquired atrioventricular block for the demonstration of the adaptation of myocardium by the new conditions.

Due to the high state of the art in microelectronics reached in recent years, multiprogrammable VVI and DDD systems are now increasingly available for physiological cardiac pacemaker treatment. It is in particular the parameters, frequency and atrioventricular delay, which require comprehensive individual function analysis of the possible settable programs. It is only in this way that the potentialities of the programmable pacemakers available can be fully utilized (1). There have been repeated attempts and noninvasive as well as invasive investigations into determining the optimal frequency and atrioventricular delay.
To our knowledge, the haemodynamic behaviour of synchronized and non-synchronized pacemaker stimulation of atrium and ventricle has been studied in a noninvasive nuclear-medical approach by Nitsch et al. only (2).

Material and methods

We have introduced a comprehensive nuclearmedical follow-up four to six weeks after surgery for patients provided with a multiprogrammable VVI or DDD pacemaker system (3).
In patients with congenital or early acquired complete atrioventricular block, this follow-up is repeated after one year for further adjustments. Irrespective of checking the variable parameters, that is

frequency and atrioventricular delay, electrocardiographic monitoring is employed to check and programme amplitude, impulse duration, sensitivity, and hysteresis.

We have applied gated radionuclide ventriculography in 41 pacemaker patients to determine optimal stimulation frequency and atrioventricular delay.

The examinations were carried out under resting conditions in programs adjustable for the Biotronik pacemaker types.

In LAO 30 to 45 degree projections, there were 30 images per cardiac cycle recorded with 1,5 million impulses per study. We determined the contractility describing parameters, amplitude, phase, longitudinal axis of the ventricle, the ratio of atrial and ventricular compartments actively involved in the contraction, the left ventricular ejection fraction, and a shape factor of the left ventricular cyclogram which (LVCF) we defined:

CYCLOGRAM SHAPE FACTOR (LVCF)

$$LVCF = K - \frac{t_{DIA} + t_{SYS}}{t_{RR}}$$

where

LVCF = Cyclogram shape factor of left ventricle
K = Empirical calibration constant (K = 1.5)
t_{DIA} = Time of diastole } of cyclogram
t_{SYS} = Time of systole } of cyclogram

Normal range: $0.98 \leq LVCF \leq 1.2$
$LVCF < 0.98$ = Shift of cyclogram
(The next pacemaker impulse is generated whilst the ventricle is being filled).

LVCF serves to describe the phase relation of enddiastole and telesystole of the left ventricular cyclogram with respect to the electrocardiographic R-wave.

Results

An example demonstrats our findings.

A 42-year-old patient with a complete atrioventricular block early acquired after myocarditis was sufficiently compensated by stroke volume adaptation. Even resting frequencies of a minimum of 12 beats per minute were tolerated without complaints.

Because of a radiologically revealed increase in heart size, a Kalos 03 VVI pacemaker was implanted in 1984 and programmed to a stimulation frequency of 31 beats per minute.

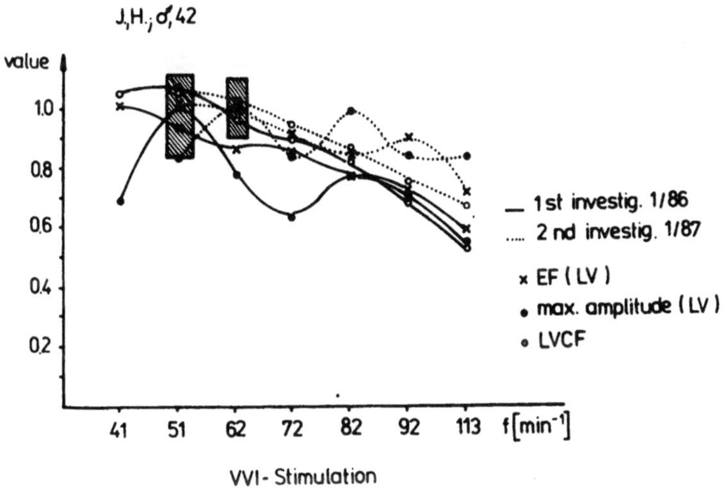

Fig.1: Response of selected parameters at the first investigation and the same one year later. (The shift of the frequency is well seen).

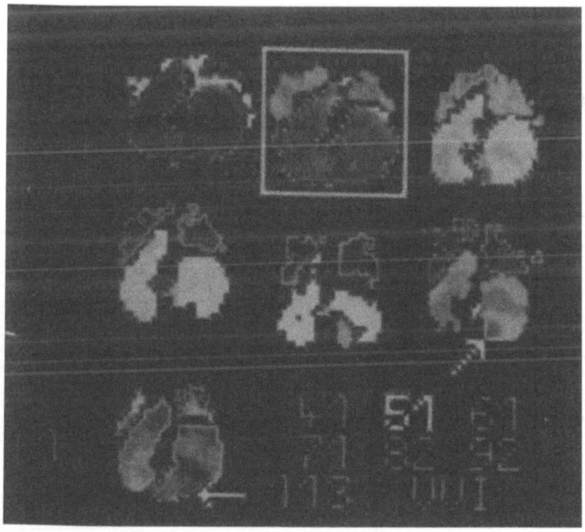

Fig.2: Phase images in depend on stimulation frequency as result of FOURIER analysis. The best homogenous pattern is seen at a frequency of 51 beats per minute. At higher ones are dyskinesias and akinesias localizable.

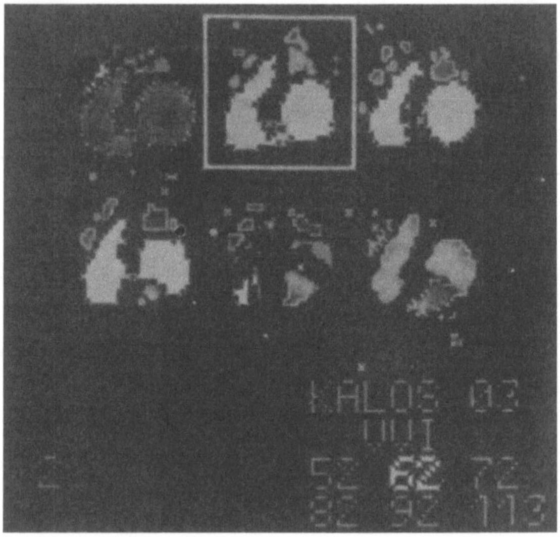

Fig.3: Phase images 1 year later. The shift to 62 bpw is very good illustrated.

The optimal pacemaker setting was determined for 41 patients, of which 22 carried a DDD system and 19 a VVI unit. The function parameters in the possible stimulation ranges were determined for all patients.
In addition, atrioventricular delays were established for those patients who carried a DDD pacemaker. Once the optimal setting had been ascertained, the pacemakers were reprogrammed in 32 of the 41 patients as demonstrated in the table.

Tab.2

	Investigated patients	Alterations after investigation		
		frequency	AV delay	frequ.and AV
DDD-System	16	11(69%)	3(20%)	2
VVI-System	25	16(64%)	0	0
total	41	27(66%)	3	2

Discussion and conclusions

Based on the results obtained to date, we believe that radionuclide ventriculography is a noninvasive technique which is well suited to determine favourable individual program settings with regard to frequency and atrioventricular delay for pacemaker patients.

We were told by all pacemaker patients that they were feeling subjectively well and in a better physical condition after the pacemakers had been reprogrammed.

Follow-up by means of the before-mentioned nuclear-cardiologic approach has appeared to be of particular value even in patients with congenital or early acquired complete atrioventricular block.

In addition to the usual parameters obtained by gated blood pool scintigraphy, it is changes in kinetics which can be derived qualitatively and semiquantitatively in particular from the parametric representations of our method and allowed for in this context.

References

1. Irnich, W.: DMW 40, 1527-1529 (1985)
2. Nitsch, I. et al.: Z. Kardiol. 72, 718 (1983)
3. Gunkel, H. et al.: Nuc-Compact 17, 186-190 (1986)

Differentiation of atrial rhythms by differentially amplified ECG

A.RUDYS, A.KIBARSKIS, V.SHILEIKIS

Department of Cardiology, Vilnius State University, Lithuania, USSR

SUMMARY. Localization of an atrial pacemaker is based on the morphology of the ECG P wave. However, it is often a low-amplitude, hardly modified element, merging with the T wave in tachycardia. The analysis of a differentially amplified ECG (DA ECG) data has permitted to establish the signs of the DA ECG atrial complexes, which were verified by atrial pacing. The shapes defined allow to locate the pacemaker in the sinus node, in the upper and lower parts of the right atrium, in the coronary sinus, in posterior lower and upper parts of the left atrium.A diagnostic algorhythm allowing to localize atrial pacemaker with high accuracy has been designed.

INTRODUCTION. Atrial rhythm, being common in young and practically healthy people, may occur in patients (pts) suffering from severe cardiovascular pathology. The diagnosis of the ectopic atrial rhythms is of great significance for evaluating the degree of the iscemic process or other myocardial damage. Their manifestation may be related to the sick sinus syndrome. The precise localization of the ectopic focus in pts with paroxysmal tachycardia acquires major importamce in surgical treatment of tachycardias, provoked by the accessory A-V junctions in particular. Revealing of atrial rhythms is built on the morphology of the P wave, which mostly constitutes a low-amplitude, hardly identified element on the stabdard ECG. Tachysystolia usually brings about its merging with the T-wave. The aim of our studies was to investigate the possibility of DA ECG atrial complex use for atrial pacemaker localization.

MATERIAL AND METHODS. A total of 65 pts with ectopic atrial rhythms aged from 14 to 67 years were investigated. 25 pts with coronary heart disease, 12 with myocarditis cardiosclerosis, 20 with neurocirculatory dystonia, 4 and 2 with rheumatic and congenital heart diseases respectively, 2 with the WPW syndrome. 31 of them manifested pacemaker shift in the atria, while the reminder (34 pts) had stable ectopic rhythm during examination. DA ECG was recorded in all pts. A bipolar lead was used, the positive electrode being placed at the sternal manubrium, the negative - at the 5th intercostal space by linea medioclavicularis dextra. The electrodes were connected with the input of a difeerential high-sensitivity amplifier supplied with the filtering system (filtering range 30-110 Hz, amplification by 50 times). The shape of an atrial complex recorded reflects both the pacemaker location as well as the atrial excitation sequence. In order to establish the shape of the DA ECG atrial complex in ectopic rhythms atrial pacing under X-ray control was performed in 61 pts from different sites of the right atrium and the coronary sinus.

RESULTS. In pacing from the ostium of the superior vena cava, i.e.from the suggested SA zone, the DA ECG atrial complex completely coincides with the atrial complex in sinus rhythm (Fig. 1), which is characterized by a peculiar shape: the first two spikes are negative (in Fig.1 they are marked as A_1 and A_2), while the terminal spike (A_3) is positive. Fig. 2 presents the DA ECG record in ectopic rhythm. The atrial complex lacks the first negative spike.Pacing the high right atrium brings about a similar complex on the DA ECG, what suggests the pacemaker to be located in this case in the upper part of tbe atrium.

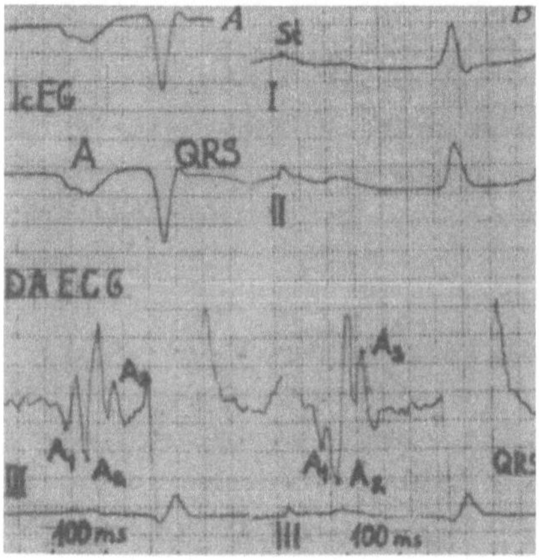

Fig. 1. Atrial complex on the DA ECG in spotaneous sinus rhythm (A), in pacing from the SA zone (B)

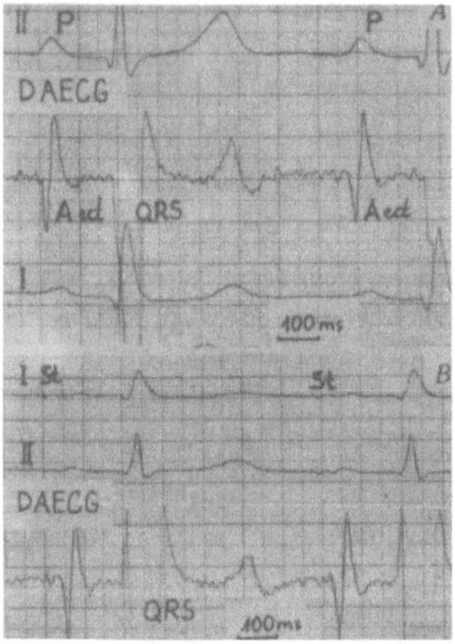

Fig. 2. Atrial complex of DA ECG in high right atrial spontaneous rhythm (A), in pacing from the upper part of the right atrium (B)

Fig. 3 illustrates a DA ECG atrial complex obtained in pacing from the low right atrium, coinciding with the atrial complex gained in the ectopic rhythm from the lower part of the right atrium. In pacing from the distal site of the coronary sinus the DA ECG reveals an atrial complex analogous to the atrial complex in spotaneous ectopic rhythm from the coronary sinus (Fig. 4).

Atrial pacing has been also performed from other sites of the right atrium and the coronary sinus. The data obtained were used for a diagnostic algorhythm děsign. Thus, the results of pacing from various sites of the right atrium and the coronary sinus allowed for differentiation of ectopic atrial rhythms according to their origin.

DISCUSSION. 65 pts with a pacemaker located in the ectopic atrial foci have been investigated. According to the atrial rhythms foci location the atrial rhythms

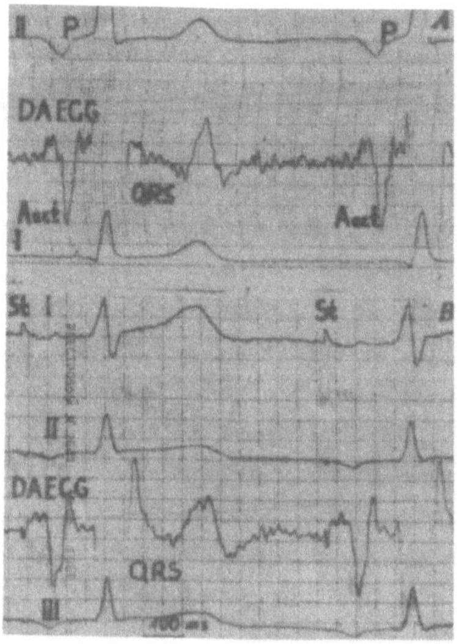

Fig. 3. Atrial complex of DA ECG in low right atrial rhythm (A), in pacing from the lower part of the right atrium (B)

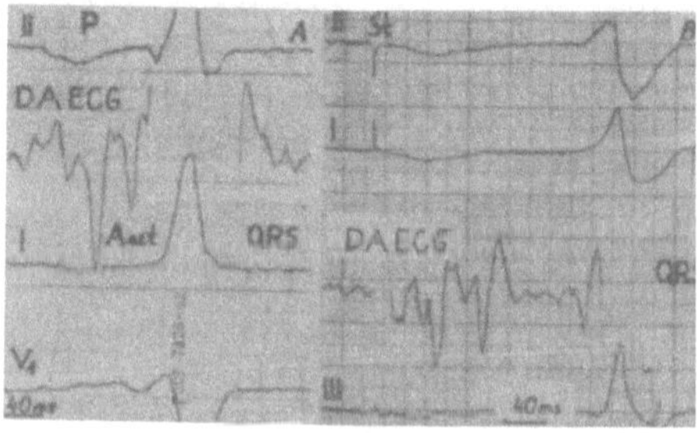

Fig. 4. Atrial complex of DA ECG in spotaneous rhythm originating from the coronary sinus (A) and in pacing from the distal end of the coronary sinus (B)

were subdivided into 5 groups, taking in consideration the findings of atrial pacing: 1) high right atrial rhythm, 2) low posterior right atrial rhythm, 3) coronary sinus rhythm, 4) high posterior left atrial rhythm, 5) low posterior left atrial rhythm. The most "active" zones from the aspect of the ectopic rhythm initiation appeared to be the upper zone of the right atrium (55.5%) and the coronary sinus ostium zone (20.0%), while the most "passive" is the left atrium (6.0%). These findings are in good relation with the data reported /1,2/. The classification of ectopic right atrial rhythms into 3 and left atrial rhythms in to 2 gourps was proved to be correct by the diagnostic algorhythm. It turned out that the usc of its informative parameters leads to a rather exact differentiation of the atrial actopic rhythms (the errors in 9-13%). The pacemaker localization by a standard ECG usually presents difficulties. It is generally accepted, that in sinus rhythm the P wave should be positive in leads I,II,aVF /3/, still, it may be positive in these leads in ectopic rhythms as well /4,5,6,7/. Leon et al. /8/ have shown the P wave to be practically the same in both pacing from the upper site of the right atrium and in sinus rhythm. The use of a DA ECG may become crucial for localizing the pacemaker in the upper part of the right atrium.

Lately, the term "the coronary sinus rhythm" has become doubtful /7,8/ as in pacing form any site of the lower part of the right atrium the P wave in the leads II,III,aVF is inverted, while the P-Q intervalduration tion depends mainly on the conduction in the A-V junction and His-Purkinje system. The negative P wave in the leads II,III,aVF may occur in pacing from the posterior part of the left atrium too, nevertheless, in this case a specific wave appears in lead V_1.

According to our data the DA ECG atrial complex, obtained in endocardial pacing from the coronary sinus ostium differs in its configuration with that revealed in pacing of the lower posterior zone of the right atrium, in the initial shape in particular. In pacing from the distal end of the coronary sinus the DA ECG curve reveals the complexes of a peculiar configuration, similar with those defined by us as belonging to the group of lower posterior left atrial rhythms.

The DA ECG recording favours a more accurate pacemaker localization , especially when a mathematical diagnostic algorhythm is employed.

The definite localization of a pacemaker in the atria may reveal the arrhythmogenic zone, induced by hypoxia in pts with coronary heart disease /9/, accessory A-V junction /10,11/ or suggest the site for endocardial pacing in order to terminate atrial ectopic tachycardia.

REFERENCES

(1) Davis L.D.Am. J. Physiol. 229, 1351 (1975)
(2) Strauss H.C. et al. Prog. in Cardiovasc. Dis., 19, 385-404 (1977)
(3) Goldberg J.M., Lynn-Johnson M.H. J.Electrocardiol,13, 209-218 (1980)
(4) Euler D.E. et al. Circulation. 59, 468 (1979)
(5) Mac Lean W.A.H. et al. Circulation, 52, 426-434 (1975)
(6) Mirowski M. et al. Am. Heart J. 81, 666-676 (1971)
(7) Waldo A.L. et al. Circulation, 42, 653-671 (1970)
(8) Leon D.F. et al. Am. J. Cardiol, 25, 6-10 (1970)
(9) Klein H.O. et al. Am. Heart J. 87, 750-756 (1974)
(10) Josephson M.E. Am. J. Cardiol, 41, 1123-1126 (1978)
(11) Watson M.M., M.E.Josephson. Am. J. Cardiol., 45, 732-741 (1980)

Controlled antiarrhythmic therapy for recurrent supraventricular arrhythmias by means of repeated transesophageal pacing

WLODZIMIERZ J.MUSIAL, JAN RUTA, HALINA BOLINSKA

Clinical Electrophysiology Laboratory, Institute of Cardiology Medical University of Lodz, Poland.

SUMMARY: Long-term results of controlled antiarrhythmic therapy in 14 pts with supraventricular arrhythmias using repeated transesophageal pacing are presented. All arrhythmias were recurrent or severe in hemodynamic consequences. After an invasive His-bundle study oral antiarrhythmic therapy was started. Its results were verified clinically, using Holter monitoring and repeated transesophageal pacing studies. In 12 cases (78%) good therapeutic results were obtained. Amiodarone was the most effective drug.

Electrophysiological studies combined with pharmacological tests are widely accepted for clinical management of patients (pts) with life threatening ventricular arrhythmias (1,2). However this invasive methods are rarely used in supraventricular tachycardias (3,4).
Transesophageal pacing (TP), a noninvasive technique can be a method of choice in this group of patients (5,6,7,8).

The purpose of our study is to present the long-term clinical results of antiarrhythmic treatment in pts with recurrent supraventricular arrhythmias. The therapy was guided using repeated TP.

MATERIAL and METHODS

Fourteen pts (8 men and 6 women) with supraventricular tachycardias were studied. In 11 of them arrhythmias were due to an overt or concealed WPW syndrome. In all cases the arrhythmias were recurrent despite of previous pharmacological treatment or severe in hemodynamic consequences. The most important clinical data are summarized in table 1.
Preliminary an invasive electrophysiological study with His bundle recording, rapid and programmed stimulation was performed. Then according to its results oral antiarrhythmic therapy was started. The wide spectrum of drugs including B-blockers, verapamil, quinidine, disopyramide, ajmaline, propafenone and amiodarone were tested. The results of therapy were verified clinically, using 24-hour Holter monitoring and repeated TP. Two to four stimulation tests were performed in each pt. The conduction capacity, refractory times and possibility of arrhythmia induction were noninvasively tested.
The typical example of serial transesophageal studies in one of our

patients is shown in fig. 1
The clinical follow up ranged from 3 to 78 month, mean 36 month.

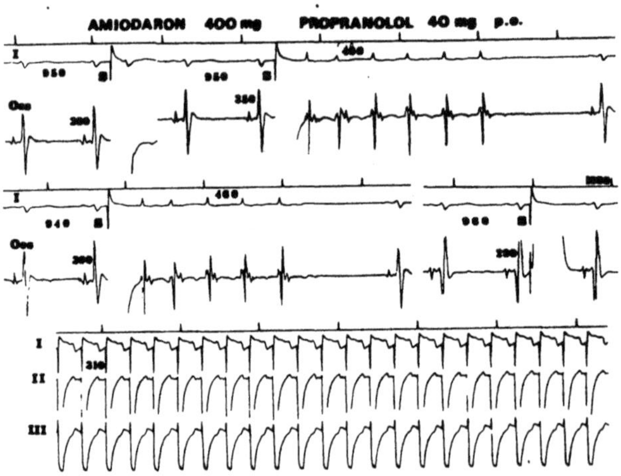

Fig. 1 Repeated TP studies in pt nr 14. 200 mg amiodarone and 40 mg propranolol p.o. was not able to prevent reentry tachycardia during programmed stimulation. On increased dose of amiodarone (up to 400 mg daily) only the short episodes of reentry are inductable.Note the prolongation of the effective refractory period of the Kent bundle and depression of antegrąde conduction capacity.Also slowing of the tachycardia rate is seen.

RESULTS

The arrhythmias were completly supressed in 9 pts and significantly reduced in another two.The total success rate was 78%.The noninvasive method permitted us to evaluate comparatively different antiarrhythmic agents.Amiodarone alone or in combination with other drugs was the most potent medicament. Good results were obtained in 8 of 10 cases (details see table 1).

No effects were obtained in 3 cases (nr 2,7,13) despite of various drug combination.One pt of this group with left lateral accessory pathway was successfully operated, another woman refused surgical treatment.In the

last case, with frequent attacks of atrial fibrillation in the begining, atrial fibrillation stabilised after several month and was well controlled with medical treatment.

The stable capture by transesophageal route (with the current strenght ranged 20-30 mA) was successfully obtained in all pts,however some of them experienced burning chest discomfort. It was easily tolerated. No other side effects were observed.

DISCUSSION

In most pts with paroxysmal supraventricular tachycardias the arrhythmia can be easily induced and terminated in the catheterization laboratory.The ability to reproduce this arrhythmia unable to study acute effects of antiarrhythmic drugs.

In 1977 Wu at all (4) propagated chronic electrophysiological studies, as a new method for evaluation the effects of antiarrhythmic agents.The same protocol used by Worum at all (3), was presented during the 10 Congress of Electrocardiology in Bratislava.

In the recent years transesophageal pacing, a noninvasive technique for diagnosis and therapy was developed (5,6,7,8).Its application has been primarily limited by either pt discomfort due to high current requirements or by the lack of constant capture.These disadvantages were reduced by wider pulse duration and interelectrode distance, which lowered pacing threshold (6).

The purpose of the present study was to examine the effects of repeated TP in treatment of pts with refractory supraventricular arrhythmias.Good therapeutic results were obtained in 78% of pts and this data were confirmed during the long clinical (mean 36 month) follow-up period.

Our study showed that repeated transesophageal pacing is a relatively simple and valuable technique that allows chronic electrophysiologic drug evaluation.The method is safe, when performed in a setting in which resuscitative procedure is readily available.It is in agreement with recently published observations (5,7).It is advantageous in comparison to the empiric drug therapy, which requires often prolonged observations with multiple hospital admittances.Also repeated invasive electrophysiological studies are sometimes difficult to perform and not accepted by all pts.The proposed protocol of combined invasive electrophysiologic studies with repeated noninvasive TP tests are especially usefull in pts with WPW syndrome in which recurrent arrhythmiasare typical in clinical picture.The performed studies allowed also to find pts with arrhythmias refractory to all drug management, who are the candidates for surgical treatment.

The obtained results have confirmed the high efficency of amiodarone therapy in pts with the preexcitation syndrome. This was previously reported by other authors (5,7).

CONCLUSIONS

1. Repeated transesophageal pacing studies are a valuable method in evaluation of chronic antiarrhythmic therapy in patients with refractory supraventricular arrhythmias.

2. Amiodarone was the most effective drug in supraventricular arrhythmias due to the WPW syndrome.

REFERENCES

(1) DiMarco, J.P., H. Garan, J.N. Ruskin: Amer. J. Cardiol. 51, 90 (1983).

(2) Horowitz, L.N., M.E. Josephson, J.A. Kastor: Progr. Cardiovasc. Dis. 23, 81 (1980).

(3) Worum, F., P. Kovacs, I. Lorincz, P. Polgar, I. Worum: In Electrocardiology 83. Cardiac Rhythm, Arrhythmias, Conduction Disturbances, ed I. Ruttkay-Nedecky, P.W. Macfarlane, Bratislava 1985, 130.

(4) Wu, D., C.R. Wyndham, P. Denes, F. Amat-y-Leon , R.H. Miller, R.C. Dhingra, K.M. Rosen: In Re-entrant Arrhythmias: Mechanism and Treatment, ed H.E. Kulbertus, MTP Press Ltd, Lancaster, 1977, 294.

(5) Critelli, G., Grassi, F. Perticone, F. Coltori, V. Monda, M. Condorelli: Amer. J. Cardiol. 51, 513 (1983).

(6) Gallagher, J.J., W.M. Smith, C.R. Kerr, J. Kasell, L. Cook, M. Reiter, R. Sterba, M. Hartle: Circulation 65, 336 (1982).

(7) Gonzalez, M.D., R.H. Guillen, O.A. Pellizzon, E.C. Raimondi: Amer. J. Cardiol. 55, 852 (1985).

(8) Prochaczek, F., J. Galecka, K. Stanek, M. Stopczyk: Stimuceur 3, 151 (1986).

Table 1

Clinical features of studied patients

PATIENT	AGE (yr)	SEX	DIAGNOSIS	TYPE of ARRHYTHMIA RSVT	AF\AFL	FOLLOW-UP (mo)	No of TPS	THERAPY *	EFFECT
1. F.M.	44	W	WPW	-	+	72	3	A,P	+
2. Z.F.	27	M	WPW	-	+	66	2		-
3. W.A.	49	M	WPW	+	-	78	3	V	+-
4. R.P.	32	M	WPW	+	-	38	3	A	+-
5. N.A.	41	M	WPW	-	+	78	3	A	+
6. J.G.	58	W	UN	-	+	78	3	A	+-
7. D.P.	38	M	UN	-	+	48	4		-
8. S.K.	31	W	conc.WPW	+	-	8	3	AJ	+
9. M.A.	20	M	WPW	+	-	6	2	A	+
10. B.W.	39	M	WPW	-	+	6	2	A	+
11. D.Cz.	54	W	BTS	+	-	8	4	V	+
12. F.W.	31	M	WPW	-	+	6	2	A	+
13. W.Z.	21	W	WPW	+	+	3	3		-
14. Ch.S.	48	W	WPW	+	+	14	3	A,BB	+-

Abbreviations: RSVT-supraventricular reentry tachycardia, AF-atrial fibrillation, AFL-atrial flutter, TPS-transesophageal pacing studies, *-only effective drugs are given, W-woman, M-man, WPW-Wolff-Parkinson-White syndrome, conc-concealed, UN-unknown, BTS-bradycardia-tachycardia syndrome, A-amiodarone, P-propafenone, V-verapamil, AJ-ajmaline, BB-betablocker, + arrhythmia fully controlled, +- improvement, - no effect

Effects of cardiac glycosides on electrical repolarization during sinus-rhythm and atrials pacing in normals and in patients with coronary artery diseases

LAUTEN, A., I. ASSMANN, and P. KASSEL
Dept. of Cardiology, Clinic of Internal Medicine, Medical School Erfurt, GDR

Summary
Global repolarization is shortened by cardiac glycosides (c.g.). We investigated following questions: 1st: Are there differences between several c.g.? 2nd: Do patients (pts.) with chronic ischemic heart disease (CIHD) respond in another way than healthy persons (HP)? 3rd: Is there a possibility for other results after partial elimination of autonomous nervous system activity? For these reasons digitoxin, digoxin, and ouabain were supplied in CIHD-pts. and HP acutely. After that we checked the effects of c.g. for global, partly for regional QT-interval in sinus rhythm and also in atrial pacing. All c.g. lead to a considerable shortening of QT-interval in sinus rhythm and atrial pacing (mean 2o - 3o ms). We observed a significant effect for ouabain in CIHD-pts.and in HP. In CIHD-pts. with raised basic values the shortening was more progressive after ouabain than in HP. There was no sure difference between CIHD-pts. and HP in surface mapping. Conclusions: We have to consider an increased influence of c.g. on the repolarization and the higher risk of ventricular ectopias in CIHD-pts.

Introduction

The electrical repolarization and its disturbances are one of the keys for understanding of ventricular tachycardias. Based on the electrical instability of the myocard - especially the ventricular fibrillation is one cause of sudden cardiac death (Aßmann, Fiehring et al.).
The mechanism of rhythm disturbances may be an inhomogenous repolarization and their influence by cardiac drugs are important under some different clinical aspects.
We investigated the influence of the cardiac glycosides: digitoxin (DT), digoxin (DG), and ouabain (OU).
The following items were of special interest:
1st: Are there differences between several c.g.?
2nd: Do patients with chronic ischemic heart disease respond in another way than healthy persons?
3rd: Is there a possibility for other results after partial elimination of autonomous nervous system activity?

Methods

Studies were performed in 33 patients aged 36 - 71 years, 22 males and 11 females with CIHD and in 32 HP (19 - 64 years, 22 males, 1o females). We investigated heart rate corrected QT-interval (QT_c) in sinus rhythm and additionally during atrial pacing (f = 9o per minute - QT_{stim}). Investigationswere performed as a complex evaluation of His-bundle-elektrogram in order to analyze several rhythm disturbances. After baseline measurements had been made, digitoxin (1,25 mg), digoxin (1,25 mg) or ouabain (o,4 mg) was given intravenously. Measurements were repeated 45 minutes after DT or DG, respectively 2o minutes after OU in the same manner.

Student's t-test for paired data was used for statistical analysis, p-values were significant at levels of 5 % or less.

In the CIHD-group we investigated the regional repolarization with body surface mapping as an enlarged precordial surface ECG with altogether 36 points. In these cases we admistered o,375 mg OU only, but no other glycosides.

Results

All c.g. led to a considerable shortening of QT-interval in sinusrhythm and atrial pacing in CIHD-patients (mean 2o - 3o ms) and in HP. We observed significant effects of all c.g.

The diminishing of the QT-values (QT_c and QT_{stim}) is very impressive after the application of OU and DG (fig. 1).

In body surface mapping after OU wie observed a similiar picture of repolarization but we did not find any signs of inhomogenous repolarization. The QT-values of all leads showed significant tendencies for diminishing (mean 15 - 24 ms) (fig. 2).

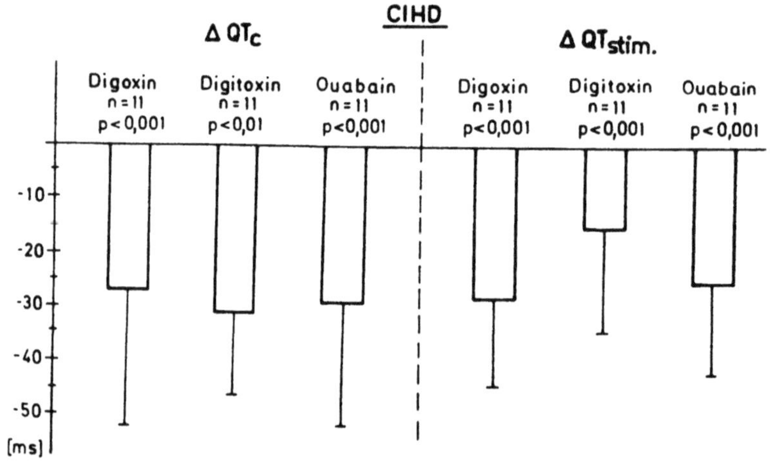

Fig. 1: CIHD and cardiac glycosides - behavior of repolarization during sinus rhythm (QT_c) and atrial pacing (QT_{stim})

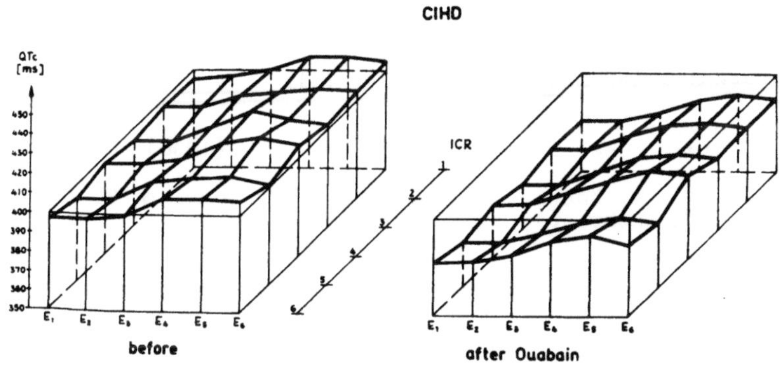

Fig. 2: QT_c before and after ouabain in body surface mapping in CIHD-patients

Discussion and conclusions

The glycoside - induced diminishing of repolarization has been known for many years; it is to be regarded as a sign of early glycoside activity (Schellong). The QT-values stated in this study demonstrated the significant shortening without clear differences between several c.g. In the same way as the sinus node function and the av-conduction (Treese,Kasper et al.;Alboni, Shanta et al.), the repolarization is mediated by the autonomous nervous system, and atrial pacing is to value as an attempt to eliminate these influence partially. We did not see any informations in connection to repolarization and atrial pacing in the literature. Our findings to this topic suggest a clear influence of DG in CIHD-patients. These relations are to be seen as pathophysiological base for treatment of ventricular ectopias (e.g."torsade-de-point"-tachycardia) caused by lengthenings or inhomogenity of the repolarization (Lauten, Aßmann). If c.g. are necessary, the priority of DG should be noted. In single cases the effect of OU to diminish the QT-time must be taken in account as an alternative therapeutical way. Despite of well known contra-argumentation against the OU-treatment, a special indication of it could be dicussed. This is of importance, if the shortening of repolarization predominates over other glycoside-effects, and if other antiarrhythmic drugs are not indicated.

References

1. Aßmann, I., H. Fiehring, K.H. Stock:
   Dt.Gesundh.-wesen 38, 336 - 342 (1983)

2. Schellong, F.:
   Verh. dtsch. Ges. inn. Med. 48, 288 - 295 (1936)

3. Treese, N., W. Kasper, H.J. Gilfrich, T. Pop, and T. Meinertz:
   Klin. Wochenschr. 61, 523 - 527 (1983)

4. Alboni, P., N. Shantha, L. Filippi, R. Pirani, S. Preziosi, A.M. Tomasi, and A. Masoni:
   Am. Heart J. 108, 1255 - 1261 (1984)

5. Lauten, A., I. Aßmann:
   Ergebn. exp. Med. 47, 215 - 227 (1987)

Are the alcoholic arrhythmias related to alcoholic cardiomypaty?

GAI V., M. SICURO, D. SAPPE', L. RISSONE

Servizio di Cardiologia, Ospedale Valdese, Pomaretto (TO), Italy

SUMMARY - 40 cronic alcoholics, males, without evidence of systemic disease not related to alcohol, were studied during alcohol free assumption with echocardiography (ECHO)and Holter monitoring (ECG-D). 10% of them showed ECHO ventricular function parameters according to a clinical diagnosis of alcoholic cardiomyopathy (CMPA). Arrhythmias prevalence was high also in the group without CMPA (CMPA-)with a 12.5% prevalence of atrial fibrillation and a 2.5% prevalence of ventricular tachicardia. A correlation was found, in the CMPA- group, between the overall presence of arrhythmias and the level of ventricular function.

INTRODUCTION - Cronic alcohol (ETOH) assumption can induce (with toxic, immunologic, deficitary mechanisms) (Rubin; Segel et al.; St. Leger et al.; Maisch et al.) different degrees of altered cardiac function with 1) cardiac output increased by hypervolemia, hypercinetic syndrome, tiamine deficiency and 2) cardiac output reduced by myopathic damage (Mathews et al.; Regan and Haider; Regan; Chavez Rivera and Barros). Alcoholic cardiomyopathy represents the overt clinical expression of impaired contractility by alcoholic myopathic damage. Furthermore ETOH can produce, by still not fully understood mechanisms, hypercinetic arrhyrhmias in prevalence supraventricular. The aim of our study is:

- to point out the circadian heart rate variation behavior, the presence of arrhythmias and of left ventricular (LVF) and right ventricular (RLF) function impairment;
- to look for possible relationships between arrhythmias and reduction of ventricular function in a group of cronic alcoholics in a free assumption phase but not in acute intoxication.

MATERIALS AND METHODS - We studied 40 cronic alcoholics, males, mean age 48 + 9.6 yrs, that daily introduce since more than 10 years some 200 grams of ETOH. They were not affected by cardiovascular diseases not related to alcohol, arterial hypertension, diabetes. All the patients underwent maximal exercise testing - in order to exclude ischemic heart disease -, 24-72 hours Holter monitoring (ECG-D), M-Mode and bidimensional echocardiogram (ECHO). At the ECG-D were evaluated: the circadian heart rate variation (ΔR/24h), the presence of supraventricular ectopic beats > 50/day (SVEB), supraventricular tachicardia (SVT), atrial fibrillation (AF), ventricular ectopic beats >30/h (VEB), ventricular tachicardia (VT), pauses and A-V conduction defects.

At the ECHO were observed: left atrial dimensions (LA); ventricular diastosistolic diameters (LVDd - LVDs), right ventricular diastolic diameter (RVDd), diastosistolic left and right ventricular volumes (LEDV-LESV; REDV-RESV), left ventricular function indexes (fractional shortening - Δ%D and ejection fraction - LEF) and right ventricular ejection fraction (REF). Results were statistically evaluated by chi-square (with Yates correction) and Student's t tests.

RESULTS - Data obtained at the ECG-D are graphically represented in fig. 1.

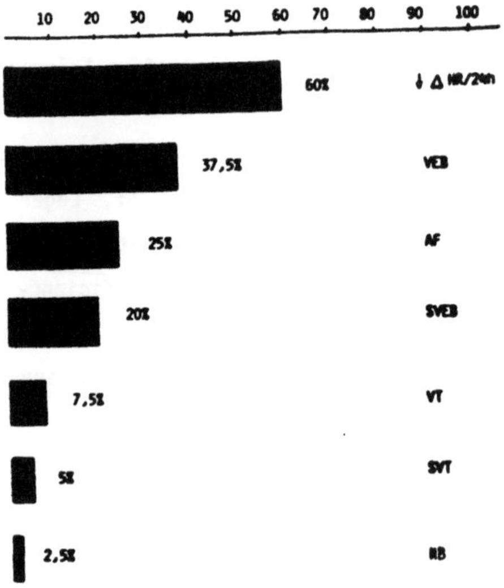

Fig. 1 - Arrytmias prevalence at the Holter monitoring. For the initials see the text.

The important reduction of circadian heart rate variation and the high prevalences of VEB, SVEB, AF, VT are evident.

ECHO revealed: LA, RVDd, REDV significantly increased (p 0.01); LVDd and LEDV limits of normality range of our laboratory. Left and right ventricular function indexes resulted altered in 4 subjects, according with a clinical diagnosis of CMPA and in normality range in the others (CMPA-); the difference in ventricular function parameters between the two groups (CMPA+/CMPA-) is statistically significant (fig. 2). AF was present in 8% of patients with normal FVS and in 75% of patients with CMPA; VT was present in 3% of CMPA- and in 50% of CMPA+. Statistical analysis (X^2)

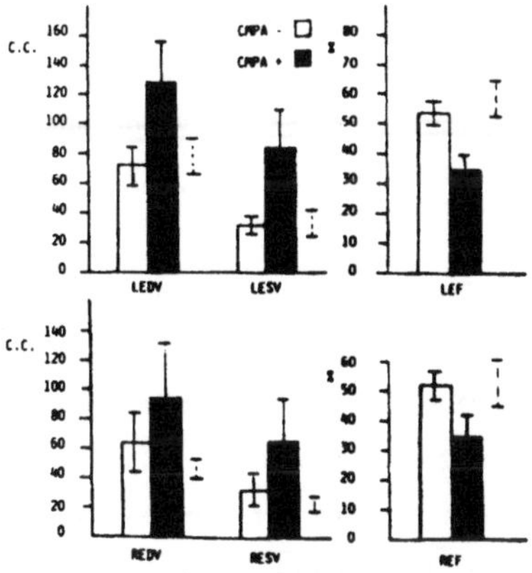

Fig. 2

Fig. 2 - 2D-ECHO values in subjects (mean ± S.D.) with (CMPA +) and without (CMPA -) alcoholic cardiomyopathy. In dotted lines reference normal values. C.C. = cubic centimeters.

LEFT VENTRICULAR FUNCTION

		A	B	
A.F.	+	3 (0.6)	3 (5.4)	6
	-	1 (3.4)	33 (30.6)	34
		4	36	40

CHI SQUARE 7.8867 p<0.01

LEFT VENTRICULAR FUNCTION

		A	B	
V.T.	+	2 (0.5)	1 (2.7)	3
	-	2 (3.7)	35 (33.3)	37
		4	36	40

CHI SQUARE 11.5716 p<0.001

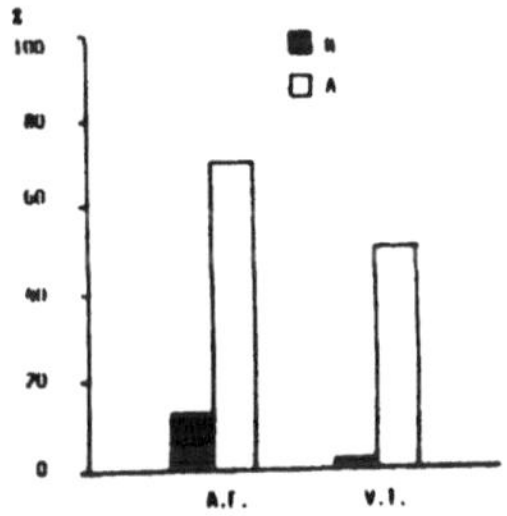

Fig. 3

Fig. 3 - Atrial fibrillation (A.F.) and ventricular tachicardia (V.T.) prevalence in subjects with normal (B) and altered (A) left ventricular function.

ARRYTMIAS:	ΔΣD
PRESENT (AR+)	32.5 ± 5.88
ABSENT (AR-)	40.4 ± 10.28
t = 2.398	0.05>p>0.02

Fig. 4 - ΔΣD value (mean ± S.D.) in subjects without cardiomyopathy that did (AR+) or did not (AR-) present arrytmias at the Holter monitoring.

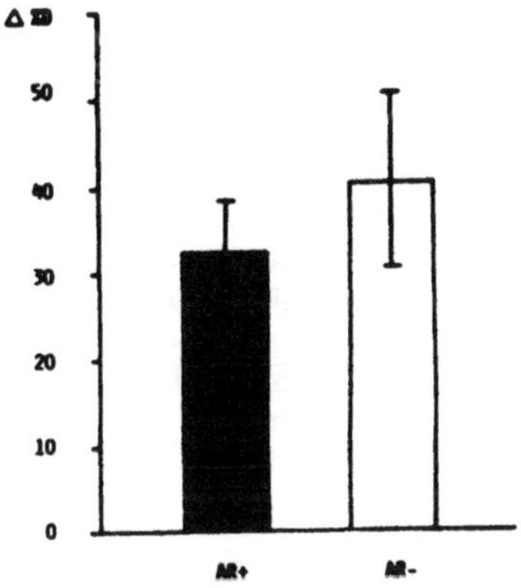

Fig. 4

showed a significant correlation respectively between AF (p 0.01) and VT (p 0.001) and impairment of left ventricular function (fig. 3). Finally dividing the patients without CMPA according to arrhythmias presence (AR+)or absence (AR-), two different levels of ventricular function are evidenced (fig. 4).

DISCUSSION AND CONCLUSIONS - The reduced circadian heart rate variation that we found could be due to an increase of hourly mean heart rate and to the presence of parasympatetic-type autonomic neuropathy ETOH induced (Khan et al.). A great number of studies, electrophysiologic too (Kelbaek et al.; Greenspon and Schaal) showed that acute ETOH introduction can provoke arrhythmias by possible direct action of ETOH as well as of its metabolis products (Regan; Chavez Rivera and Barros). In cronic alcoholic, on the other side, these mechanisms are probably associated to others immunologic, toxic, deficitary (Chavez Rivera and Barros; Khan et al.), wich are probably also underlied to CMPA. The atrial fibrillation could be correlated to hemodynamic features of this cardiomyopathy: left ventricular end diastolic pressure increased, atrial and ventricular cavities dilated. The ventricular tachicardia could be underlied to ETOH direct effect as well as to myocardial fiber damage. The high prevalence of arrhythmias in CMPA and the relation ship between arrhythmias and ventricular function levels in patients without CMPA suggest that myopathy could be underlied to CMPA - arrhythmias association. In this sense major arrhythmias could be considered an early marker of alcoholic cardiomyopathy.

REFERENCES

(1) Rubin, E.: N. England J. of Med., July 5, 28-35 (1979)
(2) Segel, L.D., S. Klausner, J. Gnadt, E. Amsterdam: med. Clin. of North Am., 68, 147-168 (1984)
(3) St. Leger, A.S., A.L. Cochrane, F. Moore: The Lancet, May 12, 1017-1020 (1979)
(4) Korararevic, Dj., D. McGee, N. Vojvodic, Z. Racic, T. Dawber, T. Gordon: The Lancet March 22, 169-172 (1980)
(5) Maisch, B., P. Deeg, G. Liebau, K. Kochsiek: Am. J. Cardiol., 52, 1072-1078 (1983)
(6) Mathews, E.C., J.M. Gardin, W.L. Henry, A.A. Del Negro, R.D. Fletcher, J.A. Snow, S.E. Epstein: Am. J. Cardiol., 47, 578-586 (1981)
(7) Regan T.J. and B. Haider: Circulation, 64 (suppl. III), 14-18 (1981)
(8) Regan T.J.: Progr. in Cardiovasc. Diseases, 28, 220-245 (1983)
(9) Chavez Rivera, I., C.L.F. Barros: Arch. Inst. Cardiol. Mex., 55, 269-287 (1983)
(10) Khan, S., D. Corelick, K. Nademanee, B.N. Singh: JACC, 9, 225A (1987)
(11) Kelbaek, H., T. Gjroup, O.J. Hertung, J. Marving, N.J. Christensen, J. Godtfredsen: Am. J. Cardiol., 59, 685-688 (1987)
(12) Greenspon, A.J., S.F. Schaal: Ann. of int. Med., 98, 135-139 (1983)

Serum potassium level in relation to malignant arrhythmias in acute myocardial infarction

BÉLA, KISS., QUI, CUONG., TIVADAR, JAKAB

Postgraduate Medical School, Budapest, Hungary

Summary

The results presented here confirm, that patients with acute myocardial infarction who are also hypokalemic have an increased risk of cardiac arrhythmias, in particular ventricular fibrillation. Primary prevention of hypokalemia and is prompt treatment are indicated in these patients

Introduction

Previous studies have indicated a close relationship between hypokalemia and development of ventricular fibrillation in acute myocardial infarction (1,2). The management of patients with acute myocardial infarction requires prevention and treatment of life threatening arrhythmias. The objective our present study was to clarify the relationship between varying levels of potassium values at hospital admission and malignant arrhythmias in patients with acute myocardial infarction.

Material and methods

Retrospective examination was performed of hospital records of 445 patients consecutively treated between 1980 and 1985 for acute myocardial infarction at the Postgraduate Medical School, Budapest. Acute myocardial infarction was documented by appropriate serum enzym elevations and serial electrocardiographic abnormalities. Plasma electrolytes were measured and patients who had potassium values of less than 3,5 mmol/l were classed as hypokalemic, those who had potassium values greater than 5,2 mmol/l were classed as hyperkalemic. Arrhythmias included in the study were as follows: atrial fibrillation (AF), ventricular fibrillation (VF), ventricular tachycardia (VT), ventricular premature beats (VPB). The association between potassium values and incidence of cardiac arrhythmias was tested using chi-square test (3).

Results

There were 285 males and 160 females included in the study. The age and sex distribution is shown in Table 1.

Table 1. Age and sex distribution of patients with AMI

AGE / SEX	< 30	30-49	50-59	60-69	> 70	TOTAL
males ♂	1	25	102	108	49	285 64%
females ♀	0	6	49	52	53	160 36%
TOTAL %	1 0,2%	31 7%	151 34%	160 36%	102 23%	445 100%

The distribution of patients having cardiac arrhythmias (AF, VT, VF) with respect to potassium values are shown in Figure 1. 35 % (19 pts) in the hypokalemic group had cardiac arrhythmias compared with 23 % (88 pts) in the normokalemic group. This difference was significant ($p < 0,05$). Increase in the prevalence of these serious arrhythmias was also significant in the hyperkalemic group ($p < 0,05$).

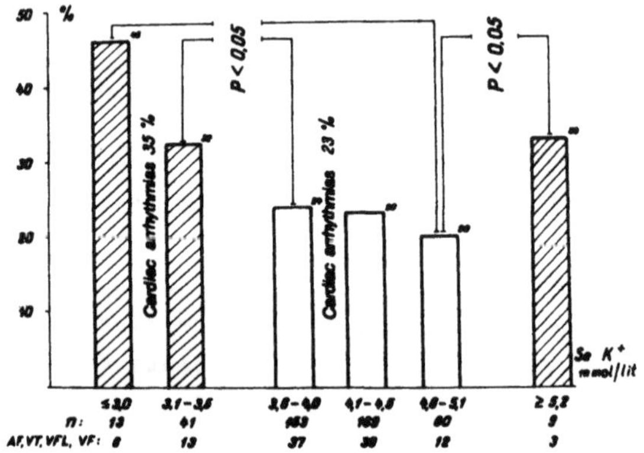

Figure 1. Incidence of AF, VT, VFL, or VF in relation to initial serum potassium levels

Regarding the incidence of premature ventricular beats 43 % (23 pts) in the hypokalemic group had premature ventricular beats compared with

35 % (133 pts) in the normokalemic group. This difference was not significant ($p > 0,05$., Fig.2).

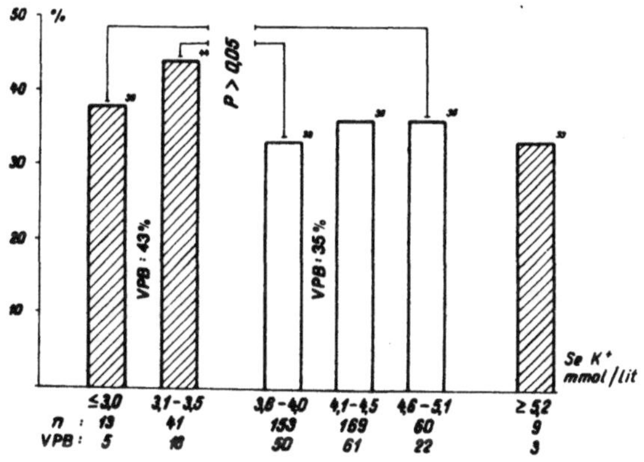

Figure 2. Incidence of PVB in relation to initial serum potassium levels

30 % (16 pts) in the hypokalemic group had ventricular tachycardia or fibrillation compared with 17 % (66 pts) in the normokalemic group. This difference was highly significant ($p < 0,01$., Fig.3).

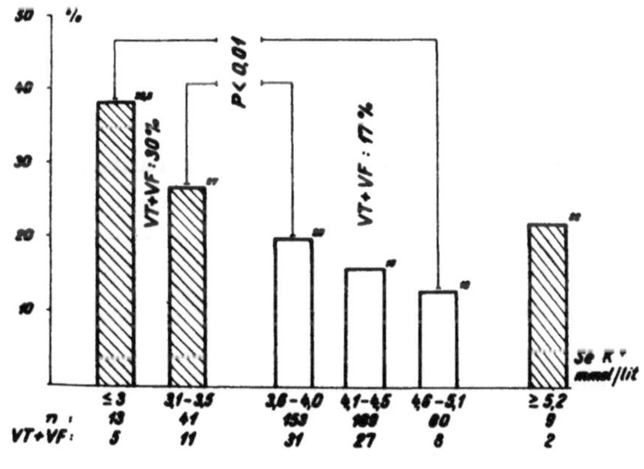

Figure 3. Incidence of VT or VF in relation to initial serum potassium levels

The incidence of ventricular fibrillation (VF) only is illustrated in Fig.4. 17 % (9 pts) in hypokalemic group had VF compared with 7 % (26 pts) in the normokalemic group. This difference was highly significant ($p < 0{,}01$., Fig.4).

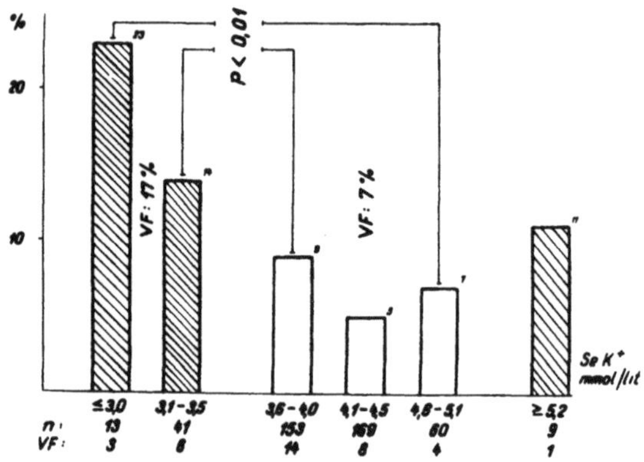

Figure 4. Incidence of VF in relation to initial serum potassium levels

Discussion

Since ischemia may produce cardiac arrhythmias we chose to study the possible role of hypokalemia in patients suffering from acute myocardial infarction (4,5,6). The incidence of life threatening ventricular arrhythmias increased with decreasing serum potassium values. It has been documented that patients with acute myocardial infarction who are also hypokalemic have an increased risk of cardiac arrhythmias, in particular ventricular fibrillation. The management of patients with acute myocardial infarction requires prevention and treatment of life threatening arrhythmias

References

(1) Stock,E., A. Goble, and G.Sloman: Brit.Med. J. 2, 719-723 (1967)
(2) Duke,M : JAMA. 43, 239-244 (1978)
(3) Juvancz, I., A.Paksy: Orvosi Biometria.Budapest. p: 69-77 (1982)
(4) Pick,A: Amer. Heart J. 72, 295-300 (1966)
(5) Fisch,C: Circulation. 47, 408-413 (1973)
(6) Gettes, L.S: Pharm. Ther. 2, 787-792 (1976)

Prognosis in ventricular tachyarrhythmia patients with coronary artery disease

RATHGEN K., K.J. ROSTOCK, D. PFEIFFER, A.SCHIRDEWAN

Central institute of cardiovascular research, Academy of Science, Wiltbergstr. 50, Berlin 1115, GDR

Summary

Ventricular tachyarrhythmias (VT) are known to be an independent prognostic factor in patients with coronary artery disease (CAD). In order to assess an effective antiarrhythmic regimen 100 consecutive patients with VT due to CAD were examined by electrophysiologic study and Holter monitoring (HM). Out of 84 patients with artificially inducible VT an effective antiarrhythmic drug therapy could be found for 61 patients, using programmed ventricular stimulation. 16 patients without inducible VT as well as 23 patients under amiodarone were controlled by HM only. All patients were provided with further dispensary care over a mean follow-up period of 40 ± 22 months (range 8 to 94 months). During this time 11 patients suffered from non-fatal VT recurrences. Two out of these underwent aneurysmectomy, another one got an automatic defibrillator. Eight out of 12 death cases occured suddenly, compaired to 2.4 % per year.

Conclusion: Intensive diagnostics and control of VT as well as dispensary care contribute to a better clinical outcome of patients with CAD.

Introduction

VT are known to be an independent prognostic factor in patients (pts.) with CAD. Programmed electrical stimulation of the heart (PES) and Holter monitoring (HM) are the widely accepted methods for investigating VT with regard to the arrhythmia substrate and trigger mechanisms. The development of antiarrhythmic management directed by PES and HM provided a decrease of sudden death rate from 40 % to 5 % per year (1 - 5).

The purpose of this study is to assess the long-term efficacy of antiarrhythmic drug therapy guided by PES and HM.

Patients and methods

The study population was selected from 178 pts., admitted to us from january 1978 to december 1986 for management of VT. One hundred of these pts. had CAD (76 male, 24 female; mean age 58 ± 10 years), with a history of myocardial infarction in 57 cases. They suffered from documented (n = 64) and suspected (n = 14) VT or syncope of unknown origin (n = 22).

All pts. underwent His bundle electrography with PES at least 5 half-lifes after discontinuation of all antiarrhythmic medication. The stimulation protocol included single and double ventricular premature

stimuli during sinus rhythm and ventricular pacing at two cycle lenghts of 600 to 400 ms and short bursts of rapid ventricular pacing (cycle lengths 400 to 250 ms). The endpoint was the induction of a sustained VT (lasting 30 sec. or longer or requiring cardioversion/ defibrillation) or nonsustained VT (lasting 6 beats to 30 sec.).
Antiarrhythmic drug testing was performed after intravenous and/or oral administration by repeating the stimulation protocol. Efficacy was defined as noninducibility of VT or in case of sustained VT when showing less than 5 beats.
Inpatient electrocardiographic monitoring was carried out over the time of hospitalization. Ambulatory HM for 24 hours was performed weekly up to every three months' in pts. without documented or induced VT and in all pts. under medication. Drug efficacy was defined as total suppression of arrhythmia and as partial suppression in case of less than three consecutive ventricular beats and decrease of ventricular premature beats by at least 50 %.
After discharge all pts. were followed up by our arrhythmia dispensary care.

Results

Out of the 100 pts., 84 had artificially inducible VT. These VT terminated spontaneously in 44 cases and by means of PES in 28 cases. In 12 pts. VT termination required DC-cardioversion or defibrillation because of hemodynamic intolerance. Out of these 84 pts. an effective antiarrhythmic drug therapy could be found for 61 pts., using PES. The remaining pts. were given amiodarone without further PES control. Sixteen pts. without inducible VT as well as 23 pts. under amiodarone were controlled by HM only.
The mean follow-up period was 40 ± 22 months (range 8 to 94 months). During this time 11 pts. suffered from non-fatal VT recurrences. Eight out of these were given another antiarrhythmic drug or combination of drugs with further PES and/or HM control. Two pts. underwent aneurysmectomy, another one got an automatic defibrillator. Twelve pts. died; 8 of these suffered from witnessed sudden cardiac death, which amounts to 2.4 % per year.

Discussion

The results of antiarrhythmic drug therapy in pts. with life-threatening VT, guided by PES and HM, prove its efficacy with regard to the decrease of the sudden death rate (2 - 4).
PES for controlling the efficacy of an antiarrhythmic drug regimen can only be applied in those pts., in whom VT is inducible . The effect of an invasive tested agent can serve as predictor for future efficacy of this drug. This approach is based on repeated stimulation tests using drugs until a single drug or a combination is found that prevent induction of VT (2 - 4). In this way an effective antiarrhythmic drug

regimen could be found for 61 pts.

In pts. without inducible VT HM is today the only available method for controlling antiarrhythmic drug efficacy. Under amiodarone we prefer HM. Taking into consideration the limitations of both methods, the combination of PES and HM seems to be highly precise for predicting antiarrhythmic drug effects.

Prognostic significance of preventing VT by an antiarrhythmic drug regimen can only be answered by long-term results: During a mean follow up period of 40 ± 22 months arrhythmic events occured as non-fatal VT in 11 % and as sudden cardiac death in 8 %, compaired to 2.4 % per year.

As against the so called empirical antiarrhythmic drug therapy of VT with a sudden death rate of up to 40 % per year the results of a controlled regimen by means of the applied methods (2 - 5) give sufficient evidence for their predictive accuracy. Therefore the risk of sudden death due to VT recurrences can be significantly reduced to less than 5 % per year.

Pts., for whom no effective medical treatment can be found, call for alternative methods like electrical ablation, surgery or antitachycardic stimulation or defibrillation with implantible devices.

On the basis of the available results by means of intensive diagnostics and controlled therapy of VT as well as dispensary care, we conclude that prognosis of pts. prone to sudden death can be improved.

References

1. Horowitz, L.N., J.Morgenroth: Am.J.Cardiol. 50, 535 - 538 (1982)
2. Horowitz, L.N., M.E.Josephson, A.Farshidi, S.R.Spielman, E.L. Michelson, A.M.Greenspan: Circulation 58, 986 - 997 (1978)
3. Mason J.W., R.A.Winkle: N.Engl.J.Med. 303, 1073 - 1077 (1980)
4. Rae, A.P., A.M.Greenspan, S.R.Spielman, N.M.Sokoloff, C.R.Webb, H.R.Kay, L.N.Horowitz: Am.J.Cardiol. 55, 1494 - 1499 (1985)
5. Vlay, S.C., C.H.Kallman, P.R.Reid: Am.J.Cardiol. 54, 87 - 90 (1984)

The control of heart rhythm in a tilt table test

KREISSIG, P., A. SKALWEIT and E. SCHUBERT

Institute of Physiology, Humboldt University, Hessische Str. 3-4, Berlin, 1040

Summary

The aim of the present study was to attain detailed information about the adaptation of the heart to orthostatic load. The investigations were performed on 34 healthy male volunteers (age 21-26 years). All subjects underwent noninvasive recordings of ECG, ICG and arterial blood pressure (BP). The chronotropic state of the heart was examined by combined analysis of heart period duration (HPD) and its variability (Δ HPD). Furthermore we analysed relative changes in stroke volume (SVF), cardiac output (COF) and total peripheral resistance (TPRF). Tilting from supine to upright position led to a decrease of HPD (-28%), Δ HPD (-58%), SVF (-33%) and COF (-23%), but to an increase of diastolic BP (+13%) and TPRF (+32%). Systolic BP remained unchanged. In the following supine period all parameters reached their initial values. The results indicate, that both parts of the vegetative nervous system participate in heart control during orthostasis. Indeed, the changes of activity of the pàrasympathicus are much larger.

Introduction

Several investigations have shown that the combined analysis of the heart rate and its spontaneous variability (sinusarrhythmia) permits an assessment of the vegetative tone of the heart (1,2).

The aim of the present study was:

- to examine the adaptation of the heart and the circulatory system to orthostasis by simultaneous analysis of various noninvasively measured parameters describing cardiovascular function;
- to attain detailed information about the changes occuring within the vegetative nervous system by using the correlation between heart period duration and sinusarrhythmia;
- to delimit psychic influences before the first test and to search for possible effects of learning after repetition of the orthostatic load test.

Material and methods

The studies were performed on 34 healthy male volunteers, aged 21 - 26 years (mean age 23,2 ± 0,23 years). All subjects underwent noninvasive recordings of ECG, impedance cardiogram (ICG) and arterial blood pressure (BP). The signal of the R- peak derived from the ECG was the basis for a continuous digital measurement of the heart period duration (HPD). From these recordings mean HPDs and corresponding spontaneous variations (Δ HPD, mean differences of consecutive HPDs) were calculated. Using the recordings of the first derivation of the ICG (dz/dt) the stroke volume factor (SVF) was calculated as the product of the maximum magnitude of the dz/dt signal, measured from the lowest to the highest value, and the corresponding time. The cardiac output factor (COF) was derived from SVF and HPD as the quotient of both parameters. Blood pressure measurement was performed a) continuously at the A. temp. using the compensation method and b) once per minute at the A. brach. using the sphygmomanometric method. The mean arterial blood pressure (MAP) was calculated as the arithmetical mean of the systolic and diastolic BP.

The quotient of MAP and COF was determined and used as a factor to characterize the total peripheral resistance (TPRF).

The orthostatic load was carried out with the help of a tilt table. After a rest period of 5 min the subjects were tilted 80 degrees upward for 3 min and then brought back to the lying position for 3 min. This orthostatic load test was performed successively for three times. All results were tested with the Wilcoxon test for paired differences and with the Wilcoxon test for independent groups. A value of $2p \leq 0,05$ was considered to be significant.

Results

The change from supine to upright position caused a decrease of HPD (-22%), Δ HPD (-58%), SVF (-30%) and COF (-23%). All of these parameters reached a minimum after 10 - 15 seconds.

The BP showed a short term decrease with its minimum after 3 seconds. After that systolic BP reached its initial value, while diastolic BP was increased (+13%), in comparison with the supine position.

Furthermore an increase of TPRF (+32%) was found.

During supine position all parameters reached their initial values.

Discussion

The observed decreases in SVF, COF and BP during orthostasis are due to the displacing of blood from the intrathoracic region to more dependent vascular structures and the resulting altered filling conditions of the heart. The lowered mean arterial blood pressure caused a reflecting increase of heart rate (decrease of HPD), diastolic BP and TPRF and a reduced sinusarrhythmia (Δ HPD).
These results confirm well those of other investigators respecting stroke volume, cardiac output, heart rate, arterial blood pressure and total peripheral resistance (3,4).

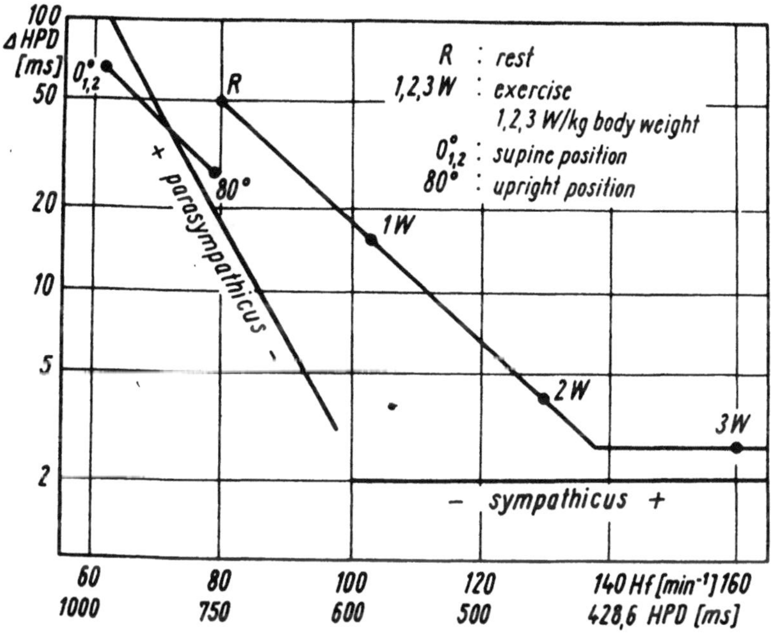

Fig. 1. Rhythm diagram - as a correlogram of HPD and Δ HPD (after (5))

The correlogram of HPD and Δ HPD (fig. 1) indicates that both parts of the vegetative nervous system are involved in the adaptation to orthostasis. The first and main part of the reaction is mediated by the withdrawal of the vagal tone and secondary by the activation of the sympathicus (HPD -28%, Δ HPD -58%). After the 5th second the

reactions are caused mainly by increasing of the sympathetic tone. The changes in HPD and Δ HPD during orthostasis are similar to those during mild bicycle exercise (2).
Our results are supported by findings that atropine influences the first part and propranolol the second part of the adjustment to orthostasis (6,7).
Each orthostatic load test brought about the same degree of reaction. Therefore prestart and learning effects can be excluded.

References

(1) Sayers, B. Mc. A.: Ergonomics 16, 17 - 32 (1973)
(2) Eckoldt, K., K. H. Bodmann, H. Cammann, B. Graichen, K. Hoppe, B. Pfeifer, V. Schwarz, and A. Wilke: Z. Physiother. 31, 277 - 283 (1979)
(3) Marees, H. de: in: Das Orthostasesyndrom. H. J. Dengler (Ed.) pp 25 - 38. Schattauer, Stuttgart - New York 1973
(4) Gauer, O. H. and H. L. Thron: in: Handbook of Physiology. Circulation, part 3. W. F. Hamilton and P. Dow (Eds.) pp 2409 - 2439. Williams and Wilkins, Baltimore 1965
(5) Schubert, E.: Dt. Gesundh.-Wesen 39, 845 - 856 (1984)
(6) Ewing, D. J., L. Hume, J. W. Campbell, A. Murray, J. M. M. Neilson, and B. F. Clarke: J. Appl. Physiol. - Respir. Environ. 49, 809 - 814 (1980)
(7) Neto, J. A. M., L. Gallo, J. C. Manco, A. Rassi, and D. S. Amorim: Cardiovasc. Res. 14, 541 - 550 (1980)

The Electrophysiologic Criteria for the Selection of Antiarrhythmic Therapy

V.N. ORLOV, A.V. SHPECTOR, V.S. SHERASHOV, V.I. MAMAEV,
G.V. KESAREV, V.A. GORSHKOW
Moscow Medicine Stomatology Institute, Moscow, USSR

We have tried to work out the electrocardiographic criteria, received through different methods of examinig the patients to select differential antiarrhythmic therapy. More than 200 patients with frequent ventricular and/or supraventricular arrhythmias were examined under the control of transesophageal electrophysiological study, the 24-hours ECG monitoring and exersice stress test. The comparative effectiveness of placebo, novocainamide, ethmozin, mexitile, dyzopyramide, neogilurytmal, bonnecor and ethacyzine - the drugs of the group of Na^{+}- channels blockers has been studied.

Among 170 patients with a coronary artery disease, which course of the illness was not complicated with different abnormalities of excitation and conductivity on the base of ECG, there were revealed, using transesophageal electrophysiological study: the disfunction of the sinus node - in 18 % of cases; the conceal atrio-ventricular blocks without prolongation of PQ interval - in 12 % and in 13 % - echo-zones of atrio-fibrillation and echo-zones of supraventricular tachycardia. According to our data, the administration of antiarrhythmic drugs in this cases should be done with care.

The use of the method of transesophageal electrophysiological examination in an acute drug test, permitted to reveal different types of conceal abnormalities in the conduction system of the heart among 37 % of patients with coronary artery disease. On the one hand, and on the other to determine diverse effects of antiarrhythmic drugs of the I class on the function of the sinus node, sino-atrial and atrio-ventricular conductivity.

In patients with a normal function of the sinus node the use of neogilurytmal and mexitile practically does not influence it. Ethacyzine and bonnecor, by all means, increase sinus node recovery time for sure.

Palpitine has a tendency to increase the automatism of the sinus node and to shorten the sino-atrial conductivity.

In cases of determined disfunction of the sinus node, neogilurytmal trustworthily increases the automatism of the sinus node; ethacyzine and bonnecor worsen it; and mexitile practically does not change it.

In patients with normal atrio-ventricular conductivity, neogilurytmal, bonnecor and ethacyzine trustworthily lower the point of Venkebach by 10 %, but that does not lead to the developement of the atrio-ventricular block. In patients with conceal atrio-ventricular block, the use of neogilurytmal and bonnecor did not significantly impair the conductivity; mexitile did not change it. That's why these drugs are not contraindicated in these patients. At the same time ethacyzine trustworthily impaired the atrioventricular conductivity in patients with hidden atrio-ventricular blockades and that's why it should be used in these cases under the control of electrophysiological study of the heart. We consider the disappearence of echo-zones of atrio fibrillation and echo zones of supraventricular tachycardia as a criterion of effectiveness of antiarrhythmic therapy in the treatement and prophilaxis of supraventricular paroxysmal arrhythmia, and therefore, impossibility in provoking arrhythmias using the stimulation of the left atrium, that was confirmed by the absence of the arrhythmia in patients during prolonged abservation.

We succeeded in achieving the disappearance of echo-zones of atrio fibrillation and supraventricular arrhythmias with aid of antiarrhythmic therapy in 70 % of the patients. Ethacyzine was the most effective drug. The results achieved with a dozed stress-test during an acute drug test confirmed the received results concerning high efficiency of ethacyzine. We have also studied the comparative effectiveness of the drugs mentioned above in patients with ventricular arrhythmias using 24-hour monitoring of ECG. The most effective ones were: ethacyzine and neogilurytmal. In case of their ineffectiveness ethmozin, dysopiramid, mexitil in the used doses never removed arrhythmia.

Besides it turned out, that all these drugs referring to Nachannels blockers help mainly one and the same group of patients.

Therefore, the patients with ventricular arrhythmias were divided into 2 groups: sensitive to the blockade of Na-channels and non-sensitive to it. There was no significant difference between these 2 groups as to their sex, age, the type of the main illness; with or without features of heart failure and basement therapy.

There was also no differense as to the initial rate of premature heart beats, the presence or abscense of paroxysms of ventricular tachycardia the initial length of the QT-interval. But one fact attracted our attention: the patients nonsensitive to neogilurytmal demonstrated significant variations of the coupling interval, though the configuration of the ectopic beats didn't change.

Among the patients nonsensitive to neogilurytmal, this electrocardiographic picture was seen in 2/3 of the patients; what exeed the number of the same cases among patients sensitive to this drug.

The same tendency was revealed during examination of the other drugs.

Therefore, the data recieved, allon to suppose, that blockators of Na^+-channels are more effective in patients with arrythmias with stable coupling interval. A question occurs: with what it is connected? As known three main mechanisms form the base of arrhythmia: re-entry, triggers activity and abnormalities of automatism.

In the first two mechanisms we have a causal connection between the sinus impulse and the ectopic beat, and the distance between them will be stable; that is the coupling interval will be stable. Another thing if the arrhythmogenic centre posesses its own automatie activity. It produces ectopic complexes with no causal connection with sinus impulse, and the coupling interval may significantly vary. The variations of the coupling interval will not be accompanied with changing of the form of the ectopic complexes, because only one centre produces them all. Based on the data recieved, we can suppose, that the blockers of Na-channels remove better the abnormalities of arrhythmias connected with re-entry mechanism and/or trigger activity, than arrhythmias produced by the automatic activity of the ectopic centre.

That's why we can formulate the following conclusions:

1. The selection of antiarrhythmic drug effective in the treatement and profilaxis of paroxisms of supraventricular arrhythmias must be done under the dynamic controle of the echo-zones of the arrhythmias.

2. Ethacyzine - was the most effective drug in the group of patients with supraventricular arrhythmia.

3. Electrophysiological controle for the condition of the conductive system of the heart is of great importance in the treatement of ventricular and supraventricular arrhythmias by ethacyzine to prevent possible complications.

4. The patients with ventricular premature beats with constant coupling interval must be treated with blockers of Na-channels which are of very high efficiency mainly in this group of patients. The most effective drugs were ethacyzine and neogilurytmal. When they areineffective the appliement of novocainamide, ethmozin, dysopyramide and mexitile is of no importance. The application of these drugs in patients nonsensitive to ethacyzine or neogilurytmal does not remove arrhythmias.

5. In patients with registrated on the ECG variations of coupling intervals more than 0,09 s, with monomophic ectopic beats, the blockers of Na-channels are less effective. It is possible, that in such cases the drugs with another mechanism of action will be the drugs of choice. For example cordarone or isoptin. But this question must be specially studied.

Cardiac rhythm and haemodynamics disturbances in patients with sick sinus syndrome and VVI pacemakers implanted

PEKARSKI V.V., GIMRIKH E.O., AKHMEDOV Sh.D., POPOV S.V., CHEKHOV A.M.
Siberian Cardiologic Centre, Tomsk, USSR

Summary

Incidence and charakter of cardiac rhythm and haemodynamics disturbances were analysed in 51 patients (pts) with sick sinus syndrome (SSS) which was reliably established according to the accepted criteria. All pts were repeatedly investigated by electrocardiographic, echocardiographic and roentgencardiometric methods. Our prospective analysis (3o months) of the clinical state of pts. shows that the VVI pacemaker implantation in pts. with SSS and the AV conduction presence is not reasonable because of frequent initiation of cardiac rhythm disturbances and risk of cardiac insufficiency development.

Introduction

About a half of pacemakers in the world are implanted for SSS. The International Symposium held in Monako (1986) recommended international cooperative investigation (Sutton P., Kenny P., 1986) to solve the problem of the most reasonable type of a pacemaker for the implantation. The aim of the study was to analyse cardiac rhythm and haemodynamics disturbances in pts with SSS and pacemakers implanted and without the pacemaker implantation in the prospective follow-up.

Material and methods

All pts (aged between 25 and 72 years) underwent the electrophysiologic study with the assessment of the sinus node recovery time (SNRT) before and after "drug denervation of the heart" (DDH) (Jose A., 1966). SSS was divided into "true" (TSSS) and "external" (ESSS) which were differentiated according to the SNRT value after DDH (Gomes J., 1985). The patients investigation included clinical examination, repeated surface and esophageal ECG recordings, roentgenocardiometry, Holter monitoring echocardiography (EchoCG).

Thirty six pts. of the I group with pacemakers implanted (29 pts. with VVI pacemakers, 7 pts with AAI ones) and 15 pts of the 2 group without the pacemaker omplantation were repeatedly investigated in a mean of 34 ± 3,6 and 39 ± 5,2 montha respectively.

Results and discussion

We revealed before the pacemaker implantation bradysystolic form of SSS in 32 pts (I type) and brady-tachy form in 4 pts (II type).All II type pts had paroxysmal atrial fibrillation (AF) with the attacks incidence of a mean 2 times in a month. In the long-term period 19 of 29 pts with VVI pacemakers implanted comllained of heart rhythm disturbances and/or intermittent dizziness. In 13 of these pts AF was documented which was permanent in 8 and paroxysmal in 5 pts. Among the pts with paroxysmal AF it arised for the first time in 4 pts with the I type

SSS and became markedly faster in 1 pt with the II type SSS. In 5 pts with the I type SSS permanent form of AF was noted for the first time and in 3 pts with the II type SSS paroxysmal AF bacame permanent. In 10 of 13 pts with AF the retrograde ventricolo-atrial (VA) conduction with the subsequent antegrade ventricular responce (VR) was documented in responce to ventricular stimulation (Fig.1). AF was induced by the

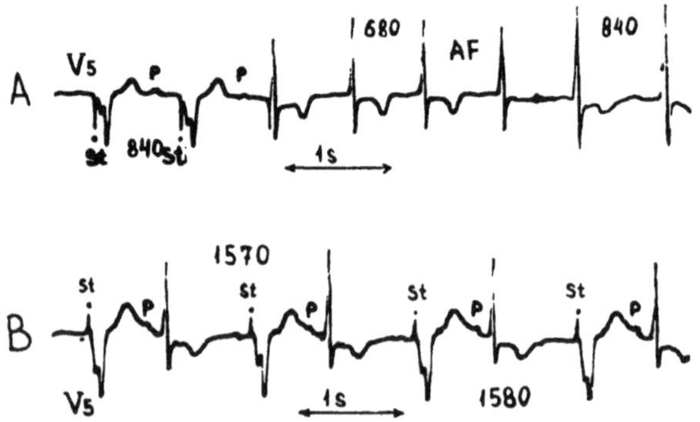

Fig. 1 A - VA conduction induces atrial fibrillation on the setting of VVI pacing; B - VA conduction with subsequent antegrade VR. St- electrical stimulus artefact.

retrograde VA conduction as assessed by Holter monitoring in 3 of 5 pts with paroxysmal AF. (Fig.1). The permanent AF developed without VA conduction in 2 pts with the II type SSS and 1 pt with the I type SSS. WE observed in another 6 pts with VVI pacemakers in the long-term period only retrograde VA conduction with haemodynamically decreased or ineffective VR. Fig. 2 is a case where our pt developed syncope 18 months after the surgery. VVI pacemaker function in this pt was normal. EchoCG recordings with the simultaneous recording of the sphygmogram and esophageal electrogram vevealed that VA conduction led to the haemodynamically ineffective VR. Thus we observed in 65% of our pts with VVI pacemakers implanted cardiac rhythm disturbances such as paroxysmal or permanent AF or retrograde VA conduction with the periodic or permanent VR. Retrograde VA conduction in the early postoperative period was recorded in 22 out of 29 pts with VVI pacemakers implanted. In the follow-up period VA conduction sustained in 11 of these 22 pts, disappeared in 3 and it was difficult to assess it in the remainder because of the permanent form of AF. Cardiac rhythm disturbances were not noted in all pts with AAI pacemakers implanted. Cardiac failure became more pronounced in the follow-up period in 12 pts with VVI pacemakers implanted. 10 of these 12 pts had VVI conduction. Eight pts developed the pacemaker syndrome. Criteria for the pacemaker syndrome assessment were cardiac failure aggravation and increasing of

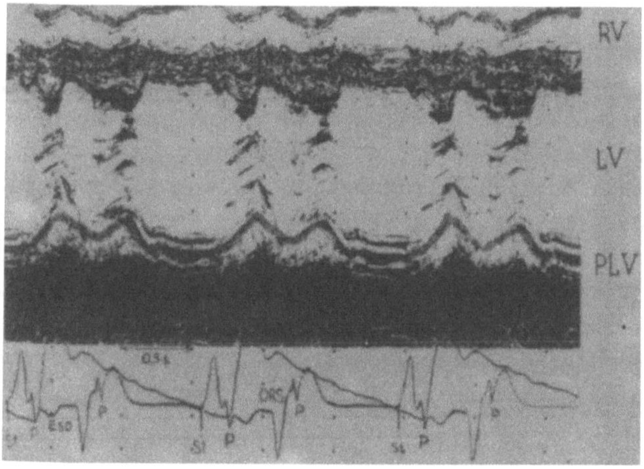

Fig.2 VA conduction leads to the haemodynamically ineffective VR. RV - right ventricle, LV - left ventricle, PLV - posterior wall of the left ventricle, Eso - esophageal electrogram

the heart size es assessed by the roentgencardiometry. Shortness of breath at exercise developed in 1 of 7 pts with AAI pacemakers, the remainder hsd no evidence of the circulation aggravation. These data suggest that the retrograde VA conduction might contribute to the cardiac failure appearance or aggravation in pts with VVI pacemakers implanted. SNRT increased in the follow-up period before DDH by a mean of 570 ms in 4 pts of the I group, did not change in 3 pts with ESSS, decreased by a mean of 2335 ms in 11 pts (31%) and in 10 pts the cessation of rapid atrial pacing led to the AV junctional rhythm development.The AV junctional rhythm development was considered as a sinus node function aggravation. Moreover 8 of 36 pts in which the cessation of rapid atrial pacing led to the AV junctional rhythm development had subsequently permanent AF. The "Wenckebach point" did not change in 4 pts and increased by a mean of10±0,9/min in the remainder. SNRT increased by a mean of 1957 ms after the DDH in 3 pts, did not change in another 3 pts with ESSS and the AV junctional rhythm appeared in the remainder (n=22). In 6 pts of the second group with TSSS and in 3 pts with ESSS SNRT increased before DDH by 567 29 ms ($p<0.05$), AV junctional rhythm was noted in 3 pts with the II type SSS in the follow-up period. The "Wenckebach point" bacame below 1203min in 1 pt, did not change in 2 pts and increased by a mean of 22 imp/min in 9 pts. SNRT increased after the DDH in 2 pts with TSSS by 3055 121 ms ($p<0.001$), did not c change in 5 pts with ESSS and 1 pt with TSSS, AV junctional rhythm was noted in 4 pts. Among 7 pts of the IIgroup with previous syncopes those sustained with the same frequency in 4 pts and stopped in 3 pts after they developed permanent AF. In 2 pts without previous syncopes those appeared in the follow-up perid.

Several investigators (Toeda T., 1986; Ryden L., 1986) recognize the role of role of atrial contraction in the cardiac output. The conclusion ofseveral investigators that in the majority of pts with SSS AV conduction is depressed as well, which may lead to the high grade AV block was the restraining factor for the wider use of AAI pacemakers (Breivik K., Ohm O., 1979; Rosen K., Loeb H., 1971). Kleinert M et al. (1983) howeever reported that h the high grade AV block was observed only in 0,6% of pts. Witte J. (1983) found AV block in 3,2% of pts. VVI pacemakers implantation in pts with TSSS as it is showm in the given work and in the reports of several investigators (Nishimura R., Gersh B., 1982; Rosenquist M., Brandt J., 1986) leads often to cardiac rhythm disturbances and/or cardiac failute aggravation because of the retrograde VA conduction presence. Thus the individual approach to such patients is needed.

References

(1) Sutton, P., and P. Kenny: PACE 9, 1110-1114 (1986)
(2) Jose, A.: Amer. J. Cardiol. 18, 476-478 (1966)
(3) Gomes, J.: Mt. Sinai J. Med. 52, 610-617 (1985)
(4) Toeda, T.: Jpn. Circ. J. 50, 385-395 (1986)
(5) Ryden, L.: PACE 9, 1131-1135 (1986)
(6) Breivik, K., O. Ohm and L. Segadal: Acta Med. Scand. 206, 153-159 (1979)
(7) Rosen, K. and H. Loeb: Circulation 43, 834-838 (1971)
(8) Kleinert, M. and H. Beckerdorf: J. Am. Coll. Cardiol. 1, 720-724 (1983)
(9) Witte, J.: PACE 6, A-* (1983)
(10) Nishimura, R. and B. Gersh: PACE 5, 903-910 (1982)
(11) Rosenquist, M., J. Brandt and H. Schuller: Amer. Heart J. 111, 292-297 (1986)

Analysis of Longtime ECG by Means of Microcomputer Including Recognition of P-waves and ST-T-segment

POLL, R., E. MEISEL, and R. HENSSGE

Medical Academy Dresden, GDR
DDR-8019 Dresden, Fetscherstraße 74

Microcomputer-aided recognition of P-waves, T-waves and of the ST-segment requires increased efficiency of automated ECG processing. A solution was found by taking into consideration the physiological-pathophysiological causality of the ECG course. Thus an efficiency is reached surpassing naked technical solutions. For ECG pattern recognition a method based on Walsh-transformation of signal segments is used. It provides recognition rates of 98.8 p.c. for R-waves and of 78.0 p.c. for a common P/T-finding. A device was installed consisting of a bedside tape-recorder and a personal computer for recording and computer-aided evaluation of three-hours-ECG in the department of cardiological functional diagnosis. The used software was completed by a second step of data processing separating P-waves and T-waves.

Recently recognition of P-waves, T-waves and of the ST-segment is demanded by physicians also in these cases only R-wave recognition is realized up to now. This fact requires increased efficiency of automated ECG processing provided by simple digital components (1).
Besides monitoring and Holter technique further tasks remain which require special solutions of microcomputer-aided ECG processing in cardiological therapy, diagnosis and research. For instance our intention was to carry out the analysis of heart rhythm more efficiently and precisely in the department of cardiological functional diagnosis by recording long strings of the ECG in rest, during exercise and during provocation tests followed by micro-aided ECG evaluation.
For this purpose a device was installed consisting of a bedside tape-recorder and a personal computer for evaluation. The mobile recording unit provides continuous tape records up to three hours using pulse-code-modulation. It may be used in the examination room or at the ward. Selectively the recorded signals are given out to a memory scope, to a customary personal computer or as an analogous signal for instance to a plotter.
Having the possibility of recording long strings, tape records of one to three hours may be obtained during a complete examination.

The computer provides feature extraction, selection of signal intervals (to be probed by the physician), time-measuring, measuring of amplitudes, counting and classification of patterns. The physician checks up the computer's findings and makes the final ECG evaluation using screen and rewritings on paper.
Such an application of the microcomputer does only pay if reliable and precise recognition of R-waves, P-waves, T-waves and ST-segments is guaranteed, also in cases of disturbances of rhythm or conduction. This can only be reached by taking into consideration the physiological-pathophysiological causality of the ECG course. The already published method of pattern recognition using Walsh-transformation of signal sections solves these tasks. It is the foundation of the procedure shown here (2,3).
The prerequisite to using this method was to remove its drawback that P-waves and T-waves were not differentiated but recognized by a common pattern (4). Here the solution is presented how to separate P- and T-waves by a second step of data processing.

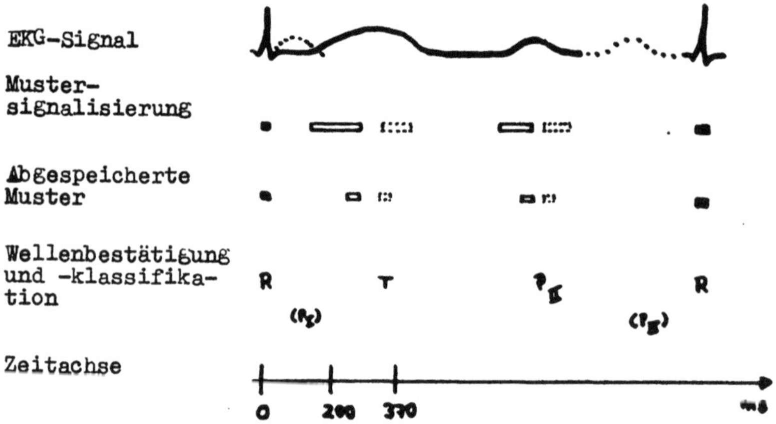

Figure 1: Principle of the separating procedure

As shown in figure 1 several waves may occur between two R-waves not fixed in time or sequence. These P-waves, T-waves, U-waves or artefacts are recognized by the first step as a common incident, called P/T-wave in this paper. By electrophysiological reason the T-wave is connected with the QRS-complex. Its connexion depends on the heart rate and shows a great variation in time.
Using the here shown method we found as a matter of experience that the recognition of nearly all T-waves was terminated in fewer than 370 ms after the preceding R-peak (5). P/T-waves occuring after this mark cannot be considered as T-waves (time-oriented recognition). If a T-wave

was recognized earlier, this mark loses its significance (incident-oriented recognition). The terminated recognition of a P/T-wave in fewer than 200 ms after the preceding R-peak has to be classified always as a P-wave. This incident is only possible, if an atrio-ventricular conduction disturbance of high degree is present. Thus these P-waves allow directly diagnostic conclusions and should be signalized as special findings. Notice, that the beginning of a T-wave may be located before this 200 ms mark.
The ECG incident searched for by the physician - i.e. P-wave, T-wave, ST-segment - is recognized by using a pattern for the beginning and a pattern for the end of the wave. Contrary to the usual ECG evaluation these patterns for computer recognition are defined in such manner that they mark parts near the top of the wave. In this way the time intervals for expecting and recognizing a single ECG wave is drastically shortened. Thus the microcomputer is enabled to classify unambiguously at least one pattern (ascending flank or descending flank) as a part of the T-wave or not. For this end two marks suffice, fixed to the R-peak independently of the heart rate (applied to heart rates between 20 and 200 beats per minute). Now T-waves and U-waves may be signalized or ignored. Further waves recognized by the common P/T-patterns are classfified as P-waves.
The time interval which the microcomputer uses for pattern recognition is shorter than the electrophysiological incident of P-wave or T-wave. For that reason all steps of computer processing, which are to be done immediately after the recognition of a wave, are carried out before a new wave may occur.
The hard- and software described here is ready for clinical use. Up to now an off-line test was carried out using 971 routine ECG. This material was already described when publishing the first step of recognition method (4,5).
The recognition ratio yielded by the first step shows table 1.

Table 1: Recognition ratio yielded by the first step

	R-wave		P/T-wave	
recognized by physician	5411	100 %	9239	100 %
computer findings	5348	98.8 %	7203	78.0 %
not recognized	63	1.2 %	2036	22.0 %
failure ratio	125	2.3 %	436	4.7 %

It is necessary to separate P-waves and T-waves in order to use this recognition method in practice. Fitted to this necessity it may be useful for other tasks of automated ECG processing under pressure, too. Table 2 shows the recognition ratio of separately indicated P-waves.

Table 2: Recognition ratio yielded by the second step

	separately indicated P-waves	
recognized by physician	4566	100 %
computer findings	3379	74.0 %
not recognized	1187	26.0 %
failure ratio	201	4.4 %
miscalculated T-waves	3	0.07 %

These results prove the premise that specially adapted algorithms taking into consideration medical foundations and the appointed clinical aim surpass naked technical solutions for pattern recognition.

(1) Poll, R. and R. Henßge: Proc. XII. Kongr. Ges. Kardiol. Angiol. DDR Rostock, Nov. 1984

(2) Poll, R. and R. Henßge: Medizintechnik 23, 20 - 24 (1983)

(3) Poll, R. and R. Henßge: Proc. X. World Congr. Cardiol. Washington, D.C., Sept. 1986

(4) Poll, R., E. Meisel, and R. Henßge: Z. Klin. Med. 41, 1133 - 1136 (1986)

(5) Poll, R. and R. Henßge: Computer methods and programs in biomed. (in the press)

Use of Microcardioanalyzer for Individualized Drug Selection in Cardiology

SIDORENKO G.I.,NIKITIN Ya.G.,YAKUBOVICH V.M.,CHIGRINOVA N.P.
Byelorussian Research Institute of Cardiology,Minsk,USSR

The experience gained from microcardioanalyzer,known as microcardio - monitor (MCM),use is shown with regard to the selection of antiar - rhythmic drugs and cardiac glycosides in 80 patients with heart rhythm disturbances.The prospects of MCM application in practical cardiology are discussed.

The portable MCM device,designated for long-time monitoring of the ECG RR wave sequences,was used for individualized antiarrhythmic and cardiac glycosides drug selection under the free-life conditions (Sidorenko G.I.et al.)The device set comprises 3 chest electrodes and ECG amplifier,30 g in weight,which is fixed to the patient's body by means of an elastic belt and,finally,MCM proper providing continuous visual indication of current values of heart rate,number of single,early and grouped premature beats and ventricular asystolia more than 2 seconds long.Sound alarm is provided additionally to the visual indication,if heart rate (HR) exceeds the preset maximal and minimal marginal limits and with occurrence of prognostically dangerous arrhythmias (Lown B.et al.)The registered parametérs may be read out by the patients themselves or by medical stuff in on-line and off-line modes.

60 patients with premature beats and 20 patients with the permanent type of atrial fibrillation (AF) were studied before and after drug prescription as well as during medication.The group under study comprised mainly patients with the ischemic heart disease and acquired valvular disease.The results of heart rhythm analyses done by MCM were compared with those,made by a physician on basis of long-time ECG recordings.The need for medication was ascertained in case of premature beat and,if antiarrhythmic drugs were prescribed,their effectiveness was evaluated. The result of the treatment was assumed to be positive,if number of premature beats was lowered by at least 70 per cent (Ivanova L.A.et al) The dynamics of HR at rest and moderate physical exercises (walking, climbing upstairs)was studied in patients with AF.

The patients were divided into 4 groups depending on the results of Holter ECG monitoring:

first group (8 patients).Premature beats were not revealed within the period of monitoring.No need for antiarrhythmic treatment.Periodic HR monitoring should be advised.

Second group (19 patients).The premature beat's occurrence is less than 30 per hour.Special antiarrhythmic treatment is not required or conducted for short periods,if premature beats cause unpleasant sensations.

Third group (20 patients).The premature beat's occurence is more than 30 per hour.Antiarrhythmic medication is required.

Fourth group (13 patients).Frequent single premature beats are observed alongside with early and grouped premature beats (of high grades). Active antiarrhythmic therapy is needed with high grade premature beat's elimination, if possible.

The results of quantitative and qualitative premature beat evaluation performed to determine the patient's relation to this or that group by means of MCM coincided in 57 of 60 cases with those, obtained by Holter ECG monitoring for the similar periods of control.

33 patients of 3rd and 4th groups were prescribed antiarrhythmic drugs, i.e. propranolol, rhythmilen or aethacizini. In those patients the number of premature beats before medication was between 30 and 2000 per hour. The number of premature beats in 24 patients was down by more than 70 per cent after 5-6 days of treatment, while that in the other 9 patients lowered only by 10 to 50 per cent which was concluded to be insufficient treatment effect and further medication was conducted with alternative antiarrhythmic drugs under the monitoring control. In evaluation of the antiarrhythmic treatment course the MCM readings coincided with the Holter monitor data in 29 of 33 patients.

20 patients with AF were studied by combined use of MCM and "Lenta MT" cardiomonitor. The MCM readings were recorded into special diares by patients themselves, who also indicated time period and type of physical activity. The number of these recordings varied from 20 to 80 for each patient during the period under control.

In practice 3 clinical forms of AF are singled out, i.e. bradysystolic with HR mainly less than 60 beats per minute, normosystolic with HR from 60 to 90 and tachysystolic with HR more than 90 beats per minute (Mazur N.A.). This assessment is based as a rule on the HR value counted at rest either by auscultation or short-time ECG recordings. Using these signs, bradysystolic AF form was revealed in 4, normosystolic in 8 and tachysystolic in 8 patients. Somewhat higher HR was observed in all patients during motor activity and food intake. It is noteworthy that value of HR increase in patients with the same clinical AF form was not similar. HR dynamics during monitoring is demonstrated in Table 1

Table 1. HR changes in patients with AF during moderate physical exercise (walking, climbing upstairs 1-2 stair-wells)

AF form	Number of patients	Resting HR	Number of patients with HR increase	
			less than 100 beats per minute	more than 100 beats per minute
Bradysystolic	4	54-60	2	2
Normosystolic	8	64-90	4	4
Tachysystolic	8	92-132	4	4
Total	20		10	10

Patients with circulatory insufficiency and lower tolerance to physical exercises received cardiac glycosides (isolanid, digoxin), their dosage being depended on HR value. 10 patients of them showed sufficiently high tolerance to moderate physical loads with little manifestation of dyspnoea and heart palpitation.In this group HR increase to physical activity was not more than 100 beats per minute,which is an indicator of adequate heart rhythm correction (Metelitsa V.I.).Complaints of quick fatigue,dyspnoea during movement,heart palpitation sensations were prevalent in the second group of patients with more significant HR increase during physical loads,i.e.up to 160 beats per minute by MCM data.HR of one patient,aged 30,with bradysystolic AF form at rest was no more than 55-60 beats per minute.He was not put on cardiac glycosides.MCM monitoring showed that great physical loads,not causing dyspnoea,lead to short-time HR increases up to 170-240 beats per minute.The control ECG,recorded on magnetic tape,revealed periods of ventricular tachycardia corresponding to sharp HR increase.

The dosage of cardiac glycosides for patients with AF,whose HR exceeded 100 beats per minute during physical loads was corrected under MCM control or additional antiarrhythmic drugs were prescribed,which contributed to higher tolerance to free-life loads.The MCM provides for individual setting of upper and lower HR marginal limits and sound alarm, which facilitates the detection of HR values beyond the preset limits. This can be caused by various reasons,glycosides intoxication including. On-line evaluation of HR changes allows the patient to make selfcontrol complying with the necessary medical recomendations (reducing physical loads,medication,etc.).

The preliminary clinical tests of portable MCM device showed that it can be used for detection of main heart rhythm disturbances and for their quantitative evaluation during antiarrhythmic treatment.The MCM use would bring special benifits for those patients,who are on long-term betablocker therapy to prevent possible side-effect.The device can also be used for screening to detect patients,requiring more detailed monitoring control.The MCM low cost and easy operation opens prospects for its use in wide-range of medical and sports institutions.

REFERENCES

(I)Сидоренко Г.И.,Никитин Я.Г.,Якубович В.М.,Малашкевич А.А.,Вахтерев Л.Ф.:Кардиология,5,5-8 (I987)
(2)Lown B.,Podrid P.I.,De Silva R.A.et al.:Curr.Probl.Cardiol.,4,1-62 (1980)
(3)Иванова Л.А.,Мазур Н.А.,Павлова Т.С.,Бугрий Е.М.,Джишамбаев Э.Д.: Кардиология,8,37-40 (I986)
(4)Мазур Н.А.:Руководство по кардиологии,3,502-537 (I982)
(5)Метелица В.И.:Справочник кардиолога по клинической фармакологии, 234 (I987)

ASSESSMENT OF THE CARDIAC FUNCTIONAL STATUS BASED ON LONG-TERM RHYTHMOGRAM RECORDING DURING SLEEP

G. Varoneckas and D. Žemaitytė

Palanga Dept., Inst. Cardiovasc. Res., 4 Vydūno St., Palanga 235720, Lithuanian SSR, USSR.

SUMMARY. An assessment of the functional cardiovascular reserve based on long-term rhythmogram recording during sleep is proposed. The method allows to evaluate baseline level of autonomic heart rate (HR) control, to detect different kind of dysrhythmias in relation with particularities of autonomic control, to choose antiarrhythmic therapy and to assess its effectiveness.

INTRODUCTION

Restriction of functional cardiovascular reserve in IHD patients is mainly conditioned by negative changes in central hemodynamics and reduced heart rate (HR) autonomic control, both resulted by coronary blood flow impairment. Heart failure and diminished protective role of parasympathetic HR control predispose, in common, to development of dangerous dysrhythmias (Schwartz et al., 1984). Because of that, an evaluation of dysrhythmias in relation to the pattern of autonomic HR control becomes important aspect while ascribing functional status of IHD patients. Autonomic HR control might be reflected by periodical HR structure and its changes during different testing conditions. Night sleep might be seen as natural testing condition with different patterns of autonomic HR control during non-REM and REM sleep, as a reflection of prevalence and reduction of parasympathetic control, correspondingly (Žemaitytė et al., 1984a).
The aim of this study was an assessment of IHD patients functional status based on long-term rhythmogram recording during sleep.

MATERIAL AND METHOD

The contingent was 800 IHD patients, aged 54.7 (SEM 1.78) yrs. The rhythmogram (a sequence of successive RR intervals) recording was done in parallel with ECG, respiration, and actogram troughout all the night in usually patient ward (Fig.1.). Recordings were switched on at 10.30-11.00 p.m. and continued till awakening in the morning. The rhythmogram continuously was fed into a Hewlett Packard computer and automatically analyzed.

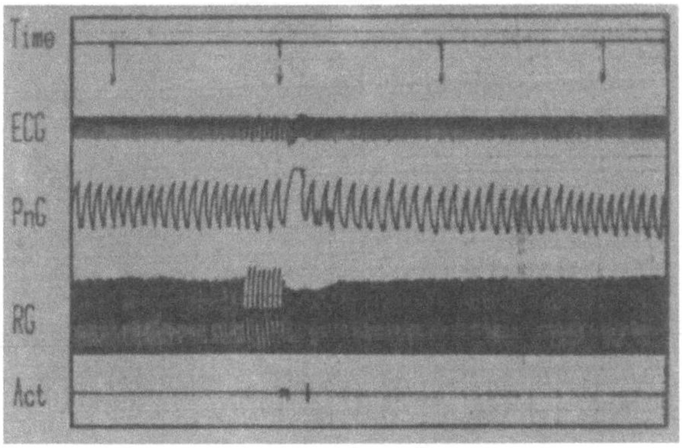

Fig.1. An example of rhythmogram recording during sleep in IHD patient.
Time, time marks from computer clock; *PnG*, nasal pneumogram; *RG*, rhythmogram; *Act*, actogram of body movements.

Respiration was recorded using nasal thermistor in respect to identify the changes of HR and its slow waves evoked by episodes of sleep apnoea (Žemaityte et al., 1984b). The actogram allows to identify the HR accelerations induced by body movements during sleep.

RESULTS

The results of rhythmogram analysis allowed to find out four main patterns of dysrhythmias corresponding to the association of their appearance with background of autonomic HR control. The patterns are following: (i) dysrhythmias appearing during REM sleep; (ii) dysrhythmias appearing during non-REM sleep; (iii) dysrhythmias associated with changes of HR frequency but independent on sleep stages; and (iv) sudden appearance of dysrhythmias without any associations ascribed above. The most unfavourable pattern is the first one, while dysrhythmias are associated with withdrawal of parasympathetic HR control and low central hemodynamics, particularly in the patients with reduced HRSP. The second pattern shows association of dysrhythmias with increase of parasympathetic control, while the others have no association with autonomic HR control directly. The investigations of HR modifications over individual sleep stages identified using EEG show that progress of sleep was followed by a decrease of HR frequency and an increase of respiratory arrhythmia, while in REM sleep an opposite HR changes were observed. This HR sleep pattern (HRSP) in IHD patients mostly was similar to the HR modifications during sleep in healthy subjects and was named typical HRSP (Žemaitytė et al, 1984b) (Fig.2.). An increase of parasympathetic HR control and a decrease of sympathetic one during non-REM sleep and controversial changes in REM sleep are responsible for those HR modifications during sleep (Žemaitytė at al., 1984a). Thus, using

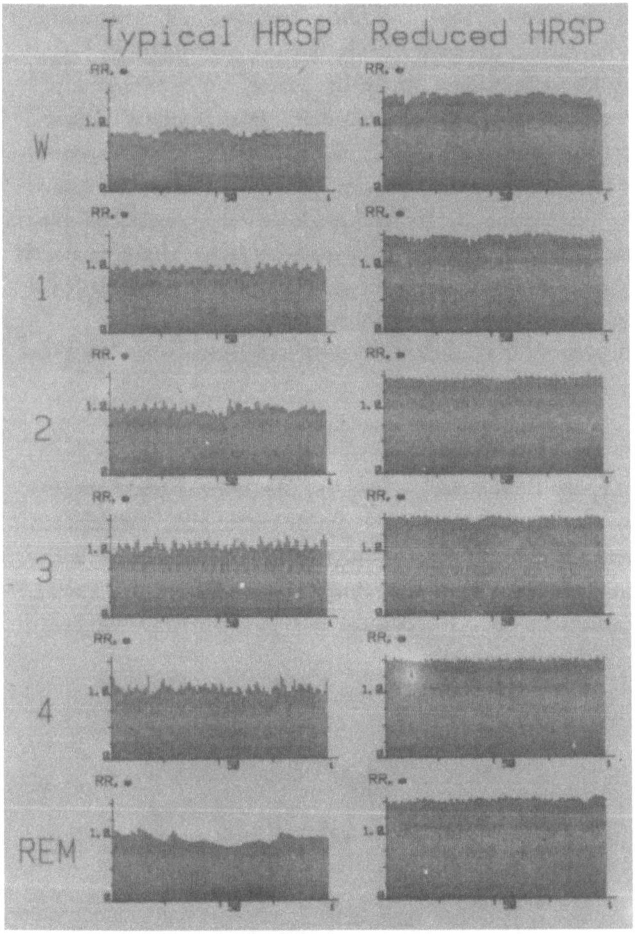

Fig. 2 . An example of typical and reduced HRSPs in IHD patients.
W, wakefulness; *1, 2, 3, 4,* and *REM*, stages of sleep.

only the changes of the HRSP, with or without computerized analysis, 3 major sleep states apart wakefulness (without involvement of EEG) might be identified: (i) light sleep (1 and 2 stages); (ii) slow wave sleep (3 and 4 stages); and (iii) REM sleep. The extent of HR changes during sleep mainly depends on the baseline level of autonomic HR control and its modification over sleep stages. A group of IHD patients characterized by a constant HR over all sleep stages and reduced baseline autonomic HR control was observed (Fig.2.). Those differences can be identified not only by computerized analysis, although using visual rhythmogram pattern. In this case, the sleep states according to the HR changes can be identified in the patients with typical HRSP, but not with reduced one. However, the fact of the reduced HRSP per se can be interpreted as negative in respect to functional cardiovascular reserve. The patients with the reduced HRSP are the ones with the worst cardiovascular functional status displaying more frequent appearance of dangerous cardiac abnormalities during sleep, especially REM sleep.

In figure 3 an example of automated HR and extrasystoles analysis during sleep in IHD patient is presented. An increase in number of extrasystoles during stage 2 and REM sleep was clearly observed.

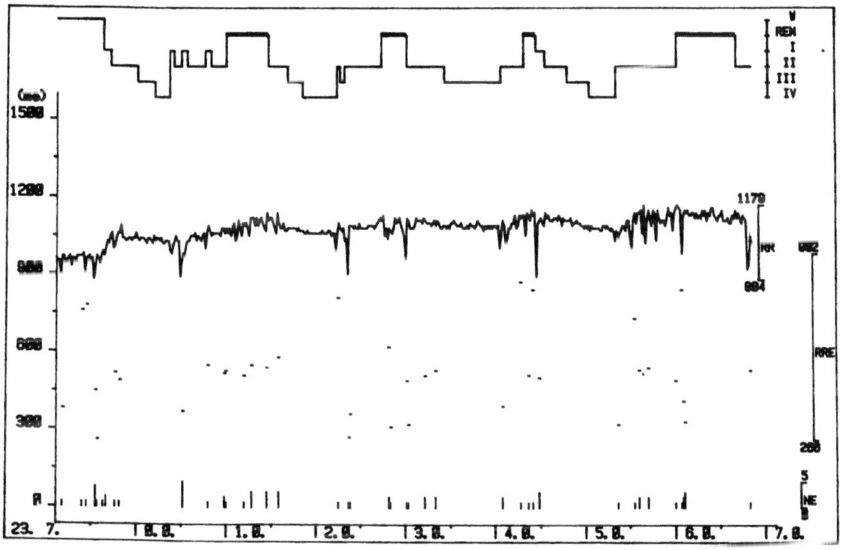

Fig. 3. An example of automated HR and extrasystoles analysis during sleep. *Abscissa,* time from the onset of experiment; *ordinate,* RR interval *(RR),* level of prematurity of extrasystoles *(RRE),* and number of extrasystoles *(NE)* averaged in 1-min periods. A hypnogram which shows scores of sleep stages (*W,* wakefulness; *I, II, III, IV,* and *REM,* stages of sleep) also is given.

Long-term rhythmogram recording makes possible detection of dysrhythmias, allows to calculate their number and identify a type of particular dysrhythmias. Some of them are presented in Figure 4, demonstrating the possibility to identifying premature beats, tachyarrhythmias, and disturbances of conduction at sinoatrial or atrioventricular levels. Thus, the long-term rhythmogram recording, using computerized analysis or only visual one, enables to evaluate quantity and quality of HR disturbances, their association with modifications of autonomic HR control reflecting functional cardiovascular reserve.

Repetitive recordings enables to control also the effectiveness of drug therapy and its side effect.

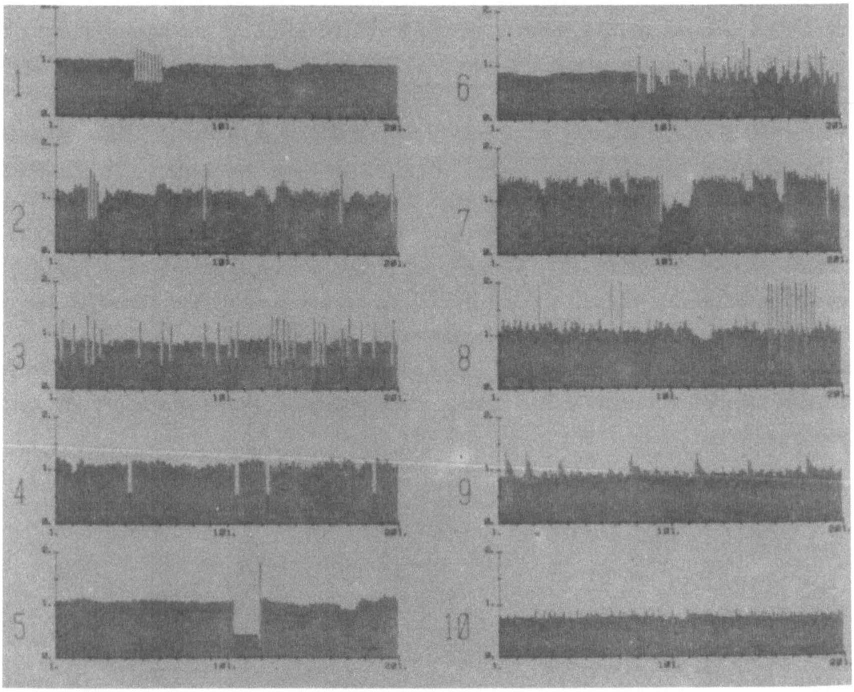

Fig. 4. Sample rhythmograms reflecting different heart rate disturbances.
1, premature atrial contractions (episode of bigeminia); *2*, premature ventricular contractions; *3*, frequent ventricular contractions with episodes of parasystolie; *4*, interpolated premature beats; *5*, paroxysm of supraventricular tachycardia; *6*, paroxysm of atrial fibrillation; *7*, episode of tachycardia on the background of the bradycardia; *8*, sinoatrial or atrioventricular blocks of the second degree; *9*, episodes of pacemaker migration outside the sinus node; *10*, premature sinus beats.

CONCLUSION

The long-term rhythmogram recording during sleep allows to identify HRSP (typical and reduced) reflecting baseline autonomic HR control and to assess functional cardiovascular reserve in IHD patients, to evaluate different kind of dysrhythmias and their relation to modifications of autonomic control, to choose antiarrhythmic therapy, to control it, and to assess its effectiveness.

REFERENCES

1. Schwartz, P.J., G.E. Billman, and H.L. Stone: Circulation 69, 790-800 (1984).
2. Žemaitytė, D., G. Varoneckas, and E. Sokolov: Psychophysiology 21, 279-289 (1984a).
3. Žemaitytė, D., G. Varoneckas, and E. Sokolov: Psychophysiology 21, 290-298 (1984b).

Autonomic nervous system control of heart rate in juvenile hypertension

ROMBERG,D.[*], SCHUBERT,E.[*], HULIN,I.[**], POPPEROVA,E.[**]

[*] Institute of Physiology, Humboldt-University, Berlin, GDR

[**] Department of Clinical Pathophysiology, Komensky University, Bratislava, Czechoslovakia

Summary

To study sympathetic and parasympathetic nerve function in juvenile hypertension the heart rate (HR) and heart rate variability (HRV) of 10 juvenile hypertensive patients and of 10 normotensive young men were examined. The HRV was calculated as the mean difference between successive RR intervals, called MSD. Average HR was observed as 65+11 beats/min (mean+SD) at the normals and 71+13 beats/min at the hypertonics. Significant differences in MSD were found between normals (65+19 ms) and hypertonics (36+13ms). These results indicate a lower parasympathetic influence on heart conrol in the juvenile hypertonics.

Introduction

Heart rate (HR) and heart rate variability (HRV) have been used in order to quantify the activities of cardiac vegetative nerves and to investigate the pathophysiology of the autonomic heart control in man. HRV was previously suggested predominantly to be affected by the parasympathetic tone whereas the HR increase resulted predominantly from the sympathetic nerves. (Eckoldt,K.et al.1973, Fouad,F.M. et al.1984). The parasympathetic and sympathetic nerve tone in patients with essential or borderline hypertension had been investigated in previous reports (Frohlich,E. et al.1971, Korner,Pl.et al.1973, Julius,S.et al.1975, Eckoldt,K.et al.1976, Alicandri et al.1985) as possible causes for hypertension.

The present study was to evalute the influence of the autonomic nervous system on HR and HRV in patients with juvenile hypertension.

Material and methods

The HR was measured out of the 2-nd Einthoven-Lead recorded in supine position in rest under normal breathing. successive RR-intervals, called mean successive difference (MSD).

The HR and MSD were calculated as the mean value of 40 beats. All values were expressed as mean + standard deviation (SD). The statistical analysis was performed by the Wilcoxon pair test and by the Wilcoxon test for independent groups.

Results

No differences in the mean age was found between the normal group and the juvenile hypertonic patients. The mean HR was significant higher in the juvenile hypertonics than in the normal subjects. A significant decrease of the MSD was found in the juvenile hypertonic patients (Table 1).

Table 1 . Mean and standard deviation of age, HR and MSD in normal and juvenile hypertonic subjects.

	normal subjects (n=10)	juvenile hypertonics (n=10)	significance
age (years)	25 + 1,2	24 + 1,4	n s
H R (beats / min)	65 + 11	71 + 13	p < 0,05
M S D	65 + 19	36 + 13	p < 0.05

The correlation between HR and MSD was only weak in the nomotensive group (r=-0,315), but more closely in the juvenile hypertonic patients (r=-0.766)..

The HR and MSD for each subject is shown in Fig. 1.

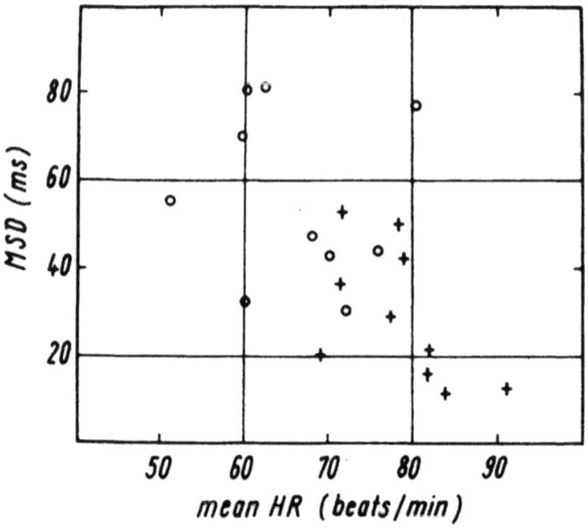

Fig.1.

Values of mean HR and MSD in 10 normotensive young men ( ) and 10 juvenile hypertonic patients ( ).

Discussion

Measures of the RR-interval have been used for the examination of the activities of cardiac vegetative nerves and the pathophysiology of the autonomic heart control in hypertension by many authors. HR is reported to be increased in some subgroups of hypertensive patients compared with normotensive subjects. The higher HR is more evident in patients with borderline hypertension (Julius,S.et al.1975), but has also been noted in patients with established hypertension (Frohlich,E.et al.1971). This increase might be determined by a higher sympathetic tone, but only a weak correlation was found between levels of HR and plasma catecholamine concentrations (Agabiti-Rosei,E.et al. 1982). On the other hand, parasympathetic activity was reported to be decreased in patients with borderline hypertension (Julius,S.et al.1971) and established essential hypertension (Eckoldt,K.et al.1976, Alicandri,C.et al.1985).

The results indicate a reduced parasympathetic and increased sympathetic nerve activity in juvenile hypertension. The modification in the parasympabthetic and sympathetic tone did not always occur simultaneously (Eckoldt,K.et al.1974, Schubert,E.et al.1981, Alicandri,C.et al.1985). In the juvenile hypertonic patients the MSD correlated more closely with HF (r=-0.766), but not in the normal group (r=-0,315).

It is not possible from these data alone to draw any conclusion about the relation between the mean HR and the MSD in the two groups, except to observe the different tightness in the correlation within these two groups. As seen in Fig.2 that only one hypertonic patient fell more than 2 SDs away from the mean value of HR for the normals, in contrast to the 6 who where more then 2 SDs below the mean MSD for the normal group. The HRV appears to be a better indicator of autonomic nerve tone than HR.

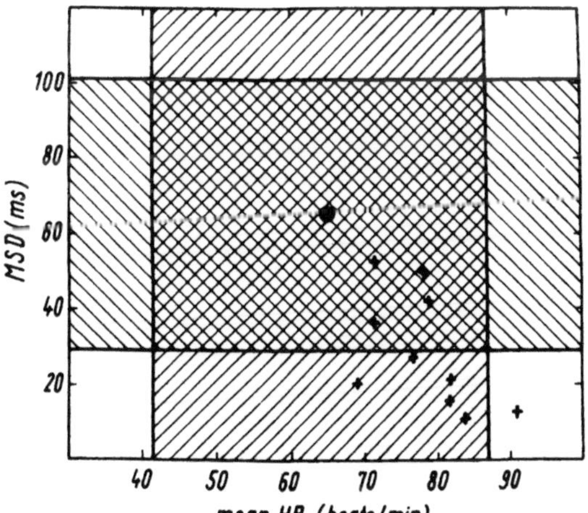

Fig.2.

Distribution of HR and MSD in juvenile hypertonic patients in comparison to the mean value of the normal group. The circle ( ) represents the mean values for the normal group.
The crosses ( ) give the MSD and HR values of the single hypertonic patients.
The hatched areas represent the mean + 2 SD of the normal subjects.

It was previously reported that the sympathetic activity (Loeffelholz et al.1985, Murthy et al.1986). According to this relation an increased sympathetic activity is assumed to be connected with the lower vagal tone observed in our group of juvenile hypertonics. This is consistent with the conclusion of previous investigations showing that the higher HR found in established hypertension was predominantly due to changes in vagal rather than cardiac sympathetic effects. (Korner,P.I.et al.1973, Eckoldt,K.et al.1976, Alicandri,C.et al.1985).

In conclusion, the results point to a modified chronotropic heart control in juvenile hypertension probably caused by an ampaired vagal function.

References

Agabiti-Rosei,E.et al.: Plasma catecholamines in essential hypertension. J.Clin.Pharmacol.Res.1982 II (suppl.1), 69-74.

Alicandri,C.et al.: Autonomic nervous system control of heart rate in essential hypertension. J.Hypertension 1985, 3:117-119.

Eckoldt,K.: Der Einfluss vegetativer Umstellungen auf die Sinusarrhythmie des Herzens. Neue Ergebnisse der Elektrokardiologie II, Jena 1974, 294-352.

Eckoldt,K.et al.: Sinus arrhythmia and heart rate in hypertonics disease. Adv.Cardiol.1976, 16:366-369.

Fonad,F.M.et al.: Assessment of parasympathetic control of heart rate by a noninvasive method. Am.J.Physiol.1982,52: 1652-1657.

Frohlich,E.et al.: Clinical-physiological correlation in the development of hypertensive heart disease. Ciculation 1971, 44: 446-455.

Julius,S.et al.: Role of parasympathetic inhibition in the hyperkinetic type of borderline hypertension. Circulation, 1971, 44: 413-418.

Julius,S.et al.: Autonomic nervous cardiovascular regulation in borderline hypertension. Am.J.Cardiol.1975, 36: 685-696.

Korner,P.I.et al.: Autonomic and non autonomic circulatory components in essential hypertension in man. Circulation 1973, 48: 107-117.

Loeffelholz,K.et al.: The parasympathetic neuroeffektor junction of the heart. Pharmacol.Rev.1985, 37: 1-25.

Murthy,S.V.et al.: Antiarrhythmic drugs and the modulation of autonomic control of heart rate in rabbits. Federation Proc.1986, 45: 2186-2190.

Schubert,E.et al.: Normal ranges and deviations of the heart rhythm regulation in man. New Frontiers of Electrocardiology, John Wiley & Sons Ltd. 1981, 409-413.

Contribution of ambulatory electrocardiographic monitoring for the diagnosis of patients with syncope.

DUKÁT A.,MIKEŠ Z.,GAVORNÍK P.,KOLESÁR J.,LIETAVA J.,GAŠPAR Ľ.,ZVONÁR J.
Clinic of Physical Medicine Comenius' University,Mickiewiczova 13, CS-813 69 Bratislava, Czechoslovakia.

Summary.

Ambulatory electrocardiographic monitoring is a non-invasive method mainly indicated for diagnosing patients with intermittent dysrhythmia, which may be related to the patient's symptoms and complaints. Transient dysrhythmia followed by cerebral ischaemia may cause changes in conductivity state,dizziness,presyncope and genuine syncope. After ruling out other causes, transient dysrhythmia can be regarded from the aspect of syncope etiology, especially so among older patients with organic heart disease. In such cases Holter electrocardiography is a useful non-invasive investigation technique, which enables to start the appropriate treatment and to monitor through serial electrocardiographic measurements, the efficiency of the started anti-arrhythmic therapy as well as the evaluating the function of implanted pacemaker.

Introduction.

Syncope is a sudden, transient loss of consciousness with inability to keep the postural tonus with later spontaneous restitution, not needed specific intervention in form of resuscitation. For the clinicians presyncope with not completely loss of consciousness is differentiated from genuine syncope. Commonly episodes of syncope have sudden beginning, short duration and are characteristic for their completely restitution during several minutes. Syncope is common and potentially dangerous problem among patients of older age groups, where the causes remain often unclear through many evaluations. Mean causes of it is: a/decrease, or loss of cerebral circulation, b/decrease of heart work and c/decrease of systemic arterial blood pressure. For these reasons now Holter electrocardiographic monitorings are common used for evaluations of symptoms of the patients. Purpose of this study was to evaluate the contribution of 24-hour ECG monitoring among symptomatic patients admitted to the clinic for the diagnosis of syncope, or presyncope.

Material and methods.

43 patients with the age of 60-82, with mean age of 68,03 years were evaluated.There were 12 men and 31 women admitted for hospitalisation with this symptom. Characteristics of the followed sample are seen at fig.1. All of them were examined at neurological department and all of them had ECG at rest and Holter ECG for 24-hour period. Dysrhythmias were evaluated after Lown's classification /1/, classes III-V were evaluated as complex forms. Method of evaluation was the same as used in other studies of the authors /2,3/..

Fig.1 Characteristics of the followed sample

Age/yrs/	60 - 82
Mean age	68,03
Males	12 = 28%
Females	31 = 72%
Symptoms	
syncope	33 = 77%
presyncope	10 =.23%
one episode	14 = 33%
repeated	29 = 67%

Fig.2 Holter monitoring among followed patients

Normal results	16 = 37%
Fibrillation	8 = 19%
Dysrhythmias	
supraventricular	27 = 62%
ventricular	36 = 84%
complex forms	14 = 33%
sy sick sinus	9 = 21%
Blocks	
atrioventricular	5 = 12%
bundle branch	3 = 7%

Fig.3 Contribution for diagnosis of syncope

Resting ECG	7 = 16%
Neurological examination	10= 23%
Biochemical examinations	5 = 12%
Holter ECG	11= 26%
Unknown origin	10= 23%
Together	43=100%

Results.

Fig.2 shows the results of Holter ECG's among followed group. Only 37% had no abnormalities during monitoring periods, 19% had atrioventrikular blocks or intraventricular ones and 19% had atrial fibrillation. Up to 91% of the patients had ectopic activity during monitorings: 62% supraventricular, from which 26% had paroxysmal supraventricular tachycardias and 84% ventricular, from which complex forms were in 33%. 21% had syndrome sick sinus. Among 86% of the patients antiarrhythmic treatment was started and among 19% implanted pacemaker abolished casdiac dysrhythmia and symptoms of the patients.
As seen from fig.3 among relatively high percentage the cause of syncope remained unclear. Resting ECG was successful for the diagnosis of cardiac origin of syncope in 16%. Neurological examinations with non-invasive and invasive techniques found out the origin in 23%. Biochemical examinations in 12% and Holter ECG was successful in another 26% of the cases as indicated for the treatment or invasive electrophysiologic testings.

Discussion and conclusions.

Syncope is quite often and potentially dangerous problem among patients of older age groups /4/.There are not many informations of their epidemiology and prognosis /5/.In older age group 10years prevalence is about 23% and 1year incidence about 7% /6/.Various patogenetic mechanisms can be involved,part of them cardiovascular diseases with transient dysrhythmias /7/.In clinical praxis for the diagnostic process many examinations are common used;one of the non-invasive techniques is Holter ECG monitoring.Offers to evaluate correlation between symptoms and rhythm or repolarisation,to predict cardiovascular risk,to evaluate therapeutical intervention and to profil the population with diseases.Main indication is for the causes of transient dysrhythmias,that may be in relation to symptoms of the patients.Such dysrhythmia with cerebral ischaemia may be the cause of changes in consciousness,dizziness,presyncope,or syncope.As for its short duration and occurence,difficult to predict,diagnosis may be done by exclusion.Correlation is necessary with symptoms of the patients after diaries and concommittant dysrhythmia on ECG.Often remains in praxis the origin of syncope uncleared as also in our group /8/.Transient dysrhythmias after exclusion other causes can be the nature and etiology of syncope,especially among older patients with already present cardiovascular disease /9/.Holter ECG monitoring is there useful and valuable non-invasive method and can indicate for causal therapeutic approach /10/.Serial ECG monitorings are useful for control of started antiarrhythmic therapy or for control of function of implanted pacemaker.

References

/1/ Lown, B., M. Wolf: Circulation 44, 363-368 /1971/.
/2/ Mikeš, Z., J. Kolesár, and A.Dukát: Čas.Lék.čes. 117, 498-503 /1978/
/3/ Arešidze, T.Ch: Metod.rekomend.MZGSSR 1, 1-18 /1984/.
/4/ Naccarelli, V.V: Med.Clin.N.Amer. 68, 1211-1230 /1984/.
/5/ Lipsitz, L.A., J.Y. Wei, J.W. Rowe: Quarterly J.Med. 55, 45-54 /1985/.
/6/ Lipsitz, L.A: Ann.Int.Med. 99, 92-105 /1983/.
/7/ Zeldis, S.M., et al.: Chest 78, 456-462 /1980/.
/8/ Bertel, O., R. Stauber, and U.C. Dubach: Schweiz.med.Wschr. 115, 439-441 /1985/.
/9/ Knight, F: Postgrad.Med. 73, 74-83 /1983/.
/10/Harrison, D.C., J.W. Fitzgerald, and R.A. Winkle: N.Engl.J.Med. 294, 373-377 /1976/.

ECG AND CARDIAC MECHANICS

CONDUCTION PROBLEMS

Correlations between ECG and echographical changes in 145 cases of hypertrophic cardiomyopathy

E.APETREI, I.COMAN, G.GEORGESCU, C.CAPRARU, D.PETRE, C.CARP
Institute of Medicine, Clinic of Cardiology, Fundeni Hospital, Bucharest, Romania.

SUMMARY

The incidence and correlations between the ECG and echographical changes have been studied in 145 cases of hypertrophic cardiomyopathy (HCM), 95 males and 5o femmales, average age 39.6 ± 13.1.
Angina was present in 59 cases (4o.6%) and syncope in 23 (15.8%).
The most frequent ECG changes were : inverted T-waves in precordial leads in 81 cases (55.8%), out of which T-waves deeper than 1o mm in 52 cases (35.8%); the LVH Sokolov-Lyon index was present in 78 (53.7%) cases; pathological Q-waves in 59 cases (4o.6%).
Variability of the inverted T-waves was present specially in cases of apical HCM.
The echographical investigation revealed an average interventricular septum (IVS) of 18.3 ± 3.1 mm and a IVS/PW ratio of 1.7 ± o.4.
Predominant/concomitant hypertrophy of the posterior wall (PW) was noted in 17 cases (11.7%).
Correlations (the χ^2 test, the Student test) point out that Q-wave patients are of smaller average age ($p < o.o5$), show a reduced incidence of angina ($p < o.o5$), while negative T-wave patients have the Sokolov positive index more frequently ($p < o.ooo5$) and the posterior wall thicker ($p < o.oo5$).
To sum up, in HCM patients global LVH and T-waves changes appear moore afton than pathological Q-waves; the association of the two ECG patterns (negative T-abnormal Q) is infrequent. Giant T-waves are relatively frequent but not characteristic of apical HCM. The ECG aspect does not correlate with the obstructive type, nor with the presence of syncope; it is rather poorly correlated with echographical and morphological findings.

MATERIAL AND METHODS

145 cases of HCM have been studied in the Clinic of Cardiology of Fundeni Hospital, Bucharest, Romania, from 1979 to 1985. The group was made up 95 males and 5o females, average age of 39.6 ± 13.1, out of which 14 patients belonged to HCM families.
The study has not included patients with acertained hypertension, or with associated coronary disease.
The echographical investigation was conducted by means of a PICKER LSC - 7ooo, or a HITACHI EUB 4o ultrasonic scanner using 2.25 and 5 MHz transducers. The measurements have been made in M-mode, from the standard transducer position, after the section plan had been selected bi-dimensionally to be perpendicular to IVS and PW;

the reccomandations of the American Echographical Society were observed; the test of amyl-nitrite was performed in 21 cases. ECG was recorded on 12 standard leads - several recordings as a rule- folowing up the possible changes in time. The investigation of the patients was made complete by anamnesis-especially on angina and syncopes. The ECG, Echo - and clinical data obtained were processed statistically, the Student test being used in comparing average values and the χ^2-test in differences of frequency.

RESULTS

Significant clinical data; presence of angina - 59 cases (4o.6%); presence of syncopes - 23 cases (15.8%).

2. Relevant ECG data : 14o cases of sinus rhythm, 23 of which showed rhythm disturbances during the follow-up (extrasystoles, paroxistical tachycardias, fibrillation or flutter); 5 cases of chronic atrial fibrillation; 5 cases with pre-excitation syndromes, 14 cases with left anterior hemiblock.

As for morphological changes 81 patients (55.8%) had negative T-waves, 52 of which (35.8%) of the total number) had T-waves over 1omm deep. The Sokolov-Lyon index>35 mm was recorded in 78 cases (53.7%); 59 (4o.6%) had pathological Q-waves. The ECG aspects, followed up over a number of years, helped acertain gradual alterations (Fig.2). We have also noted two cases of apical HCM with acute changes of T-waves during exercise testing.

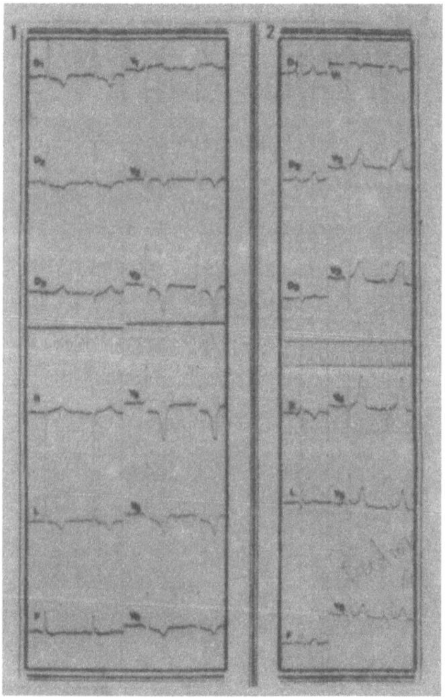

Fig.1 Most frequent ECG changes in HCM

3. Relevant echographical measurements: the average thickness of the i.v. septum was 18.3 ± 3.7 mm; the IVS/PW ratio was 1.7 ± o.4; echographical criteria for obstruction (SAM, mid-sistolic aortic valve closure) spontaneous or after amyl--nitrite- was noted in 6o cases (41.3%); 17 cases (11.7%) had predominant PW hypertrophy.

The comparativ analysis of the above-mentioned data (ECG, ECHO and clinical) has emphasized these statistically relevant correlations :

- pathological Q-waves cases : are of lower average age ($p < o.o5$); have seldom associated angina ($p < o.o5$); have seldom associated negative T-wave ($p < o.ool$) or

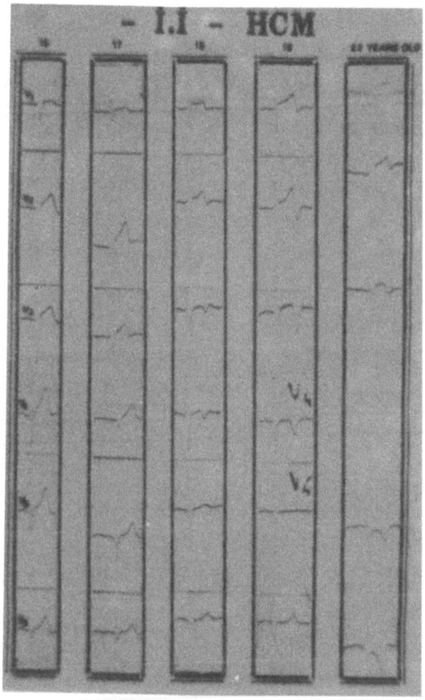

Fig.2 HCM - ECH aspect - evolution in time.

S-L index ($p < 0.0005$).

- negative T-waves cases :associate with the $^{+}$S-L index ($p < 0.0005$) much more frequently than the average; their PW is thicker than in other patients ($p < 0.005$).

12 of the 17 HCM cases with predominant/concomitant PW hypertrophy were noted to have negative T-waves. In only 3 of 11 cases of apical HCM did the T-waves prove to be over 1o mm deep.

None of the ECG changes suggestive of HCM is correlated with the echographical aspect of obstruction or with the presence of syncopes.

DISCUSSION

Without being as sensitive and specific as echography which represents the key to HCM diagnosis the ECG investigation may come up with suggestive aspects (1,4,5).

Our study was meant to establish the relevance of the ECG aspect by comparing it to the echographical data, therefore to the morphological condition.

Our results point to the predominance of global LVH aspect (with positive Sokolov index and STT changes) as well as inverted T-type ECG-both revealed in more than 5o%; contrary to previous data, the incidence of pathological Q-waves is rather smaller.

It should be noted that the two major types of changes (negativ T-waves and abnormal Q-waves) are not asociated as a rule (both being present in only 2o cases); similar findings - thought to be linked with different location of hypertrophy or different stages of the disease - have been noted (1). 25 cases were found to have no significant ECG change.

The results are somehow accounted for by the very bi-plane echo-exam which confirmed that hypertrophy is often much more extended and not limited to the IVS as clasically reported (2,6). Taking into account the assumption that LVH is the final ECG pattern in HCM(3.8) it could be possible that we examined the patients in our group at a more advanced stage of evolution of disease.

We came across the giant invered T-waves (initially described by Japanese authors in apical HCM) in only 3 cases with this type of morphological lesion; in most cases the other patients revealed

negative T-waves of less than lo mm amplitude, (9).
The data agree with the studies of Marron and col. (7).
Unlike the authors mentioned above, in our statistics the giant T-waves, without being peculiar to apical HCM are relatively frequent (35.8% of the total cases).
The angina crises, comparatively more frequent in patients with negative T-waves, can be looked upon as a further argument in the relative ischemic etiology (disproportion between muscular mass and vascular bed) of this type of alteration.
There are no statistically relevant correlations between the ECG aspects, the echographical signs of obstruction and the presence of syncopes; generally speaking, there is a rather poor predictive value of ECG changes versus echo and morphological aspects.

<u>REFERENCES</u>

1. Savage D.D., Seides S.F., Clark C.E., Henry W.L., Maron B.J., Robinson F.C., and Epstein S.E. : Circulation 58:4o2, 1978.
2. Maron B.J., Gottdiener J.S., Bonow R.O., Epstein S.E.,: Circulation 63:4o9 - 18, 1981.
3. Mc.Kenna W.J., Borggref M., England D., Deanfield J., Oakley C.M., and Goodwin J.F. : Circulation 66:1233, 1982.
4. Maron B.J., Wolfson J.K., Ciro E. and Spirito P., : Am J. Cardiol 51:189, 1983.
5. Henderson M.A., Ruddy T.D., Makowski H., and Wigle E.D., J. Am Coll. Cardiol. 1: 693, 1983.
6. Shapiro L.M., and Mc.Kenna W.J., : J Am Cardiol 2 : 437, 1983.
7. Maron B.J., Bonow R.O., Seshagiri T.N.R., Roberts W.C., and Epstein S.E., H Am J Cardiol 49;1838, 1982.
8. Silva Zelia, Brito D., Lopes Virginia, Lacerda P., Lopes M., Padua F., Madeira H., : 13-th International Congress on Electrocardiology - Abstracts.
9. Yamaguchi H., Ishimura T., Nishiyama S., Nagasaki F., Nakanishic S., Takatsu F., Nishijo T., Umeda T., and Machii K., : Am J Cardiol 44 : 4ol, 1979.

Elektrocardiotopography and two-dimensional echocardiography in the diagnosis of focal myocardial lesions associated with dilated cardiomyopathy

L.T.MALAYA et al.

310116, Kharkov, Prospekt Postysheva 2a,
Kharkov Research Institute of Therapy, USSR

SUMMARY. 57 patients with dilated cardiomyopathy /DCMP/ in the age of 32 to 56 were examined to reveal the focal alterations in myocardium in order to study possibilities of electrocardiotopography /ECTG/ and two-dimensional echocardiography /ECHO/. ECTG was registered in 108 monopolar leads and then integral topograms of the ventricle complex were built. Two-dimensional ECHO synchronized with ECG was recorded from the parasternal and apical positions in the direction of long and short axes of the left ventricle. The comparison of ECTG and ECHO data has shown the high /73,3%/ frequency of focal-cicatricial myocardial lesions in patients with DCMP. It may be related with development of the focal myocardiofibrosis. The lesion of antero-septal and antero-apical parts of left ventricle has been marked more frequently. Localization and spread of focal alterations in ECTG correspond to the extent in which myocardic segments drawing in pathologic process. They define to a considerable extent the disorder of total and regional functions of left ventricle.

In the diagnosis of dilated cardiomyopathy a great importance is attached to the complex of clinical and instrumental methods of investigation, ECG in particular. Pathologic changes of ECG are one of the significant and sometimes first manifestations of DCMP /1,3,7/.

Electrocardiographic picture of DCMP includes signs of heart muscle hypertrophy, violations of rhythm and conductivity. Signs of local myocardial lesion in the from of Q pathologic waves or QS-type complexes are frequently revealed against the background of the above changes /2,9/. At the same time these changes of ECG are not specific for DCMP and their evaluation offers diagnostic difficulties, especially for differentiating with cicatricial myocardial lesions in patients with ischemic heart disease /IHD/.

The purpose of the present work was to study a possible use of ECTG and two-dimensional ECHO for revealing focal myocardial changes in patients with DCMP.

We have examined 57 patients with DCMP /47 males and 10 females/ at the age of 32 to 56 years /their average age being 44,2 ± 2,1 years/. The diagnosis of cardiomyopathy was made on the grounds of recommendations of the WHO Experts' Committee /4/.

All the patients had chronic circulatory insufficiency which corresponded to the 3rd /in 48 patients/ and 4th /in 9 patients/ functional classes according to the classification of the New-York Heart Association /NYHA/. The control group consisted of 35 practically healthy persons.

Examination of the patients included electrocardiographic, roentgenologic and echocardiographic investigations. Registration of plural monopolar leads from 108 points on the anterior and posterior surfaces of the chest was performed by R.Z.Amirov's technique with subsequent carting of electropositivity and electronegativity by amplitude-ratio characteristics of QRS complex, ST segment and T wave.

We studied projective peculiarities and interrelations of zero zones, localization of overlaps and their area by integral topograms. Total potentials of R wave / Σ R/, balance of Σ R/ Σ Q,S total potentials, values of maxima /Rmax, Smax/ were regarded as criteria of myocardial hypertrophy. Depth and spreading of focal-cicatricial changes were evaluated by the total value of QS waves area and Q pathologic waves, sum of QS potentialis / Σ QS/ and Q waves / Σ Q/.

One-dimensional, two-dimensional and pulse Doppler ECHO were performed with the use of a Transducer which had the frequency of 3 mc and scan angle of 80°. Analysis of echocardiograms in M-mode included determination of end diastolic and systolic volumes of the left ventricle /EDV and ESV/, ejection fraction /EF/, shortening fraction /% Δ S/, mean velocity of circumferential fibres shortening /Vcf/.

Regional myocardial contractility was evaluated by the method of two-dimensional ECHO synchronized with ECG by 8 segments of the left ventricle at the projection of its short axis. Contractility of these segments was expressed in points from 1 to 3 by point scale.

As a result of analysing ECG and ECTG two main types of myocardial hypertrophy were singled out: the left ventricular hypertrophy in 12 patients /22%/ and the combined hypertrophy with prevalence of the left ventricular hypertrophy in 28 patients /48,9%/. Evaluation of the character and degree of myocardial hypertrophy was hampered in 8 patients with DCMP due to violations of intraventricular conductivity.

Topograms of 18 patients with DCMP /30,9%/ revealed zones of Qr and QS pathologic complexes which were located on the right surface of chest, mainly in its upper part. These changes were regarded as a large-focal and transmural myocardial lesion of the left ventricle posterior wall, the value of this lesion averaging 15,1 ± 1,2 by QS and 32,4 ± 1,8 by Q.

Signs of focal-cicatricial changes in anterior-septal and apical parts of the left ventricle were revealed in 24 patients/42,4%/ in the form of pathologic Qr and QS on the projection of the left lateral surface of chest in its upper and middle parts.

Side by side with a decrease of the total pump function of their heart the majority of the patients /80,6%/ developed regional violations in kinetics of the left ventricular walls.

In 27 patients with DCMP /47,3%/ the most pronounced decrease of local contractility was noted in anterior-lateral, septal and apical segments, their function being evaluated by 1,6 ± 0,16, 1,2 ± 0,12 and 1,4 ± 0,15 points correspondingly. Violations in kinetics of posterior-basal and diaphragmatic segments were observed in 19 patients /33,3%/, the level of their contractility was equal to 1,3 ± 0,13 and 1,8 ± 0,17 points.

Our attention was attracted by frequent revealing focal-cicatricial changes of myocardium by ECG and ECTG data /in 73,3% of the patients/ and corresponding disorders of regional contractility by ECHO data /in 80,6% of the patients/. This fact conforms to literature data about a high sensitivity of the ECG method in the diagnosis of focal-cicatricial myocardial lesion in cases of DCMP, the above sensitivity reaching 100% for anterior foci and 33% for lower-posterior ones in investigations performed by G.V.Riabykina et al. /2/.

We determined a direct dependence between the size of the focal lesion and the degree of violations in the contractile and pump functions of the heart, thus enabling us to single 3 groups of patients with DCMP.

Side by side with its diagnostic importance the elucidation of peculiarities of structural-functional myocardial state in cases of DCMP also enables to discover pathogenetic mechanisms of compensation and decompensation, evaluate the prognosis of the disease and approach the problems of its treating differentially.

REFERENCES

1. Mukharlyamov N.M. - Cardiology, 1984, 8, 5 - 11.
2. Mukharlyamov N.M., Popovich M.I., Zatushevskiy I.F. Dilated cardiomyopathy. - Kishinev, 1986, 158 P.
3. Sumarokov A.V., Moiseev V.S. Clinical Cardiology. - Moscow, 1986, 368 P.
4. Cardiomyopathies. Report of a WHO Expert Commitee. - Geneva, 1984, 11 - 39.
5. Evans T. - Medicine, 1979, 20 , 1042 - 1047.
6. Factor S.M., Sonnenblick E.H. - Cardiovasc.Rev.Rep., 1983, 4 , 1177 - 1182.
7. Gavazzi A., Lanzarini L., Cornalba C. et al. - G.Ital.Cardiol., 1984, 14 , 492 - 498.
8. Goodwin J.F. - Circulation, 1974, 50 , 210.
9. Goodwin J.F. - Brit.Heart J., 1982, 48 , 1 - 18.
10. Lengyel M., Kökeny M., Hajdu E. - Cor, vasa, 1982, 24 , 1 - 8.
11. Mathes P., Delius W., Sebening H. et al. - Dtsch.med.Wschr., 1976, 26 , 1.
12. Regitz V., Rudolph W. - Med.Klin., 1985, 80 , 580 - 585.

ST elevation during PTCA: role of collaterals in sudden coronary occlusion

FUMIMARO TAKATSU, TERUO NAGAYA
Division of Cardiology, Department of Internal Medicine, Anjo Kosei Hospital, 12-38, Miyuki-hommachi, Anjo, Aichi, 446 Japan

<Summary>

To clarify the role of coronary collaterals in protecting myocardium on acute coronary occlusion, 12-lead electrocardiogram (ECG) during percutaneous transluminal coronary angioplasty (PTCA) of left anterior descending coronary artery (LAD) was analysed in 68 patients. As compared with patients without angiographically visible collaterals, patients with "poor" collaterals did not show decrease in the incidence of ST elevation. However, even in these patients, the degree of ST elevation was significantly reduced. Patients with "fair" collaterals showed significant reduction both in the incidence and the degree of ST elevation. In the presence of "rich" collaterals, ST segments showed no elevation. Thus, only "rich" collaterals can protect myocardium from acute coronary occlusion surely but "poor" or "fair" collaterals also can although the protection may often be incomplete. It is also interesting that ST segment can elevate in the presence of partial coronary arterial flow supplied via collaterals.

<Introduction>

Collaterals to a coronary artery with a critical narrowing have been believed to protect myocardium from necrosis if the recipient vessel suffered from occlusion. In clinical practice, this view seems to be correct; that is, if the coronary artery giving rise to collaterals is free from significant lesions, the patient shall not have an acute infarction although he may have angina. And in such a patient, a repeat arteriogram performed several years later often discloses "silent" occlusion of the previously narrowed vessel, of which perfusion is completely replaced by well-developed collaterals. However, the role of collaterals in protecting myocardium in sudden coronary occlusion of the recipient artery remains unclear because in cases of such "silent occlusion" the stenosed vessel may have gradual progression of narrowing and not sudden occlusion. In this study, we examined ECG during PTCA of LAD in 68 patients and compared angiographical findings with incidence and degree of ST elevation.

<Methods>

All 68 patients had a critical (75% or more in luminal diameter reduction) narrowing in proximal segment of LAD. Patients having abnormal Q waves in lateral or precordial leads or severe asynergy in the anteroseptal wall on left ventriculogram were excluded. Patients showing conduction disturbances were also excluded. Collaterals were evaluated on the angiogram obtained just (several minutes) prior to PTCA after administration of isosorbide dinitrate. They were defined as "poor" when they filled only septal perforators, as "fair" when they partially filled epcardial segments of LAD and as "rich" when they filled completely LAD distal to the narrowing. The 68 study patients were subdivided into 4 groups according to the degree of development of collaterals: group 1 (33 patients); no collaterals detectable on angiogram, group 2 (12 patients); poor collaterals to LAD, group 3 (14 patients); fair collaterals to LAD, group 4 (9 patients); rich collaterals to LAD. No patients had critical narrowings in the vessels giving rise to the collaterals.

ECG: Standard 12-lead ECG was recorded at 45 to 60 seconds into the first balloon inflation. ST elevation was measured at 80 msec after the J point as compared with the control record. Sum of ST elevation was calculated by adding ST elevation in leads I, aVL and V1 through V6.

PTCA: PTCA was performed with standard technique via femoral or brachial approach. 5mg of isosorbide dinitrate was given to the target vessel before the angiogram performed several minutes prior to dilation.

<Results>

Presence or absence of ST elevation: 30 patients (91%) of group 1 showed ST elevation during balloon inflation and 11 patients (92%) of group 2 did. In group 3 patients, ST elevation appeared in 9 (64%) and in group 4 ST segment did not elevate in any case. (group 1 vs 2; NS, group 1 vs 3; $p = 0.003$, group 1 vs 4; $p << 0.0001$, group 3 vs 4; $p = 0.002$).

Degree of ST elevation: Sum of ST elevation was 9.9 ± 6.1 mV in 30 patients with ST elevation of group 1, 5.6 ± 3.6 mV in 11 patients of group 2 and 4.0 ± 3.0 mV in 9 patients of group 3 (group 1 vs 2; $p < 0.01$, group 1 vs 3; $p < 0.01$, group 2 vs 3; NS).

<Discussion>

Since the introduction of selective coronary arteriography by Dr. Mason Sones, it has been considered that ischemic myocardium was protected from necrosis if there were angiographically visible collaterals to the artery having critical stenosis from an artery without critical lesions. This traditional view seems to be proved with medical follow-up after the angiographic study. However, we could not observe what occurred at the moment when the critically narrowed vessel was finally occluded; emergency angiograms in acute myocardial infarction can visualize coronary arteries at least 30 minutes or later after the onset of chest pain and, in most cases, angiograms immediately before the acute occlusion can not be obtained. Thus, sudden occlusion of a coronary artery having a critical narrowing on balloon inflation at the very site of the narrowing could be an excellent model for very early stage of acute infarction. Flameng et al. <1> measured retrograde filling pressure on occlusion of a graft during aorto-coronary bypass surgery and observed distal filling pressure of about 40% of the aortic diastolic pressure in the presence of angiographically visible collaterals, which was only 19% in the absence of collaterals and thus suggesting functional significance of collaterals in sudden interruption of antegrade flow. However, they did not record ECG or any hemodynamical indexes of left ventricular function and thus had effects of retrograde filling remain unclear. The results of the present study indicate that incidence of ST elevation was not diminished in the presence of "poor" collaterals but even in these cases the "poor" collaterals do, to some extent, reduce degree of ST elevation, suggesting their functional efficacy if limited. Rentrop et al.<2>, by opacifying the "donor" vessel during PTCA, proved that all "poor" collaterals developed into "fair" or "rich" ones during balloon inflation and that new collaterals appeared in many patients without collaterals on films recorded prior to PTCA. Accordingly, "poor" collaterals may protect myocardium by developing into more extensive ones during balloon inflation. And, on an occlusion during natural course, they all may become "rich" in several minutes, completely protecting myocardium from necrosis and making clinical features as "silent" occlusion. However, it can not be proved because lack of ECG or other metabolic or hemodynamical data during initial several to several ten minutes during sustained occlusion of a coronary artery due to short periods of balloon inflation during PTCA. On the other hand, our results also suggest that even fair collaterals might not be able to protect myocardium completely from ischemia or necrosis at least in the initial minutes of sudden coronary occlusion because ST did elevate during balloon inflation in more than half of the patients of the group 3. Cohen et al.<3>, studying collaterals both prior and during PTCA, reported that 4 of 5 patients showing "fair" collaterals in the angiogram prior to PTCA had "rich" ones during balloon inflation and that none of the 5 patients showed ST elevation. The cause of this apparent discrepancy between their and our results is not clear although the evaluation of the degree of collaterals may be somewhat different. Another possible cause of the discrepancy might be due to the fact that 4 of their 5 patients with "fair" collaterals had critical narrowings in the right coronary artery and only one had in LAD, in which all of our 14 patients of the group 3 had a "target" lesion.

The results of this study show another interesting fact; opposite to the traditional concept that ST elevation indicates complete depletion of coronary arterial flow, ST can elevate when antegrade flow is suddenly cut off even in the presence of partial arterial blood supply from collaterals. Thus, experimental and clinical studies may be needed to elucidate the exact correlationship of ST elevation or depression with decrease of coronary arterial flow.

<Conclusions>

1. Only "rich" collaterals can protect myocardium completely and surely in the very early phase of acute coronary occlusion. However, "poor" or "fair" collaterals can do so although frequently they can only partially. 2. ST elevation can be observed in the presence of collaterals which indicate partial blood supply to the ischemic myocardium.

<References>

1. Flameng, W., Schwartz, F., Hehrlein, FW.: Am J Cardiol. 42, 187-192 (1978)
2. Rentrop, KP., Cohen, M., Blanke, H., Phillips, RA.: J Am Coll Cardiol. 5, 587-592 (1985)
3. Cohen, M., Rentrop KP.: Circulation. 74, 469-476 (1986)

Complete or incomplete right bundle branch block after coronary artery bypass surgery

F.U. HUWEZ and P.W. MACFARLANE.

University Department of Medical Cardiology, Royal Infirmary, Glasgow, Scotland.

INTRODUCTION:

Fascicular conduction defects without peri-operative myocardial infarction have, since 1974, been known (1) to complicate coronary artery bypass grafting (CABG). Later investigations (2-5) confirmed that these defects could be transient or persistent. The conduction defects involved the following: right and left bundle branch blocks (RBBB, LBBB), left anterior or posterior fasicular blocks, all with or without first degree AV block. The reported incidence of these defects varies from 4% to 25% according to different authors (1,2,5), with RBBB being the most common (2,5). There has been interest in studying the aetiology, pathogenesis and effects of these conduction defects on the morbidity and mortality after CABG. The factors so far studied in relation to their pathogenesis include the following: significant coronary artery stenosis ($\geq$ 70%), type of angina pectoris (stable, unstable or post-infarction angina), long standing hypertension, diabetes mellitus, hyperlipidemia, preoperative use of digitalis, duration of symptomatic coronary artery disease, ejection fraction, total bypass time, aortic cross clamp time, effects of cardioplegia, selective cardiac hypothermia and total body hypothermia. In view of the recent recommendations of the W.H.O. Task force on criteria for intraventricular conduction defects (7) and in particular the need for R' > R in V1 or V2 for the diagnosis of incomplete RBBB, it was decided to study those patients who developed right fascicular conduction defects following CABG.

METHODS:

From a series of consecutive computer analysed ECGs, all that exhibited incomplete or complete RBBB in patients after CABG were included in the study provided that they were not associated with intra or peri-operative myocardial infarction, which was excluded by absence of (i) pathological Q waves and (ii) rise of cardiac enzymes. 11 patients who developed such conduction defects were included (Table 1). 4 patients developed complete RBBB and 7 patients developed incomplete RBBB. The age of the patients ranged from 45-74 years with a mean of 60.5 years. They included 8 men and 3 women. All were in sinus rhythm and none had valvular, congenital or pulmonary heart disease or any other disease that might lead to bundle branch block. No patient had complete or incomplete RBBB preoperatively. The following were studied:

1. Pre-operative factors

These included long standing hypertension, previous myocardial infarction, left ventricular hypertrophy, cardiac size, left ventricular function as measured by left ventricular end-diastolic pressure, pre-operative use of digitalis and the number of vessels affected by significant stenosis ($\geq$70 %).

2. Operative factors

Operative factors included total bypass time (TBPT), aortic cross clamp time (ACCT) and the need for end-arterectomy together with CABG.

A control group of 15 consecutive patients without coronary artery disease who underwent aortic valve replacement (AVR) was used for comparison of the effects of TBPT and ACCT on the conduction system.

TABLE I	PATIENT	AGE	SEX	CONDUCTION DEFECT	TBPT (mins)	ACCT (mins)
	1	45	F	IRBBB	125	82
	2	53	M	"	90	53
	3	75	M	COMPLETE	99	62
	4	60	M	"	30	20
	5	59	M	IRBBB	90	41
	6	57	M	"	83	44
	7	72	F	"	120	65
	8	62	M	"	94	36
	9	57	M	"	111	70
	10	56	M	COMPLETE	142	98
	11	67	F	"	98	56
	Mean:	60.3			98.3	57.0

RESULTS:

No patient had pre-operative intake of digitalis, cardiomegaly or left ventricular hypertrophy. Only one patient had hypertension and this was not complicated by left ventricular hypertrophy. Three patients had an old myocardial infarction (one anterior and two inferior). Left ventricular function was normal in six patients (54%) and depressed in the other five (46%), whose left ventricular end-diastolic pressures were $\geq$ 12mm Hg. Only one patient had single vessel disease of the left anterior descending artery (LAD), five had double vessel disease of LAD and either circumflex (CX) or right coronary artery (RCA) while the remaining five patients had severe triple vessel disease. All patients had lesions involving the LAD except one who had double lesions of the CX and RCA.

The total bypass time ranged between 30-142 minutes with a mean of 98.3 $\pm$ 28.8 minutes while the aortic cross clamp time ranged between 20-98 minutes with a mean of 57 $\pm$ 21.9 minutes. The mean total bypasss time and the aortic cross times in the control group were 89.9 $\pm$ 30.3 and 67.4 $\pm$ 25.1 minutes respectively. There was no statistically significant difference between the CABG patients and the control group ($p < 0.05$) with regard to the total bypass and aortic cross clamp times. End-arterectomy was attempted on the right coronary artery in one patient but it failed.

In the control group there were two conduction defects (one complete RBBB and the other LBBB) post-operatively.

DISCUSSION:

Fascicular conduction defects after CABG have been observed in our series. RBBB is encountered more frequently than LBBB probably because the right bundle is thicker and shorter than the left bundle which makes the former more liable to trauma and ischemia than the latter. The aetiology and pathogenesis of these fascicular conduction defects are unknown but it is possible to discuss their relationship with the following factors:

1. <u>Significant coronary artery disease (> 70%)</u>.

In our series, 10 of 11 (91%) patients had multiple vessel disease almost always involving the LAD and of these 5 out of 10 had triple vessel disease. This finding is consistent with an earlier report of Wexelman et al (5) who found that post-operative fascicular conduction defects are associated with the most severe cases of coronary artery disease. That group also found a good correlation between conduction defects and significant disease of the left main stem and posterior descending artery. While Sharma et al (3) did not observe RBBB or left posterior hemiblock in their series, they found good correlation between LBBB or left anterior hemiblock and significant disease of the left anterior descending artery (LAD) either proximally or involving the first septal perforating branch.

2. <u>Prolonged total bypass and aortic cross clamp times</u>.

The mean total bypass time in the CABG patients was 98.3 minutes while in the control group it was 89.9 minutes (NS $p > 0.05$). The longer time for CABG patients is in agreement with earlier reports (2, 5). The mean aortic cross clamp time in the control group was greater (67.4 minutes) than in the CABG patients (57 minutes) but there was no statistically significant difference between the two groups ($p > 0.05$). The control group, who did not have CABG, was deliberately chosen to avoid the effects of CAD and to allow the effect of bypass or cross clamp time only to be studied. Therefore, it can concluded from these data that the development of conduction defects postoperatively is not related to total bypass or aortic cross clamp times.

3. <u>Selective hypothermic cardioplegia</u>.

In our patients only selective hypothermic cardioplegia was used and no comparison could be made with total body hypothermia. There have been conflicting reports in this respect. Selective hypothermic cardioplegia was more frequently associated with new fascicular conduction defects than total body hypothermia according to one study (4), although Zeldis (2) did not any find difference between total body hypothermia and selective cardiac hypothermia or between different types of cardioplegic solutions.

4. <u>Pre-operative use of digitalis</u>.

In the present study, there was no patient who was previously on digitalis although serum digitalis levels were not measured. Digitalis does not affect the infranodal conduction system (6), yet in two earlier studies (2,5) preoperative digitalis was significantly associated with new fascicular conduction defects after CABG.

5. <u>Long standing hypertension</u>.

In our patients only one had hypertension without left ventricular hypertrophy while in the remainder neither LVH nor cardiomegaly was found. This indirectly indicates that LV dysfunction is not important in the pathogenesis of postoperative conduction defects. In one other study only (5), long standing hypertension showed good correlation with new fascicular conduction defects post CABG. This was explained by associated LVH and myocardial fibrosis.

6. **Left ventricular dysfunction.**

Left ventricular end-diastolic pressure was $\geq$ 12mm Hg in 5 out of 11 (46%) patients in our series which is consistent with an earlier report (5) that LV dysfunction was not clearly correlated with fascicular conduction defects after CABG.

Coronary end-arterectomy was not required in 10 out of 11 (91%) of our patients. It therefore seems unlikely that end-arterectomy of the coronary arteries is the cause of fascicular conduction defects after CABG operations. However, factors such as the duration or type of angina, diabetes mellitus, hyperlipidemia, ejection fraction < 50% (5) or type of cardioplegic solutions have not been correlated with these fascicular blocks (2,4). Recently it was found (5) that new fascicular conduction defects did not affect recurrence of angina and mortality at 18 months post-operatively.

Part of the reason for undertaking the study was to utilise the new WHO criteria for incomplete Right Bundle Branch Block. These specify that the QRS duration should be < 120ms while for complete RBBB it should be in excess of this value. It seems that this value is somewhat arbitrary although, of course, it has been used in electro- cardiography for many years. Some authors favour 110 msecs. as a borderline value. A few of the ECGs reported as having incomplete Right Bundle Branch Block had a QRS duration in excess of 110ms at least as measured by the Glasgow Program. It would therefore appear to be meaningless to attach any weight to the development of complete versus incomplete Right Bundle Branch Block.

There have been arguments in the past as to whether the rSr' pattern in V1 represented a significant abnormality or whether it was simply a manifestation of basal RV depolarisation. The finding of the production of conduction defects following coronary artery surgery would lend weight to the view that incomplete RBBB is more than simply a descriptive term.

In conclusion, complete or incomplete RBBB after CABG was found to be most strongly associated with severe coronary artery disease.

REFERENCES

(1) Satinsky J., Collins J.J. Jr., Dalen R.E: Circulation. 49,50 (suppl), 170(1974).
(2) Zeldis S.M., Morganroth J., Horowitz LN et al: Am J Cardiol. 41, 860 (1978).
(3) Sharma G. J Am Coll Cardiol. 3, 529 (1984)
(4) O'Connell J.B., Wallis D., Johnson S.A. et al: Am Heart J. 103, 85 (1982).
(5) Wexelman W., Lichstein E., Cunningham J.N. et al: Am Heart J. 111, 923 (1986).
(6) Damato A.N., Lau S.H: Prog Cardiovasc. Dis. 13, 119-40 (1970).
(7) Willems J.L. et al: W.H.O. Task Force ad Hoc. JACC. 5, 1261-75 (1985).

New aspects of classifying intraventricular conduction disturbances

FLEISCHMANN, H.-J., ROSTOCK, K.-J., RATHGEN, K.
Government hospital, Scharnhorststraße 36, Berlin 1040, GDR

Programmed right atrial stimulation was applied in order to investigate the different forms of aberrant conduction. Surface ECG, His bundle electrogram and horizontal loop of the VCG (Frank method) were recorded in 101 patients. Besides all forms of usual conduction disturbances PRAS also revealed two unrecognized special disturbances. These were characterized by a prominent anterior force or by a reduced anterior force according to a posterior deviation in the horizontal loop. VCG material of apparently healthy men revealed also the same special forms of conduction disturbances. The conclusion is, that conduction disturbances do not only occur as left or right axis deviation in the frontal plane. They may also appear solely as anterior or as posterior deviation in the horizontal plane.

Some unsolved problems exist in the field of electrophysiological function of His-Purkinje-system. First it may be mentioned the discrepancy beetween anatomically and electrophysiologically postulated trifascicular structure. The concept by ROSENBAUM (1) of the left bundle branch being bifascicular, therefore appears as an oversimplification since in most cases the structure should better be termed trifascicular or fan-like (2). ECG-alterations, which would correspond to a lesion of the midseptal fascicle, more than once are described as an anterior displacement (AD) of QRS horizontal loop (3, 4, 5, 6).

The fact, that for the definition of disturbed intraventricular conduction only one plane, the frontal plane, comes into consideration, is pointed out as a second shortcoming of the actual electrophysiological concept (8). The criteria of left anterior fascicular block (LAFB) and left posterior fascicular block (LPFB) are generally established and their main criterion is represented by the axis deviation in the frontal plane (7). If intraventricular conduction is characterized as a spatial process, it is not possible to define it sufficiently by one plane only. A second plane is absolutely necessary to record all possibilities of disturbed intraventricular conduction (8).

Programmed right atrial stimulation (PRAS) was applied in order to investigate the different forms of aberrant conduction. Complete spatial recording of the intraventricular conduction is effected by surface ECG for the frontal plane and by VCG for the horizontal plane.

PRAS was applied in the usual way (8) to 101 patients (average age 48,3 years). Single premature atrial stimuli were delivered after every eight spontaneous beat at progressively decreasing 10-msec coupling intervals until effective refractory period (ERP) of the atrioventricular (AV) nodal or ventricular specialized conduction system was reached. As a second step of our investigations we searched our VCG material for analogous, unusually changed VCG loops. The same unrecognized intraventricular conduction disturbance manifest in apparently healthy men, was a prerequisite for the selection.

Table 1:

Frequency and type of induced conduction disturbances during PRAS in dependence on function of AV node

Group		n	ERP – AVN (ms) $\bar{x}$	±	s
I	not any intraventricular conduction disturbance	20	545		133
II	initial induced intraventricular conduction disturbance	33	431		58
	AD	14			
	PD	19			
III	initial and secondary induced intraventricular conduction disturbance	48	411		46
	AD → RBBB → LBBB	31			
	PD → RBBB → LBBB	17			
		101			

Intraventricular conduction disturbances were induced in 81 of 101 patients. Beginning with a prematurity of 400 $\pm$ 40 ms the first intraventricular conduction disturbances, to be characterized initialy inducible, could be triggered. The changes of intraventricular conduction were slightly, different in graduation but unequivocally recognizable by two opposite configuration in the horizontal loop of the VCG. In 45 cases an anterior deviation (AD, figure 1) of the horizontal QRS loop was obtained whilst 36 cases revealed the opposite configuration, a posterior deviation (PD, figure 2) of horizontal QRS loop. By increasingly premature atrial extrastimuli from 380 $\pm$ 60 ms in 48 cases in group III additional intraventricular conduction disturbances were induced and characterized as secondarily inducible. All the secondary induced conduction disturbances correspond to usual catergories of intraventricular blocks. The QRS

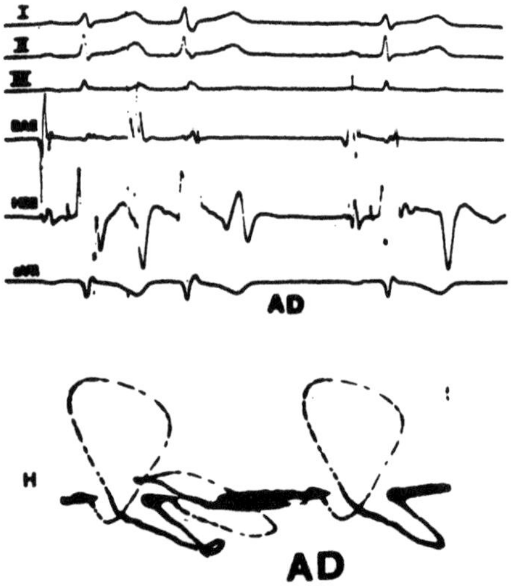

Figure 1.:

Typical example of anterior deviation (AD) during PRAS

loop of AD is characterized by an increase in amplitude and duration of the anterior forces, the left maximum horizontal vector is moved to anterior and right side, and the terminal vectors and the T loop are modified. PD is characterized by a decrease or even a loss of the anterior forces.
Furthermore we could detect in our VCG material which comprises about 3 000 VCG's, changed vector loops analogous to AD or PD, in apparently healthy men. We indentified 44 cases which correspond to AD (figure 3) and 21 cases corresponding to PD (figure 4). High R-wave in the right precordial leads and complete anterior deviation in the horizontal loop characterize AD. Loss of R in the right precordial leads and loss of anterior forces in the horizontal loop demonstrate the typical signs of PD.

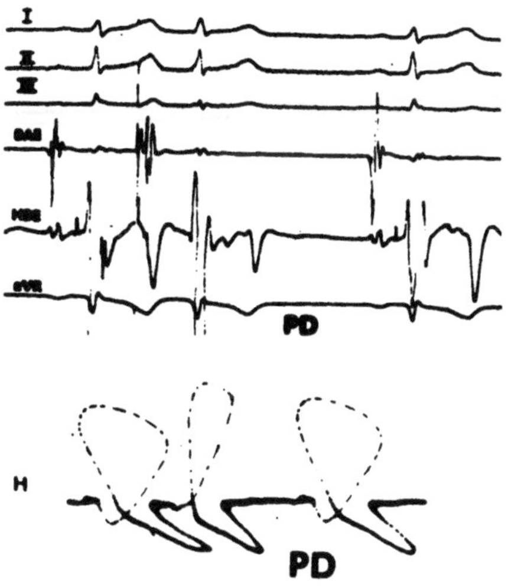

Figure 2:
Typical example of posterior deviation (PD) during PRAS

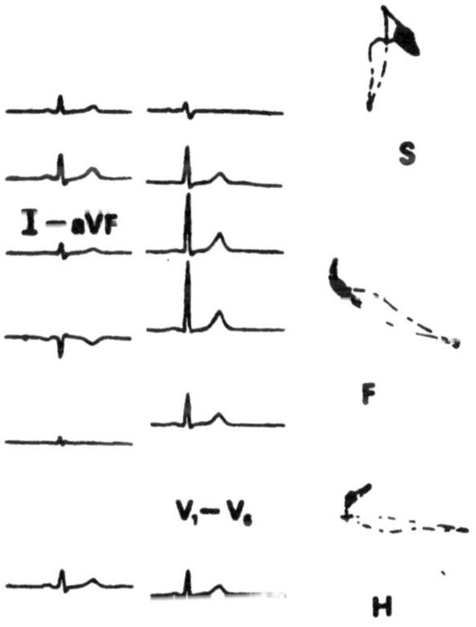

Figure 3:
Typical example of anterior deviation (AD) from a 28 years old healthy woman

- Conduction disturbances do not only occur as left or right axis deviation in the frontal plane, they may also appear solely as anterior or posterior deviation in the horizontal plane
  The frontal and horizontal plan taken into consideration when defining a disturbed intraventricular conduction will guarantee complete registration of all possibilities of disturbed intraventricular conduction within space.
- The localization of AD or PD within the conduction system is difficult. In our opinion AD is dependent on the right ventricular conduction and PD on the left ventricular conduction. That means AD is interpreted as precursor of complete right bundle branch block and PD as precursor of complete left bundle branch block.
  A delaly within the conduction system is demonstrate by a change of direction of intraventricular conduction, which could be evident independently both in

the frontal and in the horizontal plane. A block within the conduction system is demonstrated by a change of direction and time of intraventricular conduction.

- The evaluation of a high or poor R-wave in the right precordial leads may be explained not only by hypertrophy or infarction but also by a disturbed intraventricular conduction.

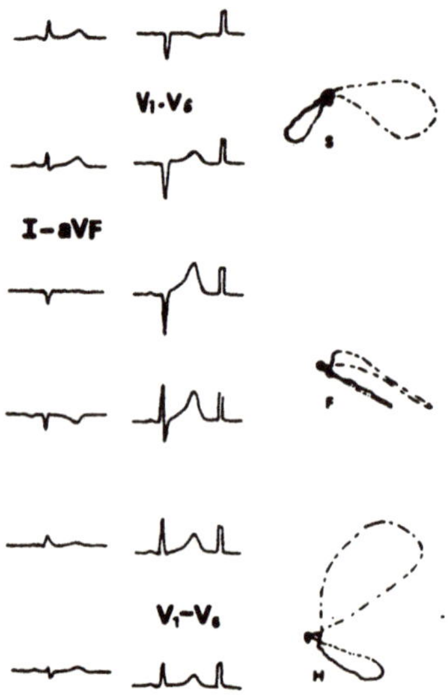

Figure 4:

Typical example of posterior deviation (PD) from a 36 years old healthy man

(1) Rosenbaum, M., M. Elizari, J. Lazzari, G. Nau, R. Levi, M. Halpern
Am. Heart J. 78, 450 - 459 (1969)

(2) Kulbertus, H., J. Demoulin
Schweiz. med. Wschr. 112, 1579 - 1584 (1982)

(3) Hoffmann, J., M. Jawahar, J. Hilsenrath, R. Hamby
J. Electrocardiol. 9, 15 - 21 (1976)

(4) Kulbertus, H., F. De Leval-Rutten, P. Casters
Br. Heart J. 38, 549 - 557 (1976)

(5) De Padua, F., D. Dos Reis, V. Lopes, J. Miguel, M. Lopes, D. Da Siva, I. De Padua
Adv. Cardiol. 21, 242 - 248 (1978)

(6) Piccolo, E., P. Delise, A. Raviele, D. D'Este, G. Totaro, B. De Piccolo, L. Autusi, R. Cazzin
J. Electrocardiol. 13, 267 - 274 (1980)

(7) Willems, J., E. De Medina et al
J. Am. Coll. Cardiol. 5, 1261 - 1275 (1985)

(8) Fleischmann, H.-J., K.-J. Rostock
Z. gesamte inn. Med. 42, 151 - 155 (1987)

Influence of quinidine versus procainamide on the QT interval

BÉLA,KISS., QUI, CUONG., TIVADAR, JAKAB

Postgraduate Medical School, Budapest, Hungary

Summary

27 patients were given quinidine and procainamide separately to evaluate whether prolongation of the QT interval by type Ia antiarrhythmic agents is a drug specific phenomenon. The increase of the QT interval was significantly greater with quinidine than with procainamide. The greater degree of QT prolongation with quinidine than with procainamide was not due to differences in sinus cycle length, QRS duration.

Introduction

An ECG pattern with long QT interval is known to be associated with ventricular arrhythmias. Such ECG changes can be due to a variety of factors such as drugs (1). Effects of different antiarrhythmic agents on the QT interval are not well understood. We have therefore investigated the comparative effects of quinidine and procainamide on the QT interval

Material and method

27 patients participated in the study. QRS duration, QT and RR intervals were measured during sinus rhythm from a standard 12-lead ECG recorded before and after giving quinidine versus procainamide. For each patient the QT interval was measured from onset of the Q wawe to the end of the T wawe which was determined by the intersection of a tangent drawn to the steepest slope of the downsloping portion of the T wawe and isoelectric base line. Doses of both drugs were close to the traditionally accepted midtherapeutic range. The QT interval was corrected for rate with Bazett's formula. Differences were analysed using a paired t test (2).

Results

In 24 of the 27 patients the increase in the corrected QT interval (QTc) was greater with quinidine than with procainamide. The control QTc interval was $0{,}431 \pm 0{,}007$ second. The QTc interval was $0{,}469 \pm 0{,}008$ second after administration of procainamide and $0{,}509 \pm 0{,}011$ second after quinidine. Mean QTc interval prolongation was $0{,}038 \pm 0{,}006$ second for procainamide and $0{,}078 \pm 0{,}010$ second for quinidine ($p < 0{,}001$). The difference between quinidine and procainamide QTc intervals was statistically significant by a paired t test ($p < 0{,}001$, Fig.1).

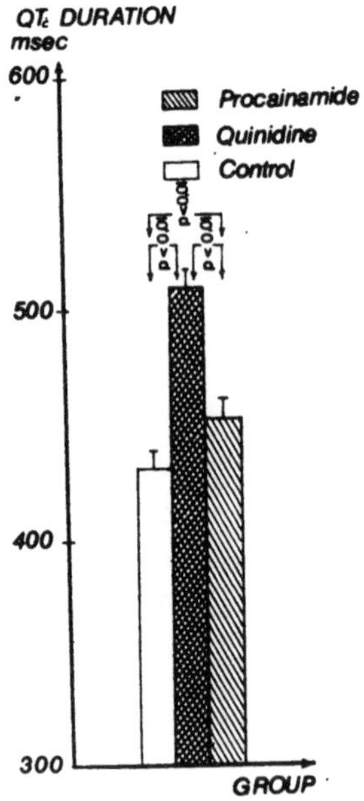

Figure 1. Corrected QT interval for all 27 patients without antiarrhythmic therapy and during therapy with procainamide and quinidine

The greater degree of QTc interval prolongation with quinidine was independent of the control QRS duration. Sinus cycle lengths were not significantly different during procainamide or quinidine administration (Fig.2).

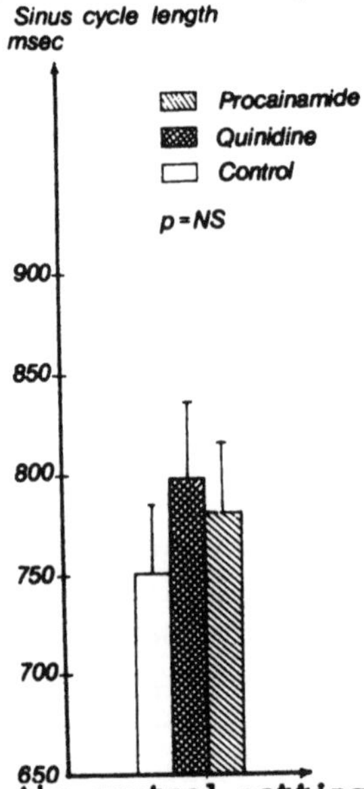

Figure 2. Sinus cycle length in the control setting and during treatment with quinidine and procainamide

Discussion

The association between prolonged QT interval and ventricular arrhythmias has been discussed in various situations. The QT interval is an electrocardiographic approximation of total ventricular depolarization and repolarization duration. The QT interval changes with a variety of factors which may be grouped into two categories. The first one is in the form of hereditary prolonged QT interval. The second category includes an aquired form of prolonged QT as caused by potassium, magnesium and calcium levels, drugs, e.g. quinidine. Quinidine is the antiarrhythmic agent most frequently associated with torsades. This arrhythmia is the principal cause of quinidine syncope (3). A similar incidence of procainamide syncope is not recognized. If the risk of torsades is related to the degree of QT interval prolongation then our study offers an explanation for the apparent lower incidence of torsades developing with procainamide

References

(1) Ward,O.C: J.Irish Med. Ass. 54, 103-109 (1964)
(2) Juvancz,I., A,Paksy: Orvosi Biometria. Budapest. p: 78-80 (1982)
(3) Reynolds,E.W., C.Vander: Mod. Concepts Cardiovasc. Dis. 45, 117-122 (1976)

S-A Block, Sinus Parasystole, S-A Dissociation
Semantics of Terms

JAROSLAV JEDLIČKA

Cardiac Laboratory, IInd Department of Medicine, Charles University
U nemocnice 2, 128 08 Prague 2, Czechoslovakia

SUMMARY: This review of S-A conduction disturbances passes criticism on the denomination "sinus parasystole" coined for parasystole-like protection of the S-A node during bidirectional S-A block. The revived notion of "S-A dissociation" and its discrimination from S-A block are presented.

The mechanism as well as nomenclature of S-A conduction disturbances are similar to those of A-V conduction disorders but their recognition may be difficult owing to the fact that sinus node activity is not registered in standard ECGs and is not possible at all in first degree S-A block. In third degree S-A block, on the other hand, the distinction between block and sinus standstill may be impracticable. The discrimination of Type I and Type II in second degree S-A block is feasible in the case of an absolutely regular sinus rhythm only.

The common diagnosis "S-A block" refers mostly to an anterograde S-A block as exemplified in Fig. 1. In Fig. 2 from the same record a premature atrial beat with a fully compensatory pause is present which indicates that sinus activity was not disturbed (shifted) by this ectopic atrial depolarization. In this situation, therefore, retrograde S-A (or A-S) block was present analogous to a protection block of an ectopic (parasystolic) focus. Finally, in Fig. 3, both anterograde and retrograde S-A block are manifested: the former causing a sinus pause equal to four P-P cycles and the latter is evidenced by the fact that retrograde atrial activation between A-V junctional escape and ventricular echo did not alter sinus rhythm; here, the diagnosis "bidirectional S-A block" is justified.

Bidirectional S-A block is a very rare phenomenon first published in 1960 (1). A similar observation from 1967 (2) suggests its denomination "sinus parasystole" which is a contradiction in terms - sinus rhythm cannot be <u>para</u>systolic (though sinus node protection in these cases is parasystole-<u>like</u>). - Retrograde S-A block is to be differentiated from simple interference of sinus and atrial ectopic (retrograde) impulses, the result being the same: a fully compensatory pause (Fig. 4).

The repetition of this event, i.e., interference of sinus impulses with normal or prolonged refractoriness of the S-A perinodal tissue in the

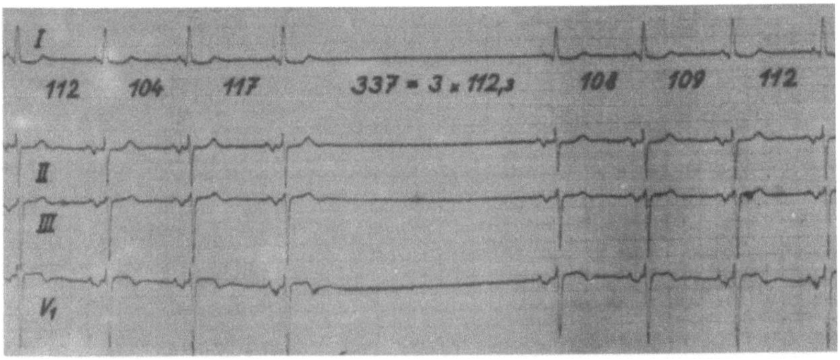

Fig. 1. Case 1. Male 59 years old with ischemic heart disease. Anterograde S-A block. Time in s/100.

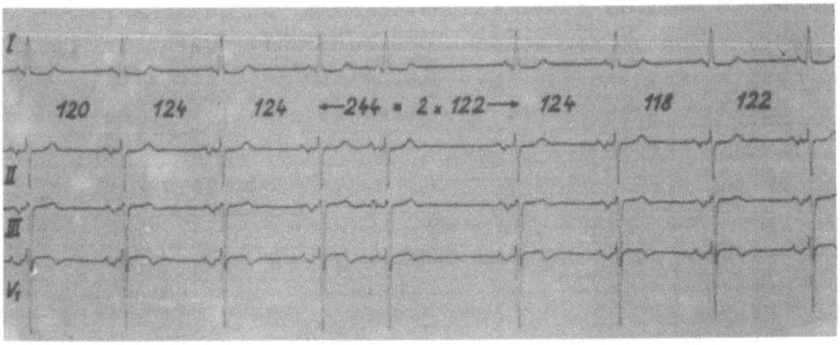

Fig. 2. Case 1. Retrograde S-A block. Time in s/100. Discussed in text.

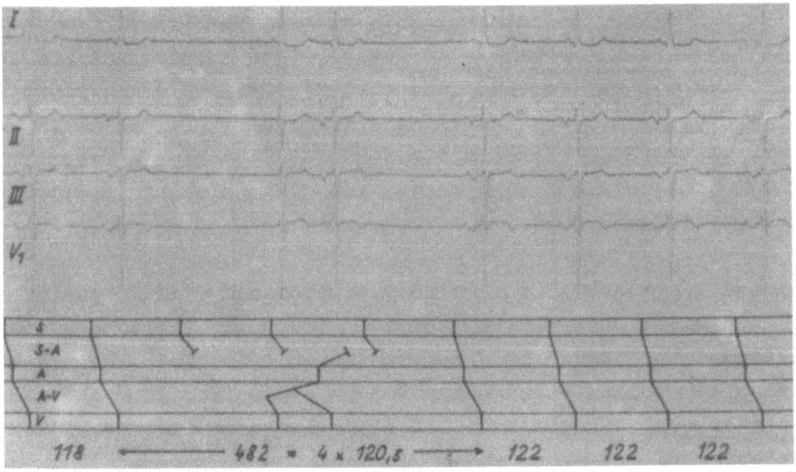

Fig. 3. Case 1. Bidirectional S-A block. Time in s/100. - See text for details.

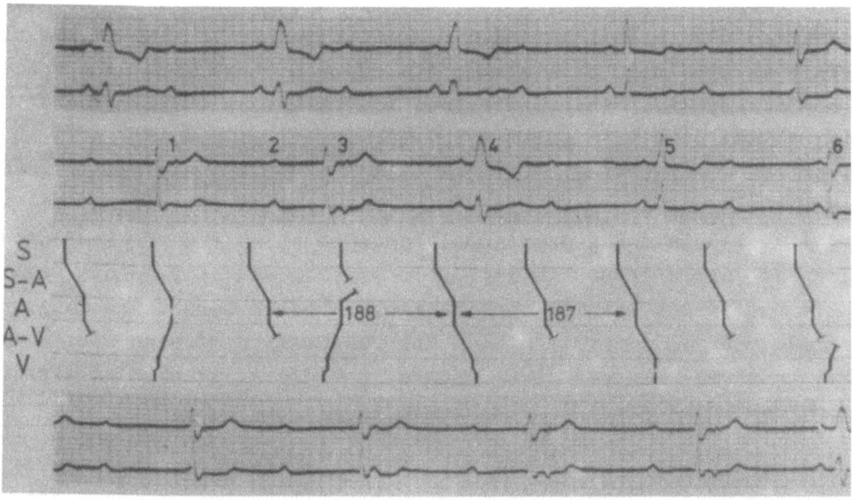

Fig. 4. Case 2. Male 75 years old with ischemic heart disease. Continuous record of Leads I and II. Advanced A-V block, LBBB of sinus beats, idioventricular rhythm of RBBB type. Note: sinus P (2) + retrograde P (3) = fusion P (1); sinus QRS (4) + idioventricular QRS (6) = fusion QRS (5). - Time in s/100. - Discussed in text.

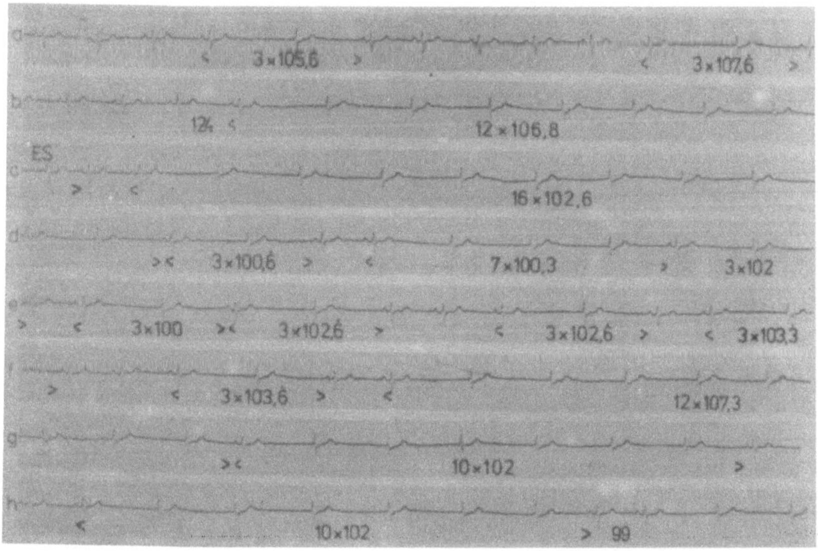

Fig. 5. Case 3. Female 41 years old with atrial septal defect. Continuous record of Lead I. Respiratory sinus arrhythmia: longest P-P (124) in b, shortest P-P (99) in h. Respiratorily induced S-A block - in addition S-A dissociation operating in longest sinus pauses. - Time in s/100. - See text for details.

wake of ectopic atrial activation, creates a condition analogous to A-V dissociation (3). Its label "S-A dissociation" is lacking in the electrocardiographic language - with one exception where used as a speculative and alternative interpretation (4). A unique observation of this pattern illustrates this point (Fig. 5). At first glance, it is an example of sinus arrhythmia with S-A block and A-V junctional escapes during sinus pauses, mostly with retrograde atrial activation. It is of interest that only those junctional escapes which are the last ones in the longest sinus pauses (multiples of 10, 12 and 16 P-P intervals) do not have retrograde atrial activation, in other words: the failure of retrograde atrial activation made the restoration of sinus rhythm possible. In these longest sinus pauses, therefore, it was S-A dissociation and not anterograde S-A block per se prolonging them.

In S-A dissociation - in contrast to A-V dissociation - only electrical and not mechanical dissociation is meant. It is self-evident that the discrimination between S-A block and S-A dissociation - similarly as between A-V block and A-V dissociation - is not only of academical, but of foremost clinical and therapeutical importance.

REFERENCES

(1) Jedlička, J.: Acta Univ. Carol. 6, 235 - 238 (1960)
(2) Schamroth, L.: Am. J. Cardiol. 3, 434 - 435 (1967)
(3) Jedlička, J.: X World Congress of Cardiol., Washington 1986. Abstract Book, p. 401
(4) Katz, L. N., and A. Pick: Clinical Electrocardiography. Part I. The Arrhythmias. Lea a. Febiger, Philadelphia 1956, p. 339

The differentiation of incomplete right bundle branch block /inc.RBBB/ and right ventricular strain /RVS/ by the spatial angular velocity

MEDVEGY,M., BALOGH,I., MAJOR,L., ANTALÓCZY,Z.

Postgraduate Medical University, 2nd Med.Dept.
Hungary-1389 Budapest, Pf.112

Summary

We state the electrical criteria in cases of systolic and diastolic overloading of right ventricle. In these cases the width of QRS remains below 0.10 sec. The right diastolic overloading is characterised by a terminal "r'" wave in V_1 lead, its absence a considerable right diastolic overloading can be excluded. If there is no diastolic overloading, the ECG sign of the systolic overloading is the "S" wave in lateral leads, whose width correlates with the right ventricular pressure /RVP/. When repolarisatical deviation can be observed in the inferior and right unipolar leads we speak of right ventricular strain /RVS/. If these cases are combined with right side intraventricular conduction defect /= inc.RBBB/, the QRS becomes wider, the terminal resultant vector significantly turns forward. The inc.RBBB can hardly be differentiated from the right ventricular /RV/ diastolic overloading on the traditional ECG, but the spatial angular velocity /saV/ curve helps to differentiate them, because in the cases of inc.RBBB the saV curve shows a high third peak, in contrast with cases without inc.RBBB, where the 3rd peak stays low.

Purpose of the study

We were studiing the electrical signs in cases of systolic and diastolic overloading of right ventricle, and in cases of their serious forms: in the RVS and inc.RBBB. The aim: to recognise and differentiate these cases and to estimate the mesurement of the RVP.

Patients and methods

106 patients with RV systolic or diastolic overloading were studied with invasive and non invasive methods. In these cases we have studied the ECG /mainly the I., III., aVL., V_1, V_2, V_6 leads/, Frank-leads, the triaxicardiogram /1/ /spatial magnitude: **M** /2/, azimuth angle: H^o, elevation angle: V^o/, spatial velocity /sV/ /3/, spatial angular velocity /saV/. The saV is a new vectorial parameter written by us. The saV curve shows the spatial angular changes of the resultant vector in each moment /4/

Results

a., We have found diastolic overloading in the following cases:
14 atrial septum defects /ASD/, the average RVP was 37/7.7 Hgmm,
6 tricuspidal insufficiencies /relative, too/ /average RVP: 61/7.5 Hgmm/.
The following electrical signs were seen: wide "S" wave in tho lateral

leads /aVL, I., V_6/, "rsr'" or"rsR" + negative "T" in the V_1 lead. The M showed two components, the second peak, wich represents the activation of the basises of left and right ventricles /5/ was lower. Its direction: H^o: 180°, V^o: -20°. The sV and saV curves had 3 peaks, two higher and a third lower ones.

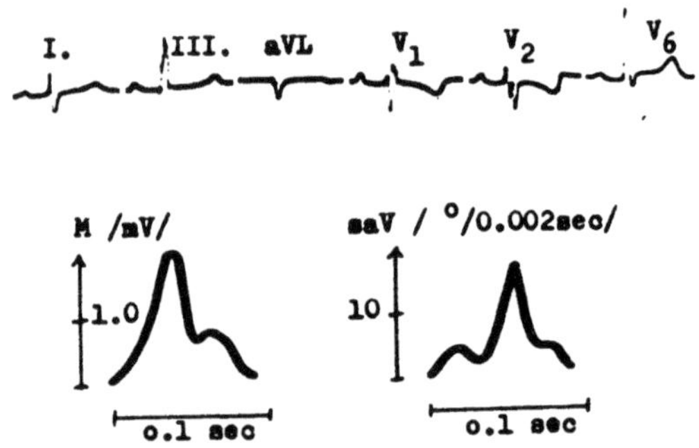

1. figure
The typical electrical picture of the RV diastolic overloading /ASD, the RVP: 36/4 Hgmm/

b., We have found middling RV systolic overloading in the following cases /the average RVP is in brackets/: 32 mitral stenosises /56/8 Hgmm/, 20 other viciums /51/9 Hgmm/, 14 ischaemical heart diseases /44/9 Hgmm/. The ECG deviation was only the "S" wave in the lateral leads. The M showed 2 peaks, the second one was lower, its direction: H^o: 160°, V^o: -20°. The sV and saV curves were similar to the diastolic overloading.

c., We could find serious form of RV systolic or diastolic overloading /=RVS/ by the following patients: 6 ASD /54/11 Hgmm/, 4 primaer pulmonal hypertonies /PPH/ /110/23 Hgmm/, 3 mitral stenosises /128/16 Hgmm/, 3 mitral stenosises + other vicium + relative tricuspidal insufficiency /118/19 Hgmm/. The electrical signs were: wide "S" wave in the lateral leads, "Rs", "rs" or + terminal "r'" or "R'" and negative "T" wave in the V_1 lead. The M showed 2 peaks, but here the second one was higher. That means: the proportion of the mass of right and left ventricles changed in favour of right ventricle, its direction: H^o: 160°, V^o: -20°.

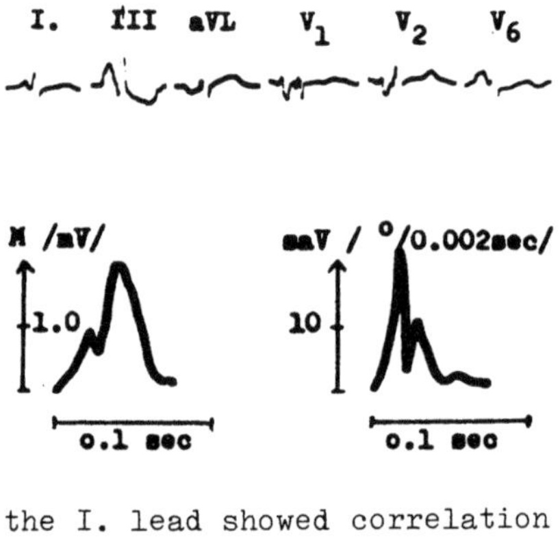

2. figure
A typical electrical picture of the RVS /Mitral stenosis, the RVP: 90/16 Hgmm/

d., The width of "S" wave in the I. lead showed correlation with the RVP in our cases. /But: time of QRS and morphology of V_1 were normal, RV diastolic overloading is out of the question/. We had 16 patients

With 0.04 or more "S" width in I. lead, the average systolic RVP was 68 Hgmm. We could not see "S" wave in every cases, especialy, where also a left ventricular overloading was with high RVP. The direction of the terminal electrical activation was backword and on the left in these cases, and rarely a break on the QRS in I. lead - a quasi positiv "S" - can be seen. This sign refers to a high RVP.

3. figure
We can see such a I. lead of ECG
/Mitral insufficiency, grad.III., RVP: 59/5 Hgmm/

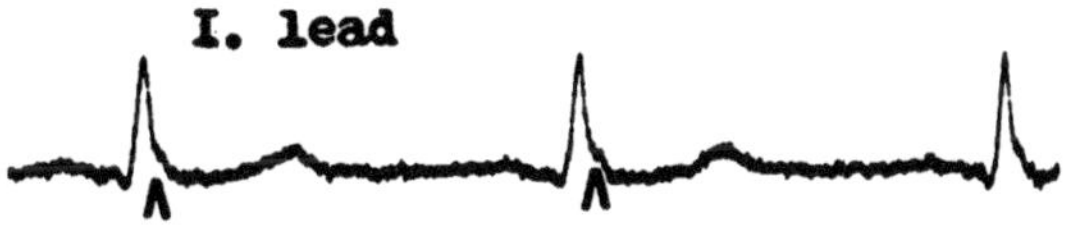

e., Among above cases we found 10 inc.RBBB / 3 ASD /52/3 Hgmm/, 3 PPH /107/15 Hgmm/, 2 mitral stenosises with other vicium + relative tricuspidal insufficiency /63/3 Hgmm/, 1 Ebstein disease /24/5 Hgmm/, 1 pulmonal emboly/. We think of the inc.RBBB, that some of the Purkinje fibres of the right Tawara bundle branch were injured due to the tightening of the RV wall. The area belonging to the blocked Purkinje fibres becomes stimulated later by myogen way, therefore terminally the resultant electrical vector moves forward to this area, and the saV curve shows a high third peak. Without intraventricular conduction defect the terminal resultant vector does not move forward, and the 3rd component of the saV curve remains low.

4. figure
The saV curve in RVS and inc.RBBB.

/The saV curves in both groups were averaged by qualitative and quantitative methods: we averaged the minimal and maximal values and the proportions of their time intervals and QRS. 12 cases of RVS, 8 cases of inc.RBBB./

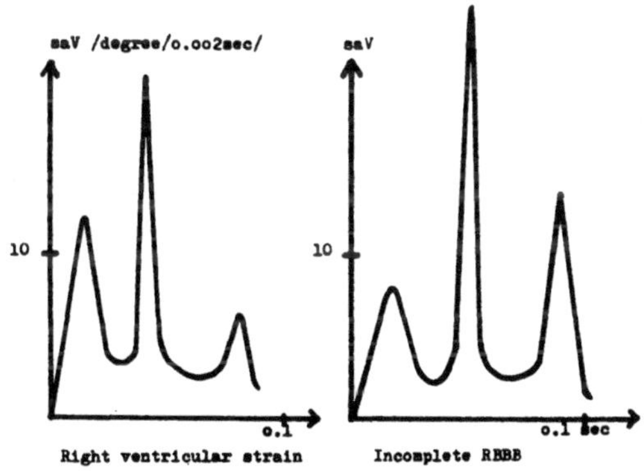

The ECG does not show a specific sign, because the picture of inc.RBBB is corresponding to the picture of the RV diastolic overloading. A wider QRS time /0.09 - 0.11 sec/ and a break of the terminal "R'" wave in V_1, or the presence of the "r'" wave in V_2 lead may sign an inc. RBBB, however the presence of the "r'" wave in V_1 does not pruve the inc.RBBB.

5. figure
A typical electrical picture of the inc.RBBB /Primaer pulmonal hypertony, the RVP: 80/25 Hgmm/

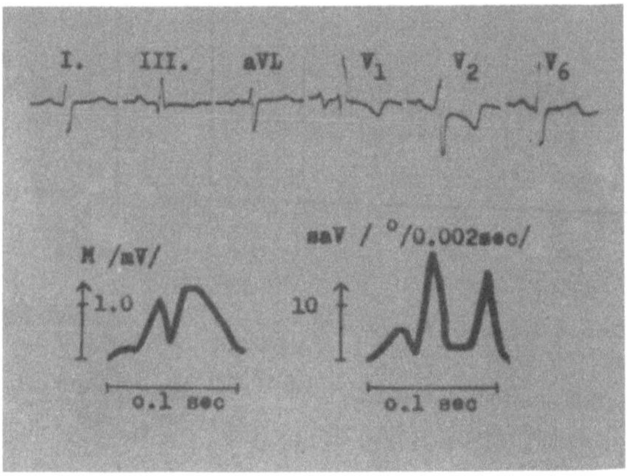

Conclusions

The importance of our study in cases of narrow QRS:

1., Terminal "r'" or "R'" wave in V_1 lead on ECG can alvays be seen in RV diastolic overloading, without this sign a significant RV diastolic overloading can be eliminated.

2., Without this sign the "S" wave in the lateral ECG leads corresponds to an increased RVP, the 0.04 sec or wider "S" wave in standard I. lead means high RVP.

3., The saV is a suitable method to differentiate the RVS and the inc.RBBB.

References

/1/ Antalóczy et al.: Magyar szabadalom 157366 /A61 b./ /1968/
/2/ Antalóczy et al.: Acta Med.Hung. 31., 201 /1974/
/3/ Medvegy et al.: Számitástechnikai 12. Neumann Kollokvium, Szeged, Előadások anyaga 254-261 /1984/
/4/ Medvegy et al.: XII. International Congress on Electrocardiology, Minsk, Abstract book 191 /1985/
/5/ Durrer, D. et al.: Circ. 41., 899-912 /1970/

HIS - ECG

LATE POTENTIALS

Late ventricular potentials and their representation on the instant topograms.

R.Z.Amirov
The Central Scientific Research Institute of Health Resort and Physical Treatment.
The Kalinin Prospect 50, Moscow, USSR.

Summary.
At the end of QRS period electrocardiotopography reveals a rapid change of the body surface potentials, which is called inversion I. At the top of T wave there is a changed charge polarity, which is called inversion II. In the patients with RBBB there is a disturbed inversion I seen as a sign of the effect of the left ventricular contractions. Inversion II is noted in acquired cardiac defects, which appears under the effect of regurgitation on the electrical field of the heart. These disturbances of the potentials are seen as late ventricular potentials. Registration of inversion of the potentials and their disturbance has become feasible by means of amplification of cardiac potentials and of use of a sum of all leads as an indifferent electrode.

Introduction. Our studies have revealed the changed shape of the cardiac electrical field, which is a spatial representation of late ventricular potentials (LVP) and which has been previously known as the disturbed inversion of potentials (1,2,3).

In the recent years a number of scientists paid attention to feasibility of registration of changes at the beginning of ST interval and at the top of T wave, which had been called late ventricular potentials (4,5,6).

The aim of this study is to show spatial characteristics of LVP and to present their interpretation.

Material and methods. Over 200 patients and healthy persons were examined by means of instant electrocardiotopography and in 60 patients late ventricular potentials were registered by means of averaging on "Neuropack physiological response recorder MEB-3102 and averager DAT-3202 Corporation Nihon Kohden.

Results. Instant topography (ECTG) allows to reveal rapid changes of the potential polarity at the end of QRS period and at the top of T wave. The first change of potentials is called inversion I and the second change seen at the top of T wave is called inversion II.

Inversion I assumes, that electronegativity seen in the anterior pericardial region at the end of QRS period is replaced rapidly by electropositivity corresponding to the beginning of ST interval. On the rest of chest surface potentials are being also changed. Inversion I shows, that in ST interval there exists a difference of potentials: electropositivity in the pericardial region and electronegativity on the rest of chest surface. Instant topography allows to to determine dislocations of ST interval in healthy persons and in patients, but not in all patients with heart disease 12-lead CG reveals displacement of ST interval. Disturbances of inversion I are seen in the patients with a ventricular hyperfunction as a transient moment and incomplete inversion of potentials. However, in the patients with RBBB disturbances of inversion I are very marked. In the patients with RBBB there is a changed relief of the electrical field seen as combination of continuing QRS period and beginning inversion of potentials at the end of QRS period. Fig.1 shows cineframes of QRS period in patient Ju. with RBBB. Frame 10 shows, that the anteriorly located electronegativity zone has acquired a positive charge caused by the left ventricular contraction (shown with an arrow).

Inversion II may have another specific feature: a) slowing and a transient moment; b) marked disturbance of a noncompleted character seen, for example, in the patients with cardiac defects; c) partial falling out in the patients with the anterior wall aneurysm.

Discussion and conclusions.

Feasibility of registration of inversion I and II of cardiac potentials and of various types of the disturbed inversions may be explained by the fact, that instant ECTG implies high amplification of potentials and that a sum of all potentials from all leads is used as an indifferent electrode. Thanks to this fact a polarity change, that is, potential inversion is registered on an instant topogram at the top of T wave and potentials are lowered on ECG with Wilson's indifferent electrode.

Registration of changes in the cardiac electrical field seen as inversions and their disturbances depends, most probably, on the effect of mechanical factors arizing during myocardial contractions. Disturbances of inversion I seen in the patients with RBBB may be explained by the effect of the beginning left ventricular contraction which changes a configuration and "dissipates" partially the electronegativity zone at the end of QRS period. Disturbances of inversion II in the patients with acquired cardiac defects result most probably from blood regurgitation in a diastole and from the delayed contraction of one of the ventricles. In the patients with the anterior postinfarction cardiac aneurysm a partial disturbance of inversion II may be explained by changes in the myocardial tension at the aneurysm site.

Conclusions: instant electrocardiotopography has allowed to reveal changes in the cardiac potentials at the end of QRS period and at the top of T wave designated as inversion I and II respectively. In the patients with heart disease various variants of disturbance of inversions have been established. Inversion of cardiac potentials and its disturbance are in essence late ventricular potentials. Instant electrocardiotopography contributes to their meticulous study.

References.

(1) Amirov, R.Z. Kardiologia,2, 55-57 (1987).

(2) Amirov, R.Z. Elektrokardiotopographie. Akademie-Verlag. Berlin, (1974).

(3) Amirov, R.Z. In: Aktuelle Probleme der Vektorkardiographie. Wien,Stuttgart Verlag Thieme, 21-27 (1968).

(4) Korsukewitz, J. et al. Z. Kardiol. 71, 697-702 (1982).

(5) Coto, C.M., Flowers,N.C. Circulation 68,suppl. III, 362-367 (1983)

(6) Erne, S.N. et al. J.Electrocardiol. 18, 315-322 (1985).

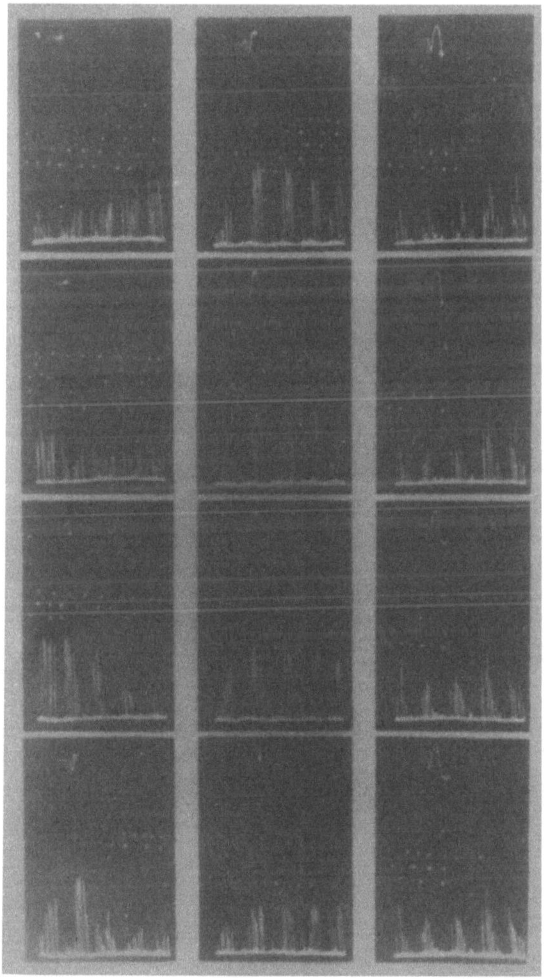

Transthoracic and transesophageal recording of cardiac micropotentials with stimulation triggered averaging

HEINKE, M. (1), H. VOLKMANN (1), H. KUEHNERT (1), G. DANNBERG (1), A. LEICHSENRING (2), M. TISCHMEYER (3), C. SCHWIND (2), R. BLAU (3)

Division of Cardiology, Department of Internal Medicine, Friedrich Schiller University, Jena, GDR (1),
Institute of Physiology, Friedrich Schiller University, Jena, GDR (2),
Department of Technical and Biomedical Cybernetics, Technical College Ilmenau, GDR (3)

Summary

12 patients with and 15 patients without vegetative blockade were examined with stimulation triggered averaging by transesophageal atrial stimulation. Heart rate variable recording of His potentials could be achieved non-invasive in 12 patients. Due to a rate proportional prolongation of the AV node conduction time, rapid atrial stimulation allowed an improved identification of the His potentials by increasing the distance between the end of the atrial potential and the onset of the His potential in the averaged ECG. Painless transesophageal atrial stimulation could be achieved by application of esophageal balloon electrodes. The increased signal to noise distance of transesophageal His potential recording might also allow a reduction of the averaging time and a beat to beat recording in a few cases.

Introduction

The application of the signal averaging technique in electrocardiology allows a non-invasive recording of His potentials (Berbari, Lazzara et al. 1973) and ventricular late potentials (El-Sherif, Gomes et al. 1985) in the high-resolution ECG.
The interval between the end of the atrial potential and the onset of the His potential restricts the transthoracic and transesophageal identification of the His bundle activity in the high-resolution ECG. The measurement of the conduction time will be possible by a sufficient interval between the end of the atrial potential and the onset of the His potential. A prolongation of this critical interval by lengthening of the AV node conduction time (AH-interval) is accessible by means of rapid atrial stimulation. Therefore we use the transesophageal atrial stimulation for the increasing of the heart rate during the non-invasive recording of the micropotentials.

Methods

For the non-invasive recording of His potentials with stimulation triggered averaging and of late potentials with QRS triggered averaging transthoracic bipolar V1V6, V1V4 and V2V6 leads are used. The bipolar ECG is amplified, high-pass filtered with a 3 dB cut off frequency of 30 Hz, 60 Hz, 90 Hz and digitally sampled with 1 ms and 512 values.
The atrial stimulation impulses of an extracardial pacemaker synchronize the summation of 100 PQ-segments of the ECG and the QRS triggers synchronize the summation of 100 ST segments of the ECG respectively. Variations of the PQ duration depending on the vegetative tonus are eliminated with a vegetative blockade with Propranolol (0,2 mg/kg) and Atropin (0,04 mg/kg). The averaged ECG is recorded with two or three filter frequencies and with a reference lead.
For the stimulation triggered averaging bipolar esophageal electrodes are used. Painless transesophageal atrial stimulation can be achieved by means of esophageal balloon electrodes (Heinke , Volkmann et al. 1986).
We use a 18-polar esophageal probe in balloon technique for the temporary transesophageal electrostimulation of the heart.

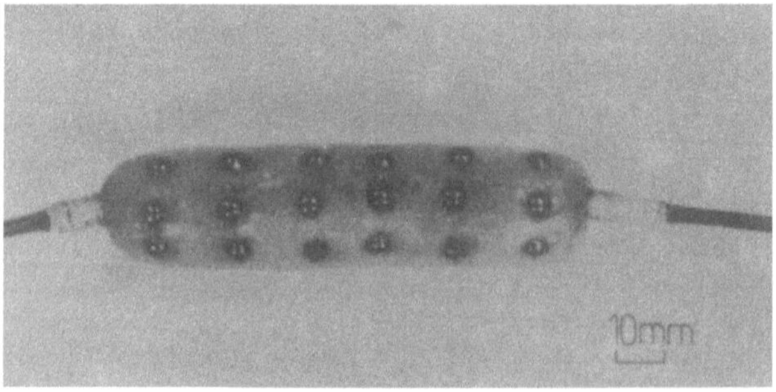

Fig. 1 18-polar esophageal probe in balloon technique for the temporary transesophageal electrostimulation of the heart.

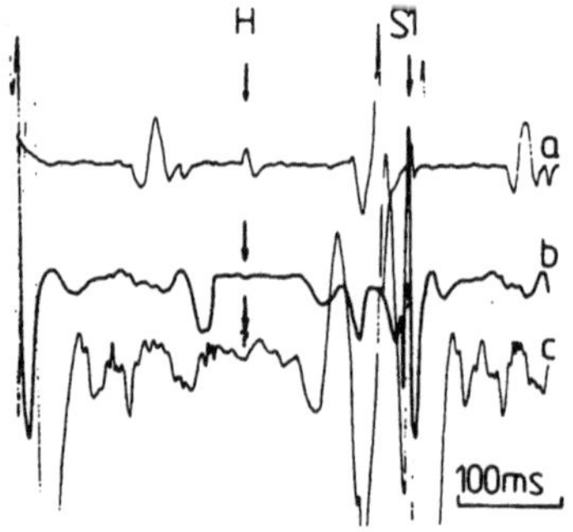

Fig. 2 Intracardiac reference lead (a), transesophageal (b) and transthoracic (c) recording of His bundle activity with 90 Hz high-pass filtering and atrial stimulation triggered averaging after vegetative blockade. Curves (b) and (c) are after 100 averagings . H= His potential, S1= stimulus, S1S1=stimulation cycle length= 375 ms.

Results

The increasing of the signal to noise distance of the transesophageal ECG compared with the transthoracic ECG is shown in figure 2. The non-invasive recording of His potentials with stimulation triggered averaging by transesophageal atrial stimulation was achieved in 75 % of the patients (9/12) with vegetative blockade and in 20 % of the patients (3/15) without vegetative blockade.

A transthoracic recording of His potentials with transesophageal atrial stimulation triggered averaging and vegetative blockade is shown in figure 3 and 4. All curves are recordings of the V1V6 lead, where (a) is a reference lead and (b) is a high-resolution ECG after 100 averagings and 60 Hz high-pass filtering.

A non-invasive recording of ventricular late potentials with QRS-triggered averaging of the ST-segment and V1V6 lead in a patient with episodes of ventricular tachycardia is shown in figure.5.

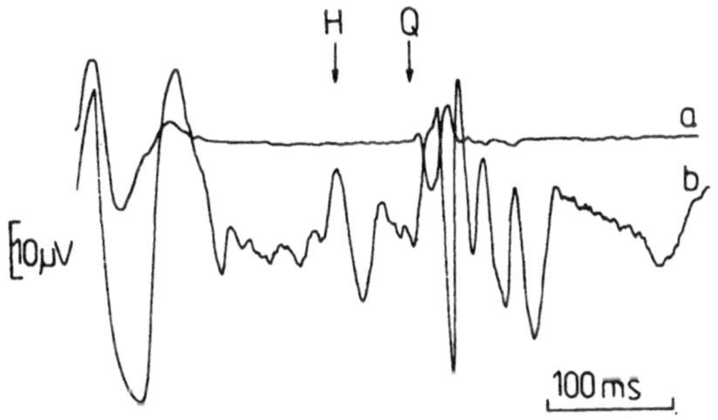

Fig. 3 Surface His bundle electrogram 10 minutes after the beginning of the vegetative blockade and S1S1= 720 ms. H= His potential, Q= QRS onset.

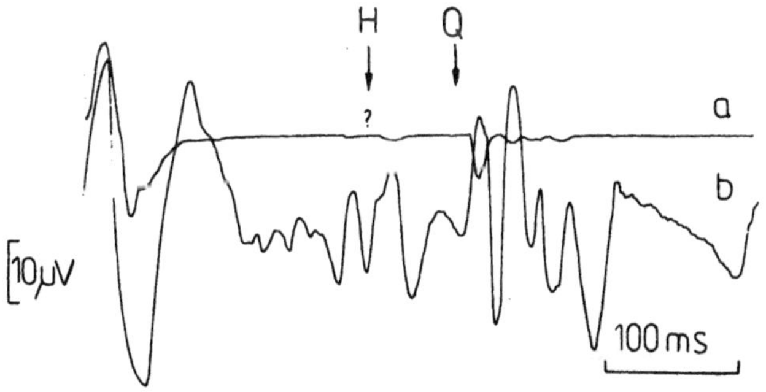

Fig. 4 Surface His bundle electrogram 25 minutes after the beginning of the vegetative blockade and S1S1= 720 ms. H= His potential, Q= QRS onset.The His potential (H) fades away, after the effect of the vegetative blockade has worn off.

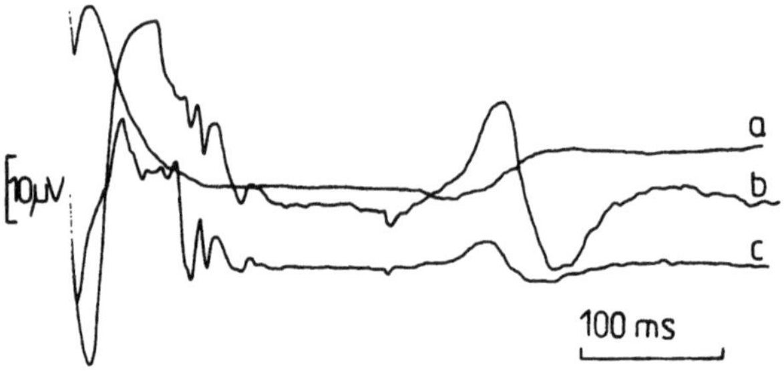

Fig. 5 Ventricular late potentials after QRS and 100 averagings, 30 Hz high-pass filtering (b) and 60 Hz high-pass filtering (c). Curve (a) is the reference lead.

Discussion

The end of the atrial potential covers the His potential in the high-resolution ECG in patients with normal and short AV-node conduction time (AH - interval) (Peper,Jonges et al. 1985). Rapid atrial stimulation prolongs the AV-node conduction time and causes the increasing of the distance between the end of the atrial potential and the beginning of the His potential in the averaged ECG.
A method for the transesophageal and transthoracic recording of the His potential is the transesophageal atrial stimulation triggered averaging with vegetative blockade. The increased signal to noise distance of transesophageal His potential recording might also allow a reduction of the averaging time and a beat to beat recording in a few cases.

References

(1) Berbari, E.J., R. Lazzara, P. Samet and B. J. Scherlag: Circulation 39, 1005-1013 (1973)
(2) El-Sherif, N., J. A. C. Gomes, M. Restivo and R. Mehra: PACE 8, 440-462 (1985)
(3) Heinke, M., H. Volkmann, M. Tischmeyer, G. Kalhoefer and R. Paliege: Z. Klin. Med. 41, 1431-1433 (1986)
(4) Peper, A., R. Jonges, T. G. Losekoot and C. A. Grimbergen: Med. & Biol. Eng. & Comput. 23, 365-376 (1985).

Frequency and significancy of ventricular late potentials in patients with myocardial infarction with and without fibrinolysis

KLEINER, H., BRUNKE, W.*, MUELLER, J.H.A.*, PECH, H., FIEHRING, H., ANDERS, G.*

Central Institute of Cardiovascular Research of the Academy of Sciences of GDR, Wiltbergstr. 50, Berlin 1115, DDR

*I. Medical Clinic of the Town Hospital "Friedrichshain", Leninallee 49, Berlin 1017, DDR

Summary

95 Patients (PTS) with definitive myocardial infarction (MI) had no fibrinolysis (FL) (reference group), 22 PTS had systemic and 36 PTS intracoronary FL. Without FL we found late potentials (LP) in anterior wall myocardial infarction (AMI) in 36%, in posterior wall myocardial infarction (PMI) in 53% and in re-MI of another coronary artery in 56% of the PTS, 16 PTS had spontaneous VT. Among the PTS with FL LP were detected in 44% in AMI and 64% in PMI. Only 4 PTS had VT.

Conclusions: FL leads to qualitative improvement of left ventricular contraction disturbances and diminuation of myocardial necrosis. The higher incidence of LP after FL may be explained by enlargement of pathomorphologically and electrically inhomogenous infarction border zone. The lower frequency of VT after FL may be attributed to higher stability against arrhythmia triggering factors.

Introduction

Electrical activity within the ST-segment has been detected by the means of high amplified and signal averaged ECG in animal experiments (1, 2, 3, 9, 10, 11, 17) and in human beings (6, 7, 8, 12, 18, 19, 20, 21, 22) in the seventies. This activity coincides with reentry VT and is regarded as an indicator of increased ventricular vulnerability (2, 5, 8, 12, 13, 14, 15, 16, 19, 21). LP have been detected in 30-65% of PTS after MI. No information about the influence of therapy during acute MI periode on frequency and significance of LP is available.

We evaluated 153 PTS with definitive MI and formed two groups: 95 PTS arrived at the hospital later than six hours after onset of MI and therefore they did not undergo FL (reference group). 58 PTS had infarction limiting therapy, i.e. 36 PTS with intracoronary and 22 with intravenous FL.

Methods: Systemic and intracoronary infusion of streptokinase has been performed as generally used. Additional antianginous therapy did not differ. Antiarrhythmics were given, if significant arrhythmias were present.

Technique: The high amplified ECG has been registered between the 4, and 52, week. We recorded 4 bipolar chest leads. After amplification (50 - 125000) and filtering (30 - 300 Hz) we averaged 100 - 200 cycles with a sampling rate of 1 kHz using an computer pdp 11/23. The trigger was set on R-peak of a limb lead. Elimination of aberrant heart beats was achieved by hard ware (prematurity) and soft ware (signaldifferences). The average window is 512 ms post trigger and measurements were made computerassisted. Noise level was below 1.5 microV after averaging.

We defined LP as electrical signals at the end of QRS within the ST-segment if the voltage was higher than twice the noise level and if the signals were present in at least two leads.

Results

Among 95 PTS without lysis (Tbl. 1) there were 39 with AMI, 47 PTS had PMI, 9 PTS had MI with re-infarction of a second coronary artery. In 46% of all PTS we registered LP and in 17% VT. The greatest incidence of LP occurred in PTS with re-infarction in a second coronary artery with 56%, followed by PMI with 53% and AMI with 36%. In this group all PTS with VT had LP too. If LP were present, VT appeared in AMI in 43%, in PMI in 36% and in re-infarction in a second coronary artery in 20%.

Table 1
Frequency of late potentials and ventricular tachycardias in patients with myocardial infarction without (n=95) and with fibrinolysis (n=58)

		without fibrinolysis				with fibrinolysis		
		with LP n (%)	with VT n (%)	without LP n (%)		with LP n (%)	with VT n (%)	without LP n (%)
AMI	(n=39)	14(36)	6 (43)	25(64)	(n=25)	11(44)	2(8)	14(56)
PMI	(n=47)	25(53)	9 (36)	22(47)	(n=33)	21(64)	2(6)	12(36)
APMI	(n= 9)	5(56)	1 (20)	4(44)				
	(n=95)	44(46)	16 (17)	51(54)	(n=58)	32(55)	4(7)	26(45)

AMI = anterior wall myocardial infarction
PMI = posterior wall myocardial infarction
APMI = re-infarction of a second coronary artery
VT = frequency of ventricular tachycardia depending on localization of MI

Table 2
Frequency of late potentials in dependence on kinetic disturbances under consideration of therapeutic management (%)

	without lysis (n=95)			systemic lysis (n=22)			local lysis (n=36)		
	LP+	LP-	K.D.(%)	LP+	LP-	K.D.(%)	LP+	LP-	K.D.(%)
Normokinesis	2		1					3	3
Hypokinesis	16	30	47	32	36	68	17	17	34
Akinesis	12	12	25	5	9	14	33	19	52
Dyskinesis	10	6	15	9	5	9	3	3	6
Aneurysm	8	5	12	5		10	6		6

LP+ = late potentials present (in %)
LP- = late potentials absent (in %)
K.D.(%) = Frequency of kinetic disturbances of the groups (%)

Among 22 PTS treated with streptokinase intraveneously there were 9 (41%) with AMI and 13 (59%) with PMI. The localization of MI in 36 PTS with intracoronary lysis is similar. There were 16 (44%) with AMI and 20 (56%) with PMI. We observed a much higher incidence of LP after FL, in AMI in 50%, in PMI in 65% (see tbl. 5). In contrast to this the frequency of VT is lower. After systemic FL there were VT in 5% and after local FL in 8% only. In the FL group there are 2 PTS with VT without LP. They had no electrophysiological examination, therefore the mechanism of VT is unknown.

PTS with LP had left ventricular contraction disturbances of qualitative higher degree compared to those without LP. If VT were additionally present, severe kinetic disturbances were dominating (Tbl. 2). The ejection fraction is in PTS with LP lower (0,4) than in PTS without (0,54). There were no correlations between frequency and degree of stenosis of involved coronary vessels and LP. The severity of kinetic disturbances correlates with the incidence, but not with the duration of LP. Alone the absence or presence and the type of VT (sustained or nonsustained) correlates with the duration and voltage of LP (tbl. 4). Nonsustained VT are characterized by short LP (20 ms) and lower voltage (ca. 5 microV).

Table 3
Late potentials in dependence on the severity of coronary artery disease (%)

	without lysis (n=95)		syst. lysis (n=22)		local lysis (n=36)	
	LP+	LP-	LP+	LP-	LP+	LP-
1-vessel-disease	20	13	14	18	12	25
2-vessel-disease	7	20	18	18	19	9
3-vessel-disease	19	21	27	5	28	6
vessels involved (average)	2.12	2.16	2.2	1.7	2.4	1.8

Table 4
Relations between duration aod amplitude of late potentials and ventricular tachycardias

	Duration (ms)	Amplitude (uV)
Patients with ventr. tachycardia	32	10
Patients without ventr. tachycardia	21	8

Table 5
Frequency of late potentials and ventricular tachycardias in dependence on localization of myocardial infarction and treatment

	systemic lysis (n=22)				local lysis (n=36)			
	n	(%)	LP+(%)	VT(%)	n	(%)	LP+(%)	VT(%)
AMI	9	41	46	5	16	44	44	3
PMI	13	59	54	0	20	56	70	5

Discussion

The highest incidence of LP has been found independently of therapeutic regimen in PTS with PMI. The electrical activation front at least reaches the basal left ventricle (6). Therefore fractionated electrical activity of the posterior wall will be perceptible as LP more frequently. It is imaginable that under special conditions LP of the anterior wall are covered by the still depolarizing posterior wall. In the reference group VT are more frequently present in AMI than in PMI. This observation is in accordance with the expectation that LP of the anterior wall can be masked by the still depolarizing posterior wall. Under this assumption LP of the anterior wall should last longer than LP of the posterior to be recognizable. Probably therefore the correlation between VT and LP is more significant in AMI. Whether the prognostic value of LP of equal duration in AMI and PMI is the same or higher in AMI needs further investigation.

The significantly higher incidence of LP after FL (tbl. 1, 2) is surprising and should not be expected at the first sight. Starting from the reference group (17% of the PTS had VT) one could calculate a probability of VT in the FL group (58 PTS) in 10 cases but there are only 4. Dyskinesias and aneurysms are more frequent in the reference group (16 resp. 13%) than in the FL groups (9 resp. 5%). After FL hypo- and akinesias are more frequent (86%) as in the reference group (70%). The therapeutic effiency of FL is obvious. Concerning the seriousness of coronary artery disease we come to the conclusion that only slightly more coronary vessels are involved if LP are present (tbl. 3). Not only the presence but also duration and voltage of LP are of more importance for their significance as risk indicator for predicting VT (tbl. 4).

Different therapy regimens influence the frequency and degree of left ventricular dysfunction, coronary artery disease, size of MI, LP and obviously also VT. In the FL groups LP are more frequently registered as in the reference group but VT are more seldom. The myocardial scare (i.e. necrosis) after MI is electrically indifferent and for the origin of LP not of direct significance. However, the infarction border zone consists of a network of morphologically and electrophysiologically normal and unnormal bundles of myocardium. These are the preconditions of asynchronous delayed depolarization and electrical fractionation that can be registered as LP from the body surface. It is imaginable that after FL the border zone is enlargee and therefore the frequency of LP is higher 85% of the PTS with VT had LP.

Surprising is the divergency of frequency of LP and VT after FL. Both groups are comparable concerning age, sex, localization of MI, number of involved cororany vessels and additional cororany therapy. The PTS with FL had a shorter time interval between onset of MI and begin of therapy, better left ventricular function and less dyskinesias and aneurysm.
The indication for antiarrhythmic drug therapy was given in PTS without FL in 21%, 3 PTS died (2 sudden deaths). In the fL group only 10% recieved antiarrhythmics, there is no death in this group. All these improvements lead to a higher stability of the myocardium against VT initiating factors.

Conclusions

1. LP are typical findings in PTS with reentry VT, 85% of these PTS had LP.
2. Thrombolysis as early as possible after onset of MI leads to an qualitative and quantitative improvement of left ventricular dysfunction.
3. Thrombolysis probably enlarges the infarction border zone as orogin of LP.
4. Although after thrombolysis a higher frequency of LP has been found,

the lesser frequency of VT obviously is due to a smaller predisposition of the myocardium to arrhythmia initiating factors.

Literature

1. Aronson, R.S.: Circ. Res. 48, 720 (1981).
2. Berbari, E.J., et al.: Am. J. Cardiology 41, 697 (1978).
3. Boineau, J.P., Cox, J.L.: Circulation 48, 702 (1973).
4. Brachmann, J.G., et al.: Circulation 67, 449 (1983).
5. Breithardt, G., Borggrefe, M.: Eur. Heart J. 7, 364 (1986).
6. Brugada, P., et al.: Am J. Cardiol. 55, 402 (1985).
7. Cain, M.E., et al.: Am. J. Cardiology 55, 1500 (1985).
8. Denes, P., et al.: Circulation 67, 1129 (1983).
9. El-Sherif, N., et al.: Circulation 55, 686 (1977).
10. El-Sherif, N., et al.: Circulation 55, 702 (1977).
11. El-Sherif, N., et al.: Circ. Res. 52, 566 (1983).
12. El-Sherif, N., et al.: Circulation 68, 644 (1983.
13. Euler. D.D., Moore, E.N.: Am. J. Cardiol. 46, 783 (1981).
14. Fontaine, G., et al., in: Masoni, A,, et al. (ed.): Cardiac electrophysiology today. Academic Press, London, New York 1982, p. 251.
15. Hoepp, H.W., et al., in: Steinbach, K. (ed.): Cardiac pacing, Proceedings of the VIIth World Symposium on Cardiac Pacing, Vienna 1983. Steinkopff-Verl., Darmstadt 1983, S. 626.
16. Hombach, V., et al.: Dtsch. Med. Wschr. 105, 1457 (1980).
17. Jospehson, M.E., et al.: Circulation 57, 659 (1978).
18. Josephson, M.E., et al.: Circulation 66, 1199 (1982).
19. Rozanski, J.J., et al.: Circulation 63, 1172 (1981).
20. Simson, M.B., et al.: Am. J. Physiol. 241, 363 (1981).
21. Simson, M.B.: Circulation 64, 235 (1981).
22. Waxman, H.L., Sung, R.J.: Circulation 62, 1349 (1980).

Intracardiac electrophysiologic testing in the postmyocardial infarction period

ASSMANN, I., A. LAUTEN, P. DITTRICH

Dept. of Cardiology
Clinic of Internal Medicine, Medical School of Erfurt, Erfurt, GDR

Summary

The prognostic value of programmed electrical stimulation (PES) was tested in 17 male survivors (age 29 - 63 years) of acute myocardial infarction (MI) 1 to 5 months after the acute event. The results were compared with other clinical and paraclinical data. In 10 patients (pts) we could initiate a nonsustained ventricular tachycardia (VT) of more than 6 echoes (mean 11 echoes, Group A), in 4 pts (Group B) the VT was sustained and turned to ventricular fibrillation (VF). An external countershock was required. In 3 pts (Group C) no VT was inducible. Contrary, in 12 pts without MI - but with sponteneours VT - we could initiate a nonsustained VT only in 3 cases. There were no correlations with the findings in the exercise test, Holter ECG or coronary arteriography, but pts wich inducible VT (Group A, B) had a worse left ventricular function, and in more than 30 % of pts VT, VF, or sudden death occurred during the follow-up. Therefore, pts with inducible VT should be observed and treated very carefully, because they are to be considered as high risk pts.

Introduction

The programmed electrical stimulation (PES) in survivors of an acute myocardial infarction (MI) is utilized for achieving prognostic informations in regard of sudden cardiac death, or occurring of ventricular tachyarrhythmia (VT) during the late post-infarction period (1-4,5). The value being controversial up to now, has induced us also to perform such examinations, and then to compare the results with other clinical and paraclinical data.

Material and Methods

In 17 male patients (pts) aged from 29 - 63 years (average age 50,8 years) - having survived MI - we carried out electrophysiological examinations 1 - 5 months after the acute event. This examination was done according to a fixed programme (Table 1).

Table:1 Electrophysiological testing, study design

Drive cycle intervals:	SR; 550-600 ms, 450-500 ms
No of extrastimuli:	2-3
Site of extrastimuli:	right ventricular apex
End point criterion:	6 Echoes
Current strength	2x Diastolic threshold
Pulse width	2 ms

Abbr. SR = sinusrhythm, MI = myocardial infarction

The results of the PES were compared with the findings of the cardiac catheterization and of the coronary arteriography, the exercise test, Holter-ECG (6 pts), and with the incidence of VT during the acute and follow-up period up to 14 months. Furthermore, we compared the results with the data of 12 pts with spontaneous VT, but without MI (Group D).

Results

In 10 pts (Group A) we could initiate nonsustained VT (7 polymorpheous, 3 monomorpheous). In 4 pts (Group B), there were sustained VT inducible which turned to ventricular fibrillation (VF) after 10 - 20 sec. External countershocks were required in these 4 cases. In 3 pts (Group C) there were no VT inducible.

Table 2: Patients with myocardial infarction (MI)

	Groups A nonsustained VT	B sustained VT VF	C normal
No.of patients/sex	10 m	4 m	3 m
Age (years)	51,8 (29-63)	49,2 (30-56)	51,0(43-60)
AMI	8	3	1
IMI	2	1	2
follow-up (months)	9 (3-13)	8 (3-14)	7 (4-12)

Abbr. AMI: anterior MI, IMI: inferior MI, VT: ventricular tachycardia, VF: ventricular fibrillation, m = male

In group D we could initiale nonsustained VT only in 3 cases with underlying coronary heart disease. 4 further pts of Group D suffered from a long QT-syndrome with spontaneous VT (torsade de pointes) during the electrophysiological testing, 8 pts of group A and 4 pts of group B suffered from VT or VF during the acute stage of MI, and 4 pts resp.1 during the follow-up. In 7 pts there occured ventricular extrasystoles (VES) Lown III, 1 patient (Group B) died suddenly. In group C only in 2 cases VES Lown III appeared during exercise (Fig. 1)

In most pts, the VT was inducible during permanent stimulation (cycle length 550 - 600 ms) and applying 2 extrastimuli. In group A, the average cycle lengths of VT were 200 - 250 ms, the number of echoes ranged between 7 and 15, mean 11. We found no significant differences between the 3 groups of MI pts with respect to other electrophysiological parameters, extent of coronary artery stenoses or exercise test. Only the left ventricular function was more depressed in group A and B (Fig.2).

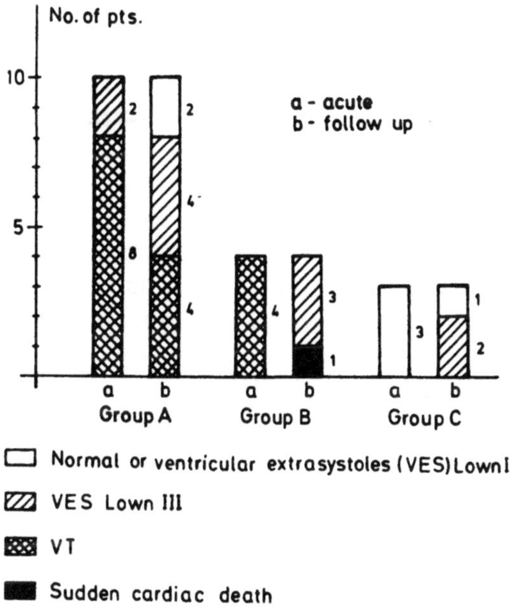

Fig.1 Incidence of ventricular tachycardia (VT), ventricular fibrillation (VF), and ventricular extrasystoles (VES) in the acute stage and during the follow-up in the different groups

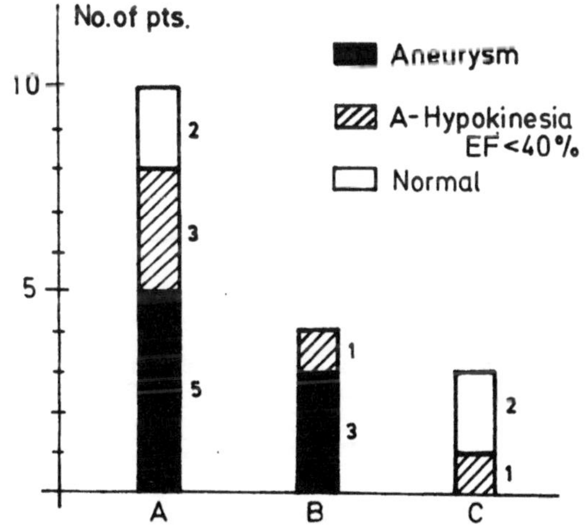

Fig.2 Left ventricular function in the different groups of patients after myocardial infarction

In 7 pts of group A and B the surgical intervention was successful in preventing VT or VF, and in 6 pts the antiarrhythmic treatment.

Discussion and conclusions

Up to now, there have not been any generally accepted criteria of the PES that have prognostic significance. This fact applies not only to end point criteria and the number of extrastimuli but also to the place and time of stimulation, or the length of drive cycle (1,2,4-6). Only one stimulus is not enough; the rate of succes is most increased if 2 or 3 extrastimuli are applied (5). We could initiate sustained or nonsustained VT after MI in more than 75 % of the unselected pts. Other authors found inducible VT in 35 - 50 % of the survivors of MI (1,6). Correlations to the severity of coronary stenoses, left ventricular function, results of exercise tests or findings in Holter-ECG were not evident (3,48). When comparing the results of PES with the occurence of VT, VF, or sudden death in the early and late MI-phase up to 1 year, there was mainly no reliable conformity to be found (1,3,6). The best results were achieved by Richard et al (quoted by 4). They found, that in 98 % of pts without inducible VT no spontaneous VT or sudden death occure while in 32 % of pts wich inducible VT such events may occur. Anyhow, this results corresponds to our experiences. In general, there may be stated, that survivors of MI with a low ejection fraction, and/or aneurysm, and inducible VT during EPS frequently develop VT or VF - or sudden death occurs. Thus, pts with inducible VT after MI should be considered as high - risk pts.

References

(1) Breithardt,G., M. Borggrefe, K.Haerten, and H.-J.Trampisch: Z.Kardiol.74, 389-396 (1985)

(2) Costard,A., M. Schlüter, K.P.Kunze, U.Wolf, and K.A. Kuck: Z.Kardiol. 75, 589-597 (1986)

(3) Roy,D., E. Marchand, P. Theroux,D.D. Waters, G.P.Pelletier, and M.G. Bourgassa: Circulation 72, 487-494 (1985)

(4) Uther,J.B., D.A.D.Richards, A.R. Denniss, and D.L. Ross: Circulation 75 (Suppl III), 161-165 (1987)

(5) Mason, J.W., P.K. Anderson, and R.A. Freedmann: Circulation 75 (Suppl III), 125-130 (1987)

(6) Morady, F., D. Hess, M.M. Scheinmann: Am.Heart J. 50, 1055-1060 (1982)

(7) Swerdlow, Ch.D., R.A. Freedman, J.Peterson, and D. Kay: Am.Heart J. 111, 433-438 (1986)

(8) Stevenson,W.G., P. Brugada, B. Waldecker, M.Zehender, and H.J.J.Wellens: Circulation 71, 1146-1152 (1985)

Multiple malformations of the conduction system of the heart in patients with paroxysmal supraventricular tachycardias

SULIMOV V.

I-st Moscow Medical Institute,Moscow,USSR

Summary.To study the incidence and possible combinations of multiple malformations of the conduction system of the heart and to find out the dependence of the efficiency of AAD therapy on the type of these congenital anomalies standard EFI including serial testing of AAD was performed in 52 p-ts with recurrent PSVT.46% of them had multiple malformations of the conduction system of the heart.The most common combinations were:coexistence of accessory AV connections,including concealed forms and concealed AN connections with discrete conduction in the AV junction.Effective AAD therapy was achived in 65% of p-ts and directly depended upon the electrophysiologic mechanism of PSVT.In cases of single or multiple accessory AV connections and concealed AN connections such AAD as rythmodan,gilurytmal and amiodaron were preferable. In cases of combinations of accessory AV connections with discrete conduction in the AV junction and in p-ts with reciprocal AV nodal PT without concealed AN connections preferable AAD were beta-blockers, calcium antagonists and aethmozin.

Introduction of the method of intracardiac electrophysiologic investigation (EFI) into clinical practice gave evidence that the majority of paroxysmal supraventricular tachycardias (PSVT) are reciprocal duc to their underlying electrophysiologic mechanism.Besides it was proved that these rhythm disturbances in many patients have a morphologic basis for their occurrence such as accessory pathways and discrete conduction in the AV junction.But these congenital anomalies are not necessarily isolated.The purpose of our research was to study the incidence and possible combinations of multiple malformations of the conduction system of the heart in patients with PSVT.We also tried to find out the dependence of the efficiency of antiarrhythmic drug (AAD) therapy on the type of these malformations.

Material and methods.

We have studied 52 patienys with recurrent PSVT proved by ECG,including 35 women and 17 men aged from 16 to 62.The frequency of PSVT varied from 10 per year to almost constant tachycardia.18 patients had ECG evidence of WPW syndrome.34 patients had no ECG evidence of any form of preexcitation syndrome.After obtaining the informed written consent and discontinuation of all AAD for 48 houres (except amiodaron) all patients underwent standard EFI including serial testing of AAD.The number of AAD tested during one EFI varied from 1 to 5,including propranolol, verapamil,amiodaron,gilurytmal,rythmodan,aethmozin,procainamid and digoxin.

Results and discussion.

Using programmed atrial and (or) ventricular stimulation PSVT were induced in all 52 patients.The analysis of the data obtained during EFI showed that all patients had one or several malformations of the conduction system of the heart,which participated in the formation of the tachycardia circuit.Out of 18 patients with ECG evidence of WPW syndrome 11 (61%) had one isolated Kent bundle:leftsided in 6 cases and rightsided in 5 cases,which participated in the formation of the retrograde limb of orthodromic AV tachycardia circuit.In 3 patients with ECG evidence of WPW syndrome type B (17%) second concealed leftsided Kent bundle was found.These patients had two types of AV tachycardia:ortodromic and antidromic.In the latter case the tachycardia circuit closed between two Kent bundles.Besides the isolated Kent bundle 4 patients with ECG evidence of WPW syndrome also had the discrete conduction in the AV junction.In these cases the tachycardia circuit was formed by slow AV nodal pathway in anterograde direction and by Kent bundle in retrograde direction.18 patients had concealed WPW syndrome:leftsided Kent bundle was found in 15 and rightsided in 3.In all these cases concealed accessory AV connection participated in the formation of the retrograde limb of AV tachycardia.8 patients (44%) had isolated Kent bundle and in 10 patients (56%) it coexisted with discrete conduction in the AV junction.Among them 2 patients had threefascicular AV nodal conduction,consisting of one fast and two slow AV nodal pathways. According to existing electrophysiological criteria AV nodal reentrant tachycardia were found in 16 patients.9 patients had dual AV nodal pathways.The AV nodal conduction curve in this group was characterized by a single discontinuation and consisted of one fast and one slow AV nodal pathway.4 patients had threefascicular AV nodal conduction,which was characterized by two discontinuations of the AV conduction curve and consisted of one fast and two slow AV nodal pathways.2 patients had quadryfascicular AV nodal conduction,which was characterized by three discontinuations of AV conduction curve and consisted of one fast and three slow AV nodal pathways.In all patients with AV nodal reentrant tachycardia the anterograde limb of the tachycardia circuit was formed by slow AV nodal pathway and the retrograde limb was formed by fast AV nodal pathway.Several patients with AV nodal reentrant tachycardia and polyfascicular mode of conduction in the AV junction showed alternation of P-R interval during tachycardia,reflecting different slow AV nodal pathways incorporated in the tachycardia circuit.Several electrophysiogical properties of the retrograde limb of the tachycardia circuit in 7 patients with AV nodal reentrant tachycardia aroused serious doubt that the retrograde limb belongs to intra nodal structures: 1.The retrograde atrial activation during the tachycardia occurred before or simul-

taneously with the begining of the ventricular activation.2.The H-A interval during the tachycardia was not more than 50 ms,that means that either the length of the retrograde limb of the tachycardia circuit is very short,or that the speed of propagation of the excitation is very high,or both.3.The H_2-A_2 interval during programmed ventricular stimulation was constant,showing the absense of decremential conduction in the AV node.4.The beta-blockers and calcium-entry blockers didn't influence the conduction in the retrograde limb of the tachycardia circuit.On the other hand,such AAD as rythmodan and gilurytmal suppressed the conduction in the retrograde limb.On the basis of these findings we came to a conclusion that in a part of patients with AV nodal reentrant tachycardia the retrograde limb of the tachycardia circuit was represented not by the AV nodal structures but by the accessory connections between the AV junctuin and the atria conducting only in retrograde direction.This form of malformation of the conduction system of the heart can be called concealed Clerc-Levy-Cristesco (CLC) syndrome.According to our data,in 44% patients with AV nodal reentrant tachycardias the discrete conduction in the AV junction coexisted with concealed accessory atrionodal (AN) connections,forming the retrograde limb of the tachycardia circuit. The results of serial testing of AAD showed the direct dependence of the effectiveness of AAD upon the electrophysiologic mechanism of PSVT. Out of 11 patients with ECG evidence of WPW syndrome and single Kent bundle the effective AAD regiment was found in 8 cases.It was rythmodan in 6 and amiodaron in 2 patients.Three patients underwent surgical correction of the WPW syndrome.For 3 patients with ECG evidence of WPW syndrome having second concealed Kent bundle no effective AAD therapy was found and in all of them the interruption of Kent bundle was performed. Among 4 patients with ECG evidence of the WPW syndrome associated with discrete conduction in the AV junction the effective AAD treatment by beta-blockers was possible in 3 cases and one patient was operated on. Out of 8 patients with isolated concealed Kent bundle the effective AAD regiment was found only in 3 cases:it was rythmodan in 2 and gilurytmal in 1.In 5 patients surgical interruption of Kent bundle was performed. Out of 10 patients with concealed WPW syndrome coexisting with discrete conduction in the AV junction the effective AAD regiment was achieved in 7 cases;verapamil in 2,amiodaron in 3 and aethmozin in 2 patients.Three patients underwent surgical interruption of Kent bundle.Out of 7 patients with AV nodal reentrant tachycardia and association of discrete conduction in the AV junction with concealed CLC syndrome the effective AAD therapy was possible in 5 cases:it was gilurytmal in 2 and rythmodan in 3 patient.In 2 cases artificial complete heart block with pacemacker implantation was performed.Out of 9 patients with AV nodal reentrant tachycardia without concealed AN connections effective AAD regiment was found in 8 cases:beta-blockers in 4,verapamil in 3 and aethmozin in 1.One patient refused the surgical correction of rhythm disturbances.
Conclusions:1.In 46% of patients with PSVT multiple malformation of the

conduction system of the heart can be find.The most common combinations are:1.Association of accessory AV connection,including concealed forms, with discrete conduction in the AV junction.2.Coexistence of discrete conduction in the AV junction with concealed accessory AN connections. 3.In cases of single or multiple accessory AV connections and concealed AN connections such AAD as rythmodan,gilurytmal and amiodaron are preferable.4.In cases of the combination of accessry AV connections with discrete conduction in the AV junction and in cases of AV nodal reentrant tachycardias without concealed AN connections the preferable AAD are bete-blockers,calcium antagonists and aethmozin.

The first derivative of the electrocardiogram.

MAKOLKIN V.I., MOROZOVA N.S.

1-st Moscow Medical Institute, Moscow, USSR.

Summary. The first derivative of the ECG was used to determine the time parameters of the repolarisation period. It was found the dependence on the heart rate of some periods such as: the terminal phase of the repolarisation,the Q-T interval, the interval between the maximal QRS and T vectors and also of the period correspondent to the ST segment.This dependence allows to lead out the regression equation in order to calculate the proper values of the time parameters.It was not found the dependence on the heart rate of the medium period of the repolarisation correspondent to the middle part of the third phase of the cardiac action potential.

As it is well known the duration of the repolarisation period is oscillated greatly even in healthy persons. Probably becouse of this fact it is not used in practical electrocardiography. Howerever,in investigations of Lepeschkin E.,Suravicz B.,Nagao T.,Sano T. the attention was payed on changeable duration of the T wave and ST segment in some patological statesments.Therefore, the more detale investigation of the duration of the repolarisation period with the help of first derivative of ECG is of great interest.

Material and methods: the first derivative of the ortogonal leads of McFee system was registered on the "Nihon-Kohden" cardiopolygraph.50healthy persons without any cardiac desease were examined.

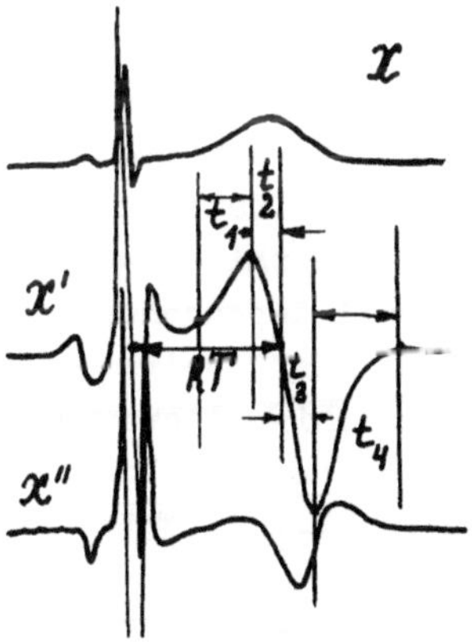

The following parameters were the subject of the analysis:

1.Four time periods of the T wave (t_1,t_2,t_3,t_4).

2.The time between the maximal QRS and T vectors(the so-called RTperiod).

3.The period RT-t_2(greatly correspondent to the ST segment).

4.Q-T interval.

Results and discussion: The received dates are shown on the table 1.

The duration of the time intervals of the 1-st derivative of the ECG.

	t_1	t_2	t_3	t_4	RT	$RT-t_2$	QT
X	0,04-0,10 0,07 ± 0,002	0,03-0,05 0,04± 0,001	0,03-0,06 0,04 ± 0,001	0,06-0,11 0,09 ± 0,002	0,20-0,34 0,26 ± 0,004	0,16-0,30 0,22 ± 0,003	0.36-0.54 0,44 ± 0,006
Y	0,04-0,09 0,06 ± 0,002	0,03-0,05 0,04 ± 0,001	0,03-0,05 0,04 ± 0,001	0,05-0,11 0,08 ± 0,002	0,20-0,38 0,27 ± 0,004	0,18-0,33 0,23 ± 0,004	0,36-0,54 0,45 ± 0,005
Z	0,03-0,09 0,06 ± 0,002	0,03-0,06 0,04 ± 0,001	0,04-0,06 0,05 ± 0,001	0,06-0,11 0,09 ± 0,002	0,22-0,36 0,26± 0,004	0,16-0,30 0,22 ± 0,004	0,36-0,54 0,45 ± 0,005

It becomes clear the great variability of some intervals: t_1 and t_4 are oscillated within the limits 0,06 sec., while t_2 and t_3 are oscillated whithin the limits 0,02-0,03 sec. The big limits of oscillation are also noted for RT and $RT-t_2$ intervals. The correlation analysis revealed the dependence of these intervals on heart rate.

The correlation rates of time periods of the 1-st derivative on heart rate.

	t_1	t_4	RT	$RT-t_2$	Q-T
X	0,41 ± 0,12	0,42 ± 0,12	0,80 ± 0,05	0,75 ± 0,06	0,80 ± 0,05
Y	-	0,47 ± 0,11	0,72 ± 0,07	0,70 ± 0,07	0,81 ± 0,05
Z	-	0,41 ± 0,12	0,76 ± 0,06	0,73 ± 0,07	0,79 ± 0,06

According to our investigations the bigest correlation rate was found for the t_4 period and the smallest for the t_2 and t_3 periods. Only in "z" lead this rate was rather big for the t_3 period as it was for the t_1 period in "x" lead. We assumed that the big dependence of t_1 on heart rate was due to non exact determination of its begining. This leads to the including of the part of heart rate dependent ST period to this interval. This was proved by the fact, that we found the greate dependence of the period $RT-t_2$ on heart rate (the correlation rate is 0,7). The received dates shows that the duration of the cardiac action potential is mostly dependent on heart rate in "plato" phase and also in terminal phase. The duration of the third phase in its medium part (rapid repolarisation) shows the small dependence on heart rate. The heart rate dependence of some periods of 1-st derivative allows to receive the equation of regression for them. This allows to estimate the alteration of time periods of repolarisation in pathological statesments (hypertrophy of ventriculars, bundle bunch blocks) which is rather difficult on standart ECG.

While examining the duration of the Q-T interval it was found that it was longer on the 1-st derivative than on the standart ECG. In order to create this fact the tracing was written with greate intensification and speed and then the 1-st derivative was received with computer. After that we saw, that both tracings were finished at the same time. Therefore, on standart ECG with usual intensification and speed the Q-T period becomes artificially shorter.

References:

(1) Lepeschkin E., Surawicz B. :Amer.Heart Journal. 46, 9-20 (1953)
(2) Surawicz B. :Advances in Electrocardiography. 377 (1972)
(3) Nagao T. : Japanese Circulation Journal. 39 (1975)
(4) Sano T. et al. : Japanese Circulation Journal. 32 (1968)

Reliability of noninvasive His bundle recordings.

J.BYTEŠNÍK, J.LEXA, J.FABIÁN

Institute for Clinical and Experimental Medicine, Vídeňská 800,
140 00 Prague 4, Czechoslovakia

SUMMARY

The authors present their own experience with noninvasive recording of the bundle of His electrogram using the technique of computer-assisted averaging of the signal coming from the thorax surface. Several progressive design features have been used in an effort to diminish the effect of disturbing electrical activity. A total od 140 patients were examined noninvasively and invasively at an interval of 24 hours at most. The noninvasive technique yielded an assesable bundle of His electrogram in 22 out of the 39 patients in whom the electrogram had been obtained also invasively, ie, in 56%.

Comparison of the values of the H-V interval (ie, conduction by the distal His-Purkinje system) in the above 22 subjects revealed a close correlation between both procedures (r = 0.92).

The noninvasive His bundle electrogram seems to be a promising screening method for more detailed estimation of atrio-ventricular and intraventricular conduction. A further technical improvement is needed as well the combination of this method with some stress tests.

INTRODUCTION

In differential diagnosis of heart rhythm disturbances, a major role is played by the His bundle electrogram (HBE). There are, however, limitations to the invasive nature of intracardiac recording. In the 1970s, the technique of noninvasive recording of the HBE was developed (Berbari,E.J. et al., 1973, Flowers, N.C. et al., 1974). This technique, however, involves a number of complex technical problems. The present article shows our own experience with noninvasive HBE recording and offers a comparison of findings obtained from the use of both - invasive and noninvasive - technique.

MATERIAL AND METHODS

We carried out a comparison of noninvasive and invasive HBE recordings in 40 subsequent patients (36 men and 4 women) aged 18-78. Most frequently, the diagnoses in this group of patients included: coronary disease with ventricular extrasystole or ventricular tachycardia (13 patients), ventricular preexcitation (7 patients), bifascicular block (6 patients), atrioventricular block type I - III (5 patients). Selective coronary angiography and left ventricular angiography were performed in 38 patients of the group.

Invasive HBE was recorded by the standard technique according to Sherlag (Byteŝník,J. et al., 1982). The recording rate was 100 mm/s. The conduction intervals were determined with an accuracy of 5 ms.

Noninvasive HBE recording was carried out using an apparatus developed at IKEM. A detailed technical description of its operation was published former (Lexa,J. et al., 1985, Lexa,J., Stupka,J.,1986, Lexa,J. et al.,1987)

Noninvasive HBE recording was performed within 1-24 hours before or after invasive examination while excluding any possible effect of drugs that might affect atrioventricular or intraventricular conduction intervals. Antiarrhythmic drugs were withdrawn for a period of a least 5 half-lives of the elimination phase. In two cases, simultaneous noninvasive and invasive HBE recording was carried out. The H-V interval was measured from the beginning of the spike H (bundle of His depolarization) to the start of ventricular depolarization, defined as the beginning of the Q wave (or the QRS complex) on a simultaneous conventional ECG recording. The H-V interval was determined with an accuracy of 5 ms. Assessment of the noninvasive H-V interval recording was done independently by two reviewers, out of whom at least one was unaware of the invasive H-V value. For the noninvasive HBE recording to be regarded as assesable, a distinct H wave, identically determined by both reviewers, had to be present, and the H-V value, subtracted by both reviewers, had to be identical or differ by 5 ms at most. When subtracting two H-V values differed by 5 ms, the noninvasive value closer to that determined invasively was considered for comparison with the H-V value measured invasively.

RESULTS

Of a total of 40 subjects examined in this group, the spike H could not be distinguished in the resting recording of an invasive HBE in one patient with ventricular pre-excitation. Noninvasive HBE recording failed to yield a distinct H wave in 18 patients (Tab.1). This means that, in a randomized group of patients with various brady- and tachyarrhythmias, while using the noninvasive technique, we were able to obtain an assessable HBE recording in 56% of patients in whom bundle activity was demonstrable by invasive investigation. Having excluded from our group ten subjects in whom already surface ECG had shown that the noninvasive averaging technique would not be capable of HBE recording (in cases such as frequent extrasystole hindering the averaging process, or marked pre-excitation with an extremely short P-R segment), the success rate was substantially higher (out of 30 patients, a noninvasive HBE recording was obtained in 22, ie, in 73% of patients).

Tab.1. Comparison of H-V intervals (in ms) subtracted from noninvasive (n-HBE) and invasive (i-HBE) electrogram recording of the bundle of His in 40 patients (N=nonevaluable)

Patient	H-V (n-HBE)	H-V (i-HBE)	Patient	H-V (n-HBE)	H-V (i-HBE)
1.	50	50	21.	30	30
2.	N	70	22.	35	30
3.	60	60	23.	40	40
4.	N	40	24.	40	45
5.	N	35	25.	35	35
6.	40	45	26.	50	50
7.	40	40	27.	45	50
8.	40	45	28.	N	60
9.	30	30	29.	N	55
10.	55	50	30.	N	40
11.	N	40	31.	N	60
12.	35	35	32.	N	50
13.	50	50	33.	40	40
14.	N	55	34.	N	N
15.	35	34	35.	N	50
16.	N	50	36,	N	70
17.	N	40	37.	N	60
18.	N	45	38.	40	40
19.	30	35	39.	45	40
20.	N	70	40.	45	50

A comparison of recordings using both techniques showed that the values of the H-V interval, determined invasively and non-invasively, were virtually identical. The relationship of both values compared by linear regression can be expressed as: $y = 0.898 \cdot x + 5.110$,
in which y is the value of the H-V interval obtained in invasive HBE, and x is the H-V value from noninvasive HBE recordings.

The correlation coefficient of the relationship of the H-V interval values yielded by noninvasive and invasive recordings was 0.92. The mean H segment amplitude in the noninvasive HBE was 1.2 uV, with a range between 0.6 uV and 2.5 uV. Fig.1 shows an example of a noninvasive HBE recording.

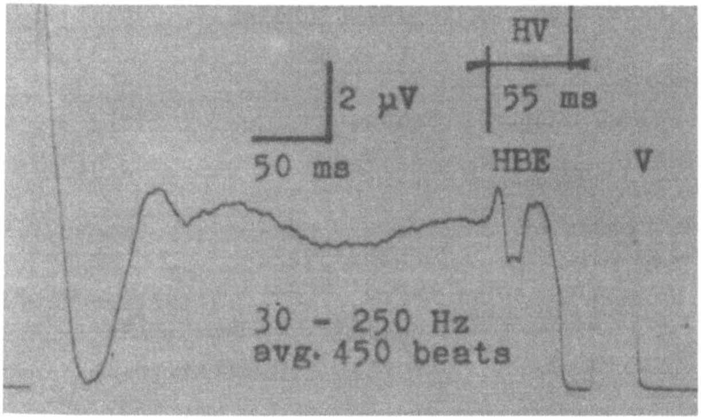

DISCUSSION AND CONCLUSIONS

To improve the quality of noninvasive HBE recordings we used a special isolation amplifier with very small dimensions enabling its incorporation into the input cable. Another progressive design feature was the application of fibre optics instead of the original shielded cable. To perform averaging, we used a special modification of the technique of synchronized recording of part of the cardiac cycle that ensures a higher stability of the synchronization point (Lexa,J. et al.,1985).

Using the above technique, we obtained assessable His bundle electrograms in 56%.

Some studies in the world literature report attempts at a comparison of H-V interval values obtained from invasive and noninvasive HBE recordings (Vincent,R. et al.,1978, Abboud,S. et al., 1983, McKenna,W.H. et al., 1981). In our comparison the correlation coefficient was 0.92. Our group was, at the same time, one of the largest and, compared with a series also containing more than 20 patients, the interval between both recordings was relatively shorter in our group. This fact renders our findings less questionable.

The results show that the noninvasive technique of HBE using averaging of more cardiac cycles enables to obtain comparable data in approximately a half of the patients examined. This makes it a suitable screening technique to evaluate conduction through the His-Purkinje system (e.g. in patients with bifascicular block) and to assess, the effect of drugs on atrioventricular conduction. We believe that further development of this technique, in combination with oesophageal atrial stimulation, will enable this noninvasive technique to replace a significant proportion of invasive electrophysiological procedure in the future.

REFERENCES:

(1) Berbari,E.J., Lazzara,R., Samet,P., Scherlag,B.J.: Circulation, 48, 1005-1013 (1973)

(2) Flowers,N.C., Hand,R.C., Orander, P.C., Miller,K.B., Walden,M.O., Horan,L.G.: Amer. J. Cardiol. 33, 383-389 (1974)

(3) Bytešník,J., Fabián,J., Pavlovič,J., Roháč,J.: Prakt.Lék. 62, 85-90 (1983)

(4) Lexa,J., Bytešník,J., Stupka,J.: Lék. a Techn.,16, 20-30 (1985)

(5) Lexa,J., Stupka,J.: Lék. a techn. 17, 28-31 (1986)

(6) Lexa,J., Bytešník,J., Stupka,J.: Acta Facult.Med.Univ.Brunensis, Nr.92, Brno, 247-253 (1987)

(7) Abboud,S., Belhassen,B., Pelleg,A., Lamado,S., Sadeh,D.: J.Electrocardiology, 16, 397-402 (1983)

(8) Vincent,R., Stroud,N.P., Jenner,R., English,M.J., Wollons,D.J., Chamberlein,D.A.: Brit.Heart J., 49, 124-130 (1978)

(9) McKenna,W.J., Rowland,E., Mortara,D., Divers,T., Krikler,D.M.: PACE, 4, 281-288 (1981).

Role of AV system electrophysiologic changes in the pathogenesis of paroxysmal atrial fibrillation

CHEKHOV A.M., GIMRIKH E.O., POPOV S.V., PEKARSKI V.V.
Siberian Cardiologic Centre, Tomsk, USSR

Summary

The contribution of AV system to the atrial fibrillation initiation was studied. The AV system is shown may be an area of atrial fibrillation initiation with subsequent sustaining of paroxysms. Patients (pts) with paroxysmal atrial fibrillation (PAF) reveal electrophysiologic disturbances of intra- and interatrial conduction and of AV node conduction.

Introduction

Mechanism of PAF development was considered as a result of the left atrium cavity increasing (Chauvin M. et al., 1983; Boineau J., 1985), electrophysiologic changes of atria (Chauvin M. et al.; Josephson M. et al.) and metabolic and vegetative innervation of the heart disturbances (Priest M., et al.). We attempted to show in our work role of AV node and AV conduction in the pathogenesis of PAF.

Material and methods

The intracardiac electrophysioligic study was performed in 115 pts (mean age 48±1 years) with documented PAF. The mean incidence of atrial fibrillation paroxysms was 14±4,7 times a month. Neither pts have rheumatic or other genesis of valvular heart disease or thyreotoxicosis. The electrophysiologic study was performed without preliminary antiarrhythmic therapy (Josephson M. et al.; Smetnev A. et al.). We analysed in this study together with the accepted criteria the effective refractory period of AV system (ERP) and its dispersion (the difference between the confirmed minimum and maximum values of ERP at several values of St_I and St_2), the duration and amplitude disturbances via His bundle branches, the duration of the tachycardia zone. The control group consisted of 18 pts without the organic heart disease but with ventricular extrasystole without PAF and ventricular tachycardia. Results of the study are processed according to Students criteria.

Results

All pts had typical A_2H_2 increasing with St_ISt_2 increasing as assessed by the programmed stimulation (Fig.1). The vulnerable period was revealed in 87 pts and its duration was 49±5 ms at A_2H_2 values exceeding 191±16,3 ms. In 46 cases A_2H_2 values exceeded 250 ms, incidentally the repeated atrial responce was obtained before the ventricular potential. The programmed stimulus induced paroxysms of more than 1 minute duration in 64 out of 87 pts (74%). We succeeded to document the ERP of AV system in 92 pts; its value was 287±8,8 ms. In the remaining 23 pts ERP of AV system was less than of atria. Dispersion of

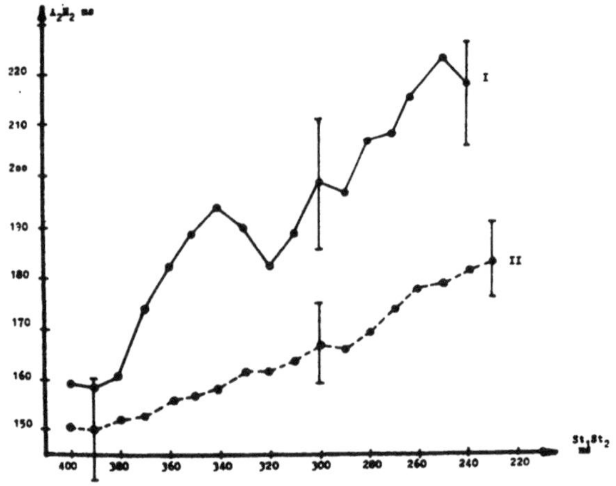

Fig.1 Values of A_2H_2 interval at St_1St_2 during the programmed atrial stimulation: I - in pts without PAF, II - in control group

AV system ERP was revealed in 86 pts (75%) and was a mean of 55,6±5,4 ms (20-150 ms). Conduction disturbances through the His bundle arised at a_2V_2 interval values of more than 250 ms in 74 cases.

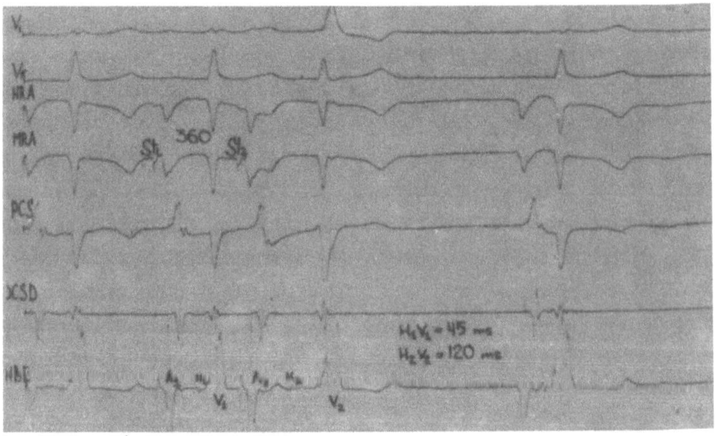

Fig.2 The conduction disturbance through the His bundle and bundle branches during the programmed atrial stimulation in a patient with PAF

These distirbances were characterized by decreasing of H_2 potential amplitude (p 0.05), the increasing of H duration (p 0,01) and of H_2V_2 interval duration (p 0.001), (Fig.2). The mean maximum H_2V_2 value was 63,9±4,5 ms during the programmed atrial stimulation which was reliably (p 0.001) more than that of H_IV_I. Conduction disturbances through His bundle branches at initial rhythm were observed in 6 pts, during the spontaneous paroxysms in 18 pts and during the programmed stimulation in 81 pts (71%). Among these 71 pts the right bundle branch block in 6% and intermittent right and left bundle branch block in 15% of cases developed.

Discussion

Electrophysiologic study data suggest that the possibility of reentry initiation in the AV system as a result of its longitudinal dissosiation (Boineau J., Pop T. et al.; Ritland D.). The initiation of this kind of tachycardias is characterized either by "breakdown" of the AV conduction curve or by critical lengthening of the A_2H_2 interval (Smetnev A. et al.; Ritland D.).

The critical increasing of A_2H_2 interval in the most pts of our study was a typical electrophysiologic sign. We suggest therefore that there are basic prerequisits for the development of reentry circuit in the AV system with the formation of the repeated excitation wave and its input into atria. Electrophysiologic disturbances present in atria might contribute to the development of atrial fibrillation. The ERP instability in AV system in pts with PAF is an additional evidence of PAF development possibility from the AV system. This fact suggests the presence in AV system several pathways refractoriness of which changes continuously.

Thus there are three basic electrophysiologic criteria which allow to suggest that PAF might initiate not only in atria but in the AV system: 1) gradual exponential lengthening of the A_2H_2 interval with the shortening of the testing stimulus delay; 2) dispersion of the AV system ERP; 3) the presence of conduction disturbances in the area of His bundle and bundle branches.

Conclusion

The AV system might be an area of atrial fibrillation initiation with subsequent sustaining of paroxysms due to pathogenetic links in atria. Patients with PAF have electrophysiologic disturbances of intra- and intercardiac conduction and conduction through the AV node.

References

(1) Chauvin M., C.Brechenmacher and J.Voegtlin: Arch. Mal Coeur, 76, 1020-1030 (1983)
(2) Boineau J.: Circulation, 72, 249-257 (1985)
(3) Josephson M., D. Scharf and J. Kastor: Amer. J. Cardiol. 39, 972-981 (1977)
(4) Priest M., T. Cooper: Circulation, 4, 254-259 (1979)
(5) Pop T., D. Fleischmann and S. Effert: Klin. Wschr., 57, 31-36
(6) Smetnev A., S. Golitsin and S. Sokolov: Kardiologiya, 5, 38-41
(7) Fricke G., B. Bartsch and H. Mattern: Herz-Kreislauf, 9, 395-406 (1977)
(8) Ritland D.: Ann. Intern. Med., 65, 328-331 (1966)
(9) Josephson M., S. Seides: Clinical Electrophysiology. Techniques and interpretations. Philadelphia, (1979)
(10) Rosen K., P. Denes and D. Wu: In: The Conduction System of the heart. Ed. by H.J.J. Wellens et al. Hague, (1978).
(11) Sulimov V., V. Makolkin and A. Syrkin: Kardiologiya, 5, 17-25 (1984)

Is the HV interval dependent on the recording site of His bundle electrogram?

POPOV S.V., CHEKHOV A.M., GIMRIKH E.O., PEKARSKAYA M.V.
Siberian Cardiologic Centre, Tomsk, USSR

Sommary

The HV interval change depending on the recording site of intracardiac His bundle electrogram is studied. Measurements were performed in 15 patients with paroxysmal tachycardias and arrhythmias but without conduction disturbances on the electrocardiogram. The HV interval was recorded in the areas close to the His bundle. The HV interval value is shown to be measured and assessed at a maximum amplitude of H-potential.

Introduction

The development of the method for His bundle electrogram recording and its practical use allowed to verify the mechanism of a number of cardiac rhythm and conduction disturbances. However a large controversy exists in the literature to date regsrding to the interpretation of the HV interval value for the individual patient. The aim of the present study was to investigate the dependence of the HV interval value on the His bundle electrogram recording site.

Matérial and methods

The study population consisted of 15 patients (8 males and 7 females) aged between 18 and 39 years (mean 32,7 1,9 years) with paroxysms of tachycardias and arrhythmias who underwent intracardiac electrophysiologic study for the proper choice of antiarrhythmic therapy. The 4-pole electrode (USCI) was inserted via one of the femoral veins and placed under the X-ray control into the right ventricle to the interventricular septum for His bundle electrogram recording. The initial registration of His bundle potential was performed from the electrode poles 2-3. Then the electrode was slowly withdrawn under the intracaddiac electrogram control via the tricuspid valve to the position where the His bundle potential of a maximum amplitude was recorded f from the electrode poles 2-3. Thereafter before the antiarrhythmic agents administration His bundle electrogtam was recorded in the setting of sinus rhythm in the bipolar lead from 1-2 (I positinn), 2-3 (II position), 3-4 (III position) poles simultaneously with the paper speed of 100 and 250 mm/s. Values of AH, AV, HV intervals and amplitude of H-potential were assessed in each of the abovementioned positions according to the accepted criteria (Sherlag B., Lau S. et al., 1969; Roberts N., 1973; Narula O., 1975;). The results obtained are procecced with the use of Student´s criteria.

Results

The intracardiac electrophysiologic study data have not confirmrd the presence of intraventricular conduction disturbances in any patient.

Results of the study are presented in the table.

Table I. Values of the intervals AH, HV and of the H-amplidude measured during the intracardiac electrophysiologic study in 15 pts

	HBE recording site								
	I		II		III		P_{I-II}	P_{II-III}	P_{I-III}
H mV	0,13	0,01	0,22	0,03	0,12	0,03	0,02	0,05	NS
AH ms	102	3,0	99	5,0	84	2,5	NS	0,02	0,01
HV ms	34	4,1	46	2,9	58	3,1	0,05	0,05	0,05

HBE - His bundle electrogram, I,II,III - endocardial electrode positions, NS - npt significant

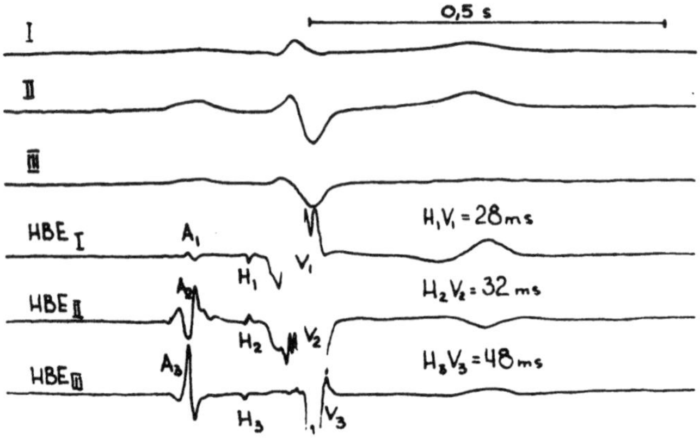

Fig.1 Patient F., 28 years. A part of electrophysiologic study recording. I,II,III - surface ECG leads; HBE_I, HBE_{II}, HBE_{III} - distal (I), mean (II) and proxomal (III) electrode positions

Discussion

A number of investigators (Sherlag B., Lau S. et al, 1969; Damato A., Patton R. et al, 1969; Roberts N., 1975; Herbinger W., 1981; Sherlag B., Samet P. et al., 1972) report that the AV interval amplitude fluctuates from 37 5 to 51 6 ms. Our data obtained in patients without intracardiac conduction disturbances support thei results. We noted however that in individuals of our patients the HV interval value could fluctuate from 30 to 70 ms while in the same patient the fluctuation range was 20 ms in several registration points of His bundle electrogram (Fig.1). This suggests that HV interval values are to be measured and assessed in relation to the His bundle potential amplitude to exclude errors in their interpretation specifically if one suspects the presence of anomalous conducting pathways.

Conclusion

The HV interval value is not a strongly fixed quantity and is to be measured and assessed at a maximum amplitude of the His bundle potential.

References

(1) Sherlag B., S. Lau and R. Helfant: Circulation, I, 39-48 (1969)
(2) Roberts N.: His bundle electrocardiography in children. M.D. Thesis, Cambridge (1973)
(3) Narula O.: His bundle electrocardiography and clinical electro - physiology F.S. Davies Company, Philadelphia (1975)
(4) Damato A., R. Patton and C. Steiner: Circulation, 40, 61-72 (1969)
(5) Bekheit J. and P. Murtagh: Br. Heart J., 33, 719-725 (1971)
(6) Roberts N.: The cardiac conducting system and the His bundle electrogram. New York, Appleton Century Crofts (1975)
(7) Herbinger W.à Temporare Elektrostimulation des Herzens. New York (1981)
(8) Sherlag B., P. Samet and R. Helfant: Circulation, 46, 601-612

System for detection of micropotentials

A. VOSS, U. BUHSS, B. REIME

Academy of Sciences of the GDR
Central Institute of Cardiovascular Research
Wiltbergstr. 50, Berlin, 1115

Summary

One common problem in diagnostics and therapy of heart and cardiovascular diseases is to discern those patients threatened by heavy rhythm disturbances. Under certain unfavourable conditions, ventricular late potentials caused by ischemically damaged areas of the heart muscle may release single premature cardiac actions. But in the more unfavourable case they might cause life-threatening tachycardias, which may lead to much feared sudden heart death. With high probability the occurence of such delayed potentials in patients with coronary heart diseases is an indicator of increased risk for ventricular tachycardias or at the worst for a sudden death.
These ventricular late potentials can be registered from the body surface only by the averaging technique (temporal and spatial).
The application of modern procedures of signal processing allows us to improve the recovery rate of late potentials or to reduce the influence of technical and biological artifacts.
With the help of our new three-channel signal averager, which is equipped with two microprocessors, we have created the basis for reliable recognition of electrical instability and inhomogeneity of the heart.

Physiological aspects

Regular micropotentials of the heart are potentials from the cardiac conduction system that are required physiologically and are therefore necessary for proper functioning of the myocardium. Such micropotentials are for example the sinus-node potential, the potential of the AV-node and the His-bundle potential.
Irregular micropotentials are an expression of pathological changes of excitatory conduction and represent ventricular delayed depolarization potentials (late potentials). Therefore, they may be an indicator of serious electrical instability and inhomogeneity of the heart.
In a more general sense, the occurence of such pathological signals could be conceived as a massive disturbance in the complex system cell-conduction pathway-myocardium. Considering the complicated

processes associated with the release of action potentials, one can well imagine the sensibility of this system to milieu alterations (e.g. impaired substrate supply, deteriorated energy conversion, electrolyte shifts).
Under certain conditions these late potentials may elicit either single premature actions of the heart (ventricular ectopic beats) or, in the less favourable case, provoke life-threatening ventricular tachycardias. This mechanism is characterized as reexcitation of healthy myocardial areas by the same process of excitation, and presupposes an unidirectional block in part of the working muscle and a delayed conduction velocity in another area.
It can be assumed that the delayed depolarization potentials may directly elicit ventricular tachycardias, whose coupling interval to the preceding QRS complex is larger then 200 to 220 ms.

Technical solution and examples

For the detection of micropotentials of the heart from body surface we use the method of linear averaging with the help of microcomputers (Fig. 1).

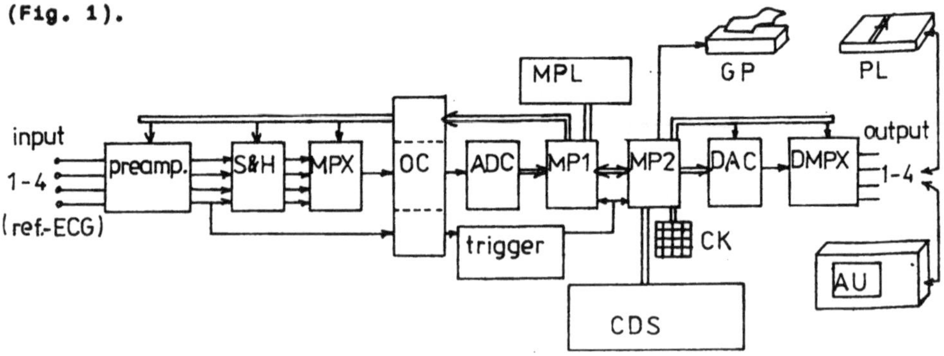

Fig. 1 Schematic diagram of the system
(S&H - sample-and-hold circuit, MPX - multiplexer
OC - opto-coupler, ADC - analog digital converter,
MP1 - microprocessor 1, MP2 - microprocessor 2,
DAC - digital analog converter, DMPX - demultiplexer)

The signals from three ECG leads are preamplified by means of low noise preamplifier and submitted to a band-pass filter (high-pass filter with programmable frequency 30/80 Hz, low-pass filter 250 Hz for anti-aliasing). The signal from the fourth lead is the so called reference-ECG for the triggering procedure. The trigger itself is able to work in two ways, the estimation of R peak maximum or the estimation of the maximum of the first derivation. The signals are now sampled (sample-and-hold stage) simultaneously with 1000 Hz. The multiplexer selects one of the channels and passes it to the opto-

coupler for potential separating. The first microcomputer, which is responsible for the above-mentioned procedures, works in real time as a three-channel non-recursive digital filter and transmits the results to the second microprocessor. This microprocessor effects linear temporal signal averaging to improve the signal-noise-ratio. the number of averaging steps has to be choosen before starting the measurement.
The observation interval of the QRS-complex extends from 256 ms before the trigger point (R-wave) to 576 ms after the trigger point. Thus, we can record irregular pathological and regular normal micro-potentials simultaneously.
To further increase the signal-noise-ratio, strongly noised complexes, arrhythmias and those complexes imediately following the rejected activities are excluded from averaging. These complexes whose heart rate variance exeeds a fixed level are ignored too. For that reason the RR interval and the area below the ECG signal curve (the integral) are calculated and pattern formed from some averaged ECG complexes. By keyboard input the investigator may determine the maximum deviation of the single ECG complex from the calculated pattern values. During every heart beat the deviation of the actual ECG complex from the averaged pattern is examined and if the difference is higher then the determined maximum, the complex is excluded from averaging.
The results of averaging are displayed on a grafic printer and/or on analogue curve monitor or ECG strip chart recorder.
Fig. 2 and Fig. 3 show examples of regular (His-bundle potential) and irregular (late potential) micropotentials.

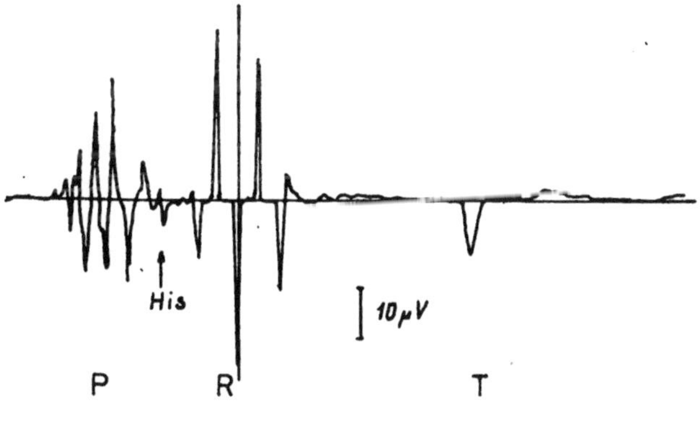

Fig. 2 Regular micropotential - His-bundle potential (differentiated signal)

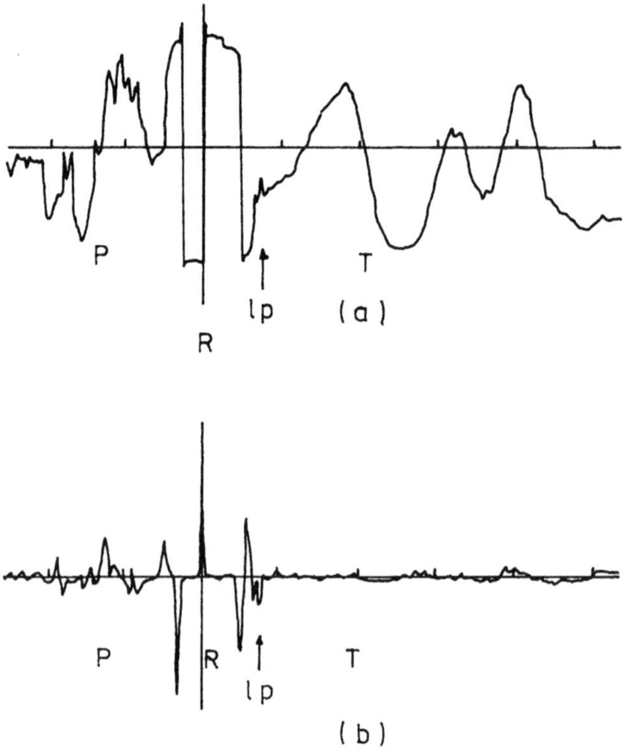

Fig. 3 Irregular micropotential - late potential
(a) filtered 30-300 Hz
(b) differentiated signal

Conclusions

For optimization of the recovery rate of late potentials the use of modern procedures of signal processing is required. This includes a high accuracy of ECG triggering and survaillance of heart period duration and the filtering of signals with non-ringing, phase-stabile digital filters. Additional programs have to be developed, in order to eliminate possibly unrecognized trigger errors or overlooked arrhythmias. To solve some of these problems we have developed the above mentioned signal averager.

References

(1) W.Craelius, M.Restivo, M.A. Assadi, N.El-Sherif
Criteria for optimal averaging of cardiac signals,IEEE Trans. on biomed. engn. 33, 957-966 (1986)
(2) G.Breithardt, R.Becker, L.Seipel, R.-R. Abendroth
Nichtinvasive Registrierung ventrikulärer Spätpotentiale-Methodik und erste Erfahrungen, Z.Kardiol. 70, 1-7 (1981)
(3) Fiehring,H., H.-J.Kleiner, A.Voß, B.Reime
Entwickeltes System zur Erfassung und Verarbeitung von Mikropotentialen des Herzens, research report Berlin, ZIHK, 1986

The Clinical Evaluation of the Late Potentials in Patients with Ventricular Arrhythmias

SHUJI YAKUBO, M.D., YUKIO OZAWA, M.D., NAOSHI TANIGAWA, M.D., MASAKI NAGASAWA, M.D., RYUSUKE KOJIMA, M.D., KAZUHIKO·JINNO, M.D., HARUMI MAKI, M.D., ICHIRO WATANABE, M.D., SATOSHI SAITO, M.D., AND MICHINOBU HATANO, M.D.

The Second Department of Internal Medicine, School of Medicine, Nihon University
30-1, Ohyaguchikamimachi, Itabashi-ku, Tokyo 173, Japan

SUMMARY

We investigated the recognition of late potentials (LPs) in patients with and without organic heart diseases and spontaneous ventricular arrhythmias. LPs in patients with idiopathic cardiomyopathy were noted frequently in the dilated type with high grades of ventricular arrhythmias. Patients with old myocardial infarctions had a higher rate of LPs recognition in cases of sudden death or ventricular tachycardias. We concluded LPs must be evaluated in each of the different groups of organic heart diseases to estimate the clinical value of ventricular arrythmias.

PURPOSE OF THE STUDY

Recent studies have shown late potentials (LPs) may predict the development of reentrant ventricular arrhythmias and sudden cardiac electrical death.[1-4] These signals may be a new independent maker to evaluate ventricular arrhythmias incomparison with long term electrocardiography (ECG) or electrical stimulation methods. At the present time, we have studied the recognition of LPs for evaluating spontaneous ventricular arrhythmias in patients with and without organic heart disease.

MATERIALS AND METHODS

We studied 418 cases classified into 6 groups (Table 1). All of premature ventricular contractions (PVCs) have been observed by standard ECG, long term ECG and/or ECG monitoring. The evaluation of PVCs was done by using a modification of Lown's classification; Grade I is within 1440 PVCs/day, Grade II is more than 1440 PVCs/day, Grade III is multiple PVCs, Grade IVa is coupled PVCs and Grade IVb is continuous repetitive PVCs less than 5 beats, and Grade V is R on T. We also classified ventricular tachycardia (VT) as being continuously more than 6 beats. If a patient had many grades of PVCs in the classifications mentioned above, we evaluated each of III, IVa, IVb, V grades and VT, and in the same patients the highest classification graded was selected among 0, I and II.

Signal averaging ECGs were recorded by means of a high resolution MAC-1 unit (Marquette Electronics) to estimate LPs non-invasively. The MAC-1 unit uses three electrodes six leads are generated from. We evaluated LPs, averaged 1024 beats, at band pass filter setting from 100 (or 80), 200 to 300 Hz, and diagnosed LPs as signals outlasting the standard QRS complex by more than 20 msec in at least three or more leads and exceeding twice the amplitude of base line noise.

We also investigated the effects of aneurysmectomy for LPs and VT.

TABLE I PATIENTS POPULATION AND THE RECOGNITION OF LATE POTENTIALS

		Age Mean SD(Range)	LP(%)
1) Normal subjects	60(M:36,F:24)	41.2 ±15.6(15-68)	0
2) PVCs without organic heart disease	45(M:20,F:25)	43.4 ±16.4(12-68)	0
3) PVCs with organic heart disease	64(M:38,F:26)	52.9 ±14.4(16-77)	7.8
4) Idiopathic VT	9(M:5,F:4)	44.4 ±15.0(23-67)	0
5) Idiopathic cardiomyopathy DCM	15(M:10,F:5)	47.8 ±14.1(24-68)	46.7
HCM	8(M:5,F:3)	44.4 ±16.2(23-66)	12.5
6) Myocardial infarction Acute (within 4 weeks)	65(M:53,F:12)	60.0 ±10.1(32-81)	39.3
Old (over 4 weeks)	152(M:115,F:37)	61.7 ±11.2(35-83)	42.1

LP; late potential, PVCs; premature ventricular contraction, VT; ventricular tachycardia, DCM; dilated cardiomyopathy, HCM; hypertrophic cardiomyopathy

RESULT

1) Normal subjects.

No LPs were recorded in 60 normal subjects.

2) PVCs without organic heat disease.

In 45 patients, LPs have not been observed.

3) PVCs with organic heart disease (excluding OMI and idiopathic cardiomyopathy).

LPs were recorded for 7.8% of this group. In four of the 5 patients with LPs, PVCs of a higher grade than IVa were observed.

4) Idiopathic VT.

In 9 cases of patients with idiopathic VT estimated by electrical stimulation and long term ECG, LPs were not seen.

5) LPs and ventricular arrhythmias in patients with idiopathic cardiomyopathy.

23 patients of this group were divided into dilated cardiomyopathy (DCM) and hypertrophic cardiomyopathy (HCM). In the former group of 15 patients, LPs were observed in 46.7%. One of 8 cases in the latter group showed LPs and high grade (II, III, IVa and IVb) of PVCs. In patients with DCM, LPs in each grade of PVCs showned 100% in IVb and VT (Fig.1). While LPs were not recorded in 72.7% of patients without VT, IVa and IVb.

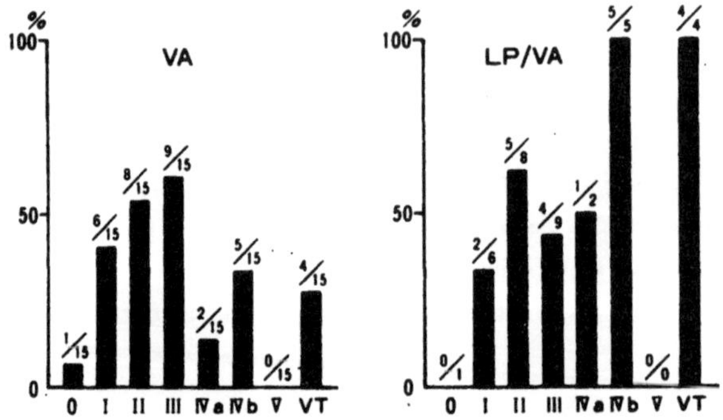

Fig.1. VA and LP in 15 patients with DCM.
VA=ventricular arrhythmia; LP=late potential; DCM=dilated cardiomyopathy

6) LPs and PVCs in patients with acute myocardial infarction (AMI).

In 65 cases, LPs were recognized in 39.3% within 7 days, in 42.2% at second and third week, and in 43.1% at fourth week from onset. In patients with a higher grade of PVCs (IVb, V and VT), LPs were frequently recorded (Fig.2).

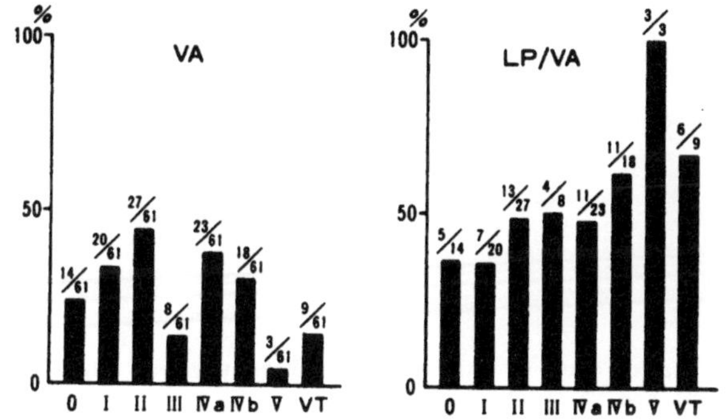

Fig.2. VA and LP in 61 patients with AMI.
VA=ventricular arrhythmia; LP=late potential; AMI=acute myocardial infarction

7) LPs and PVCs in patients with OMI (Fig.3).

In 152 patients, LPs were recorded in 42.1%, and found in all 14 cases of VT, ventricular fibrillation or sudden cardiac death. We observed LPs more frequently in higher grades of PVCs in the classification.

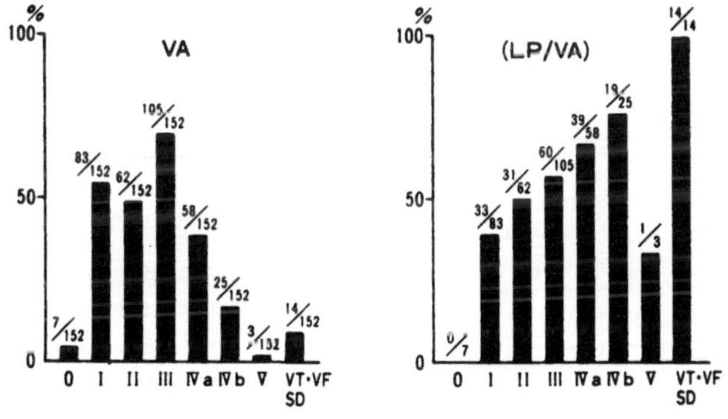

Fig.3. VA and LP in 152 patients with OMI.
VA=ventricular arrhythmia; LP=late potential; OMI=old myocardial infarction; SD=sudden death

8) The effects of aneurysmectomy for LPs in patients with VT and ventricular aneurysm (Fig.4).

In 3 patients with OMI, ventricular aneurysm and VT, LPs were found before aneurysmectomy. After operation, LPs had disappeared with VT.

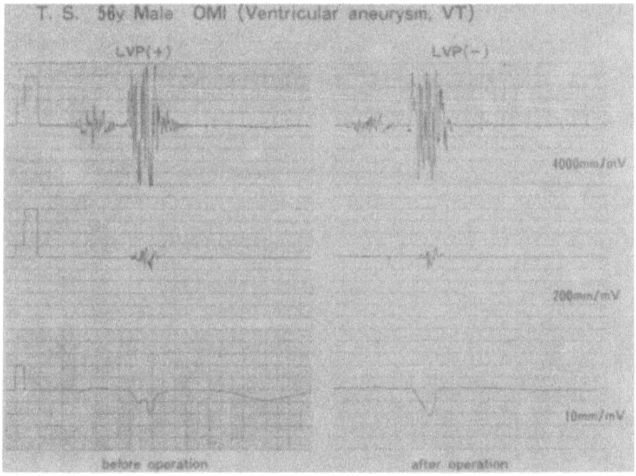

Fig.4. Disappearance of LP and VT after LV anéurysmectomy in this patients with MI and VT.
LP=late potential; VT=ventricular tachycardia; LV=left ventricular; MI=myocardial infarction

CONCLUSION

We studied the recognition of LPs by body surface signal averaging ECG in patients with spontaneous ventricular arrhythmias.

1) LPs have not been recorded in normal subjects, in patients with PVCs only and in patients with idiopathic VTs.

2) Patients with PVCs and organic heart disease showed a low rate of the recognition of LPs.

3) In patients with idiopathic cardiomyopathy, the recognition of LPs were more frequent in DCM than in HCM, and in those with high grades of ventricular arrhythmias.

4) In spite of the evidence of a high gade of ventricular arrhythmias, the recognition of LPs were at lower rate in AMI than OMI.

5) The patients with OMI have shown a high rate of recognition of LPs in cases with sudden cardiac death or VT.

6) The evaluation of changes of LPs for treatment of ventricular arrhythmias remains obscure. However, the effects of aneurysmectomy for the ventricular electrical instability can be estimated by the disappearance of LPs after operation.

We concluded LPs must be evaluated in each of the different groups of organic heart diseases to estimate the clinical value of ventricular arrhythmias.

REFERENCE

1. BREITHARDT G, BECKER R, SEIPEL L, ABENDROTH RR, OSTERMEYER J: Noninvasive detection of late potentials in man, a new marker for ventricular tachycardia. Eur Heart J 2:1 (1981)
2. ROZANSKI JJ, MORTARA D, MYERBURG RJ, CASTELLANOS A: Body surface detection of delayed depolarization in patients with recurrent ventricular tachycardia and left ventricular aneurysm. Circulation 63:1172 (1981)
3. SIMSON MB: Use of signals in the terminal QRS complex to identify patients with ventricular tachycardia after myocardial infarction. Circulation 64:235 (1981)
4. DENES P, SANTARELLI P, HAUSER RG, URETZ EF: Quantitative analysis of the high-frequency component of the terminal portion of the body surface QRS in normal subjects and in paients with ventricular tachycardia. Circulation 67:1129 (1983)

Escape pacemaker characteristics following catheter-induced ablation of the atrioventricular junction

KÁROLY ZÁMOLYI, ZOLTÁN ANTALÓCZY, ÁDÁM SZÉKELY, EDE KÉKES

Postgraduate Medical University, POB 112 H-1389 Budapest, Hungary

Summary

Closed-chest electrical ablation of the His-bundle was performed in 18 patients/pts/ for controlling their drug resistant paroxysmal supraventricular tachyarrhythmias /atrial fibrillation and flutter in 14 pts, AV nodal reentrant tachycardia in 2 pts, AV reciprocating tachycardia - concealed WPW - in 2 pts/. Our purpose was to study the escape rhythms in the immediate and longterm follow-up periods /up to 27 months/ following this procedure. The escape rhythms appeared in 1-20 minutes after delivery of the shock with a mean cycle length/CL/ of 2106 ± 965 ms in 15/18 pts. The QRS morphology showed a RBBB pattern in 9 pts, a LBBB in 1 pt, both configurations in 7 pts and narrow QRS in 1 pt. In early postablation period an acceleration of the escape frequency was observed. On the first days the mean escape CL was 1124 ± 193 ms in 11/18 pts. Later on the escape CL gradually increased and showed no substantial change during the long-term follow-up period /mean CL: 1577 ± 137 ms/. Permanent 2° and 3° AV block was produced in 13 pts with a normal escape QRS pattern in 6 pts and with RBBB in 6 pts. One of the pts has not any escape rhythm.
In conclusion, QRS pattern of the escape rhythm does not indicate the place of the induced lesion immediately following the shock. Stable right bundle-branch-block escape QRS complexes are frequent.

Introduction

The often occuring and recurrent supraventricular tachyarrhythmias significantly decreases the quality of the patients' life and a part of those are refractory to all the known and used antiarrhythmic drugs. There is a new therapeutical approach to solve this problem from 1982. Gallagher and Scheinman elaborated a catheter technique for closed-chest disruption of atrioventricular conduction. Using this procedure synchronized electrical shock by direct-current is given using a catheter electrode on the His-bundle and producing AV block. The purpose of this study is to investigate the characteristics of the escape rhythms having occured after His-bundle ablation.

Patients

18 patients, 10 male and 8 female, aged 38-72/mean 55/ years were treated by high-energy shocks delivered to the atrioventricular conduction system from a conventional transvenous pacing catheter/Gallagher method/ /3/.

The primer arrhythmias were as follows:paroxysmal atrial fibrillation and atrial flutter/13 pts/, permanent atrial flutter/1 pt/, AV nodal reentrant tachycardia/2 pts/, AV reciprocating tachycardia/concealed WPW/ /2 pts/. All patients had so symptomatic paroxysmal arrhythmias which proved refractory to multiple drug therapy. The duration of their histories varied from 2 years to 26 years. Only 6 patients had organic heart disease/mitral valve disease 1 pt, coronary artery disease 5 pts/.

Method

After the ablation we followed by ECG the features:

1/ Onset time of the escape beats

2/ The escape QRS morphology and its alteration

3/ The cycle lengths of the escape rhythms

4/ The escape recovery time/when permanent pacing was transiently discontinued/

5/ The AV conduction

A continuous monitoring was performed after ablation for a minimal 24 up to a maximal 72 hours. Moreover, we followed daily the ECG for at least 10-18 days. The control points in time were the first month after ablation and then in every 3 months. All patients have remainded free of arrhythmia, without medication, for follow-up periods of 2 to 27 months.

Results

Table 1. Electrophysiologic data

Patient	Onset time of the escape beat	Postablation AV conduction		Postablation QRS morphology	
		early	late	early	late
1	20 min	CHB	CHB	LBBB RBBB	normal
2	1 min	CHB	CHB	LBBB RBBB	normal
3	2 min	CHB	normal	RBBB	normal
4	1 min	CHB	CHB	RBBB	RBBB
5	1 min	CHB	CHB	LBBB	normal
6	5 min	1°+RBBB	CHB	RBBB	normal
7	2 min	CHB	CHB	normal	normal
8	5 min	CHB	CHB	RBBB LBBB	normal
9	4 min	CHB	normal	LBBB RBBB	normal
10	1 min	CHB	CHB	RBBB LBBB	no QRS
11	3 min	CHB	CHB	RBBB LBBB	RBBB
12	3 min	CHB	CHB	RBBB	RBBB
13	2 min	CHB	2°block	LBBB RBBB	RBBB
14	1 min	CHB		RBBB	
15	3 min	CHB	CHB	RBBB	RBBB
16	5 min	CHB	normal	RBBB	RBBB
17	8 min	CHB	2° block	RBBB	RBBB
18	3 min	CHB	1° block	RBBB	RBBB

RBBB=right bundle branch block,LBBB=left bundle branch block, CHB= complete heart block

The Table I. offers all the electrophysiologic data in each patients in terms of the onset time of the escape beats after ablation, as well as the degree of the AV block in the early and late follow-up periods and the QRS morphology of the escape rhythms. AV junction was interrupted immediately after ablation in all patients. The escape beats appeared in 1-20 minutes after delivery of the shock with right bundle branch block QRS morphology in 9 patients, left bundle branch block in one patient, both configuration in 7 patients and narrow QRS in one patient. Permanent second degree and complete AV block was produced in 13 patients with a normal escape QRS pattern in 6 patients and with right bundle branch block in 6 patients. One of the patients has not any escape rhythm. The AV conduction resumed within 24 hours in patient number 3 and 16, within 2 days in patient number 9. The patient number 14 died on the 13th days after the urgent ablation. Cause of death was not related to this procedure.

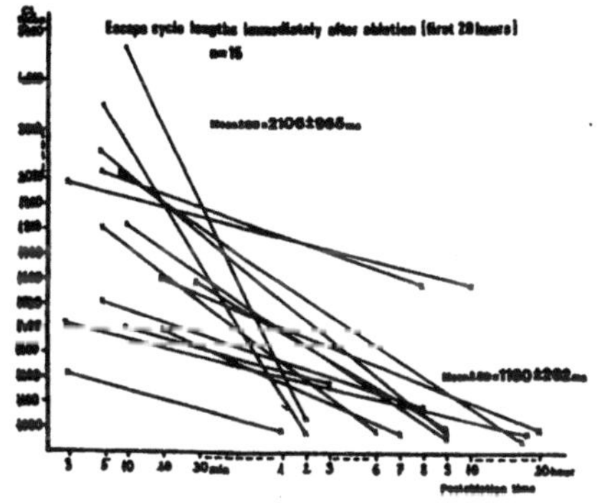

Figure 1

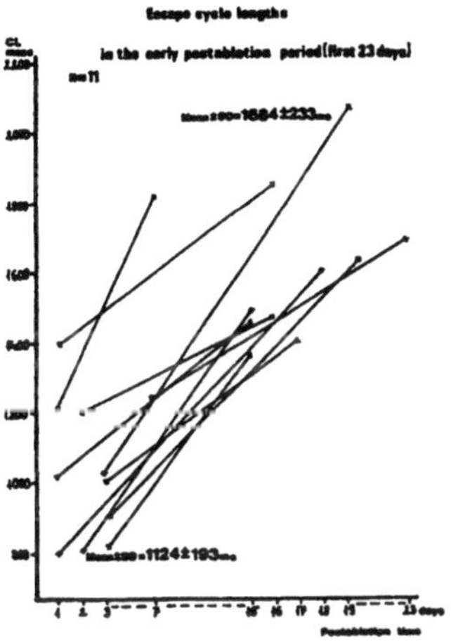

Figure 2

The first figure demonstrates the cycle lengths in msec immediately after ablation. The results clearly showed the significant shortening. In early postablation period an acceleration of the escape frequency was observed, however later on the cycle lengths of the escape rhythms gradually increased as it is can observed on figure 2. Later on the escape cycle lengths showed no substantial change during the long-term follow-up period. The mean steady escape cycle length was: 1577$\pm$137 msec.
The Table 2. summarizes the escape recovery time in milliseconds of 12 patients and total time of follow-up periods when the patients were observed. The escape recovery time increased in each patients during the follow-up when permanent pacing was transiently discontinued.

Table 2. Recovery time of the escape rhythms

Patient No.	Recovery time/msec/		Follow-up period
1	2000	4200	27 months
2	1800	1920	25 "
4	1840	3920	22 "
5	1520	1680	20 "
6	1600	2040	19 "
7	1640	1920	18 "
8	1520	2000	18 "
10	1840	PM dependence	14 "
11	2000	4000	10 "
12	1560	3120	7 "
13	1000	1160	9 "
15	1920	3200	5 "

Discussion

Recently a catheter technique for closed-chest ablation of AV conduction has been described/3,6/. This new technique is simple to perform, safe, and avoids the need for open heart surgery. Complete AV block is achieved in 95% of the patients, but a normal conduction is recovered in 20-25% of them/1,5/. Short-term results suggest that a good subsidiary escape rhythm can be preserved in most patients, although this does not preclude the development of pacemaker-dependence at a later date in consequence of late scarring of the lesion/4/. In the first days the cardiac rate is high and variable, the escape rhythms are made up of WRS of various morphologies and widths.Later on the escape rhythm tends to stabilize as the rate decreaes and there is a tendency towards a reduction in the multifarious QRS morphologies /2/.

Conclusions

1/The AV conduction recovers within 1 hour or latest few days, 2/after an early acceleration the escape frequency gradually decreases during 10-18 days and then no significant alteration occurs, 3/the escape rhythm may dissapear then can recur, 4/it can happen that in the beginning there seems to be an unsuccesful intervention but hours later the complete AV block turn up, 5/immediately after ablation all patients had evidence of a subsidiary escape rhythm with wide QRS morphology, 6/stable right bundle branch block escape QRS complexes are frequent, 7/the QRS morphology indicates the starting location of the escape rhythm only later on, 8/after the ablation the recovery time of the escape rhythms gradually increases.

References

/1/ Davis M.J.et al: Aust.NZ J.Med. 14,479-486 /1984/
/2/ Fabra J.M.et al: In Gómez F.P,ed.: Cardiac Pacing,1560-1567 /1985/
/3/ Gallagher J.J.et al: N.Engl.J.Med. 306,194-200 /1982/
/4/ Gallagher J.J.et al: In Josephson M,ed.: Tachycardias:Mechanisms Diagnośis Treatment 271-285/1984/
/5/ Nathan A.W. et al: Lancet 1,1280-84, /1984/
/6/ Scheinman M.M et al: JAMA 248, 851-55 /1982/

Registration of cardiac micropotentials from body surface - a possibility to diagnose myocarditides

PRIES, W.; NOWAK, R.; WERNER, G.; BLUNK, L.

Internal Clinic of the Military Medical Academy, Bad Saarow, GDR

Summary: Myocarditis can occur as a so-called accompanying disease in or after general infections. Cases of a clinically mild course are often not diagnosed. The experience of clinicians leads one to assume that conventional electrocardiography relatively often fails to diagnose such courses.

Therefore, we were interested in the precision of the method of the continuous registration of cardiac micropotentials from body surface.

Fifteen patients with a feverish Angina tonsillaris were included in our study series.

We simultaneously recorded cardiac micropotentials and a conventional ECG on the first, seventh and fourteenth day of the disease.

Electrode placement was adjusted to the optimal registration of regular micropotentials (His potentials, pre-P potentials).

A change in time intervals has so far not been observed in amplified body surface ECG either.

Investigations will be continued and more patients included.

First results of a study covering a relatively long period and dealing with the incidence of the so-called accompanying myocarditis or infectious-allergic myocarditis are presented, which can occur in all cases of infectious diseases.

From this study only the courses of this disease which showed no clinical and electrocardiographic signs of a myocarditis are described here.

These investigations are based on the suspicion that mild courses of the disease can perhaps not be recorded by conventional electrocardiography.

An answer to this question appears to be of great importance, since especially the present feverish general disease makes the clinical diagnosis more difficult.

The method of the continuous registration of cardiac micropotentials from body surface could be a great help.

First some remarks on the device system we set up and used.

Long time, for biophysical and technical reasons it was regarded as impracticable to measure bioelectric potential differences originating only from activities of the impulse fromation and conduction system on body surface.

At present it is internationally considered to be proved that cardiac micropotentials (pre-P potentials, His bundle potentials and ventricular late potentials) can be led from body surface with appropriate equipment.

Cardiac micropotentials reach signal amplitudes of 2-20 microvolt on body surface and are superimposed by biological and technical noise voltages with considerably higher voltage values. Therefore they can't be registered with conventional ECG recording devices and nor after corresponding amplification either.
The problem is to differentiate signal from noise. In most cases the signal averaging technique is used to improve the signal-to-noise ratio. Using this technique of summation and averaging of several hundred cardiac cycles, however, dynamic changes during the recording period are lost.
This is probably the most important disadvantage, if we disregard the very expensive aspect of the averaging technique.
An improvement of the signal-to-noise ratio can not only be achieved by time-related and event-related averaging, respectively, but by spatial averaging too.
Our working group concentrates its efforts on the latter method, since by a possible continuous recording all dynamic signal changes are registered.
A new ECG amplifier was therefore developed which realizes the principle of spatial averaging.
An amplification ($V \sim 10^6$) and variable band-pass filtering allow the continuous registration of cardiac micropotentials with a customary ECG recording system.
A Faraday cage is not necessarily required. Sixteen specially made electrodes were used for the lead.
We developed a new bipolar arrangement of electrodes.
Figure 1 shows the multielectrode arrangement we used.

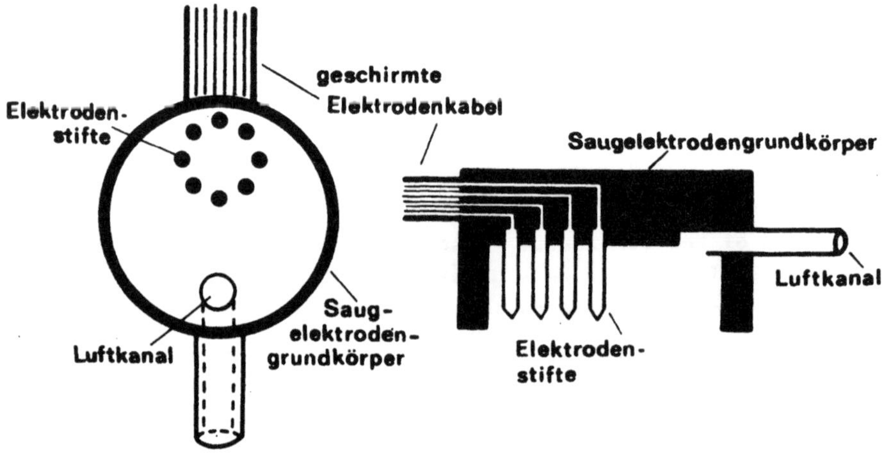

Fig. 1. The multielectrode arrangement
In a suction electrode body covering an area of 2 cm^2, there are 8 gold-plated electrode pins being 3 mm apart from each other. These electrode pins are applied without electrode paste.

Due to the small sectional area of the electrodes and the low pressure produced by the suction electrode pins are virtually sucked in the epidermis. The effective electrode surface is about 6 - 8 mm^2.
In addition to this, there is a better regional cutaneous circulation caused by low pressure.
With this electrode we attain transition resistances of less than 5 kiloohm on the pretreated skin after an application time of 1 - 2 minutes.
By averaging these 8 bipolar ECG leads it is possible to continuously record micropotentials with an amplitude of 5 microvolt. We used this device system not only to register regular and irregular cardiac micropotentials, but to record the fetal electrocardiogram transabdominally.
Fifteen (11 male and 4 female) patients at a mean age of 28.5 $\pm$ 6.6 years with a feverish Angina tonsillaris were included in the study.
The diagnosis was proved by clinical, microbiological and laboratory-chemical findings.
Parallel to these patients we examined a control group of 15 clinically healthy probands.
Regular cardiac micropotentials and a conventional ECG (standard leads by Einthoven, Goldberger and Wilson) were recorded on the first, seventh and fourteenth days of the disease.
Examinations have always been made at the same time and in the same room. Only one person interpreted the curves.
We placed the electrodes on thorax so that there were optimal conditions for the registration of His potentials in all probands of the control group (100 per cent) in all three examinations. In addition, a pre-P potential could be recorded in 2 probands. In the patient group His potentials could also be recorded in the first two examinations in 100 per cent of the cases, but in the third examination only in 14 patients.
The pre-P potential was consistently recorded in 6 patients.
A change in time intervals has so far not been observed in the patient group and nor in the control group either.
As the investigations are at present, we conclude that a period of 14 days surely doesn't allow a final decision.
Investigations will be continued up to the sixth week after the onset of the disease for the present.
More patients will be included.
There are some Figures showing the curves.

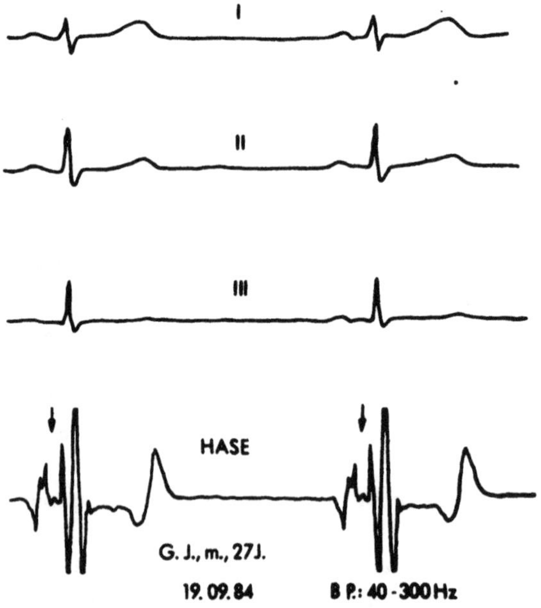

Fig. 2. The curve of a patient with a His bundle potential

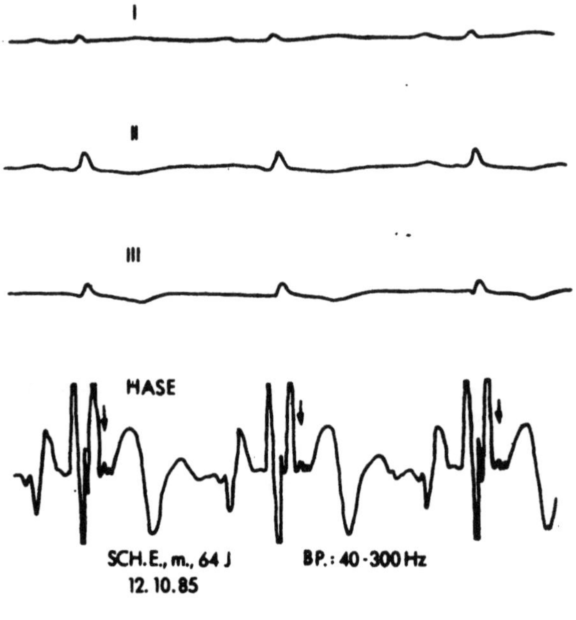

Fig. 3. The late potential in a patient

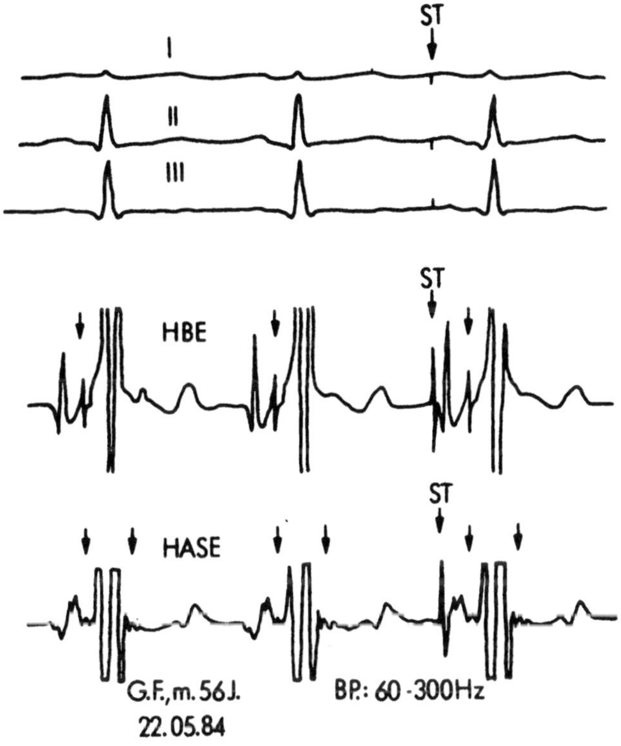

Fig. 4. Late potential and a His bundlepotential

AUTHORS INDEX